MATERNAL-NEWBORN NURSING

The Critical Components of Nursing Care

MATERNAL-NEWBORN NURSING
The Critical Components of Nursing Care

Linda Chapman, RN, DNSc
Clinical Associate Professor
University of Arizona College of Nursing
Tucson, Arizona
Professor Emeritus
Samuel Merritt University
Oakland, California

Roberta F. Durham, RN, PhD
Professor
Department of Nursing and Health Sciences
California State University, East Bay
Hayward, California
Professor Alumnus
Samuel Merritt University
Oakland, California

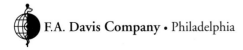
F.A. Davis Company • Philadelphia

F. A. Davis Company
1915 Arch Street
Philadelphia, PA 19103
www.fadavis.com

Printed in the United States of America

Last digit indicates print number: 10 9 8 7 6 5 4 3

Publisher, Nursing: Lisa B. Deitch
Developmental Editor: Shirley Kuhn
Director of Content Development: Darlene D. Pedersen
Senior Project Editor: Padraic J. Maroney
Design and Illustration Manager: Carolyn O'Brien
Cover Photo: Courtesy of Baby Jane-Hope Hallowell

As new scientific information becomes available through basic and clinical research, recommended treatments and drug therapies undergo changes. The author(s) and publisher have done everything possible to make this book accurate, up to date, and in accord with accepted standards at the time of publication. The author(s), editors, and publisher are not responsible for errors or omissions or for consequences from application of the book, and make no warranty, expressed or implied, in regard to the contents of the book. Any practice described in this book should be applied by the reader in accordance with professional standards of care used in regard to the unique circumstances that may apply in each situation. The reader is advised always to check product information (package inserts) for changes and new information regarding dose and contraindications before administering any drug. Caution is especially urged when using new or infrequently ordered drugs.

Library of Congress Cataloging-in-Publication Data

Chapman, Linda, 1949-
 Maternal-newborn nursing : the critical components of nursing care / Linda Chapman, Roberta F. Durham.
  p. ; cm.
 Includes bibliographical references and index.
 ISBN-13: 978-0-8036-1754-4
 ISBN-10: 0-8036-1754-2
 1. Maternity nursing. I. Durham, Roberta F. II. Title.
 [DNLM: 1. Maternal-Child Nursing. WY 157.3 C466m 2010]
 RG951.C43 2010
  618.92'01--dc22   2009040283

To our mothers ... June Henderson
and Virginia "Ducky" Durham

Preface

Maternal-Newborn Nursing: The Critical Components of Nursing Care is a basic maternity textbook focusing on evidence-based practice for all levels of nursing programs. We designed this book to address the contemporary needs of both faculty and students.

As maternal-newborn professors, we have had numerous students tell us that they do not have enough time to prepare for class or clinical and also fulfill their other responsibilities of taking care of their children or working to finance their education. Because we realize that today's students lead complex lives and must juggle multiple roles as student, parent, employee, and spouse, we developed this textbook, with its accompanying electronic ancillaries, to present the critical components of maternity nursing in a clear and concise format that lends itself to ease of comprehension while maintaining the integrity of the substantive content. It may be particularly useful for programs designed to present the subject of maternity nursing in an abbreviated or condensed way.

ORGANIZATION

This evidence-based text utilizes theory and clinical knowledge of maternity nursing. The conceptual framework is Family Developmental Theory, and substantive theory that forms the foundation for maternity care is presented. It is organized according to the natural sequence of the perinatal cycle, pregnancy, labor and birth, postpartum and neonate. We have taken a bio-psycho-social approach dealing with the physiology, psychological adaptation, and social and cultural influences impacting childbearing families with emphasis on nursing actions and care of women and their families. We believe childbirth is a natural, developmental process.

Maternal-Newborn Nursing: The Critical Components of Nursing Care reflects current trends in maternity services including a trend towards higher levels of intervention in maternity care. These trends are reflected in our inclusion of a chapter on tests during the antepartal period, as well as a chapter devoted to fetal assessment and electronic fetal monitoring. We have devoted one chapter to the care of cesarean birth families, since nearly one third of births in the United States are cesarean births.

FEATURES

This textbook presents the critical components of maternity in a pragmatic condensed format by using the following features:

- Information presented in a bulleted format for ease of reading.
- Flow charts, diagrams, tables, clinical pathways, and concept maps used to summarize information.
- Case studies used to assist with integration of knowledge.

Audio Book

In an effort to help students manage their time more effectively, each book comes with a CD containing audio recorded abridged versions of selected chapters for students to listen to at any time or while commuting to and from classes and clinical. Students can use these audio files to reinforce the content in the text, to refresh their reading before class, or to review for an exam. The audio files provide another way of learning in one product.

Critical Components

This textbook focuses on the critical components of maternity nursing. Critical components are the major areas of knowledge essential for a basic understanding of maternity nursing. The critical components were determined from the authors' combined 45 years of teaching maternity nursing in both traditional and accelerated programs and years of clinical practice in the maternity setting. This focus is especially evident when discussing complications or deviations from the norm.

The focus of the text is on normal pregnancy and childbirth. Chapters on low-risk antenatal, intrapartal, postpartal, and neonatal are followed by chapters on high-risk and complications in each area. Common complications germane to the nursing domain and childbearing population focus on understanding and synthesizing the critical elements for nursing care.

Chapter on Care of Cesarean Birth Families

Approximately 30% of births in the United States are by cesarean section. In response to this increased trend in cesarean births, a chapter is dedicated to the intrapartum and postpartum care of the cesarean birth families.

Chapter Format

This textbook clusters physiological changes, nursing assessment, and nursing care content in a single chapter. Typically a chapter is divided into systems where the physiology, nursing care including assessment and interventions, expected outcomes and common deviations of one subsystem are presented. Psychosocial and cultural dimensions of nursing care are highlighted within the chapter.

Flow Charts, Diagrams, Tables, and Clinical Pathways

We use flow charts, tables, and clinical pathways as avenues for presenting vast amounts of information in a condensed format. These teaching/learning aides allow us to present content in a clear and concise format.

Case Studies

We introduce two case studies, one low-risk and one high-risk, in the units on antepartal care and carry them forward and develop them further in subsequent chapters. These case studies are presented at the end of each chapter as a strategy to summarize the key elements of the chapter, to assist the students in their development of critical thinking skills, and to help them integrate the content into clinical practice.

The development of the case studies over multiple content areas, antepartum, intrapartum, and postpartum allows students to critically analyze the assessment data in relationship to nursing care. This type of teaching/learning activity aids in bringing the content "to life" for students as they synthesize new knowledge.

Review Questions

Review questions appear at the end of each chapter to facilitate student review of key chapter content.

Special Features

We have used a variety of boxes throughout the chapters to highlight information.

- Critical Component boxes highlight critical information in maternal-newborn nursing
- Medication boxes highlight the commonly administered medications used during pregnancy, labor and birth, postpartum, and neonatal period.
- Cultural Consideration boxes stress the importance of awareness of cultural factors in nursing care.
- Evidence-Based Practice boxes highlight current research and practice guidelines related to nursing care.
- Standards of Care and Professional Position Statement boxes highlight key perinatal nursing issues from professional organizations such as AWHONN.

Glossary

The text contains a glossary of terms related to maternal-newborn nursing for ease of looking up definitions for boldface terms used in the book.

Appendices

The appendices include:

- Common and standard laboratory values for pregnant and non-pregnant women as well as for the neonate
- AWHONN Quick Guide for Neonatal Skin Care
- AWHONN Quick Guide to Breastfeeding
- Conversion table
  - *Approximate temperature equivalents*
- Cervical Dilation Chart

IMPORTANT FEATURES OF THE INSTRUCTOR'S RESOURCE DISK

The nursing shortage has resulted in the widespread development and expansion of nursing programs. Many nursing programs, which can be as short as 12 months in length, typically teach maternity nursing in a compact or abbreviated format. Faculty are challenged to develop courses with fewer credit units that are taught in 5 weeks or less. This requires a critical analysis to identify essential components of the subject area and the appropriate teaching–learning resources. Maternity nursing textbooks are not designed for current approaches to nursing education at the associate, traditional baccalaureate, accelerated baccalaureate, or entry level master's nursing programs. This textbook addresses the reality of nursing education

today and presents the critical components of maternity in a pragmatic, condensed format with ancillary course materials to facilitate students' learning and faculty teaching of maternity nursing.

Current nursing students are a diverse group and many are older, more mature learners. They may enter a nursing program with prior degrees and work experience in fields outside of nursing. Most students want materials presented in a clear and concise format that allows them to use their critical thinking skills to integrate the new knowledge into their previous knowledge base and life experiences. Because some nursing students have completed their transition to adulthood they are believed by education experts to be better poised to master the knowledge they need and arrive at clinical judgments and ethical and moral decisions inherent in nursing practice. Utilization of critical components, concept mapping, evidence-based practice guidelines, and focused activities will satisfy the needs of these specialized learners who are intolerant of "busy work" and extraneous material.

The theme for the new millennium in nursing education is "we can no longer teach as we were taught." That includes teaching in a shorter time frame for both theory and clinical, and teaching for understanding of critical elements. This book responds to innovations in nursing curricula and the new population of nursing students.

Our ancillary products respond to needs and learning styles of current students. For example, some nursing students are already college graduates with academic, life, and work experience contributing to their critical thinking and ability to synthesize complex information and seek evidence-based solutions to clinical problems. In the research literature, current students are described as widely diverse, highly motivated, mature, autonomous, and excellent learners who actively pursue learning opportunities. The ancillary resources allow them to utilize a variety of technology-based resources rather than the outdated, more traditional approaches used in other maternity textbooks.

Supplemental instructor aids for theory class include:

- An 8-week syllabus guide
- Detailed classroom activities for each content area
- PowerPoint slides with graphics
- Image bank
- Over 500 NCLEX type questions in Brownstone format with NCLEX descriptors.
- Activities using Internet resources

Supplemental instructor materials for clinical include:

- Detailed clinical syllabus for inpatient and community-based perinatal settings
- Clinical integration activities with critical thinking activities and directions from authors on implementation including:
  - *Family study: format and directions for a community-based postpartum home family study for clinical students*
  - *Guidelines for simulations*
  - *Topics for clinical integration seminars*
  - *Expectant parent interview activity*
  - *Teaching cards for use with postpartum families*
  - *Medication cards*
  - *Skills laboratory exercises*
  - *Chart review exercise*
  - *Clinical preparation tools*

- Antepartal data collection worksheet
- NICU data collection worksheet
- Postpartum data collection worksheet
- Labor and delivery data collection worksheet
- Newborn assessment worksheet
- Nursing care plans for postpartum and labor and delivery

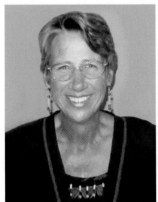

Linda Chapman

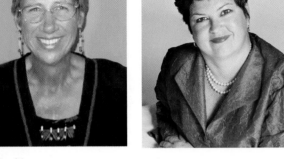

Roberta F. Durham

Contributors

Susan M. Cantrell, MSN, RNC
Assistant Professor
Samuel Merritt University
Oakland, California
Chapter 7

Mabel Choy-Bland, RN, BS
Emergency Department
Kaiser Permanente Hospital
Hayward, California
Research Assistant on chapter development

Deanna Luz Reyes Delgado, RN, BS
Neonatal Intensive Care Unit
Children's Hospital and Research Center Oakland
Oakland, California
Research Assistant on chapter development and NCLEX questions

Sylvia Fischer, RN, MSN, CNM
Clinical Assistant Professor
University of Arizona College of Nursing
Tucson, Arizona
Chapter 13

Melissa M. Goldsmith, PhD, RNC
Clinical Associate Professor
University of Arizona College of Nursing
Tucson, Arizona
Chapter 17

Stefanie Hahn, RN, BS
Perinatal Staff Nurse
Alta Bates Medical Center
Berkeley, California
Research Assistant on Interactive Computer Exercises

Sarah Hampson, RN, MS
Assistant Professor
Samuel Merritt University
Oakland, California
Chapter 5

Megan Levy
Research Assistant
Baccalaureate Nursing Student
California State University, East Bay
Hayward, California

Vivian Chioma Nwagwu, RN, MSN
Health Facilities Evaluator
State of California Department of Public Health
Licensing & Certification Program
San Jose, California
Research Assistant on PowerPoint development

Corrine Marie Smith, RN, MS, ANP-C
Nurse Practitioner
Olivetan Benedictine Sisters
Holy Angels Convent
Jonesboro, Arkansas
Chapter 8

Nora Webster, CNM, MSN
Course Faculty
Frontier School of Midwifery and Family Practice
Tucson, Arizona
Chapter 4

Reviewers

Marie Adorno, APRNC, MN
Associate Professor
Our Lady of Holy Cross College
New Orleans, Louisiana

Betty J. Beard, RN, PhD
Professor of Nursing
Eastern Michigan University
Ypsilanti, Michigan

Deborah F. Campagna, RN, MS, LCCE, FACCE
Associate Nursing Faculty
Hudson Valley Community College
Troy, New York

Patty Donlin, RN
Labor & Delivery Staff Nurse
Alta Bates Medical Center
Berkeley, California

Denise M. Fitzpatrick, RNC, MSN
Course Coordinator
Dixon School of Nursing
Willow Grove, Pennsylvania

Brenda Gleason, RN, MSN
Assistant Nursing Professor
Iowa Central Community College
Fort Dodge, Iowa

Bobbe Ann Gray, RNC, PhD
Assistant Professor
Wright State University
Dayton, Ohio

Marilyn Johnessee Greer, RN, MS
Associate Professor
Rockford College
Rockford, Illinois

Marilyn Hardy-Bougere, RN, MSN
Instructor of Nursing
Jacksonville State University
Jacksonville, Alabama

Marlene Huff, RNC, PhD
Associate Professor
University of Akron
Akron, Ohio

Nancy Hula, RN, MSN
Assistant Professor, Level Coordinator
Bryan LGH College of Health Sciences
Lincoln, Nebraska

Linda E. Jensen, RN, PhD
Assistant Professor
University of Nebraska
Kearney, Nebraska

Holly K. Kailani, RN, DNP(C)
Assistant Professor of Nursing
Hawai'i Pacific University
Honolulu, Hawaii

J. Mari Beth Linder, RN, PhD
Associate Professor, Director of Nursing Department
Missouri Southern State University
Joplin, Missouri

Ann Lowenkron, DNS, MA, BS
Associate Professor Emerita
Indiana University Purdue University Indianapolis
Indianapolis, Indiana

Sandy Ludwig, RN, MSN, NNP
Nursing Instructor
Eastern Arizona College
Thatcher, Arizona

Maria A. Marconi, RN, MS
Assistant Professor of Clinical Nursing
University of Rochester
Rochester, New York

Randee L. Masciola, RN, MS, CNP
Women's Health Nurse Practitioner, Clinical Instructor
Ohio State University
Columbus, Ohio

Kathleen Matta, RN, MSN, CNS, IBCLC
Director, Department of Nursing
Santa Fe Community College
Santa Fe, New Mexico

Barbara McClaskey, RNC, PhD, ARNP
Professor
Pittsburg State University
Pittsburg, Kansas

Debra Migues, RN, MSN, CD
Associate Professor
Louisiana College
Pineville, Louisiana

Carrie Mines, RN, MSc(T), PhD
Level 1 Coordinator Mohawk McMaster BScN Program
Mohawk College
Hamilton, Ontario, Canada

Janet Young Newcamp, RNC, MN, CNS, CCE
Assistant Professor
Edinboro University of Pennsylvania
Edinboro, Pennsylvania

Linda Pasto, RN, MSN
Professor of Nursing and Health
Tompkins – Cortland Community College
Dryden, New York

Lois A. Pine, RN, MS, ICCE, CLC
Assistant Lecturer
University of Wyoming
Laramie, Wyoming

Christine Ratto, RN, MS
Staff Nurse III
Labor & Delivery
University of California, San Francisco
San Francisco, California

Jacquelyn Reid, CNM, EdD, CNE
Associate Professor
Indiana University Southeast
New Albany, Indiana

Linda L. Rider, RNC, MS
Interim Chair, Department of Nursing
University of Central Oklahoma
Edmond, Oklahoma

Melodie Rowbotham, RN, MSN
Clinical Assistant Professor
University of Missouri – St. Louis
St. Louis, Missouri

Mileva Saulo–Lewis, RN, EdD
Associate Professor
Samuel Merritt University
Oakland, California

Christine L. Sayre, RN, MSN
Auxiliary Faculty, Clinical Instructor
Ohio State University
Columbus, Ohio

Marilyn J. Simons, RNC, DNS, FNE, IBCLC
Professor
Indiana Wesleyan University
Marion, Indiana

Nancy Someson, RN
Antenatal Testing
University of California, San Francisco
San Francisco, California

Brent Sommer, CRNA, MPHA
Assistant Professor
Clinical Coordinator, CRNA Program
Samuel Merritt University
Oakland, California

Cordia A. Starling, RN, EdD
Professor, Division Chair of Nursing
Dalton State College
Dalton, Georgia

Suzanne Stewart, RN, BS
Faculty
Community College of Denver
Denver, Colorado

Darice Taylor, RNC, MSN
Clinical Assistant Professor
University of Arizona
Tucson, Arizona

Barbara Tewell, RNC, BSN
Perinatal Staff Nurse
Naval Medical Center San Diego
San Diego, California

Acknowledgments

We are grateful for the following people who helped us turn an idea into reality:

Our husbands, Chuck Chapman and Douglas Fredebaugh, for their support and love

Our colleagues at Samuel Merritt University who helped us develop from novice to expert teachers

Our current colleagues at the University of Arizona, College of Nursing and California State University, East Bay Department of Nursing and Health Sciences for their suggestions and support

Our teachers and mentors Katharyn A. May, RN, DNSc, FAAN and Ramona T. Mercer, RN, PhD, FAAN

Sylvia Fischer, RN, MSN, CNM who coordinated the photo shoots and for her family for sharing their cesarean birth

David VanGelder, our outstanding photographer

University Medical Center and Tucson Medical Center nursing staff who facilitated our photo sessions

Our F. A. Davis team, Lisa Deitch, Shirley Kuhn, and Padraic Maroney for their guidance

Kathleen Rehak for technical document support at key intervals

Our contributors for sharing their expertise

Contents in Brief

Table of Contents

Maternity Nursing Overview

Trends and Issues

OBJECTIVES

On completion of this chapter, the student will be able to:

☐ Define key terms.
☐ Discuss current trends in the management of labor and birth.
☐ Discuss the current trends in maternal and infant health outcomes.
☐ Identify leading causes of infant deaths.
☐ Discuss current maternal and infant health issues.
☐ Identify the primary maternal and infant goals stated in *Healthy People 2010*.

TRENDS

During the past 100 years, maternity nursing has undergone numerous changes in response to advances in technology, medicine, and nursing and to the individual desires of childbearing couples (Table 1-1).

The present trend in an increase in both cesarean births and induction of labor is a significant change in the approach to labor and birth. Management of labor and birth has moved from the low use of obstetrical interventions in the natural childbirth era that began in the 1960s to high use of obstetrical interventions and to a more controlled event. The impetus for this shift has been a childbearing generation whose members embrace technology and who have a desire to control when and how their children are born. The scheduling and method of childbirth are also influenced by physicians' preferences.

Changes have also occurred in fertility and birth rates, preterm rates, neonatal birth weight rates, infant mortality rates, and maternal death and mortality rates.

Fertility and Birth Rates

The National Center for Health Statistic (NCHS) defines **fertility rate** as "the total number of live births, regardless of age of mother, per 1,000 women of reproductive age, 15–44 years" (Centers for Disease Control and Prevention [CDC], 2007). **Birth rate** is the number of live births per 1,000 people (CDC, 2007). It is estimated that in 2008 the United States birth rate was ranked number 151 out of 224 countries (CIA, 2008b). The following is a sample ranking of other countries:

■ Niger is ranked no. 1 with a rate of 49.62.
■ Mexico is ranked no. 104 with a rate of 20.04.
■ The United States is ranked no. 151 with a rate of 14.18.
■ New Zealand is ranked no. 153 with a rate of 14.9.
■ The United Kingdom is ranked no. 183 with a rate of 10.65.
■ Canada is ranked no. 192 with a rate of 10.29.
■ Hong Kong is ranked no. 224 with a rate of 7.37 (CIA, 2008b).

In the United States, there was a 50% decrease in both the fertility and birth rates between 1910 and 2007 (Table 1-2). During this period, the fertility rate decreased from 126.8 to 69.5 live births per 1,000 women between the ages of 15 and 44. The birth rate during this same period decreased from 30.1 to 14.3 live births per 1,000. The decline in fertility and birth rates from 1910 to 2007 may be attributed to:

■ Availability of a variety of contraceptive methods with a high effectiveness rate
■ Increased numbers of women delaying and/or limiting pregnancy/children to focus on careers
■ Legalization and availability of elective abortions
■ Rising cost of raising children

TABLE 1–1   PAST AND PRESENT TRENDS

PAST TRENDS	PRESENT TRENDS
Obstetrical Nursing: Focus on physiological changes and needs of the mother and infant.	Family-Centered Maternity Nursing: Focus on both the physiological and psychosocial changes and needs of the childbearing family.
Primarily home births	Primarily hospital births
Women labored in one room and delivered in another room.	Women labor, deliver, and recover in the same room.
Delivery rooms "cold and sterile."	Birthing rooms "warm and homelike"
Expectant fathers and family excluded from the labor and birth experience.	Expectant fathers and family/friends involved in the labor and birth experience.
Expectant fathers excluded from cesarean births	Expectant fathers or family members in the operating room during cesarean births.
Labor pain management: Amnesia or "twilight sleep" to natural childbirth.	Labor pain management: Analgesics and epidurals
Hospital postpartum stay of 10 days.	Hospital postpartum stay of 48 hours.
Infant mortality rate of 58.1 per 1,000 live births in 1933 (Kochanek & Martin, 2004)	Infant mortality rate of 6.3 per 1,000 live births in 2008 (CIA, 2008a)
Maternal mortality rate of 619.1 per 100,000 live births in 1933 (Hoyert, 2007)	Maternal mortality rate of 12.1 per 100,000 live births in 2003 (Hoyert, 2007)
Induction of labor rate of 9.5% in 1990 (Martin et al., 2006)	Induction of labor rate of 21.2% in 2004 (Martin et al., 2006)
Cesarean section rate of 20.7% in 1996 (Martin et al., 2006)	Cesarean section rate of 31.1% in 2006 (Hamilton et al., 2007)
Low probability of infants surviving who were born at or before 28 weeks of gestation.	Increased survival rates of infants born between 24 weeks and 28 weeks of gestation.

TABLE 1–2   BIRTH AND FERTILITY RATES 1910–2007 (RATES PER 1,000 LIVE BIRTHS)

YEAR	1910	1930	1950	1970	1980	1990	1995	2000	2005	2006	2007
BIRTH RATE	30.1	21.3	24.1	18.4	15.9	16.7	14.6	14.4	14.0	14.2	14.3
FERTILITY RATE	126.8	89.2	106.2	87.9	68.4	70.9	64.6	65.9	66.7	68.5	69.5

Source: Hamilton et al. (2003, 2006, 2007, 2009).

TABLE 1–3   BIRTH RATES BY AGE OF MOTHER (PER 1,000)

AGE OF MOTHER	15–19	20–24	25–29	30–34	35–39	40–44	45 +
1990	59.9	116.5	120.2	80.8	31.7	5.5	0.2
2005	40.4	102.2	115.6	95.9	46.3	9.1	0.6
2006	41.9	105.9	116.8	97.7	47.3	9.4	0.6
BIRTH RATE INCREASE 2005–2006	3%	4%	1%	2%	2%	3%	—

An interesting trend is noted for the 15-year period from 1990 to 2005 (Table 1-3). The birth rates decreased for women age 15 to 29, but increased for women age 30 to 45 and older. There was a 19% increase in birth rate for women age 30 to 34 years, a 46% increase for women 35 to 39 years; a 65% increase for women 40 to 44 years; and a 300% increase for women older than 45 years. These increases may reflect the option of women choosing to delay pregnancy and motherhood until they are established in their careers.

In the United States in 2006, there were a total 4,265,996 births. The percentages of these births by race, as reported by CDC, are as follows:

- Non-Hispanic white: 54%
- Hispanic: 24%
- Non-Hispanic black: 14%
- Asian or Pacific Islanders: 6%
- American Indian or Alaska Native: 1%

These percentages reflect the multicultural population of the United States and present an exciting challenge to health care workers to adapt their care to reflect an understanding of the health care beliefs and cultural practices of a wide variety of childbearing families.

Preterm Births

- **Very premature:** Neonates born at less than 32 weeks' gestation
- **Moderately premature:** Neonates born between 32 and 34 weeks' gestation
- **Late premature:** Neonates born between 34 and 36 weeks' gestation (Hamilton, Martin, & Ventura, 2006).

The number of premature births rose from 10.6% of live births in 1990 to 12.8% in 2006 (Hamilton, Martin, & Ventura, 2007) (Table 1-4), reflecting a 21% increase over this time period.

- The greatest increase was in late premature births (Hamilton et al., 2006).
- The 2005 percentages of premature births based on race of mother are:
  - *Non-Hispanic black: 18.4*
  - *American Indian or Alaska Native: 14.1*
  - *Hispanic: 12.1*
  - *Non-Hispanic white: 11.7*
  - *Asian or Pacific Islander: 10.8 (Hamilton et al., 2006).*

The increase in preterm birth rate is alarming in that it has an impact on:

- The emotional well-being of parents
- The length and quality of life for the preterm infant:
  - *A shorter gestational period increases the risk of complications related to immature body organs and systems that can have life-long negative effects.*
  - *68.6% of all infant deaths occur in preterm infants (MacDorman & Mathews, 2008).*
- The increased cost related to health care of preterm infants.

The increase in preterm birth may have a relationship to the increase of birth rates in women 35 years and older. As they age, women are at greater risk for complications during pregnancy such as gestational diabetes and hypertensive disorders. These complications can have an impact on the length of the pregnancy and the overall well-being of the developing fetus.

TABLE 1–4 PERCENTAGE OF PRETERM BIRTHS

	1990	2005	2006
VERY PRETERM	1.9	2.0	2.04
MODERATELY PRETERM	1.4	1.6	1.62
LATE PRETERM	7.3	9.1	9.14

Source: Hamilton et al. (2006, 2007).

Neonatal Birth Weight Rates

Neonatal birth weight rates are reported by the CDC in three major categories of low, normal, and high. Normal birth weight is between 2,500 and 3,999 grams; high birth weight is 4,000 grams or greater; low birth weight is below 2,500 grams. Low birth weight is divided into two categories:

- **Low birth weight (LBW)** is defined as birth weight that is less than 2,500 grams, but greater than 1,500 grams.
- **Very low birth weight (VLBW)** is defined as a birth weight that is less than 1,500 grams.

The National Vital Statistics Reports for 2006 birth data states that:

- The percentage of LBW neonates has increased from 7.0 in 1990 to 8.3 in 2006.
- The percentage of VLBW neonates has increased from 1.27 in 1990 to 1.48 in 2004 (Hamilton et al., 2007).

The weight of neonates at birth is an important predictor of future morbidity and mortality rates (Martin et al., 2006). VLBW neonates are 100 times more likely to die during the first year of life than neonates with birth weights greater than 2,500 grams; whereas neonates with birth weights between 4,000 and 4,999 grams have the lowest mortality rate during the first year of life (Martin et al., 2006).

Infant Mortality Rates

Infant mortality is defined as a death before the first birthday. Infant mortality rates in the United States have significantly decreased from 47.0 per 1,000 live births in 1940 to 6.3 in 2008 (Table 1-5). This decrease is related to:

- Improvement and advances in the knowledge and care of high-risk neonates.
  - *Advances in medical technology such as extracorporeal membrane oxygenation therapy (ECMO) that is used for respiratory distress in preterm infants (see Chapter 17)*
- Medical treatments such as exogenous pulmonary surfactant

Although this is a significant decrease, the infant mortality rate remains too high for a nation with the amount of available wealth and health care resources. The 10 major causes of infant deaths are listed in Table 1-6.

- Between 1994 and 2006, there was a significant decrease in infant deaths related to sudden infant death syndrome (SIDS) and respiratory distress syndrome of newborns (RDS).
  - *The decrease in SIDS can be attributed to instructing parents to place their infants on their backs to sleep versus on their stomachs.*
  - *The decrease in deaths related to RDS reflects advances in medical and nursing care of preterm infants.*

TABLE 1–5   INFANT MORTALITY RATES (RATES PER 1,000 LIVE BIRTHS)

YEAR	1940	1950	1960	1970	1980	1990	1992	1994	1996	1998	2000	2004	2008
RATE	47.0	29.2	26.0	20.0	12.6	9.2	8.5	8.0	7.3	7.2	6.9	6.76	6.3

Sources: CIA (2008a); Kochanek (2004); Minino (2006).

■ The CDC, and the Health Resources and Service Administration in *Healthy People 2010*, have set a goal to decrease infant mortality rate to 4.5 per 1,000 live births by 2010.

CRITICAL COMPONENT

Infant Mortality

The infant mortality rate is highest for:
■ Mothers 16 years and younger related to socioeconomic status and being biologically immature.
■ Mothers older than 44 years of age related to an increased risk of complications due to age, such as gestational diabetes and hypertensive disorders.

Maternal Death and Mortality Rates

The Department of Health and Human Services classifies maternal deaths as follows:

■ **Maternal death** is defined by the World Health Organization (WHO) as the death of a woman during pregnancy or within 42 days of termination of pregnancy. The death is related to the pregnancy or aggravated by pregnancy or management of the pregnancy. It excludes death from accidents or injuries.
■ **Direct obstetric death** is a death resulting from complications during pregnancy, labor/birth, and/or postpartum, and from interventions, omission of interventions, or incorrect treatment.

■ **Indirect obstetrical death** is defined as a death that is due to a preexisting disease or a disease that develops during pregnancy that does not have a direct obstetrical cause, but its likelihood is aggravated by the changes of pregnancy.
■ **Late maternal death** is defined as a death that occurs more than 42 days after termination of pregnancy from a direct or indirect obstetrical cause.
■ **Pregnancy-related cause** is defined a maternal death during pregnancy or within 42 days of termination of pregnancy regardless of cause of death (Hoyert, 2007).

Maternal mortality rates have significantly decreased from 607.9 per 100,000 live births in 1915 to 7.1 in 1998 (Hoyert, 2007). In 1999, there was a change in the International Classification of Diseases (ICD) that added late maternal death and pregnancy-related causes to the ICD-10. Since the addition of these two classifications, the reported maternal mortality rate has increased from 9.9 per 100,000 in 1999 to 12.1 per 100,000 in 2003 (Table 1-7).

Worldwide there are more than 500,000 maternal deaths per year. Ninety-nine percent of these deaths occur in developing countries (World Health Organization [WHO], 2007).

Primary causes of maternal deaths worldwide are:

■ Severe hemorrhage: 25%
■ Infections: 13%
■ Eclampsia: 12%
■ Obstructed labor: 8%
■ Complications of abortions: 13%
■ Other causes, such as anemia, HIV/AIDS and cardiovascular disease: 29% (WHO, 2007)

TABLE 1–6   LEADING CAUSES OF INFANT DEATHS AND MORTALITY RATES (RATES PER 100,000 LIVE BIRTHS)

CAUSE OF DEATH	1994 RATE	2006 RATE
Congenital malformations and chromosomal abnormalities	173.4	136.6
Disorders related to short gestation and low birth weight	107.6	113.5
Sudden infant death syndrome	103.0	50.3
Newborn affected by maternal complications of pregnancy	32.8	39.7
Newborns affected by complications of placenta, cord, and membranes	24	26.3
Accidents	21.7	26.2
Respiratory distress of newborns	39.6	18.8
Bacteria sepsis of the newborn	18.7	18.4
Neonatal hemorrhage	Not reported	14.0
Disease of the circulatory system	24.1	12.6

Sources: Heron, Hoyert, Xu, & Tejada-Vera (2008); Kochanek (2004).

TABLE 1–7	MATERNAL MORTALITY RATES 1915–2003 (RATES PER 100,000 LIVE BIRTHS)									
DATE	1915	1925	1935	1945	1955	1965	1975	1985	1995	2003
RATE	607.9	647.1	582.1	207.2	47.0	31.6	12.8	7.8	7.1	12.1

Source: Hoyert (2007).

ISSUES

Primary issues affecting the health of mothers and infants are births rates for teenagers, tobacco use during pregnancy, substance abuse during pregnancy, and health disparities.

Birth Rate for Teenagers

The birth rate for teenaged women in the United States has significantly decreased since 1991 (Table 1-8) but is still higher than in other developed countries, with a reported 2004 birth rate of 41.1 per 1,000 women 15 to 19 years of age compared to 4.6 rate in the Netherlands (Table 1-9). Teen births not only affect teen mothers, but also have a long-term effect on their children and present a variety of issue for both the teen parents and society:

- Poverty and income disparities
  - *Approximately 50% of teen mothers begin receiving welfare within 5 years of the birth of their first child (The National Campaign to Prevent Teen Pregnancy, 2007).*
  - *Approximately 25% of teen mothers will have a second child within 24 months, which further decreases their ability to complete school and qualify for a well-paying job (The National Campaign to Prevent Teen Pregnancy, 2007).*
- Health issues for teen mothers
  - *Teen mothers are at higher risk for sexually transmitted illnesses and HIV.*
  - *Teen mothers are at higher risk for hypertensive problems during pregnancy.*
- Health issues of infants born to teen mothers
  - *Infants born to teen mothers are at greater risk for health problems that include prematurity and/or low birth weight (The National Campaign to Prevent Teen Pregnancy, 2007).*
  - *Prematurity and/or low birth weight places the infant at higher risk for infant death, respiratory distress syndrome, intraventricular bleeding, visional problem, and intestinal problems (The National Campaign to Prevent Teen Pregnancy, 2007).*

CRITICAL COMPONENT

Teen Pregnancies

- The average related cost for teen pregnancies to federal, state, and/or local government in 2004 was $1,430 per teen mother or an overall cost of $9.1 billion.
- The decrease in teen birth rates by one-third between 1991 and 2004 had an estimated cost savings to governmental agencies of $6.7 billion.

(The National Campaign to Prevent Teen Pregnancy, 2007)

- Educational issues
  - *Only 40% of teen mothers graduate from high school (The National Campaign to Prevent Teen Pregnancy, 2007).*
  - *Children of teen mothers are at higher risk for not completing high school and they have lower scores on standardized tests.*
- Teen fathers
  - *Teenage males without an involved father are at a higher risk for dropping out of school, abusing alcohol and/or drugs, and being incarcerated (The National Campaign to Prevent Teen Pregnancy, 2007).*
  - *Unmarried teen fathers pay less than $800 a year in child support (The National Campaign to Prevent Teen Pregnancy, 2007).*

TABLE 1–8	BIRTH RATES FOR TEENAGE WOMEN (RATES PER 1,000 LIVE BIRTHS)		
AGE	1991	2005	CHANGE
10–14	1.4	0.7	↓ of 50%
15–17	38.6	21.4	↓ of 45%
18–19	94.0	69.9	↓ of 26%

Source: Hamilton et al. (2006).

TABLE 1–9	INTERNATIONAL TEEN BIRTH RATE FOR 2004
NATION	RATE PER 1,000 WOMEN AGE 15–19
Netherlands	4.6
Switzerland	5.2
Japan	5.6
Denmark	5.7
Sweden	5.9
Norway	8.2
Germany	11.0
Canada	14.5
Portugal	19.6
United Kingdom	19.6
United States	26.8

Source: United Nations Statistics Division (2004).

Tobacco Use During Pregnancy

Tobacco use during pregnancy is associated with an increase risk of LBW, intrauterine growth restriction, miscarriage, abruptio placenta, premature birth, SIDS, and respiratory problems in the newborn.

■ Cigarette smoking during pregnancy declined from 19.5% in 1989 to 12.9% in 1998, but increased to 16.3% in 2004 (CDC and the Health Resources and Service Administration, 2000; Martin et al., 2006).

■ Medical costs for birth complications attributed to smoking during pregnancy were estimated at $1.4 billion to $2.0 billion (CDC and the Health Resources and Service Administration, 2000).

■ Women who smoke during pregnancy are less likely to breast-feed their infants.

■ The National Vital Statistics Reports for 2004 states that:

■ *The percentage of smoking during pregnancy has increased from 12.9% in 1998 to 16.3% in 2004.*

■ *Based on educational level, the highest percentage of smokers are women with some high school education and the lowest are women who are college graduates.*

■ *Based on race, the highest percentages of smokers are American Indian and Alaskan Natives and the lowest are Asian or Pacific Islanders (Martin, 2006) (Table 1-10).*

Substance Abuse During Pregnancy

The use of alcohol and illicit drugs during pregnancy can have a profound effect on the developing fetus and the health of the neonate.

■ Exposure to alcohol during pregnancy places the developing fetus at higher risk for fetal death, low birth weight, intrauterine growth retardation, mental retardation, and fetal alcohol syndrome (CDC and the Health Resources and Service Administration, 2000).

■ Exposure to illicit drugs such as cocaine during pregnancy is associated with incidences of preterm birth and abruptio placenta as well as drug withdrawal for the neonate.

■ Health care cost for complications in the neonate related to substance abuse is estimated at:

■ *$75 million to $9.7 billion for fetal alcohol syndrome*

■ *$500 million for infants exposed to cocaine during pregnancy (CDC and the Health Resources and Service Administration, 2000).*

Health Disparities

The topic of health disparities addresses the differences in access, use of health care services, and health outcomes for various factors such as age, race, ethnicity, socioeconomic status, and geographic groups and health status of these populations.

■ The largest health disparity occurs in people of low income regardless of their race or ethnicity (Agency for Healthcare Research and Quality, 2007).

■ People of low income are less likely to receive comprehensive primary health care and have higher rates of avoidable hospitalization (Agency for Healthcare Research and Quality, 2007).

CRITICAL COMPONENT

Prenatal Care

Low-income women are less likely to seek early and continuous prenatal care. These health care behaviors place both the woman and her unborn child at higher risk for complications during pregnancy, labor and birth, and postpartum.

■ The percentages of women who begin prenatal care during the first trimester and those who begin prenatal care late in the pregnancy or receive no prenatal care based on race are listed in Table 1-11.

CRITICAL COMPONENT

Infant Mortality

The 2003 mortality rate for infants of mothers who began prenatal care after the first trimester or did not receive prenatal care was 8.96 per 1,000 live births. This rate is 45% higher than mortality rates for infants of mothers who began prenatal care during the first trimester.

(Mathews & MacDorman, 2006)

■ Disparities exist in birth outcomes as measured by percentages of premature births and low birth weight (Table 1-12).

■ Disparities exist in infant mortality rates based on race (Table 1-13).

These disparities can partially be attributed to barriers to access to health care for low-income families. Examples of barriers to access to health care are limited finances, lack of transportation, difficulty with dominant language, and attitudes of the health care team.

TABLE 1–10 SMOKING DURING PREGNANCY FOR 2004	
RACE	PERCENTAGE
American Native and Alaskan Native	18.2
Non-Hispanic white	13.8
Non-Hispanic black	8.4
Hispanic	2.6
Asian or Pacific Islanders	2.2

Source: Martin et al. (2006).

TABLE 1–11 2004 REPORTED PERCENTAGES FOR PRENATAL CARE		
RACE	PERCENTAGE BEGINNING PRENATAL CARE DURING FIRST TRIMESTER	PERCENTAGE OF LATE OR NO PRENATAL CARE
WHITE	88.9	2.2
BLACK	76.5	5.7
HISPANIC	77.5	5.4

Source: Martin et al. (2006).

TABLE 1–12 2004 REPORTED PERCENTAGES OF PRETERM BIRTH AND LOW BIRTH WEIGHT BY RACE

	VERY PRETERM (>32 WEEKS)	PRETERM (LESS THAN 37 WEEKS)	VERY LOW BIRTH WEIGHT (>1500 GRAMS)	LOW BIRTH WEIGHT (>2500 GRAMS)
ALL RACES	2.01	12.5	1.48	8.1
WHITE	1.63	11.5	1.20	7.2
BLACK	4.05	17.9	3.15	13.7
HISPANIC	1.77	12.0	1.20	6.8

Source: Martin et al. (2006).

TABLE 1–13 2003 INFANT MORTALITY RATES BY RACE FOR THE FIVE LEADING CAUSES OF DEATH (RATES PER 100,000 LIVE BIRTHS)

CAUSE OF DEATH	NON-HISPANIC WHITE	NON-HISPANIC BLACK	AMERICAN INDIAN	ASIA OR PACIFIC ISLANDER	HISPANIC
ALL CAUSES OF DEATH	569.7	1,360.7	872.9	482.9	564.5
CONGENITAL MALFORMATIONS, DEFORMITIES, AND CHROMOSOMAL ABNORMALITIES	128.0	167.5	187.6	117.2	144.2
DISORDERS RELATED TO SHORT TERM GESTATION AND LOW BIRTHWEIGHT	79.5	313.7	112.6	86.9	94.7
SUDDEN INFANT DEATH SYNDROME	50.5	108.8	124.0	27.7	25.6
NEWBORN AFFECTED BY MATERNAL COMPLICATIONS OF PREGNANCY	33.6	94.1	Not reported	26.7	30.4
NEWBORN AFFECTED BY COMPLICATIONS OF PLACENTA, CORD, AND MEMBRANES	23.4	51.6	Not reported	14.3	21.0

Source: Mathews & MacDorman (2006).

MATERNAL AND CHILD HEALTH GOALS

The health of a nation is reflected in the health of expectant women and their infants (CDC and Health Resources and Service Administration, 2000). Diseases and illness related to complications during pregnancy and the neonatal period can have a life-long impact on the health of that individual. Low birth weight and premature neonates are at higher risk for chronic respiratory diseases and abnormalities in neurological development. The CDC and Health Resources and Services have set national health goals that are published in *Healthy People 2010* (Table 1-14). Improving the health of women before and during pregnancy and the health of infants will have life-long effects on the health of the nation.

TABLE 1–14   *HEALTHY PEOPLE 2010* MATERNAL AND INFANT HEALTH GOALS

OBJECTIVES	BASELINE	2010 TARGET
Reduction in fetal and infant deaths:		
▪ Fetal deaths at 20 or more weeks of gestation	6.8 per 1,000	4.1 per 1,000
▪ Fetal and infant deaths during the perinatal period	7.5 per 1,000	4.5 per 1,000
Reduction of infant deaths:		
▪ All infant deaths (within 1 year)	7.2 per 1,000	4.5 per 1,000
▪ Neonatal deaths (within the first 28 days)	4.8 per 1,000	2.9 per 1,000
▪ Postnatal deaths (between 29 days and 1 year)	2.4 per 1,000	1.2 per 1,000
Reduction in infant deaths related to birth defects	1.6 per 1,000	1.1 per 1,000
Reduction of death from sudden infant death syndrome (SIDS)	0.72 per 1,000	0.25 per 1,000
Reduction of maternal deaths	7.1 per 100,000 live births	3.3 per 100,000 live births
Reduction of maternal illness and complications	31.2 per 100 deliveries	24 per 100 deliveries
Increase of maternal prenatal care:		
▪ Care beginning in first trimester	83% of live births	90% of live births
▪ Early and adequate prenatal care	74% of live births	90% of live births
Increase the proportion of very low birth weight (VLBW) infants born at level III hospitals or subspecialty perinatal centers	73%	90%
Reduction of cesarean births		
▪ Women giving birth for the first time	18%	15%
▪ Prior cesarean birth	72%	63%
Reduce low birth weight (LBW) and very low birth weight (VLBW):		
▪ Low birth weight	7.6%	5.0%
▪ Very low birth weight	1.4%	0.9%
Reduction of preterm births	11.6%	7.6%
Increase the percentage of healthy full-term infants who are put down to sleep on their backs	35%	70%
Reduction in developmental disabilities in children:		
▪ Mental retardation	131 per 10,000	124 per 10,000
▪ Cerebral palsy	32.2 per 10,000	31.5 per 10,000
Increase of pregnancies begun with optimum folic acid levels:		
▪ Median RBC folate levels among nonpregnant women age 15–44 years	160 ng/mL	220 ng/mL
Increase abstinence from alcohol, cigarettes, and illicit drugs among pregnant women:		
▪ Alcohol	86%	94%
▪ Binge drinking	99%	100%
▪ Cigarette smoking	87%	99%
▪ Illicit drugs	98%	100%
Increase in mothers who breastfeed:		
▪ In early postpartum	64%	75%
▪ At 6 months	29%	50%
▪ At 1 year	16%	25%

Source: CDC and Health Resources and Service Administration (2000).

■ ■ ■ **Review Questions** ■ ■ ■

1. The population with the lowest birth rate, but highest premature birth rate is:
   A. Non-Hispanic white
   B. Non-Hispanic black
   C. American Indian or Alaska Native
   D. Asian or Pacific Islanders
   E. Hispanic

2. Moderately premature neonates are neonates born:
   A. At less that 28 weeks' gestation
   B. Between 28 weeks and 30 weeks' gestation
   C. Between 30 and 32 weeks' gestation
   D. Between 32 and 34 weeks' gestation
   E. Between 34 and 36 weeks' gestation

3. The two most important predictors of an infant's health and survival after birth are:
   A. Gestational age and birth weight
   B. Gestation age and early prenatal care
   C. Gestational age and complication during labor and birth
   D. Gestational age and Apgar score

4. Which of the following health care issues has the greatest related cost to federal, state, and/or local governments?
   A. Teen pregnancies
   B. Tobacco use during pregnancy
   C. Substance abuse during pregnancy
   D. Sexually transmitted diseases during pregnancy

5. A primary maternal and infant goal stated in *Healthy People 2010* is:
   A. Reduce labor induction to 25%.
   B. Reduce cesarean birth for first-time mothers to 15%.
   C. Reduce high birth weight neonates to 10%.
   D. Reduce neonatal blindness by 5%.

References

Agency for Healthcare Research and Quality. (2007). *National Healthcare Disparities Report 2005*. Retrieved from www.ahrq.gov/qual/nhdr05/nhdr05.htm (Accessed August 17, 2009).

Centers for Disease Control and Prevention (CDC). (2007). *NCHS Definitions* [online]. Retrieved from www.cdc/gov/data/series/sr_21_008acc.pdf (Accessed August 17, 2009).

Centers for Disease Control and Prevention, and Health Resources and Service Administration. (2000). *Healthy People 2010* [online]. Retrieved from www.healthypeople.gov/Document/HTML/Volume2/16MICH.htm (Accessed August 17, 2009).

Centers for Disease Control and Prevention, and Health Resources and Service Administration. (2001). *2001 Surgeon General's Report – Women and Smoking* [online]. Retrieved from www.cdc.gov/tobacco/data_statistics/sgr_2001 (Accessed August 17, 2009).

Central Intelligence Agency (CIA). (2008a). *Rank Order – Infant Mortality Rates.* Retrieved from www.CIA.gov/library/publications/the-world-factbook/rankorder/2091rank.html (Accessed August 17, 2009).

Central Intelligence Agency (CIA). (2008b). *Rank Order of Birth Rates.* Retrieved from www.CIA.gov/library/publications/the-world-factbook/rankorder/2054.html (Accessed August 17, 2009).

Hamilton, B., Martin, J., and Ventura, S. (2006). *Births: Preliminary data for 2005. Health E-Stats.* [online – released November 21, 2006]. Retrieved from www.cdc/gov/nchs/products/pubs/pubd/hestats/prelimbirths05/prelimbirths05.htm (Accessed August 17, 2009).

Hamilton, B., Martin, J., and Ventura, S. (2007). Preliminary data for 2006. *National Vital Statistics Reports, 56*, 1–28 [online]. Hyattsville, MD: National Center for Health Statistics. Retrieved from www.cdc.gov/nchs/data/nvsr/nvsr56/nvsr56_07.pdf (Accessed August 17, 2009).

Hamilton, B., Martin, J., and Ventura, S. (2009). Preliminary data for 2007. *National Vital Statistics Reports, 57*, 1–23. Hyattsville, MD: National Center for Health Statistics.

Hamilton, B., Sutton, P., and Ventura, S. (2003). Revised birth and fertility for 1990's and new rates for Hispanic populations 2000 and 2001: United States. *National Vital Statistics Report, 51*, 1–95 [online]. Retrieved from www.cdc.gov/nchs/data/nvsr/nvsr51/nvsr51_12.pdf (Accessed August 17, 2009).

Heron, M., Hoyert, D., Xu, J., & Tejada-Vera, B. (2008). Death: Preliminary data for 2006. *National Vital Statistics Report, 56*, 1–52.

Hoyert, D. (2007). Maternal mortality and related concepts. *National Center for Human Statistics. Vital Health Stat, 3*, 1–13.

Kochanek, K., & Martin, J. (2004). *Supplemental analyses of recent trend infant mortality. Health E-Stats* [online]. Retrieved from www.cdc.gov/nchs/products/pubs/pubd/hestats/infantmort/infantmort.htm (Accessed August 17, 2009).

MacDorman, M., & Mathews, T. (2008). *Recent trends in infant mortality in the United States.* NCHS data brief no. 9. Hyattsville, MD: National Center for Health Statistics. Retrieved from www.cdc.gov/nchs/data/databriefs/db09.htm (Accessed August 17, 2009).

Martin, J., Hamilton, B., Sutton, P., Ventura, S., Menacker, F., & Kirmeyer, S. (2006). *Final data for 2004. National vital statistics reports, 55*, 1–20. Retrieved from www.cdc.gov/nchs/data/nvsr/nvsr55/nvsr545_11.pdf (Accessed August 17, 2009).

Mathews, J., & MacDorman, F. (2006). Infant mortality statistics from 2003 period linked birth/death data set. *National Vital Statistics Report, 54*, 1–32. Retrieved from www.cdc.gov/nchs/data/nvsr/nvsr54/nvsr54_16.pfd (Accessed August 17, 2009).

Minino, A., Heron, M., & Smith, B. (2006). *Deaths: Preliminary data for 2004. Health E-Stats* [online]. Retrieved from www.cdc.gov/nchs/products/pubs/pubd/hestats/prelimimdeaths04/prelimdeaths04.htm (Accessed August 17, 2009).

The National Campaign to Prevent Teen Pregnancy. (2007). *Why it matters.* Retrieved from www.thenationalcampaign.org (Accessed Auguest 17, 2009).

National Center for Health Statistics. United Nations Statistics Division. (2004). *Demographic yearbook 2004.* New York: United Nations.

World Health Organization (2007). *Maternal mortality in 2005.* Retrieved from www.who.int/reproductive-health/publications/maternal_mortality_2005/mme_2005.pdf (Accessed August 17, 2009).

Ethics and Standards of Practice Issues

2

OBJECTIVES

On completion of this chapter, students will be able to:
- ☐ Define key terms.
- ☐ Debate ethical issues in maternity nursing.
- ☐ Explain standards of practice in maternity nursing.
- ☐ Describe legal issues in maternity nursing.
- ☐ Examine concepts in evidence-based practice.

*I*NTRODUCTION

Maternity nursing is an exciting and dynamic area of nursing practice. With that excitement come issues related to ethical challenges, high rates of litigation in obstetrics, and the challenge of practicing safe and evidence-based nursing care that is responsive to the needs of women and families. This chapter presents the foundational principles set forth by the American Nurses Association (ANA) Code of Ethics and specialty practice standards from the Association for Women's Health, Obstetric and Neonatal Nurses (AWHONN) that outline duties and obligations of obstetric and neonatal nurses. Ethical principles are reviewed within the context of perinatal dilemmas and ethical decision making. Common issues in litigation in maternity nursing are presented. Evidence-based practice and challenges in research use in the perinatal setting are explored.

*E*THICS IN NURSING PRACTICE

The study of ethics is based in philosophical discussions of ancient Greek scholars about the nature of good and evil or right and wrong. Ethics is an integral part of nursing practice and represents the ideal of social order. The ethical tradition of nursing is self-reflective, enduring, and distinctive. Nurses' moral and ethical responsibility to do the right thing is discussed in the ANA Code of Ethics for Nurses (2001).

ANA Code of Ethics

The ANA Code of Ethics makes explicit the primary goals, values, and obligations of the profession of nursing (ANA, 2001). The code of ethics for nursing serves as:

- A statement of the ethical obligations and duties of every nurse
- The profession's non-negotiable ethical standard
- An expression of nursing's own understanding of its commitment to society

The ANA Code of Ethics for Nurses describes the most fundamental values and commitments of the nurse; boundaries of duty and loyalty; and aspects of duties beyond individual patient encounter (Table 2-1).

Ethical Principles

Ethical and social issues affecting the health of pregnant women and their fetus are increasingly complex. Some of the complexity arises from technological advances in reproductive technology, maternity care, and neonatal care. Nurses are autonomous professionals who are required to provide ethically competent care. Some ethical principles related to patient care include (Lagana & Duderstadt, 2004):

- **Autonomy:** The right to self determination
- **Respect for others:** Principle that all persons are equally valued
- **Beneficence:** Obligation to do good
- **Nonmaleficence:** Obligation to do no harm
- **Justice:** Principle of equal treatment of others or that others be treated fairly
- **Fidelity:** Faithfulness or obligation to keep promises
- **Veracity:** Obligation to tell the truth
- **Utility:** The greatest good for the individual or an action that is valued

Ethical Approaches

Clinical situations arise where ethical principals conflict with each other. For example, the patient's right to self-determination, autonomy, includes the right to refuse treatment that may be beneficial to the pregnancy outcome for the fetus. Consideration of ethical approaches can help nurses as they encounter ethical dilemmas. There are a variety of ethical approaches. Two key approaches are:

- The Rights Approach: The focus is on the individual's right to choose, and the rights include the right to privacy, to know the truth, and to be free from injury or harm.
- The Utilitarian Approach: This approach posits that ethical actions are those that provide the greatest balance of good over evil and provides for the greatest good for the greatest number.

TABLE 2–1   AMERICAN NURSES ASSOCIATION CODE OF ETHICS

PROVISION 1	The nurse, in all professional relationships, practices with compassion and respect for the inherent dignity, worth, and uniqueness of every individual unrestricted by consideration of social or economic status, personal attributes, or nature of the health problems.
PROVISION 2	The nurse's primary commitment is to the patient, whether an individual, family, group, or community.
PROVISION 3	The nurse promotes, advocates for, and strives to protect the health, safety, and rights of the patient.
PROVISION 4	The nurse is responsible and accountable for individual nursing practice and determines the appropriate delegation of tasks consistent with the nurse's obligation to provide optimum care.
PROVISION 5	The nurse owes the same duties to self as to others, including the responsibility to preserve integrity and safety, to maintain competence, and to continue personal and professional growth.
PROVISION 6	The nurse participates in establishing and maintaining health care environments and conditions of employment conducive to the provision of quality health care and consistent with the values of the profession through individual and collective action.
PROVISION 7	The nurse participates in the advancement of the profession through contributions to practice, education, administration, and knowledge development.
PROVISION 8	The nurse collaborates with other health professionals and the public in promoting community, national, and international efforts to meet health needs.
PROVISION 9	The profession of nursing, as represented by associations and their members, is responsible for articulating nursing values, for maintaining the integrity of the profession and its practice, and for shaping social policy.

Source: American Nurses Association. (2001). *Code of ethics for nurses with interpretive statements.* Silver Spring, MD: American Nurses Publishing. Retrieved from http://www.nursingworld.org

One can see how these two approaches could result in ethical dilemmas when decisions are made in clinical situations where the individual's right to choose may be in conflict with the greatest good for society.

Ethical Dilemmas

An **ethical dilemma** is a choice that has the potential to violate ethical principles (Lagana & Duderstadt, 2004). In nursing it is often based on the nurse's commitment to advocacy. Action taken in response to our ethical responsibility to intervene on behalf of those in our care is patient **advocacy**. Advocacy also involves accountability for nurses' responses to patients' needs (Lagana, 2000). A unique aspect of maternity nursing is that the nurse advocates for two individuals, the woman and the fetus. The maternity nurse's advocacy role is more clearly assigned for the pregnant woman than for the fetus, yet the needs of the mother and fetus are interdependent (Lagana & Duderstadt, 2004). Examples of ethical dilemmas in clinical practice are presented in Box 2-1.

Ethics in Neonatal Care

Ethics involves determining what is good, right, and fair (Pierce, 1998). The role of nurses in the neonatal intensive care unit (NICU) requires a dual role for nurses to protect the well-being of vulnerable infants as well as supporting and respecting parental decisions. According to the ANA Code of Ethics (2001), nurses have an obligation to safeguard the well-being of patients, but they also have the obligation to avoid inflicting harm. One example of a situation in which ethical decision making conflicts can arise is in the care of infants with extreme prematurity. Pierce (1998) suggests three categories for neonates in the NICU:

■ Infants in whom aggressive care would probable be futile, where prognosis for a meaningful life is extremely poor or hopeless

BOX 2–1   CLINICAL EXAMPLES OF PERINATAL ETHICAL DILEMMAS

■ Court-ordered treatment
■ Withdrawal of life support
■ Harvesting of fetal organs or tissue
■ In vitro fertilization and decisions for disposal of remaining fertilized ova
■ Allocation of resources in pregnancy care during the previable period
■ Fetal surgery
■ Treatment of genetic disorders or fetal abnormalities found on prenatal screening
■ Equal access to prenatal care
■ Maternal rights versus fetal rights
■ Extraordinary medical treatment for pregnancy complications
■ Using organs from an anencephalic infant
■ Genetic engineering
■ Cloning
■ Surrogacy
■ Drug testing in pregnancy
■ Sanctity of life versus quality of life for extremely premature or severely disabled infants
■ Substance abuse in pregnancy
■ Borderline viability: to resuscitate or not
■ Fetal reduction
■ Preconception gender selection

■ Infants in whom aggressive care would probably result in clear benefit to overall well-being, where prevailing knowledge and evidence indicate excellent chances for beneficial outcomes and meaningful interactions
■ Infants in whom the effect of aggressive care is mostly uncertain (Fig. 2-1).

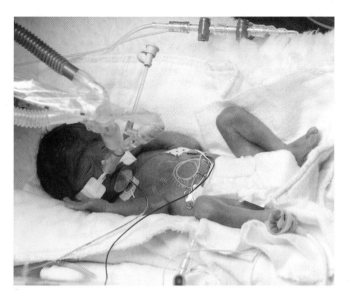

Figure 2-1 Extremely premature baby in NICU.

Caring for infants in the face of prognostic uncertainty can present ethical dilemmas for nurses as they balance the needs of the infant's well-being with the parent's rights to make decisions. Nurses must continually involve parents in ongoing assessment of infant's overall well-being. This may be challenging as parents deal with the loss of a "dream" child, the shock of a critically ill neonate, or an unexpected pregnancy outcome. Nurses must report data and perceptions clearly to parents and actively listen to their concerns and understanding of current clinical reality and long-term prognosis. Team conferences with physician, nurses, parents, and social workers can be crucial to developing plans of care. Lack of consensus about a plan of care can result in profound harms for the infants, families, the health care team, and society (Penticuff, 1998) and can include needless suffering of the infant, psychological distress and conflict between the family and providers, and inappropriate expenditure of societal resources. Penticuff (1998) proposes that moral responsibility for the good and harm that comes to an infant in the NICU is not borne exclusively by either the parents or the health care team. Nurses and all health care providers are obligated to both respect parental wishes and uphold ethical standards. Legal and ethical precedent suggests that parents ought to be the chief decision makers (*Nurse's Legal Handbook*, 2004). However, parents often lack the expertise required to make decisions yet are ultimately required to care for the long-term needs of the child.

Collaboration among parents and professionals is essential to work for the infant's good when making treatment decisions for infants in the NICU. Collaborative working relationships encompass working together with mutual respect for the accountabilities of each profession to the shared goal of quality patient outcomes (Asokar, 1998). **Paternalism** is a system under which an authority makes decisions for others.

Society holds the sanctity of life in high regard, as without life other values are irrelevant (*Nurse's Legal Handbook*, 2004). Questions emerge about the quality of life when caring for critically ill neonates. A method to organize clinical data and some questions have been proposed, the Four Topics Method, which works with every kind of clinical situation to facilitate clinical decision making (Jonsen, Siegler, & Winslade, 2006).

Four Topics Method

Three ethicists (Jonsen, Siegler, and Winslade) developed a method with which to work through difficult clinical situations with ethical dilemmas. While it has deep philosophical roots, clinicians use this method as it is in keeping and fits with how they normally think about challenging clinical situations. The authors have identified four "topics" that are basic and intrinsic to every clinical encounter. Focusing discussion around these four topics is one a way to organize the facts of the particular clinical situation:

- Medical Indications: A review of diagnosis and treatment options
- Patient Preferences: Clinical patients' values preferences are integral to all clinical situations.
- Quality of Life: Objective is to improve, or at least address, quality of life for the patient.
- Contextual Features: In the wider societal context beyond care providers and patient, to include family, the law, hospital policy, insurance companies, and so forth

No one topic bears more weight than the others. Each is evaluated from the perspective of the facts of the situation at hand. Details of a situation can be outlined according to the four topics (using the four boxes), and there are a series of questions that the clinician should ask related to each topic. The questions and topics may assist the nurse to clarify ethical dilemmas and conflicts in clinical situations. In Table 2-2, the Four Topics Method is presented highlighting issues in the NICU related to an infant with extreme prematurity.

Nurses must first be clear about their moral and ethical perspective to be effective as part of the collaborative health care team. Nurses spend more time at the bedside providing care for neonates and interacting with parents than any other health professional. Central concepts in nursing are advocacy and caring. Nurses assume a key role in ethical decision making because of their unique position in all perinatal settings. Ethical sensitivity in professional practice develops in contexts of uncertainty; client suffering and vulnerability; and through relationships characterized by receptivity, responsiveness, and courage on the part of professionals. A little dose of practical wisdom goes a long way.

STANDARDS OF PRACTICE

In addition to a Code of Ethics from the ANA (2001), practice standards help to guide professional nursing practice. The Association of Women's Health, Obstetric and Neonatal Nurses (AWHONN), the professional organization for maternity nurses, has developed practice standards. The standards summarize what AWHONN (2003) believes is the nursing profession's best judgment and optimal practice based on current research and clinical practice. AWHONN believes that these standards are helpful for all nurses engaged in the functions described. As with most or all such standards, certain qualifications should be borne in mind (Tables 2-3 and 2-4).

- These standards articulate general guidelines; additional considerations or procedures may be warranted for particular patients or settings. The best interest of an individual patient is always the touchstone of practice.
- These standards are but one source of guidance. Nurses also must act in accordance with applicable law, institutional rules and procedures, and established interprofessional arrangements concerning the division of duties.

TABLE 2–2 THE FOUR TOPICS METHOD

MEDICAL INDICATIONS	PATIENT PREFERENCES
The Principles of Beneficence and Nonmaleficence	**The Principle of Respect for Autonomy**
1. What is the patient's medical problem? History? Diagnosis? Prognosis? 2. Is the problem acute? Chronic? Critical? Emergent? Reversible? 3. What are the goals of treatment? 4. What are the probabilities of success? 5. What are the plans in case of therapeutic failure? 6. How can this patient be benefited by medical and nursing care, and how can harm be avoided? ■ In the NICU, in the case of extreme neonatal prematurity, decisions related to viability related to gestational age and probability of survival are central.	1. Is the patient mentally capable and legally competent? Is there evidence of incapacity? 2. If competent, what is the patient stating about preferences for treatment? 3. Has the patient been informed of benefits and risks, understood this information, and given consent? 4. If incapacitated, who is the appropriate surrogate? Is the surrogate using appropriate standards for decision making? 5. Has the patient expressed prior preferences, e.g., Advance Directives? 6. Is the patient unwilling or unable to cooperate with medical treatment? If so, why? 7. Is the patient's right to choose being respected to the extent possible in ethics and law? ■ In the NICU, parents are surrogate decision makers for the neonate and need to be fully informed of risks and benefits of treatment options.
QUALITY OF LIFE	CONTEXTUAL FEATURES
The Principles of Beneficence and Nonmaleficence and Respect for Autonomy	**The Principles of Loyalty and Fairness**
1. What are the prospects, with or without treatment, for a return to a normal life? 2. What physical, mental, and social deficits is the patient likely to experience if treatment succeeds? 3. Are there biases that might prejudice the provider's evaluation of the patient's quality of life? 4. Is the patient's present or future condition such that his or her continued life might be judged undesirable? 5. Is there any plan and rationale to forgo treatment? 6. Are there plans for comfort and palliative care? ■ In the NICU, quality of life and the potential for the neonate to achieve meaningful human interactions, long-term prognosis for disabilities are key issues in decision making.	1. Are there family issues that might influence treatment decisions? 2. Are there provider (physicians and nurses) issues that might influence treatment decisions? 3. Are there financial and economic factors? 4. Are there cultural or religious factors? 5. Are there limits on confidentiality? 6. Are there problems of allocation of resources? 7. How does the law affect treatment decisions? 8. Is clinical research or teaching involved? 9. Is there any conflict of interest on the part of the providers or the institution? ■ In the NICU, parents are key decision makers. Conflicts between parental desires and institutional or provider can arise related to initiation of treatment and continuation of treatment.

■ These standards represent optimal practice. Full compliance may not be possible at all times with all patients in all settings.

■ These standards serve as a guide for optimal practice. They are not designed to define standards of practice for employment, licensure, discipline, reimbursement, or legal or other purposes.

■ These standards may change in response to changes in research and practice.

■ The standards define the nurse's responsibility to the patient and the roles and behaviors to which the nurse is accountable. The definition of terms delimits the scope of the standards.

LEGAL ISSUES IN DELIVERY OF CARE

Maternity nursing is the most litigious of all the areas of nursing. Contributing to this is the complexity of caring for two patients, the mother and the fetus. There are five clinical situations that account for a majority of fetal and neonatal injuries and litigation in obstetrics (Feinstein, Torgersen, & Atterbury, 2003):

■ Inability to recognize and/or inability to appropriately respond to intrapartum fetal compromise

■ Inability to effect a timely cesarean birth (30 minutes from decision to incision) when indicated by fetal or maternal condition

■ Inability to appropriately initiate resuscitation of a depressed neonate

■ Inappropriate use of oxytocin or misoprostol leading to uterine hyperstimulation, uterine rupture, and fetal intolerance of labor and/or fetal death

■ Inappropriate use of forceps/vacuum and/or preventable shoulder dystocia

The number of obstetric malpractice claims represents only about 5% of all malpractice claims, but the dollar amount for the claims represents up to 35% of the total financial liability of a hospital or health care system (Simpson & Creehan, 2008). The literature indicates that

TABLE 2–3 STANDARDS FOR PROFESSIONAL NURSING PRACTICE IN THE CARE OF WOMEN AND NEWBORNS

STANDARDS OF CARE
STANDARD I. ASSESSMENT The nurse collects health data about women and newborns.
STANDARD II. DIAGNOSIS The nurse analyzes the assessment data in determining diagnoses and identifying problems of women and newborns.
STANDARD III. OUTCOME IDENTIFICATION The nurse identifies expected outcomes individualized to the woman or newborn.
STANDARD IV. PLANNING The nurse develops a plan of care that prescribes interventions to attain expected outcomes for women or newborns.
STANDARD V. IMPLEMENTATION The nurse implements the interventions identified in the woman's or newborn's plan of care.
STANDARD VI. EVALUATION The nurse evaluates women's and newborns' progress toward expected outcomes.

STANDARDS OF PROFESSIONAL PERFORMANCE
STANDARD I. QUALITY OF CARE The nurse systematically evaluates the quality and effectiveness of nursing practice and implements measures to improve the quality of care for women and newborns.
STANDARD II. PERFORMANCE APPRAISAL The nurse evaluates her or his own nursing practice in relation to professional practice standards and relevant statutes and regulations.
STANDARD III. EDUCATION The nurse acquires and maintains current knowledge in maternal, newborn, and/or women's health nursing practice.
STANDARD IV. COLLEGIALITY The nurse contributes to the professional development of peers, colleagues, and other health care providers.
STANDARD V. ETHICS The nurse's decisions and actions on behalf of women and newborns are determined in an ethical manner.
STANDARD VI. COLLABORATION The nurse collaborates with women, families, significant others, and health care providers in providing care.
STANDARD VII. RESEARCH The nurse integrates research findings in practice.
STANDARD VIII. RESOURCE UTILIZATION The nurse considers factors related to safety, effectiveness and cost in planning and delivering care to women and newborns.
STANDARD IX. PRACTICE ENVIRONMENT The nurse promotes a safe and therapeutic environment for women, newborns, family, significant others, and care providers.
STANDARD X. ACCOUNTABILITY The nurse is professionally and legally accountable for her or his practice.

Source: Association for Women's Health, Obstetric and Neonatal Nurses (AWHONN). (2003). *Standards for professional nursing practice in the care of women and newborns* (6th ed.). Washington, DC: Author.

patients who are more dissatisfied with the interpersonal interaction with health care providers are more likely to pursue litigation (Lagana, 2000). It has also been suggested that increased use of technology may interfere with a nurse's ability to engage with women and families in a therapeutic and caring interaction.

Fetal Monitoring

One clinical issue that is often a key element of litigation is related to interpretation of fetal heart rate (FHR) monitoring and is related to the nurse's ability to recognize and appropriately respond to intrapartal fetal compromise. For that reason, this is the focus of this section and serves as an example of how nursing standards, guidelines, and policies should be the foundation of safe practice. Common allegations related to fetal monitoring are:

■ Failure to accurately assess maternal and fetal status
■ Failure to appreciate a deteriorating fetal status
■ Failure to treat a nonreassuring FHR
■ Failure to correctly communicate maternal/fetal status to the care provider
■ Failure to institute the chain of command when there is a clinical disagreement

TABLE 2–4   TERMS RELATED TO STANDARDS

TERM	DEFINITION
ASSESSMENT	A systematic, dynamic process by which the nurse, through interaction with women, newborns and families, significant others, and health care providers, collects, monitors, and analyzes data. Data may include the following dimensions: psychological, biotechnological, physical, sociocultural, spiritual, cognitive, developmental, and economic, as well as functional abilities and lifestyle.
CHILDBEARING AND NEWBORN HEALTH CARE	A model of care addressing the health promotion, maintenance, and restoration needs of women from the preconception through the postpartum period; and low-risk, high-risk, and critically ill newborns from birth through discharge and follow-up, within the social, political, economic and environmental context of the mother's, her newborn's, and the family's lives.
DIAGNOSIS	A clinical judgment about the patient's response to actual or potential health conditions or needs. Diagnoses provide the basis for determination of a plan of nursing care to achieve expected outcomes.
DIVERSITY	A quality that encompasses acceptance and respect related to but not limited to age, class, culture, disability, education level, ethnicity, family structure, gender, ideologies, political beliefs, race, religion, sexual orientation, style, and values.
EVALUATION	The process of determining the patient's progress toward attainment of expected outcomes and the effectiveness of nursing care.
IMPLEMENTATION	The process of taking action by intervening, delegating, and/or coordinating. Women, newborns, families, significant others, or health care providers may direct the implementation of interventions within the plan of care.
OUTCOME	A measurable individual, family, or community state, behavior, or perception that is responsive to nursing interventions.
STANDARD	Authoritative statement enunciated and promulgated by the profession and by which the quality of practice, service or education can be judged.
STANDARDS OF CARE	Authoritative statements that describe competent clinical nursing practice for women and newborns demonstrated through assessment, diagnosis, outcome identification, planning, implementation, and evaluation.
STANDARDS OF NURSING PRACTICE	Authoritative statements that describe the scope of care or performance common to the profession of nursing and by which the quality of nursing practice can be judged. Standards of nursing practice for women and newborns include both standards of care and standards of professional performance.
STANDARDS OF PROFESSIONAL PERFORMANCE	Authoritative statements that describe competent behavior in the professional role, including activities related to quality of care, performance appraisal, resource utilization, education, collegiality, ethics, collaboration, research, and research utilization.

Source: Association for Women's Health, Obstetric and Neonatal Nurses (AWHONN). (2003). *Standards for professional nursing practice in the care of women and newborns* (6th ed.). Washington, DC: Author.

Nurses are accountable for safe and effective FHR assessment and failure to do so contributes to claims of nursing negligence (Gilbert, 2007; Mahlmeister, 2000). AWHONN (2000) provides a position statement on fetal assessment that states:

■ AWHONN strongly advises that nurses should complete a course of study that includes physiological interpretation of electronic fetal monitoring (EFM) and its implications for care in labor.
■ Each facility should develop a policy that defines when to use EFM and auscultation of FHR and that specifies frequency and documentation based on best available evidence, professional association guidelines, and expert consensus.

Timely communication and collaboration with care providers is essential to ensure indeterminate or normal (non-reassuring) FHR patterns are managed appropriately. Organizational resources and systems should be in place to support timely interventions when FHR is indeterminate or normal (Simpson & Knox, 2003). Uniform FHR terminology and interpretation are necessary to facilitate appropriate communication and legally defensible documentation (Feinstein, Torgersen, & Atterbury, 2003).

Interpretation of FHR data can sometimes result in conflict. There may be agreement about ominous patterns and normal patterns but often care providers encounter patterns that fall between these extremes (Freeman, 2002). Some issues of conflict in the clinical setting cannot be resolved between the caregivers immediately involved, yet need to be resolved quickly.

1. The nurse must initiate the course of action when the clinical situation is a matter of maternal or fetal well-being.
2. In a case of a primary care provider not responding to an abnormal FHR or a deteriorating clinical situation, the nurse should use the chain of command to resolve the situation, advocate for the patient's safety, and seek necessary interventions to avoid a potentially adverse outcome.
3. At the first level, notify the immediate supervisor to provide assistance. Further steps are defined by the structure of the institution, and a policy outlining communication for the chain of command should be present (Fig. 2-2).

Risk Management

Risk management is a systems approach to the prevention of litigation. It involves the identification of systems problems, analysis, and treatment of risks before a suit is brought (Gilbert, 2007). There are two key components of a successful risk management program:

■ Avoiding preventable adverse outcomes to the fetus during labor requires competent care providers who use consistent and current FHR monitoring language and who are in practice environments with systems in place that permit timely clinical intervention.
■ Decreasing risk of liability exposure includes methods to demonstrate evidence that appropriate timely care was provided that accurately reflects maternal fetal status before, during, and after interventions occurred.

Not all adverse or unexpected outcomes are preventable or are result of poor care. Authors suggest (Simpson & Creehan, 2008; Simpson & Knox, 2003) the risk of liability can be reduced and injuries to mothers and neonates can be reduced when all members of the perinatal team follow two basic tenets:

■ Use applicable evidence and/or published standards and guidelines as the foundation of care.
■ Make patient safety a priority over convenience, productivity, and costs.

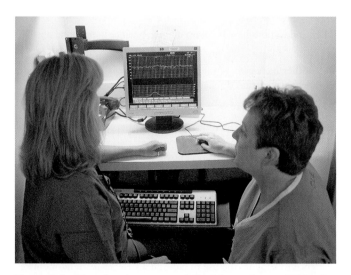

Figure 2-2   Together the nurse and physician review an EFM strip.

EVIDENCE-BASED PRACTICE

Health care professions are moving toward thinking that practice decisions ought to be made with the best available knowledge or evidence. Evidence-based practice (EBP) and terms such as evidence-based medicine (EBM) and evidence-based nursing (EBN) reflect a very important global paradigm shift in how to view health care outcomes, how the discipline is taught, how practice is conducted, and how health care practices are evaluated for quality (Milton, 2007).

In the early 1990s in the United States, the Agency for Health Care Policy and Research (AHCPR) was established with interdisciplinary teams to gather and assess available research literature and develop evidence-based clinical guidelines. Nurses were prominent members of the interdisciplinary teams who performed this early work. In the mid-1990s, AHCPR was changed to the Agency for Healthcare Research and Quality (AHRQ) and it now has a clearinghouse for clinical guidelines (http://www.guidelines.gov).

Many health professionals have chosen to view the EBP movement as a systematic approach to determine the most current and relevant evidence upon which to base decisions about patient care (Melnyk & Fineout-Overholt, 2005). Rigorously conducted research that reports findings that are "good evidence" may not always translate to the "right" decisions for an individual patient. Most authors and clinicians have extended the definition of **evidence-based practice (EBP)** to include the integration of best *research evidence*, *clinical expertise*, and *patient values* in making decisions about the care of patients (Reilly, 2004). Clinical expertise comes from knowledge and experience over time. Patient values are the unique circumstances of each patient and should include patient preferences. Characteristics of best research evidence is quantitative evidence such as clinical trials and laboratory experiments, evidence from qualitative research, and evidence from experts in practice.

Evidence-Based Practice Research: Cochrane Review

An important resource for evidence-based practice is systematic reviews. One such source is Cochrane Reviews (http://www.cochrane.org). The Cochrane review is an international consortium of experts who perform systematic reviews and meta-analysis on all available data, evaluating the body of evidence on a particular clinical topic for quality of study design and study results. These reviews look at randomized clinical trials of interventions related to a specific clinical problem and after assessing the findings from rigorous studies make recommendations for clinical practice. They consider the randomized controlled trial (RCT) as the gold standard of research evidence.

Although not absolute, a hierarchy of evidence can be helpful when evaluating research evidence. When considering potential interventions, nurses should look for the highest level of available evidence relevant to the clinical problem. A hierarchy of strength of evidence for treatment decisions is presented in Box 2-2, indicating unsystematic clinical observations as the lowest level and systematic reviews of RCTs as the higest level of evidence.

BOX 2–2   HIERARCHY OF STRENGTH OF EVIDENCE
                FOR TREATMENT DECISIONS

Systematic reviews of randomized clinical trials (i.e., Cochrane Reviews)

↑

Single randomized trial (individual RCT research)

↑

Systematic review of observational studies addressing patient important outcomes

↑

Single observational studies addressing patient important outcomes

↑

Physiological studies (i.e., studies of indicators such as blood pressure)

↑

Unsystematic clinical observations (clinical observations made by practitioners over time)

(DiCenso, Ciliska, & Guyat, 2005)

Evidence-Based Nursing

Evidence based nursing (EBN) has become an internationally recognized, although sometimes contested part of nursing practice (Flemming, 2007). EBN is central to the knowledge base for nursing practice. Critics of EBN dislike the central role that randomized controlled trials (RCTs) take in providing evidence for nursing, claiming that the context and experience of nursing care are removed from evaluation of evidence. One of the principles of evidence-based health care has been driven by requirements to deliver quality care within economically constrained conditions (Critical Component: Evidence-Based Nursing).

CRITICAL COMPONENT

Evidence-Based Nursing

To practice EBN, a nurse is expected to combine the best research evidence with clinical expertise while taking into account the patients' preferences and their situation in the context of the available resources. Evidence-based decision making should include consideration of the patients' clinical state, clinical setting, and clinical circumstances.

(DiCenso, Ciliska, & Guyatt, 2005)

Some nurses have adopted a predominantly medical model of evidence, with RCTs as the central, methodological approach to define good evidence. EBN has been criticized for this stance, focusing on the lack of relevance of RCTs for nursing practice. Criticisms stem from the fact that RCTs are given an illusionary stance of credibility, when there may not be credible evidence relevant to nursing practice.

Utilization of Research in Clinical Practice

To enhance EBP and support the choices of childbearing women and families, we must find a way to utilize qualitative research findings in practice (Durham, 2002). Although nursing has developed models for assisting a practitioner in applying research findings in practice (Cronenwett, 1995; Stetler, 1994; Titler & Goode, 1995), these models only assist in applying quantitative research.

Qualitative research, like quantitative research, should be of value and used in practice settings. Qualitative researchers investigate naturally occurring phenomena and describe, analyze, and sometimes develop a theory on the phenomena. They also describe the context and relationships of key factors related to the phenomena. This kind of work is conducted in the "real world," not in a controlled situation, and yields important findings for practice. Practitioners may not be aware of qualitative research findings, or, if they are, they may not be able to apply the findings. Reports of qualitative research should be more readily understood by persons in practice as they are conveyed in language that is more understandable to the practitioner. Story lines from qualitative research are often a more compelling and culturally resonant way to communicate research findings, particularly to staff, affected groups, and policymakers (Sandelowski, 1996). Despite the fact that qualitative research is conducted in the "real world" and is more understandable to many practitioners, as with quantitative research utilization, a gap exists between the world of qualitative research and the world of practice. A creative bridge between these worlds is needed. Some guidelines for bridging that gap are outlined by Swanson, Durham and Albright (1997) and include evaluating the findings or proposed theory for its context, generalizability, and fit with one's own practice, evaluating the concepts, conditions, and variation explained in the findings, and evaluating findings for enhancing and informing one's practice.

In the current era of cost containment, nurses must know what is going on in the real world of their patients because practitioners are limited to interacting with clients within an ever-smaller window of time and space. Qualitative research can assist in bringing practitioners an awareness of that larger world and its implications for their scope of practice (Swanson, Durham, & Albright, 1997). Qualitative research describes and analyzes our patients' realities. The research findings have the capacity to influence conceptual thinking and cause practitioners to question assumptions about a phenomenon in practice (Cronenwett, 1995). Incorporating qualitative research as evidence to support research-based practice has the capacity not only to enhance nursing practice, but also to resolve some of the tensions between art and science with which nurses sometimes find themselves struggling (Durham, 2002).

Research Utilization Challenges

Many innovations have become common practice in perinatal nursing:

■ Fetal monitoring
■ Mother/baby care
■ Early postpartum discharge

These changes in care were influenced by:

■ Social context of the time
■ Medical and technological innovations
■ Families' desires for the best possible care

How nurses respond to the increasing use of technology during birth, threats of litigation, and providing the best care under time and cost constraints are the realities facing current perinatal nursing care today (Martell, 2006).

Continuous electronic fetal monitoring in labor is one of the most common interventions during labor. However, there is little evidence to support the use of continuous electronic fetal monitoring, particular with low-risk patients. A Cochrane review compared the efficacy and safety of routine continuous EFM of labor with intermittent auscultation (Thacker, Stroup, & Chang, 2006). The reviewers concluded that use of routine EFM has no measurable impact on infant morbidity and mortality.

Although EBP is the goal of nursing care and has become the standard of care in the United States, the evidence about EFM has not been used in practice (Wood, 2003). Research evidence does not support the use of continuous EFM. Despite this, many reasons contribute to its continued use such as habit, convenience, liability, staffing, and economics (Woods, 2003). It is no longer acceptable for nurses to continue doing things the way they have always been done, by tradition without questioning whether or not it is the best approach.

■ ■ ■ Review Questions ■ ■ ■

1. The organization that publishes standards and guidelines for maternity nursing is the:
   A. National Perinatal Association
   B. American Nurses Association
   C. American Academy of Pediatrics
   D. Association of Women's Health, Obstetrics and Neonatal Nursing

2. Autonomy is defined as the right to:
   A. Do good
   B. Equal treatment
   C. Self-determination
   D. Be valued

3. Ethics involves determining what is:
   A. Correct, fair, and just
   B. Correct
   C. Just, voluntary, and respect
   D. Just, good, and true

4. Evidence-based decision making should include consideration of:
   A. Patient's clinical state, clinical setting, and clinical circumstances
   B. Patient's clinical state, acuity, and financial considerations
   C. Clinical setting, acuity, and resources
   D. Patient's clinical state, clinical resources and financial considerations

5. Risk management is an approach to the prevention of:
   A. Morbidity and mortality
   B. Litigation
   C. Staff conflicts
   D. Poor care

References

American Nurses Association (ANA). (2001). *Code of ethics for nurses with interpretive statements.* Silver Spring, MD: American Nurses Publishing. Retrieved from http://www.nursingworld.org/ethics/ecode.htm (Accessed June 7, 2009).

Aroskar, M. (1998). Ethical working relationships in patient care: Challenges and possibilities. *Nursing Clinics of North America, 33*(2), 287–293.

Association for Women's Health, Obstetric and Neonatal Nurses (AWHONN). (2000). *Fetal Assessment Clinical Position Statement.* Washington, DC: Author.

Association for Women's Health, Obstetric and Neonatal Nurses (AWHONN). (2003). *Standards for professional nursing practice in the care of women and newborns* (6th ed.). Washington, DC: Author.

Cronenwett, L. (1995). Effective methods for disseminating research findings to nurses in practice. *Nursing Clinics of North America, 30*(3), 429–438.

DiCenso, A., Ciliska, D, & Guyatt, G. (2005). Introduction to evidence-based nursing. In: A. DiCenso, G. Guyatt, & D. Ciliska (Eds.), *Evidence-based nursing: A guide to clinical practice* (pp. 3–19). St. Louis, MO: Elsevier Mosby.

Durham, R. (2002). Women, work and midwifery. In R. Mander & V. Flemming (Eds), *Failure to progress* (pp. 122–132). London: Routledge.

Feinstein, N., Torgersen, K., & Atterbury, J. (2003). *AWHONN's fetal heart monitoring principles and practices* (3rd ed.). Washington, DC: Association of Women's Health, Obstetric and Neonatal Nurses.

Flemming, K. (2007). The knowledge base for evidence-based nursing: A role for mixed methods research? *Advances in Nursing Science, 30*(1), 41–51.

Freeman, R. (2002). Problems with intrapartal fetal heart rate monitoring interpretation and patient management. *American Journal of Obstetrics and Gynecology, 100*(4), 813–816.

Gilbert, E. (2007). *Manual of high risk pregnancy and delivery.* St. Louis, MO: C. V. Mosby.

Jonsen, A., Siegler, M., & Winslade, W. (2006). *Clinical ethics: A practical approach to ethical decisions in clinical medicine* (6th ed.). New York: McGraw-Hill.

Lagana, K. (2000). The "right" to a caring relationship: The law and ethic of care. *Journal of Perinatal & Neonatal Nursing, 14*(2), 12–24.

Lagana, K., & Duderstadt, K. (2004). *Perinatal and neonatal ethics: Facing contemporary challenges.* White Plains, NY: March of Dimes.

Mahlmeister, L. (2000). Legal implications of fetal heart rate assessment. *JOGNN, 29,* 517–526.

Martell, L. (2006). From innovation to common practice: Perinatal nursing pre 1970 to 2005. *Journal of Perinatal & Neonatal Nursing, 20*(1), 8–16.

Melnyk, B. M., & Fineout-Overholt, E. (2005). *Evidence-based practice in nursing and healthcare: A guide to best practice.* Philadelphia: Lippincott Williams & Wilkins.

Milton, C. L. (2007). Evidence-based practice: Ethical questions for nursing. *Nursing Science Quarterly, 20*(2), 123–126.

Nurse's Legal Handbook (5th ed.) (2004). Philadelphia: Lippincott, Williams & Wilkins.

Penticuff, J. (1998). Defining futility in neonatal intensive care. *Nursing Clinics of North America, 33*(2), 339–352.

Pierce, S. F. (1998). Neonatal intensive care: Decision making in the face of prognostic uncertainty. *Nursing Clinics of North America, 33*(2), 287–293.

Reilly, B. (2004). The essence of EBM. *British Medical Journal, 329,* 991–992.

Sandelowski, M. (1996). Using qualitative methods in intervention studies. *Research in Nursing and Health, 19,* 359–364.

Simpson, K., & Creehan, P. and Association of Women's Health, Obstetrics and Neonatal Nursing. (2008). *Perinatal nursing* (3rd ed.). Philadelphia: Lippincott Williams & Wilkins.

Simpson, K., & Knox, E. (2003). Common area of litigation related to care during labor and birth: Recommendations to promote patient safety and decrease risk exposure. *Journal of Perinatal and Neonatal Nursing, 17*(2), 110–125.

Stetler, C. (1994). Refinement of the Stetler/Marram model for application of research findings to practice. *Nursing Outlook, 42,* 15–25.

Swanson, J., Durham, R., & Albright, J. (1997). Clinical utilization/application of qualitative research. In J. Morse (Ed.), *Completing a qualitative project: Details and dialogue* (pp. 253–282). Thousand Oaks, CA: Sage.

Thacker, S., Stroup, D., & Chang, M. (2006). *Continuous electronic heart rate monitoring for fetal assessment during labor.* (Cochrane Review). In: The Cochrane Library Issue 1, 2006. Oxford: Update Software

Titler, M., & Goode, C. (1995). Research utilization. *Nursing Clinics of North America, 30*(3), xv.

Woods, S. (2003). Should women be given a choice about fetal assessment in labor? *The American Journal of Maternal/Child Nursing, 28*(5), 292–298.

Antepartal Period

Genetics, Conception, Fetal Development, and Reproductive Technology

3

OBJECTIVES

On completion of this chapter, students will be able to:

- ☐ Define key terms.
- ☐ Discuss the relevance of genetics within the context of the care of the childbearing family.
- ☐ Identify critical components of conception, embryonic development, and fetal development.
- ☐ Describe the development and function of the placenta and amniotic fluid.
- ☐ List the common causes of infertility.
- ☐ Describe the common diagnostic tests used in diagnosing causes of infertility.
- ☐ Describe the most common methods used in assisted fertility.
- ☐ Discuss the ethical and emotional implications of assisted reproductive therapies.

GENETICS AND THE CHILDBEARING FAMILY

Genetics is the branch of science that focuses on the knowledge of heredity and variations of organisms.

Genes

- Genes are composed of DNA (hereditary material) and protein.
- They are the basic functional and physical units of heredity.
- There are approximately 30,000 genes in the human genome.
- The **genome** is an organism's complete set of DNA.
- Numerous genes are located on each human chromosome.
  - *Each human cell contains 46 chromosomes.*
  - *There are 22 homologous pairs of chromosomes and one pair of sex chromosomes (XX or XY).*
- **Genotype** refers to a person's genetic makeup.
- **Phenotype** refers to how the genes are outwardly expressed, (i.e., eye color, hair color, height).

Dominant and Recessive Inheritance

- Genes are either dominant or recessive. When there is both a dominant and a recessive gene in the pair, the traits of the dominant gene present.

- The traits of the recessive gene are present when both genes of the pair are recessive.
- Genetic diseases or disorders are usually related to a defective recessive gene and present in the developing human when both pairs of the gene have the same defect.
  - *Examples of common recessive genetic disorders are cystic fibrosis, sickle cell anemia, thalassemia, and Tay-Sachs disease (Table 3–1).*
  - *A person who has only one recessive gene for a disorder is known as a carrier and does not present with the disorder.*
  - *Genetic disorders related to a dominant gene are rare.*

Sex-Linked Inheritance

- Also referred to as X-linked inheritance or traits (see Table 3-1)
- These are genes or traits that are located only on the X chromosome. These genes can be either recessive or dominant. The Y chromosome does not have the corresponding genes for some of the X chromosome's genes.
- A male child who receives an X chromosome with a disorder of one or more of its genes presents with the disorder when the Y chromosome does not carry that gene; the gene, even though it may be recessive, becomes dominant.
- Female children who have one X chromosome with a sex-linked trait disorder do not present with the trait, but are carriers of the trait.

TABLE 3–1   GENETIC DISEASES

DISEASE (PATTERN OF INHERITANCE)	DESCRIPTION
SICKLE-CELL ANEMIA (R)	The most common genetic disease among people of African ancestry. Sickle-cell hemoglobin forms rigid crystals that distort and disrupt red blood cells (RBCs); oxygen-carrying capacity of the blood is diminished.
CYSTIC FIBROSIS (R)	The most common genetic disease among people of European ancestry. Production of thick mucus clogs in the bronchial tree and pancreatic ducts. Most severe effects are chronic respiratory infections and pulmonary failure.
TAY-SACHS DISEASE (R)	The most common genetic disease among people of Jewish ancestry. Degeneration of neurons and the nervous system results in death by the age of 2 years.
PHENYLKETONURIA OR PKU (R)	Lack of an enzyme to metabolize the amino acid phenylalanine leads to severe mental and physical retardation. These effects may be prevented by the use of a diet (beginning at birth) that limits phenylalanine.
HUNTINGTON'S DISEASE (D)	Uncontrollable muscle contractions between the ages of 30 and 50 years, followed by loss of memory and personality. There is no treatment that can delay mental deterioration.
HEMOPHILIA (X-LINKED)	Lack of factor VIII impairs chemical clotting; may be controlled with factor VIII from donated blood.
DUCHENNE'S MUSCULAR DYSTROPHY (X-LINKED)	Replacement of muscle by adipose or scar tissue, with progressive loss of muscle function; often fatal before age 20 years due to involvement of cardiac muscle.

R = recessive; D = dominant.
Source: Scanlon & Sanders (2007).

Relevance of Genetics in the Care of the Childbearing Family

■ The scientific knowledge of genetics is rapidly increasing with the desire that gene therapy will be used to correct genetic disorders such as heart disease, diabetes, and Down's syndrome.

■ The Human Genome Project, a 13-year international, collaborative research program that was completed in 2003, has provided the scientific community with valuable information that is being used in the diagnosis, treatment, and prevention of genetically linked disorders.

■ Ten percent of all abnormalities of the developing human are due to genetic factors (Sadler, 2004).

■ Couples who have a higher risk for conceiving a child with a genetic disorder include:
  ■ *Maternal age older than 35*
  ■ *History of previous pregnancy resulting in a genetic disorder or newborn abnormalities*
  ■ *Man and/or woman who has a genetic disorder*
  ■ *Family history of a genetic disorder*

■ Perinatal genetic testing, such as amniocentesis, allows for the early detection of genetic disorders, such as trisomy 21, hemophilia, and Tay-Sachs disease.

■ Diagnosis of genetic disorders during pregnancy provides parents with options to:
  ■ *Continue or terminate the pregnancy*
  ■ *Prepare for a child with this genetic disorder*
  ■ *Use gene therapy when available*

■ Making a decision to maintain a pregnancy or terminate a pregnancy based on the outcomes of genetic testing is very stressful for the couple.
  ■ *Nurses can be supportive by answering questions and clarifying information and options.*

■ *Nursing actions for couples who elect to terminate the pregnancy are:*
  ■ Explain the stages of grief they will experience.
  ■ Inform the couple that grief is a normal process.
  ■ Encourage the couple to communicate with each other and share their emotions.
  ■ Refer the couple to a support group if available in their community

■ *Nursing actions for couples who elect to continue the pregnancy are:*
  ■ Provide them additional information about the genetic disorder.
  ■ Refer them to support groups for parents who have children with the same genetic disorder.
  ■ Provide a list of Web sites that contain accurate information about the disorder.
  ■ Explain that they will experience grief over the loss of the "dream child" and this is normal.
  ■ Encourage them to talk openly to each other about their feelings and concerns.

■ A general understanding of genetics and the possible effects on the developing human are necessary for nurses, especially those practicing in the obstetrical or pediatric areas. Nurses may need to:
  ■ *Explain/clarify diagnostic procedures used in genetic testing (i.e., purpose, findings, and possible side effects).*
  ■ *Clarify or reinforce information the couple received from their health care provider or genetic counselor.*

■ Maternal–child nurses need to have knowledge and information regarding:
  ■ *Genetic counseling services available in the parents' community*
  ■ *Access to genetic services*
  ■ *Procedure for referral to the different services*
  ■ *The information or services these agencies provide*

TERATOGENS

- **Teratogens** are defined as any drugs, viruses, infections, or other exposures that can cause embryonic/fetal developmental abnormality (Table 3-2).
- Birth defects can occur from genetic disorders or be the result of teratogen exposure.
- The degree or types of malformation vary based on length of exposure, amount of exposure, and when it occurs during human development.
- The developing human is most vulnerable to the effects of teratogens during organogenesis, which occurs during the first 8 weeks of gestation. Exposure during this time can cause gross structural defects (American College of Obstetricians and Gynecologists [ACOG], 1997).
- Exposure to teratogens after 13 weeks of gestation may cause fetal growth restriction or reduction of organ size (ACOG, 1997).

CRITICAL COMPONENT

Teratogens

The developing human is most vulnerable to the effects of teratogens during the period of organogenesis, the first 8 weeks of gestation.

CRITICAL COMPONENT

Toxoplasmosis

- Can cause fetal demise, mental retardation, and blindness when the embryo is exposed to *Toxoplasma* during pregnancy (see Table 3-2).
- *Toxoplasma* is a protozoan parasite found in cat feces and uncooked or rare beef and lamb.
- Pregnant women or women who are attempting pregnancy need to avoid contact with cat feces (i.e., changing a litter box).
- Pregnant women or women who are attempting pregnancy should avoid eating rare beef or lamb.

MENSTRUAL CYCLE

A woman's menstrual cycle is influenced by the ovarian cycle and endometrial cycle (Fig. 3-1).

Ovarian Cycle

The **ovarian cycle** pertains to the maturation of ova and consist of three phases:

- The **follicular phase** begins the first day of menstruation and last 12 to 14 days. During this phase, the graafian follicle is maturing under the influence of two pituitary hormones: luteinizing hormone (LH) and follicle-stimulating hormone (FSH). The maturing graafian follicle produces estrogen.
- The **ovulatory phase** begins when estrogen levels peak and ends with the release of the oocyte (egg) from the mature graafian follicle. The release of the oocyte is referred to as ovulation.
  - *There is a surge in LH levels 12 to 36 hours before ovulation.*
  - *There is a decrease in estrogen levels and an increase in progesterone levels before the LH surge.*
- The **luteal phase** begins after ovulation and last approximately 14 days. During this phase, the cells of the empty follicle undergo changes and form into the corpus luteum.
  - *The corpus luteum produces high levels of progesterone along with low levels of estrogen.*
  - *If pregnancy occurs, the corpus luteum continues to release progesterone and estrogen until the placenta matures and assumes this function.*
  - *If pregnancy does not occur, the corpus luteum degenerates and results in a decrease is progesterone and the beginning of menstruation.*

Endometrial Cycle

The **endometrial cycle** pertains to the changes in the endometrium of the uterus in responses to the hormonal changes that occur during the ovarian cycle. This cycle consist of three phases:

- The **proliferative phase** occurs following menstruation and ends with ovulation. During this phase, the endometrium is preparing for implantation by becoming thicker and more vascular. These changes are in response to the increasing levels of estrogen produced by the graafian follicle.
- The **secretory phase** begins after ovulation and ends with the onset of menstruation. During this phase, the endometrium continues to thicken. The primary hormone during this phase is progesterone which is secreted from the corpus luteum.
  - *If pregnancy occurs, the endometrium continues to develop and begins to secrete glycogen.*
  - *If pregnancy does not occur and the corpus luteum begins to degenerate and the endometrial tissue degenerates.*
- The **menstrual phase** occurs in response to hormonal changes and results in the sloughing off of the endometrial tissue.

CONCEPTION

Conception, also known as fertilization, occurs when a sperm nucleus enters the nucleus of the oocyte (Fig. 3-2).

- Fertilization normally occurs in the outer third of the fallopian tube.
- The fertilized oocyte is called a **zygote** and contains the diploid number of chromosomes (46).

Cell Division

- The single-cell zygote undergoes mitotic cell division known as **cleavage.**
  - *Mitotic cell division or mitosis occurs when a cell (parent cell) divides and forms two daughter cells that contain the same number of chromosomes as the parent cell.*
- Three days after fertilization, the zygote has formed into a 16-cell, solid sphere that is called a **morula.**
- Mitosis continues, and around day 5 the developing human is known as the blastocyst and enters the uterus.
- The **blastocyst** is composed of an inner cell mass known as the **embryoblast,** which will develop into the embryo, and an outer cell mass known as the **trophoblast,** which will assist in implantation and become part of the placenta.

TABLE 3–2   TERATOGENIC AGENTS

AGENT	EFFECT
Drugs And Chemicals **ALCOHOL**	Increased risk of fetal alcohol syndrome occurring when the pregnant woman ingests six or more alcoholic drinks a day. No amount of alcohol is considered safe during pregnancy. Newborn characteristics of fetal alcohol syndrome include: ■ Low birth weight ■ Microcephaly ■ Mental retardation ■ Unusual facial features due to midfacial hypoplasia ■ Cardiac defects
ANGIOTENSIN-CONVERTING ENZYME (ACE) INHIBITORS	Increased risk for: ■ Renal tubular dysplasia that can lead to renal failure and fetal or neonatal death ■ Intrauterine growth restriction
CARBAMAZEPINE (ANTICONVULSANTS)	Increased risk for: ■ Neural tubal defects ■ Craniofacial defects, including cleft lip and palate ■ Intrauterine growth restriction
COCAINE	Increased risk for: ■ Heart, limbs, face, gastrointestinal tract, and genitourinary tract defects ■ Cerebral infarctions ■ Placental abnormalities
WARFARIN (COUMADIN)	Increased risk for: ■ Spontaneous abortion ■ Fetal demise ■ Fetal or newborn hemorrhage ■ Central nervous system abnormalities
Infections/Viruses **CYTOMEGALOVIRUS**	Increased risk for: ■ Hydrocephaly ■ Microcephaly ■ Cerebral calcification ■ Mental retardation ■ Hearing loss
HERPES VARICELLA (CHICKEN POX)	Increased risk for: ■ Hypoplasia of hands and feet ■ Blindness/cataracts ■ Mental retardation
RUBELLA	Increased risk for: ■ Heart defects ■ Deafness and/or blindness ■ Mental retardation ■ Fetal demise
SYPHILIS	Increased risk for: ■ Skin, bone and/or teeth defects ■ Fetal demise
TOXOPLASMOSIS	Increased risk for: ■ Fetal demise ■ Blindness ■ Mental retardation

Sources: American College of Obstetricians and Gynecologists (ACOG; 1997); Scanlon & Sanders (2007).

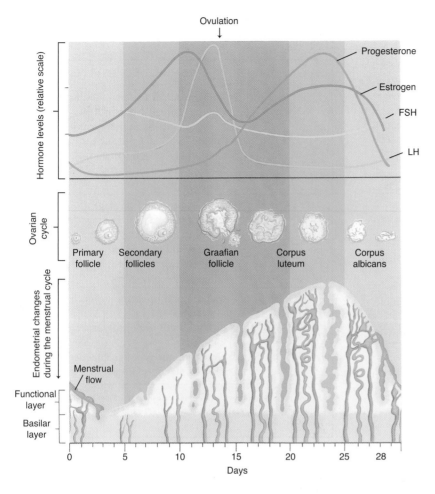

Figure 3-1 The menstrual cycle. The levels of the major hormones are shown in relationship to one another throughout the cycle. Changes in the ovarian follicle are depicted. The relative thickness of the endometrium is also shown.

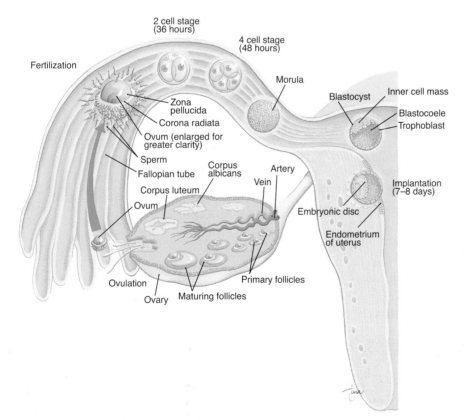

Figure 3-2 Ovulation, fertilization, and early embryonic development. Fertilization takes place in the fallopian tube, and the embryo has reached the blastocyst stage when it becomes implanted in the endometrium of the uterus.

- **Multiple gestation** refers to more than one developing embryo such as twins and triplets.
  - *Twins can be either monozygotic or dizygotic.*
  - *Monozygotic twins, also referred to as identical twins, are the result of one fertilized ovum splitting during the early stages of cell division and forming two identical embryos. These developing fetuses are genetically the same.*
  - *Dizygotic twins, also referred to as fraternal twins, are the result of two separate ova being fertilized by two separate sperm. These developing fetuses are not genetically the same.*

Implantation

- **Implantation**, the embedding of the blastocyst into the endometrium of the uterus, begins around day 5 or 6.
- Progesterone stimulates the endometrium of the uterus, which becomes thicker and more vascular in preparation for implantation.
- Enzymes secreted by the trophoblast, now referred to as the chorion, digest the surface of the endometrium in preparation for implantation of the blastocyst.
- Implantation normally occurs in the upper part of the posterior wall of the uterus.

EMBRYO AND FETAL DEVELOPMENT

Embryo

The developing human is referred to as an **embryo** from the time of implantation through 8 weeks of gestation. **Organogenesis**, the formation and development of body organs, occurs during this critical time of human development.

- Primary germ layers begin to develop around day 14 (Table 3-3).
- These germ layers, known as the ectoderm, mesoderm, and endoderm, form the different organs, tissues, and body structure of the developing human.
  - *The **ectoderm** is the outer germ layer.*
  - *The **mesoderm** is the middle germ layer.*
  - *The **endoderm** is the inner germ layer.*
- The heart forms during the 3rd gestational week and begins to beat and circulate blood during the 4th gestational week.
- By the end of the 8th gestational week the developing human has transformed from the primary germ layers to a clearly defined human that is 3 cm in length with all organ systems formed (Fig. 3-3).

Fetus

The developing human is referred to as a **fetus** from week 9 to birth. During this stage of development, organ systems are growing and maturing (Table 3-4).

Fetal Circulation

- The cardiovascular system begins to develop within the first few weeks of gestation.
- The heart begins to beat during the 4th gestational week.
- Unique features of fetal circulation are (Fig. 3–4):
  - *High levels of oxygenated blood enter the fetal circulatory system from the placenta via the umbilical vein.*

TABLE 3–3   STRUCTURES DERIVED FROM THE PRIMARY GERM LAYERS

LAYER	STRUCTURES DERIVED*
ECTODERM	Epidermis; hair and nail follicles; sweat glands Nervous system; pituitary gland; adrenal medulla Lens and cornea; internal ear Mucosa of oral and nasal cavities; salivary glands
MESODERM	Dermis; bone and cartilage Skeletal muscles; cardiac muscles; most smooth muscles Kidneys; adrenal cortex Bone marrow and blood; lymphatic tissue; lining of blood vessels
ENDODERM	Mucosa of esophagus, stomach, and intestines Epithelium of respiratory tract, including lungs Liver and mucosa of gallbladder Thyroid gland; pancreas

*These are representative lists, not all-inclusive ones. Most organs are combinations of tissues from each of the three germ layers.
Source: Scanlon & Sanders (2007).

- *The **ductus venosus** connects the umbilical vein to the inferior vena cava. This allows the majority of the high levels of oxygenated blood to enter the right atrium.*
- *The **foramen ovale** is an opening between the right and left atria. Blood high in oxygen is shunted to the left atrium via the foramen ovale. After delivery, the foramen ovale closes in response to increased blood returning to the left atrium. It may take up to 3 months for full closure.*
- *The **ductus arteriosus** connects the pulmonary artery with the descending aorta. The majority of the oxygenated blood is shunted to the aorta via the ductus arteriosus with smaller amounts going to the lungs. After delivery, the ductus arteriosus constricts in response to the higher blood oxygen levels and prostaglandins.*

PLACENTA, MEMBRANES, AMNIOTIC FLUID, AND UMBILICAL CORD

Placenta

- The placenta is formed from both fetal and maternal tissue (Fig. 3-5).
  - *The chorionic membrane that develops from the trophoblast along with the chorionic villi form the fetal side of the placenta. The **chorionic villi** are projections from the chorion that embed into the decidua basalis and later form the fetal blood vessels of the placenta.*
  - *The endometrium is referred to as the decidua and consists of three layers: decidua basalis, decidua capsularis, and decidua vera. The **decidua basalis**, the portion directly beneath the blastocyst, forms the maternal portion of the placenta.*

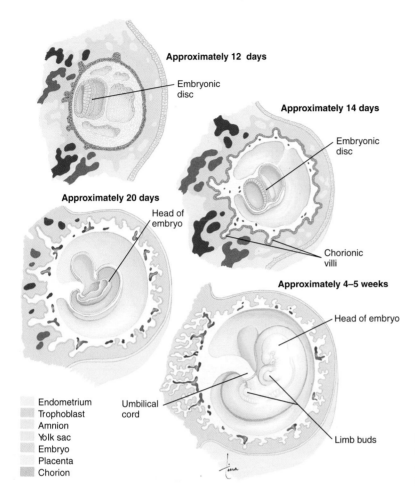

Approximately 12 days
— Embryonic disc

Approximately 14 days
— Embryonic disc

Approximately 20 days
Head of embryo

Chorionic villi

Approximately 4–5 weeks
— Head of embryo

Umbilical cord

Limb buds

Endometrium
Trophoblast
Amnion
Yolk sac
Embryo
Placenta
Chorion

Figure 3-3 Embryonic development at 12 days (after fertilization), 14 days, 20 days, and 4–5 weeks. By 5 weeks, the embryo has distinct parts but does not yet look definitely human.

■ The maternal side of the placenta is divided into compartments or lobes known as **cotyledons**.

■ The placental membrane separates the maternal and fetal blood and prevents fetal blood mixing with maternal blood, but allows for the exchange of gases, nutrients, and electrolytes.

Function of the Placenta

■ Metabolic and gas exchange: In the placenta, fetal waste products and CO_2 are transferred from the fetal blood into the maternal blood sinuses by diffusion. Nutrients, such as glucose and amino acids, and O_2 are transferred from the maternal blood sinuses to the fetal blood through the mechanisms of diffuse and active transport.

■ Hormone production: The major hormones the placenta produces are progesterone, estrogen, human chorionic gonadotropin (hCG), and human placental lactogen (hPL), also known as human chorionic somatomammotropin.

  ■ *Progesterone facilitates implantation and decreases uterine contractility.*

  ■ *Estrogen stimulates the enlargement of the breasts and uterus.*

  ■ *Human chorionic gonadotropin (hCG) stimulates the corpus luteum so that it will continue to secrete estrogen and progesterone until the placenta is mature enough to secrete these hormones. This is the hormone assessed in pregnancy tests. hCG rises rapidly during the first trimester and then has a rapid decline.*

■ Human placental lactogen (hPL):

  ■ *Promotes fetal growth by regulating glucose available to the developing human.*

  ■ *Stimulates breast development in preparation for lactation.*

■ Viruses, such as rubella and cytomegalovirus, can cross the placental membrane and enter the fetal system and cause fetal death or defects.

■ Drugs can cross the placental membrane. Women should consult with their health care provider before taking any medication/drugs. Drugs with an FDA pregnancy category C, D, or X should be avoided during pregnancy or when attempting pregnancy.

■ The placenta becomes fully functional between the 8th and 10th weeks of gestation.

■ By the ninth month, the placenta is between 15 and 25 cm in diameter, 3 cm thick, and weighs approximately 600 g.

CRITICAL COMPONENT

Medications

Women who are pregnant or attempting pregnancy should consult with their health care provider before taking any prescribed or over-the-counter medications, as medications can cross the placental membrane.

TABLE 3–4   SUMMARY OF FETAL DEVELOPMENT

GESTATIONAL WEEK	LENGTH* AND WEIGHT	FETAL DEVELOPMENT/CHARACTERISTICS
12	8 cm 45 g	Red blood cells are produced in the liver. Fusion of the palate is completed. External genitalia are developed to the point that sex of fetus can be noted with ultrasound. Eyelids are closed. Fetal heart tone can be heard by Doppler device.
16	14 cm 200 g	Lanugo is present on head. Meconium is formed in the intestines. Teeth begin to form. Sucking motions are made with the mouth. Skin is transparent.
20	19 cm 450 g	Lanugo covers the entire body. Vernix caseosa covers the body. Nails are formed. Brown fat begins to develop.
24	23 cm 820 g	Eyes are developed. Alveoli form in the lungs and begin to produce surfactant. Footprints and fingerprints are forming. Respiratory movement can be detected.
28	27 cm 1300 g	Eyelids are open. Adipose tissue develops rapidly. The respiratory system has developed to a point that gas exchange is possible, but lungs are not fully mature.
32	30 cm 2100 g	Bones are fully developed. Lungs are maturing. Increased amounts of adipose tissue are present.
36	34 cm 2900 g	Lanugo begins to disappear. Labia majora and minora are equally prominent. Testes in upper portion of scrotum
40	36 cm 3400 g	Fetus is considered full term at 38 weeks. All organs/systems are fully developed.

*Length is measured from the crown (top of head) to the rump (buttock). This is referred to as the CRL.
Sources: Sadler (2004); Scanlon & Sanders (2007).

Embryonic Membranes

■ Two membranes (amnion and chorion) form the amniotic sac (also referred to as the bag of waters).
■ The chorionic membrane (outer membrane) develops from the trophoblast.
■ The amniotic membrane (inner membrane) develops from the embryoblast.
■ The embryo and amniotic fluid are contained within the amniotic sac.
■ The membranes stretch to accommodate the growth of the developing fetus and the amniotic fluid.

Amniotic Fluid

■ Amniotic fluid is the fluid contained within the amnion (Fig. 3-6).
■ Amniotic fluid is clear and is mainly composed of water. It also contains proteins, carbohydrates, lipids, electrolytes, fetal cells, lanugo, and vernix caseosa.

■ Amniotic fluid during the first trimester is produced from the amniotic membrane. During the second and third trimesters, the fluid is produced by the fetal kidneys.
■ Amniotic fluid increases during pregnancy and peaks around 34 weeks at 800 to 1,000 mL and then decreases to 500 to 600 mL at term.

Function of Amniotic Fluid

■ Acts as a cushion for the fetus when there are sudden maternal movements
■ Prevents adherence of the developing human to the amniotic membranes
■ Allows freedom of fetal movement which aids in symmetrical musculoskeletal development
■ Provides a consistent thermal environment

Abnormalities

■ **Polyhydramnios** or hydramnios refers to excess amount of amniotic fluid (1,500–2,000 mL). Newborns of mothers who

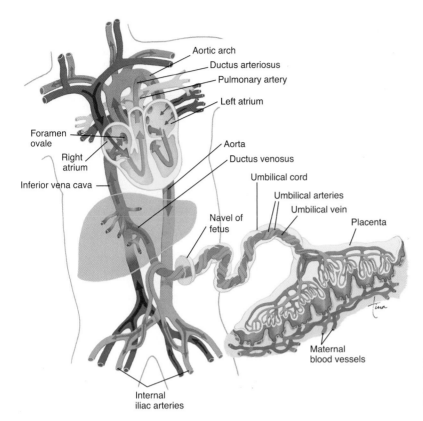

Figure 3-4 Fetal circulation. Fetal heart and blood vessels are shown on the left. Arrows depict direction of blood flow. The placenta and umbilical vessels are shown on the right.

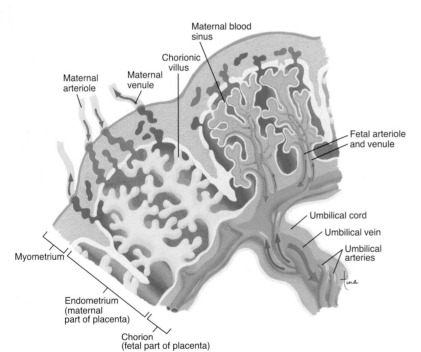

Figure 3-5 Placenta and umbilical cord. The fetal capillaries in the chorionic villi are within the maternal blood sinuses. Arrows indicate the direction of blood flow in the maternal and fetal vessels.

experienced polyhydramnios have an increased incidence of chromosomal disorders and gastrointestinal, cardiac, and/or neural tube disorders.

■ **Oligohydramnios** refers to decrease amount of amniotic fluid (<500 mL at term or 50% reduction of normal amount), which is generally related to a decrease in placental function. Newborns of mothers who experienced oligohydramnios have an increased incidence of congenital renal problems.

Umbilical Cord

■ Connects the fetus to the placenta
■ Consist of two umbilical arteries and one umbilical vein
  ■ *Arteries carry deoxygenated blood.*
  ■ *The vein carries oxygenated blood.*
■ The vessels are surrounded by **Wharton's jelly**, a collagenous substance, which protects the vessels from compression.

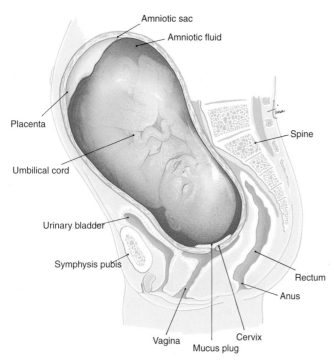

Amniotic sac
Amniotic fluid
Placenta
Spine
Umbilical cord
Urinary bladder
Symphysis pubis
Rectum
Anus
Vagina
Cervix
Mucus plug

Figure 3-6   Fetus, placenta, umbilical cord, and amniotic fluid.

■ Usually inserted in the center of the placenta.
■ Average length of the cord is 55 cm.

CRITICAL COMPONENT

Umbilical Vessels

■ After delivery of the newborn, assess the number of vessels in the cord.
■ Newborns with two vessels (one artery and one vein) have a 20% chance of having a cardiac or other vascular defeat.
■ Document the number of vessels present in the newborn. Record and report abnormalities to the pediatrician or pediatric nurse practitioner.

INFERTILITY AND REPRODUCTIVE TECHNOLOGY

Infertility affects the physical, social, psychological, sexual, and economical dimensions of the couple's lives. More than 5 million couples experience difficulties in conceiving (Storment, 2006). In approximately 80% of these couples, a cause can be identified. **Infertility** is defined as the inability to conceive and maintain a pregnancy after 12 months (6 months for woman older than 35 years old age) of unprotected sexual intercourse.

Causes

One third of the causes are related to female factors alone, one third to male factors alone, and one third to a combination of male and female factors (Frey & Patel, 2004).

■ Male causative factors are classified into five categories: endocrine, spermatogenesis, sperm antibodies, sperm transport, and disorders of intercourse (Porche, 2006).

■ *Endocrine: Pituitary diseases, pituitary tumors, and hypothalamic diseases may interfere with male fertility. Low levels of luteinizing hormone (LH), follicle-stimulating hormone (FSH), or testosterone can also decrease sperm production.*

■ *Spermatogenesis is the process in which mature functional sperm are formed. Several factors can affect the development of mature sperm. These factors are referred to as gonadotoxins and include:*

   ■ Drugs (e.g., chemotherapeutics, calcium channel blockers, heroin, alcohol, and nicotine)
   ■ Infections (e.g., contracting mumps after puberty, prostatitis, and sexually transmitted illnesses)
   ■ Systemic illness
   ■ Heat exposure: Prolonged heat exposure to the testicles (e.g., use of hot tubs, wearing tight underwear, and frequent bicycle riding)
   ■ Pesticides
   ■ Radiation to the pelvic region

■ *Sperm antibodies are an immunological reaction against the sperm that causes a decrease in sperm motility. This is seen mainly in men who have had either a vasectomy reversal or experienced testicular trauma.*

■ *Sperm transport factor addresses the structures related to the male reproductive anatomy that might be missing or blocked, thus interfering with the transportation of sperm. These causes can include vasectomy, prostatectomy, inguinal hernia, and congenital absence of the vas deferens.*

■ *Disorders of intercourse include erectile dysfunction (inability to achieve and maintain an erection), ejaculatory dysfunctions (retrograde ejaculation), anatomical abnormalities (hypospadias), and psychosocial factors that can interfere with fertility.*

■ Female causative factors are classified into three major categories: ovulatory dysfunction, tubal and pelvic pathology, and cervical mucus factor (Frey & Patel, 2004).

   ■ *Ovulatory dysfunction includes anovulation or inconsistent ovulation. These factors affect 15% to 25% of couples experiencing infertility and have a very high success rate with appropriate treatment (Storment, 2006).*

   ■ *Tubal and pelvic pathology include (1) damage to the fallopian tubes most commonly related to previous pelvic inflammatory disease or endometriosis and (2) uterine fibroids, benign growths of the muscular wall of the uterus, which can cause a narrowing of the uterine cavity and interfere with embryonic and fetal development causing a spontaneous abortion.*

   ■ *Cervical mucus factors include (1) cervical surgeries such as cryotherapy, a medical intervention use to treat cervical dysplasia and (2) infection. These may interfere with the ability of sperm to survive or enter the uterus.*

Diagnosis of Infertility

When a couple is experiencing difficulty in conceiving, both the man and the woman need to be evaluated. Initial screening for the female partner can be provided by her gynecologist (history, physical examination, and pelvic examination; Table 3-5). Initial screening for the male partner should be performed by a urologist and include history and physical (Table 3-6). The couple may be referred to a reproductive specialist after this initial screening.

Common Diagnostic Tests

■ Screening for sexually transmitted illnesses (STIs)
■ Laboratory test to assess hormonal levels (TSH, FSH, LH, and testosterone)

TABLE 3–5 AREAS OF FOCUS FOR THE MEDICAL HISTORY OF THE FEMALE PARTNER

HISTORY COMPONENTS	FOCUS OF ASSESSMENT
MEDICAL HISTORY AND REVIEW OF SYSTEMS	Abnormal hair growth Weight gain Breast discharge Hypothyroid or hyperthyroid symptoms History of diabetes mellitus or current symptoms of DM Current medical problems and medications Vaccination history Allergies
SURGICAL HISTORY	Fallopian tube surgery Ectopic pregnancy Appendectomy Other pelvic surgeries
MENSTRUAL CYCLE AND DEVELOPMENTAL HISTORY	Age of menarche Breast development Dysmenorrhea History of sexually transmitted illnesses Use of prior contraception History of diethylstilbestrol (DES) exposure History of abnormal results from Papanicolaou smear and subsequent treatment
SEXUAL HISTORY	Frequency of sexual intercourse Timing of intercourse with basal body temperature charting or ovulation predictor kits Dyspareunia (painful intercourse) Use of lubrications Previous births
INFERTILITY HISTORY	History of infertility treatment in pregnancy Duration of current infertility
SOCIAL HISTORY	Use of alcohol, tobacco, caffeine, recreational drugs Exposure to chemotherapy or radiation Excessive stress
FAMILY HISTORY OF GENETIC DISEASES	Ancestry-based genetic diseases, i.e., cystic fibrosis, sickle cell disease and thalassemia

Source: Frey & Patel (2004).

■ Semen analysis
- ■ *The male partner abstains for 2 to 3 days before providing a masturbated sample of his semen.*
- ■ *Specimens are either collected at the site of testing or brought to the site within an hour of collection.*
- ■ *The semen analysis includes volume, sperm concentration, motility, morphology, white blood cell count, immunobead, and mixed agglutination reaction test.*
- ■ *Several semen analyses may be required because sperm production normally fluctuates.*

■ Assessing for ovulatory dysfunction
- ■ *Basal body temperature (BBT): The female partner takes her temperature each morning before rising using a basal thermometer and records her daily temperature. Ovulation has occurred if there is a rise in the temperature by 0.4°F for 3 consecutive days.*
- ■ *Ovarian reserve testing: On day 3 of the menstrual cycle a serum FSH and estradiol test is performed. Further evaluation is needed by a reproductive specialist when the FSH is greater than 10 IU/L (Frey & Patei, 2004).*
- ■ *Detecting LH surge: There is a rapid increase in LH 36 hours before ovulation that is referred to as the LH surge and can be tested with urine or serum. The urine test can be performed at home and be used to assist in identifying the ideal time for intercourse when pregnancy is desired.*

■ **Hysterosalpingogram** is radiological examination that provides information about the endocervical canal, uterine cavity, and the fallopian tubes. Under fluoroscopic observation, dye is slowly injected through the cervical canal into the uterus. This examination can detect tubal problems such as adhesions or occlusions; and uterine abnormalities such as fibroids, bicornate uterus, and uterine fistulas.

■ **Endometrial biopsy** is performed to assess the response of the uterus to hormonal signals that occur during the cycle. The biopsy is performed at the end of the menstrual cycle. The procedure is performed in the clinical or medical office.

TABLE 3–6   AREAS OF FOCUS FOR THE MEDICAL HISTORY OF THE MALE PARTNER

HISTORY COMPONENTS	FOCUS OF ASSESSMENT
MEDICAL HISTORY AND REVIEW OF SYSTEMS	General health Erectile function Degree of virilization History of sexually transmitted illnesses Testicular infections (mumps), genital trauma or undescended testicle Pubertal development History of exposure to high temperatures (hot tubs) or recent fever Current medical problems and medications such as calcium channel blockers Vaccination history Allergies
SURGICAL HISTORY	History of hernia or testicular or varicocele surgery
SEXUAL HISTORY	Previously fathered a pregnancy History of contraception use History of infertility in a previous relationship Excessive use of lubricants
FAMILY HISTORY OF GENETIC DISEASES	Ancestry-based genetic diseases, i.e., cystic fibrosis, sickle cell disease and thalassemia Family history of male infertility

Source: Frey & Patel (2004).

Treatment

■ Treatment for the male partner ranges from lifestyle changes to surgery.
  - ■ *Treatment for endocrine factors may include hormonal therapy.*
  - ■ *Treatment for abnormal sperm count may focus on lifestyle changes such as stress reduction, improved nutrition, elimination of tobacco, and elimination of drugs known to have an adverse effect on fertility.*
  - ■ *Treatment for sperm antibodies is corticosteroids to decrease the production of antibodies.*
  - ■ *Treatment for infections of the genitourinary tract may include antibiotics.*
  - ■ *Treatment for sperm transport factor may include repair of varicocele or inguinal hernia.*
  - ■ *Treatment for disorders related to intercourse may include surgery such as transurethral resection of ejaculatory ducts.*
■ Treatment for the female partner also ranges from lifestyle changes to surgery.
  - ■ *Treatment for anovulation can focus on lifestyle changes such as stress reduction, improved nutrition, elimination of tobacco, and elimination of drugs known to have an adverse effect on fertility. Treatment also includes the use of a variety of medications that stimulate egg production. The most common medication used is clomiphene citrate.*
  - ■ *Treatment for tubal abnormalities may include surgery to open the tubes.*
  - ■ *Treatment for uterine fibroids may include surgical removal of the fibroids known as a* **myomectomy**.

■ *Treatment for cervical factor related to infection is antibiotics.*

Medication

Clomiphene Citrate

- ■ Indication: Anovulatory infertility
- ■ Action: Stimulates release of FSH and LH which stimulates ovulation
- ■ Common side effects: Hot flashes, breast discomfort, headaches, insomnia
- ■ Route and dose: PO; 50–200 mg/day from cycle day 3–7.

(Data from Deglin & Vallerand, 2009)

Common Methods of Assisted Fertility

When the previously mentioned treatments are not successful the couple is usually referred to an infertility expert. This is an obstetrician who has specialized in infertility. Additional testing is done, and based on the outcome there are a variety of procedures that can be used to assist in fertility (Table 3-7).

Emotional Implications

■ Couples experience a "roller coaster" effect during diagnosis and treatment. Each month they become excited and hopeful that they will conceive and then the woman has a period and their excitement and hopes turn to sadness and possibly depression.

TABLE 3–7 COMMON ASSISTED FERTILITY TECHNOLOGIES

TECHNOLOGY	PROCEDURE
ARTIFICIAL INSEMINATION (AI): Intracervical Intrauterine Partner's sperm Donor sperm	Sperm that has been removed from semen is deposited directly into the cervix or uterus using a plastic catheter. The sample is collected by masturbation and the sperm is separated from the semen and prepared for insemination. Sperm can be from the partner or from a donor when the male partner does not produce sperm. Examples of fertility conditions where this procedure is used include (1) poor cervical mucus production as a result of previous surgery of the cervix, (2) anti-sperm antibodies, (3) diminished amount of sperm, and (4) diminished sperm motility.
TESTICULAR SPERM ASPIRATION	Sperm are aspirated or extracted directly from the testicles. Sperm are then microinjected into the harvested eggs of the female partner. Examples of fertility conditions where this procedure is used is with men who (1) had an unsuccessful vasectomy reversal, (2) have an absence of vas deferens, and (3) have an extremely low sperm count or no sperm in their ejaculated semen.
IN VITRO FERTILIZATION (IVF)	IVF is a procedure in which oocytes are harvested and fertilization occurs outside the female body in a laboratory.
ZYGOTE INTRAFALLOPIAN TRANSFER (ZIFT)	In ZIFT, a zygote is placed into the fallopian tube via laparoscopy 1 day after the oocyte is retrieved from the woman and IVF is used.
GAMETE INTRAFALLOPIAN TRANSFER (GIFT)	In GIFT, sperm and oocytes are mixed outside of the woman's body and then placed into the fallopian tube via laparoscopy. Fertilization takes place inside the fallopian tube. Examples of fertility conditions in which these procedures are used is (1) a history of failed infertility treatment for anovulation, (2) unexplained infertility, and (3) low sperm count.
EMBRYO TRANSFER (ET)	ET is when through IVF an embryo is placed in the uterine cavity via a catheter. Example of fertility condition in which this procedure is used is when the fallopian tubes are blocked.

■ Infertility can be seen as a crisis in the couple's lives and relationship (Sherrod, 2004).
■ Diagnosis and treatment of infertility can cause:
   ■ *Stress, anxiety, and depression for both the female and/or male partner. One or both partners may experience guilt and blame him- or herself or the partner for the inability to conceive.*
   ■ *Strain between the partners. Sexual activity becomes prescribed due to the type of testing required and the method of treatment, causing sexual dysfunction (Read, 2004).*
   ■ *Strain within the extended family. The couple may avoid family gatherings, especially those that involve children because they remind them of their infertility problems.*
■ Social isolation
   ■ *Some couples withdraw from social interaction because it is too painful to be around other couples who have children.*
   ■ *Some couples do not share with others that they are experiencing problems with fertility; thus, they do not have people who can be supportive during diagnosis and treatment.*
■ Self-esteem
   ■ *The individual's self-esteem can be affected by infertility.*
   ■ *The woman may feel less like a woman because she cannot conceive or the man may feel less like a man when he cannot impregnate his partner.*
   ■ *The man or woman may feel like he or she has a defective body and is ashamed of it.*

Research Box

Olshanky, E. (2003). A theoretical explanation for previously infertile mothers' vulnerability to depression. *Journal of Nursing Scholarship, 35,* 263–268

Since the 1980s, the focus of the research of Ellen Olshanky, DNSc, RNC has been on the psychosocial effects of infertility. In this article, Dr. Olshanky synthesized the results of several grounded theory studies on the experience of infertility and summarized her theory of identity as infertility. According to her theory:

■ Women who are distressed by their infertility become consumed with concerns about the infertility and often neglect their relationships with friends, spouse, or family members. This can lead to social isolation.
■ Infertility becomes the focus of the marriage or couple relationship and other aspects of the relationship are often ignored. This can lead to a dysfunctional marriage or couple relationship.
■ Career women may experience a sense of loss of self due to the shift of focus from career to infertility. This also contributes to social isolation.
■ Once pregnancy has been achieved, the women often have difficulty perceiving themselves as pregnant women.

- Counseling
  - *Most couples can benefit from counseling during the time of diagnosis and treatment and after treatment has stopped.*
  - *Ideally, counseling should start before treatment begins. Couples may have too high expectations regarding reproductive technology and may not want to recognize that treatment may not be successful.*
  - *Counseling includes:*
    - Discussion on how treatment may have an effect on them as a couple, as an individual, and as a family
    - Discussion on the different treatment measures and any ethical dilemmas that might be related to these treatments
    - Discussion on the effects, consequences, and resolution of treatment
    - Discussion on when to stop treatment
    - Discussion on adoption

Ethical Implications

Assisted reproductive technologies (ART) have created numerous ethical dilemmas. The primary one is what to do with the "surplus" embryos. This refers to the embryo produced from hyperstimulation of the ovaries that occurs when IVF technologies are being used. Several eggs from the woman may be harvested and fertilized using IVF, but only two or three are returned to the woman's body. The "surplus" embryos are either frozen for future use or allowed to perish. This has raised the question of when life begins and the rights of the embryo. Other ethical questions that arise are:

- Who owns the embryos – the woman or the man?
- Who decides what will happen with the "surplus" embryos?
- Who has access to ART, as health insurance providers may not pay for the costs of ART?
- At what point should the health care provider tell the couple to stop using ART?
- When artificial insemination with donor sperm is used, do you tell the child and if so when?
- Does the sperm donor have any rights or responsibilities regarding the child produced from his donation?

The Nurse's Role

- The role of the nurse varies based on where he or she interfaces with the couple who is experiencing infertility.
- Nurses who work in an infertility clinic take on a variety of roles (e.g., counseling, teaching, supporting and assisting in the procedures).
- Nurses, whether they work in acute care settings or in clinics, need to be aware of the emotional impact infertility has on the individual as well as the couple. Couples become frustrated when they work with health care professionals who do not understand the effect infertility has on their lives (Sherrod, 2004).

CRITICAL COMPONENT

Infertility

- The experience of infertility has an effect on the individual as well as the couple's emotional well-being.
- Nurses' awareness of how infertility affects all aspects of the individual and of the couple's relationship will enhance the effectiveness of the nursing care provided to these couples or individuals.

■ ■ ■ Review Questions ■ ■ ■

1. Your patient delivered a full-term baby 12 hours ago. The woman and her husband, who are in their early 20s, have just been informed by their pediatrician that their baby has trisomy 21 (Down syndrome). This is their first child and they did not have prenatal genetic testing. Your nursing care will include (select all of the correct nursing actions):
   A. Explaining that they will go through a grieving process over the loss of their "dream" child.
   B. Explaining the importance of talking openly to each other about their feelings and concerns regarding their child.
   C. Explaining they will benefit from seeing a genetic counselor.
   D. Explaining that they should direct questions regarding the baby's diagnosis to their pediatrician.

2. The developing human is most vulnerable to teratogens during
   A. The first 4 weeks of gestation
   B. The first 8 weeks of gestation
   C. The first 12 weeks of gestation
   D. The first 16 weeks of gestation

3. You are a nurse working in a prenatal clinic. Your patient, an 18-year-old woman, is in her 10th gestational week. She wants to know when her baby's heart started to beat. You inform her that it usually begins to beat around:
   A. The second week of gestation
   B. The third week of gestation
   C. The fourth week of gestation
   D. The fifth week of gestation

4. Which placental hormone is responsible for regulating glucose availability to the fetus?
   A. Progesterone
   B. Estrogen
   C. hCG
   D. hPL

5. You are a nurse in a family planning clinic. Your patient has been married five years. She used an IUD which was removed 12 months ago. She informs you that she and her husband have been trying to get pregnant for the past 12 months. Initial screening to determine the cause of infertility includes (select all of the correct answers):
   A. Sperm analysis
   B. Testicular biopsy
   C. Assessing for ovulation
   D. Hysterosalpingogram

References

American College of Obstetricians and Gynecologists (ACOG). (1997). *Teratology* (educational bulletin no. 236). Washington, DC: Author.

Deglin, J., & Vallerand, A. (2009). *Davis's drug guide for nurses* (11th ed.). Philadelphia: F. A. Davis.

Frey, K., & Patel, K. (2004). Initial evaluation and management of infertility by primary care physician. *Mayo Clinical Proceedings, 79,* 1439–1443.

Olshansky, E. (2003). A theoretical explanation of previously infertile mothers' vulnerability to depression. *Journal of Nursing Scholarship, 35,* 236–268.

Porche, D. (2006). Male infertility: Etiology, history, and physical assessment. *JNP, 2,* 226–228.

Read, J. (2004). Sexual problems associated with infertility, pregnancy, and ageing. *BMJ, 329*, 559–561.

Sadler, T. W. (2004). *Langman's medical embryology*. Philadelphia: Lippincott Williams & Wilkins.

Scanlon, S., & Sanders, T. (2007). *Essentials of anatomy and physiology* (5th ed.). Philadelphia: F. A. Davis.

Sherrod, R. (2004). Understanding the emotional aspects of infertility: Implications for nursing practice. *Journal of Psychosocial Nursing and Mental Health Services. 42*, 40–47.

Storment, J. (2006). Infertility and recurrent pregnancy loss. In Curtis, M., Overholt, S., & Hopkins, M. *Glass' office gynecology* (6th ed.). Philadelphia: Lippincott Williams & Wilkins.

Physiological Aspects of Antepartum Care

4

OBJECTIVES

On completion of this chapter, students will be able to:

- ☐ Define key terms.
- ☐ Identify the major components of preconception health care.
- ☐ Describe methods for diagnosis of pregnancy and determination of estimated date of delivery.
- ☐ Identify the progression of anatomical and physiological changes over the course of a pregnancy.
- ☐ Link the anatomical and physiological changes of pregnancy to signs and symptoms and common discomforts of pregnancy.
- ☐ Describe appropriate interventions to relieve common discomforts of pregnancy.
- ☐ Identify the critical elements of assessment and nursing care during initial and subsequent prenatal visits.
- ☐ Describe the elements of patient education and anticipatory guidance appropriate for each trimester of pregnancy.

Nursing Diagnosis

- Knowledge deficit related to physiological changes of pregnancy
- Knowledge deficit related to nutritional requirements during pregnancy
- Altered health maintenance related to knowledge deficit regarding self-care measures during pregnancy
- Knowledge deficit of warning signs of pregnancy.
- Sleep pattern disturbance related to discomforts of late pregnancy
- Constipation related to changes in gastrointestinal tract during pregnancy

Nursing Outcomes

- The pregnant woman will report eating a diet following food pyramid guidelines with the recommended calorie intake and will achieve the recommended weight gain throughout pregnancy.
- The pregnant woman will verbalize understanding of self-care needs in pregnancy such as posture/body mechanics, rest and relaxation, personal hygiene, and activity and exercise.
- The pregnant woman will verbalize an understanding of expected anatomical and physiological changes of pregnancy in contrast to warning signs of pregnancy, will verbalize an understanding of when to implement measures for relieving discomforts associated with normal physical changes versus when to notify her care provider, and will report experiencing a reduction in anxiety.
- The pregnant woman will verbalize an understanding of strategies for constipation management in pregnancy and will resume normal bowel function.

INTRODUCTION

The scope of this chapter is nursing care and interventions in normal pregnancy based on an understanding of the physiological aspects of pregnancy. Chapter 5 addresses the psychosocial and cultural components of the antepartum period. The **antepartum (antepartal) period**, also referred to as the prenatal period, begins with conception and ends with the onset of labor.

The focus of antepartum nursing care during prenatal care is:

- Regular assessment of the health of the pregnancy
- Regular assessment and screening of risk factors for potential complications
- Implementation of appropriate interventions based on risk status or actual complications
- Inclusion of significant others/family in care and education to promote pregnancy adaptation
- Education on health promotion and disease prevention

PRECONCEPTION HEALTH CARE

Preconception care is defined as a set of interventions that aim to identify medical, behavioral, and social risks to a woman's health or pregnancy outcome through prevention and management (Centers for Disease Control and Prevention [CDC], 2006). Preconception care consists of health promotion, risk screening, and implementation of interventions for childbearing-aged women before a pregnancy with the goal of modifying risk factors that could negatively impact a pregnancy (CDC, 2006; Table 4-1). This care is critical because several risk behaviors (i.e., smoking) and exposures negatively affect fetal development and pregnancy outcomes (Critical Component: Preconception Health Care). In addition, because almost half of pregnancies are unintended (i.e., mistimed or unwanted at the time of conception), preconception care optimizes a woman's health for potential pregnancy (Martin, Hamilton, Menacker, Sutton, & Mathews, 2007).

CRITICAL COMPONENT

Preconception Health Care

Assessing a woman for risk factors and implementing interventions when appropriate can positively impact her current or future health as well as the health of any future pregnancies, resulting in better health outcomes for women and families.

(CDC, 2006)

Routine Physical Examination and Screening

Two of the primary components of a preconception health care visit are a physical examination and relevant health screening in the form of laboratory or diagnostic testing (see Table 4-1).

- The physical examination includes:
  - *Comprehensive physical examination*
  - *Breast examination*
  - *Pelvic examination*
- Laboratory and diagnostic tests include:
  - ***Papanicolaou smear (Pap smear),*** *a screening test for cervical cancer*
  - *Blood type and Rh factor*
  - *Blood count*
  - *Serum cholesterol*
  - *Serum glucose*
  - *Urinalysis*
  - *HIV*
  - *Syphilis*
  - *Sexually transmitted disease (STD) cultures*
- Additional testing may be ordered based on history and physical examination findings.

Anticipatory Guidance and Education

Anticipatory guidance is the provision of information and guidance to women and their families that enables them to be knowledgeable and prepared as the process of pregnancy and childbirth unfold. Anticipatory guidance and education in the childbearing-aged population spans topics from health maintenance, self-care, and lifestyle choices to contraception and safety behaviors. The nurse is key in providing this aspect of care. It is imperative that a woman's age, sexual orientation, culture, religion, and additional values and beliefs are acknowledged and respected, and that this information is incorporated appropriately into the nurse's teaching plan (Critical Component: Preconception Education).

CRITICAL COMPONENT

Preconception Education

The goal of preconception education is to provide a woman with information she can use to enhance her health before becoming pregnant. When a woman seeks care specifically because she is planning for a future pregnancy, more emphasis is placed on counseling and anticipatory guidance related to preparation and planning for a pregnancy.

Anticipatory guidance and teaching include:

- Nutrition
- Prenatal vitamins
- Exercise
- Self-care
- Contraception cessation
- Timing of conception
- Modifying behaviors to reduce risks

Nutrition

Maintaining a healthy weight with a normal BMI is especially important prior to pregnancy. Eating nutritious foods with an emphasis on fresh fruits and vegetables, lean protein sources, low-fat or non-fat dairy foods, whole grains and small amounts of healthy fats (see Fig. 4-8).

- Referring women who are either significantly underweight or overweight for dietary counseling and planning in order to achieve a healthier weight before conception.
- Maintaining a healthy weight prior to and during pregnancy reduces a woman's risk for adverse perinatal outcomes.

Maternal obesity is associated with increased perinatal morbidity and mortality from a variety of causes such as:

- Complications during childbirth due to large for gestational age (LGA) infants and macrosomia
- Prolonged labor
- Postpartum hemorrhage
- Poor wound healing following a cesarean birth.
- Increased risk for antepartum complications such as hypertension, preeclampsia, gestational diabetes, thromboembolism, and urinary tract infections.
- Poor perinatal outcomes can also result from inadequate maternal weight during pregnancy such as small for gestational age (SGA) infants and preterm birth.

Prenatal Vitamins

Many women planning a pregnancy begin taking a prenatal vitamin supplement. Prenatal vitamins contain a wide range of vitamins and minerals important for good health during pregnancy:

- Folic acid supplementation: Decreases risk of neural tube defects (Critical Component: Folic Acid Supplements).
- Calcium, magnesium, and vitamin D: Contribute to bone health and osteoporosis prevention throughout the lifespan, including during the childbearing years.
- Iron supplementation is commonly prescribed during pregnancy, although there is some controversy about the benefit of this practice as a routine recommendation.

TABLE 4–1 COMPONENTS OF HEALTH HISTORY AND RISK FACTOR ASSESSMENT IN PRECONCEPTION CARE

COMPONENT	PURPOSE AND ACTIONS
IDENTIFYING INFORMATION Age, gravida/para, address, race/ethnicity, religion, marital/family status, occupation, education	To determine specific risks based on sociodemographic characteristics ■ Provide education and anticipatory guidance To identify psychosocial resources and available sources of support ■ Refer for social services, counseling services, spiritual support
HISTORY Prior and present health status	To determine past and present health status: ■ Provide education and anticipatory guidance. ■ Refer for additional testing/procedures. ■ Refer to physician specialist, counseling services, substance abuse treatment, genetic counseling, dietician, social services as indicated. ■ Administer rubella and/or hepatitis vaccines as indicated. ■ Refer to cessation programs as appropriate (e.g., smoking).
MEDICAL History of or current medical conditions/diseases Surgeries (including blood transfusions) History of physical/sexual abuse Medication use (prescription, OTC, complementary) Allergies Immunizations	To identify any components in medical history that may increase risk in the well-woman population ■ Initiate actions to minimize risks.
FAMILY MEDICAL Current health status Genetic Medical conditions/diseases	To determine both modifiable and non-modifiable risk factors related to family and genetic history ■ Initiate actions to minimize risks.
REPRODUCTIVE Menstrual Obstetric Gynecological Contraceptive Sexual	To ascertain details about menstrual cycles, past pregnancies and their outcomes, any gynecological disorders including infertility, past or present contraceptive use, history of sexually transmitted infections, sexual orientation, past or present sexuality issues, use of safer sex practices.
SELF-CARE/LIFESTYLE/SAFETY BEHAVIORS	To determine frequency of health maintenance visits (well-woman and dental), nutrition and bowel patterns, sleep patterns, exercise history, stress management To identify tobacco, alcohol, and substance use/abuse, caffeine use To identify use of complementary and alternative medicine (CAM) modalities To identify spiritual or religious practices To determine safety practices such as use of seat belts, sunscreen, smoke alarms and carbon monoxide detectors, gun safety ■ Initiate actions to minimize risks
PSYCHOSOCIAL Mental health Social	To ascertain past and present psychological and emotional health To identify social patterns and sources of emotional and social support in family and friends ■ Refer to mental health providers as needed
CULTURAL Beliefs/values Practices Primary language	To identify cultural practices and beliefs/values impacting health ■ Incorporate knowledge of beliefs and practices in care. To determine need for translation ■ Obtain translation assistance as needed. ■ Provide educational materials in woman's primary language.
ENVIRONMENTAL Home Workplace	To identify past and current exposure to environmental or occupational hazards/toxins ■ Refer for environmental exposure counseling, genetic counseling when indicated.
FINANCIAL Basic needs Resources Health insurance	To determine adequacy of resources to meet basic ongoing needs ■ Refer for social services, economic support services as indicated

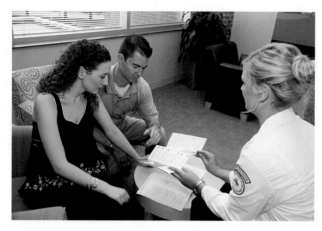

Figure 4-1 Nurse providing anticipatory guidance and education on self-care.

■ A woman who is anticipating a short time period between pregnancies is at risk for iron-deficiency anemia. Iron supplementation may be prescribed and she is encouraged to include iron-rich foods in her diet in between pregnancies since she is likely to have reduced iron stores and may also be anemic from the previous recent pregnancy.

■ Mega-doses of vitamins and minerals are not recommended, as they may be toxic to the developing fetus.

CRITICAL COMPONENT

Folic Acid Supplements

In 1992, the CDC began recommending daily folic acid supplementation of 0.4 mg daily for childbearing-aged women after folic acid was shown to reduce the incidence of neural tube defects (NTDs) such as spina bifida, with an expected reduction in NTD incidence in the United States of 50%. The beneficial impact of folic acid supplementation is greatest between 1 month before pregnancy and through the first trimester, the period of neural tube development.

Exercise

A program of regular exercise positively impacts a woman's health and may generally be continued once she has conceived. It is best to implement such a program several months in advance of conception so that when pregnancy occurs, regular exercise is already comfortable and routine.

■ Some form of aerobic activity, including regular weight-bearing exercise such as walking or running, as well as stretching exercises and some type of weight work/muscle strengthening together provide overall body conditioning.

■ The weight-bearing exercise and weight/strengthening work also enhance bone health and help prevent osteoporosis.

Self-Care

Most women are pregnant for at least 2 weeks before being aware of their pregnancy. For this reason, it is helpful to counsel the preconception woman to decrease risk behaviors and eliminate exposure to substances that are known or suspected to be harmful during gestation as soon as she stops using contraception or begins trying to become pregnant (Fig. 4-1). The woman should avoid:

■ Alcohol

■ Tobacco

■ Second-hand smoke
■ Excessive use of caffeine
■ Illicit drugs
■ Medications contraindicated in pregnancy (prescription, over-the-counter, and herbal supplements)
■ Environmental toxins

The woman should be encouraged to:

■ Use safer sex practices to prevent STDs
■ Use seat belts in a car
■ Ensure that smoke alarms and carbon monoxide detectors are in working order
■ Apply sunscreen when outdoors
■ Maintain adequate relaxation and sleep
■ Maintain optimal oral health as periodontal disease has been associated with adverse pregnancy outcomes including preterm birth and low birth weight (CDC, 2006).
■ Treat periodontal disease before a pregnancy eliminates poor oral health as a risk factor for adverse pregnancy outcomes.
■ Discuss the use of complementary or alternative medicine modalities, such as acupuncture, herbal supplements, homeopathy, and massage, with her primary health care provider. Some of these interventions may need to be discontinued before a pregnancy for safety reasons.

Contraception Cessation

Before conception, it is ideal for a woman to have at least two or three normal menstrual periods. For all women planning a pregnancy, discontinuation of contraception and tracking of menstrual cycles will aid in facilitating conception and subsequently in dating the pregnancy once conception is achieved.

■ Women using some form of hormonal contraception need to stop hormonal contraception and begin the use of a barrier method of birth control or fertility awareness family planning techniques for the next few months before conception.
■ Women using Depo-Provera for contraception need to be informed that it may take from several months up to more than a year to conceive after discontinuing injections.
■ Women using an intrauterine device (IUD) need to have the device removed.

Timing of Conception

Many women are interested in learning more about their menstrual cycles in order to gain more control over their ability to conceive.

■ Preconception counseling can include basic information about the menstrual cycle, when in the cycle a woman is able to conceive, signs of ovulation, the lifespan of ovum and sperm, and how to time sexual intercourse in order to increase the likelihood of conception.
■ Women who have used fertility awareness family planning principles are familiar with these concepts and can simply reverse the behaviors they practiced when using the method to avoid conception.

Modifying Behaviors to Reduce Risk

With each topic of conversation in preconception counseling, women gain information allowing them to positively affect their overall health and reduce perinatal risk. Several factors contribute to risk reduction or elimination by modifying risk factors related to preexisting medical conditions, high-risk behaviors, and self-care and safety behavior deficits to improve outcomes of future pregnancies (Evidence-Based

Practice: Recommendations to Improve Preconception Health and Health Care in the United States).

Nursing Actions in Preconception Care

■ Provide comfort and privacy.
■ Use therapeutic communication techniques.
■ Obtain the health history.
■ Conduct a review of systems.
■ Assist with physical and pelvic exams.
■ Assist with obtaining specimens.
■ Provide teaching about procedures.
■ Provide antepartum guidance related to plan of care and appropriate follow-up.
■ Assess the patient's understanding.
■ Provide education, recommendations, and referrals to help woman make appropriate behavioral, lifestyle, or medical changes based on history or physical examination.

Evidence-Based Practice: Recommendations to Improve Preconception Health and Health Care in the United States

Centers for Disease Control and Prevention. (2006). Recommendations to improve preconception health and health care—United States. *MMWR Recommendations and Reports*, 55(RR-6); 1–23.

The CDC reviewed the literature and consulted with national experts to develop a list of 10 recommendations that will, when implemented consistently, improve preconception health and health care nationally. The result will be improved perinatal outcomes in the United States. The recommendations focus on improving public awareness of the importance of preconception care, providing access to preconception care including health insurance coverage and particularly for women with a previous adverse pregnancy outcome, screening for risk, following up with appropriate interventions for identified risks, providing health promotion and risk reduction education, expanding research efforts in the areas of preconception care, and monitoring improvements and outcomes. These efforts are intended to contribute to the achievement of the *Healthy People 2010* objectives.

DIAGNOSIS OF PREGNANCY

The diagnostic confirmation of pregnancy is based on a combination of the presumptive, probable, and positive changes/signs of pregnancy. This information is obtained through history, physical and pelvic examinations, and laboratory and diagnostic studies.

Presumptive Signs of Pregnancy

The **presumptive signs** of pregnancy include all subjective signs of pregnancy (i.e., physiological changes perceived by the woman herself):

■ **Amenorrhea:** Absence of menstruation
■ Nausea and vomiting: Common from week 2 to 12
■ Breast changes: Changes begin to appear at 2 to 3 weeks
  ■ *Enlargement, tenderness, and tingling of breast*
  ■ *Increased vascularity of breast*
■ Fatigue: Common during the first trimester
■ Urination frequency: Related to pressure of enlarging uterus on bladder; decreases as uterus moves upward and out of pelvis

■ **Quickening:** A woman's first awareness of fetal movement; occurs around 18 weeks' gestation

All of these changes could have causes outside of pregnancy and are not considered diagnostic.

Probable Signs of Pregnancy

The **probable signs** of pregnancy are objective signs of pregnancy and include all physiological and anatomical changes that can be perceived by the health care provider.

■ **Chadwick's sign:** Bluish-purple coloration of the vaginal mucosa, cervix, and vulva seen at 6 to 8 weeks
■ **Goodell's sign:** Softening of the cervix and vagina with increased leukorrheal discharge; palpated at 8 weeks
■ **Hegar's sign:** Softening of the lower uterine segment; palpated at 6 weeks
■ Uterine growth and abdominal growth
■ Skin hyperpigmentation
  ■ *Melasma (chloasma), also referred to as the mask of pregnancy: Brownish pigmentation over the forehead, temples, cheek, and/or upper lip*
  ■ *Linea nigra: Dark line that runs from the umbilicus to the pubes*
  ■ *Nipples and areola: Become darker; more evident in primigravidas and dark-haired women*
■ **Ballottement:** A light tap of the examining finger on the cervix causes fetus to rise in the amniotic fluid and then rebound to its original position; occurs at 16 to 18 weeks
■ Positive pregnancy test results
  ■ *Laboratory tests are based on detection of the presence of human chorionic gonadotropin (hCG) in maternal urine or blood.*
  ■ *The tests are extremely accurate, but not 100%. There can be both false-positive and false-negative results. Because of this, a positive pregnancy test is considered a probable rather than a positive sign of pregnancy.*
  ■ *A urine pregnancy test is best performed using a first morning urine specimen, which has the highest concentration of hCG, and becomes positive about 4 weeks after conception.*
  ■ *A maternal blood pregnancy test can detect hCG levels before a missed period.*
  ■ *Home pregnancy tests are also accurate (but not 100%) and are simple to perform. These urine tests use enzymes and rely on a color change when agglutination occurs, indicating a pregnancy. The home tests can be performed at the time of a missed menstrual period. If a negative result occurs, the instructions suggest that the test be repeated in one week if a menstrual period has not begun.*

All of these changes could also have causes other than pregnancy and are not considered diagnostic. The presumptive and probable signs of pregnancy are important components of assessment in confirming a pregnancy. Early in gestation, before any positive signs of pregnancy, a combination of presumptive and probable signs is used to make a practical diagnosis of pregnancy.

Positive Signs of Pregnancy

The **positive signs** of pregnancy are the objective signs of pregnancy that can only be attributed to the fetus:

■ Auscultation of the fetal heart, by 10 to 12 weeks
■ Observation and palpation of fetal movement by the examiner
■ Sonographic visualization of the fetus: Cardiac movement noted at 4 to 8 weeks

Sonographic Diagnosis of Pregnancy

Ultrasound visualization of a pregnancy has increasingly become a routine and expected part of prenatal care. The gestational sac can be seen at 5 weeks' gestation and fetal cardiac activity can be observed between 6 and 7 weeks' gestation. Indications for ultrasound examination of an early pregnancy for purposes of diagnosis include:

■ Pelvic pain or vaginal bleeding in the first trimester
■ History of repeated pregnancy loss or ectopic pregnancy (the implantation of a fertilized ovum outside the uterus)
■ Uncertain menstrual history
■ Discrepancy between actual size and expected size of pregnancy based on history

Calculation of Due Date

An important piece of information to share with a newly pregnant woman and her family is her "due date" or estimated date of birth (EDB). It is more commonly known now as estimated date of delivery (EDD). This date represents a best estimation as to when a full-term infant will be born. The original term used for this date was the "estimated date of confinement" (EDC).

Calculation of the EDD is best accomplished with a known and certain last menstrual period date (LMP). Other tools are used to determine the most accurate EDD possible if the LMP is not known and are used throughout the pregnancy to confirm EDD based on an LMP. These tools are:

■ Physical examination to determine uterine size
■ First auscultation of fetal heart rate with a **Doppler** and/or a fetoscope (stethoscope for auscultation of fetal heart tones)
■ Date of quickening
■ Ultrasound examination

Naegele's Rule

Naegele's rule is the standard formula for determining an EDD based on an LMP. The formula is: First day of LMP – 3 months + 7 days.

Formula for Naegele's Rule

LMP	April 27
	–3 months
	January 27
	+7 days
EDD	February 3

It is important to remember that the EDD as determined by Naegele's rule is only a best guess of when a baby is likely to be born. Two factors influence the accuracy of this rule:

■ Regularity of woman's menstrual cycles
■ Length of a woman's menstrual cycles

Naegele's rule relies on the following for accuracy:

■ Regular menstrual cycles for its accuracy
■ 28-day menstrual cycle with 14 days between onset of menses and ovulation and 14 days between ovulation and onset of the subsequent menses

Most women give birth within the time period of 3 weeks before to 2 weeks after their EDD. The window for **term gestation** is 5 weeks from 37 to 42 weeks of gestation.

Weeks of Gestation

Once an EDD has been determined, a pregnancy is counted in terms of weeks of gestation beginning with the first day of the LMP and ending with 40 completed weeks (the EDD). A useful tool for quickly and easily calculating gestational age throughout the pregnancy is the gestational wheel (Fig. 4-2), but it is less reliable than Naegele's rule due to variations of up to a few days between wheels. It is best to calculate a due date initially using Naegele's rule and then employ a gestational wheel to determine weeks and days of gestation using the Naegele's rule-based EDD.

To use this device, the first day of the LMP date on the outside circle is lined up with the beginning of the pregnancy designation on the inside circle. The EDD is then read as the date on the outside circle that lines up with 40 completed weeks on the inside circle.

Trimesters

A pregnancy is also counted in terms of trimesters roughly divided into 3-month segments:

First trimester: First day of LMP through 12 completed weeks
Second trimester: 13 weeks through 27 completed weeks
Third trimester: 28 weeks through 40 completed weeks

PHYSIOLOGICAL PROGRESSION OF PREGNANCY

Pregnancy results in maternal physiologic adaptations involving every body system. Every change has either the maintenance of the pregnancy, the development of the fetus, or preparation for the labor and birth as its basis and is protective of the woman and/or the fetus. To both understand a woman's experience of normal pregnancy and be effective in identifying deviations from normal, the nurse must have a basic foundation in the physiology of pregnancy.

This understanding is critical not only for risk assessment and implementation of appropriate nursing interventions to reduce risk, but also for providing effective patient education and anticipatory guidance grounded in knowledge of the physiological basis for the normal physical changes in pregnancy and their resulting common, and normal, discomforts. The next sections present the changes that occur in each system, and Table 4-2 summarizes the major physiological changes and factors that influence these changes.

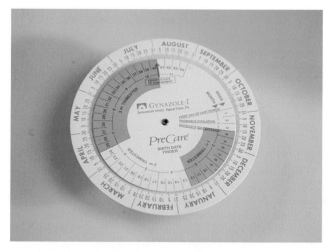

Figure 4-2   Gestational wheel.

TABLE 4–2 PHYSIOLOGICAL CHANGES IN PREGNANCY

PHYSIOLOGICAL CHANGES	CLINICAL SIGNS AND SYMPTOMS
REPRODUCTIVE SYSTEM—BREASTS	
Increase of estrogen and progesterone levels: Initially produced by the corpus luteum and then by the placenta Increased blood supply to breasts Increase of prolactin: Produced by the anterior pituitary	Tenderness, feeling of fullness, and tingling sensation Increase in weight of breast by 400 g Enlargement of breasts, nipples, areola, and Montgomery follicles (small glands on the areola around the nipple) Striae: Due to stretching of skin to accommodate enlarging breast tissue Prominent veins due to a twofold increase in blood flow Increased growth of mammary glands Increase in lactiferous ducts and alveolar system Production of colostrum, a yellow secretion rich in antibodies, begins to be produced by end of 16th week of gestation
REPRODUCTIVE SYSTEM—UTERUS	
Increased levels of estrogen and progesterone Enlargement of uterus to accommodate developing fetus and placenta Expanded circulatory volume leads to increased vascular congestion. Acid pH of vagina	Hypertrophy of uterine wall Softening of vaginal muscle and connective tissue in preparation for expansion of tissue to accommodate passage of fetus through the birth canal Uterus contractibility increases in response to increased estrogen levels, leading to Braxton-Hicks contractions. Hypertrophy of cervical glands leads to formation of mucus plug which serves as a protective barrier between uterus/fetus and vagina Hypertrophy of vaginal glands leads to increase in leukorrhea Cessation of menstrual cycle (amenorrhea) and ovulation Increase in uterine size to 20 times that of nonpregnant uterus Weight of uterus increases from 70 g to 1,000 g. Blood flow to the uterus is 500–600 mL/min at term. Goodell's sign: Softening of the cervix Hegar's sign: Softening of the lower uterine segment Chadwick's sign: Bluish coloration of cervix, vaginal mucosa, and vulva Acid environment inhibits growth of bacteria. Acid environment allows growth of *Candida albicans*, leading to increased risk of candidiasis (yeast infection).
CARDIOVASCULAR SYSTEM	
Decrease in peripheral vascular resistance Increase in blood volume by 40%–50% Increase in cardiac output by 30%–50% Increase in RBC count by 30% Increase in RBC volume by 17%–30% Increase in WBC count Increased demand for iron in fetal development Hypercoagulability Increased venous pressure and decreased blood flow to extremities due to compression of iliac veins and inferior vena cava	Decrease in blood pressure Hypervolemia of pregnancy Increased heart rate of 15–20 bpm Increased stroke volume of 30% Systolic murmurs, load and wide S1 split, load S2, obvious S3 Increase in heart size Increase in peripheral dilation Physiological anemia of pregnancy Hemodilution is caused by the increase in plasma volume being relatively larger than the increase in RBCs, which results in decreased hemoglobin and hematocrit values. Values up to 15,000 mm^3 in the absence of infection Iron-deficiency anemia: Hemoglobin <11 g/dL and hematocrit <33% Plasma fibrin increase of 40% Fibrinogen increase of 50% Decrease in coagulation inhibiting factors Protective of inevitable blood loss during birth Edema of lower extremities Varicosities in legs and vulva Hemorrhoids

Continued

TABLE 4–2   PHYSIOLOGICAL CHANGES IN PREGNANCY—CONT'D

PHYSIOLOGICAL CHANGES	CLINICAL SIGNS AND SYMPTOMS
RESPIRATORY SYSTEM	
Hormones of pregnancy stimulate the respiratory center and act on lung tissue to increase and enhance respiratory function Increase of oxygen consumption by 15%–20% Estrogen, progesterone, and prostaglandins cause vascular engorgement and smooth muscle relaxation. Upward displacement of diaphragm by enlarging uterus Estrogen causes a relaxation of the ligaments and joints of the ribs.	Increase in tidal volume by 30%–40% Slight increase in respiratory rate Increase in inspiratory capacity Decrease in expiratory volume Slight hyperventilation Slight respiratory alkalosis Dyspnea Nasal and sinus congestion Epistaxis Shift from abdominal to thoracic breathing Chest and thorax expand to accommodate thoracic breathing and upward displacement of diaphragm. Slight decrease in lung capacity
RENAL SYSTEM	
Increased progesterone levels, which cause a relaxation of smooth muscles Pressure of enlarging uterus on renal structures Alterations in cardiovascular system (increased cardiac output and increased blood and plasma volume) lead to increased renal blood flow of 50%–80% in first trimester and then decreases. Decreased renal flow in third trimester Increased vascularity	Dilation of renal pelvis and ureters leads to increased risk of urinary tract infections (UTI). Ureters become elongated with decreased motility, leading to increased risk of UTI. Decreased bladder tone with increased bladder capacity leads to urinary frequency and incontinence and increased risk of UTI. Displacement of bladder in third trimester leads to urinary frequency and nocturia. Increased glomerular filtration rate leads to increased urinary output. Increased renal excretion of glucose and protein leads to glucosuria and proteinuria. Dependent edema Hyperemia of bladder and urethra
GASTROINTESTINAL SYSTEM	
Increase levels of hCG and altered carbohydrate metabolism Increased progesterone levels lead to decreased muscle tone and slowing of digestive processes. Increased progesterone levels lead to decreased muscle tone of gallbladder, resulting in prolonged emptying time. Changes in senses of taste and smell Displacement of intestines by uterus Increased levels of estrogen lead to increased vascular congestion of mucosa.	Nausea and vomiting during early pregnancy Constipation Delayed stomach emptying leads to heartburn Increased risk of gallstone formation and cholestasis Increase or decrease in appetite Nausea Pica: Abnormal; craving for and ingestion of nonfood substances such as clay or starch Flatulence, abdominal distension, abdominal cramping, and pelvic heaviness Gingivitis, bleeding gums, increase risk of periodontal disease
MUSCULOSKELETAL SYSTEM	
Increased progesterone and relaxin levels lead to softening of joints and increased joint mobility, resulting in widening and increased mobility of the sacroiliac and symphysis pubis. Distension of abdomen related to expanding uterus, reduced abdominal tone, and increased breast size Increased estrogen and relaxin levels lead to increased elasticity and relaxation of ligaments. Abdominal muscles stretch due to enlarging uterus	Altered gait: "Waddle" gait Facilitates birthing process Pelvic tilts forward, leading to shifting of center of gravity that results in change in posture and walking style, increasing lordosis Increased risk of falls due to shift in center of gravity and change in gait and posture Round ligament spasm Increase risk of joint pain and injury Diastasis recti

TABLE 4–2   PHYSIOLOGICAL CHANGES IN PREGNANCY—CONT'D

PHYSIOLOGICAL CHANGES	CLINICAL SIGNS AND SYMPTOMS
INTEGUMENTARY SYSTEM	
Estrogen and progesterone levels stimulate increased melanin deposition, causing light brown to dark brown pigmentation.	Linea nigra Melasma (chloasma) Darken of nipples, areola, vulva, scars, and moles
Increased blood flow, increased basal metabolic rate, progesterone-induced increase in body temperature, and vasomotor instability	Hot flashes, facial flushing, alternating sensation of hot and cold Increased perspiration
Increased action of adrenocorticosteroids leads to cutaneous elastic tissues becoming fragile.	Striae gravidarum (stretch marks) on abdomen, thighs, breast, and buttocks
Increased estrogen levels lead to color and vascular changes.	Angiomas (spider nevi) Palmar erythema: Pinkish-red mottling over palms of hands
Increased androgens lead to increase in sebaceous gland secretions.	Increased oiliness of skin and increase of acne
ENDOCRINE SYSTEM	
Decreased follicle-stimulating hormone	Amenorrhea
Increased progesterone	Maintains pregnancy by relaxation of smooth muscles, leading to decreased uterine activity, which results in decreased risk of spontaneous abortions Decreases gastrointestinal motility
Increased estrogen	Facilitates uterine and breast development Facilitates increases in vascularity Facilitates hyperpigmentation Alters metabolic processes and fluid and electrolyte balance
Increased prolactin	Facilitates lactation Stimulates uterine contractions
Increased oxytocin	Stimulates the milk let-down or ejection reflex in response to breastfeeding
Increased human chorionic gonadotropin (hCG)	Maintenance of corpus luteum until placenta becomes fully functional
Human placental lactogen/human chorionic somatomammotropin	Facilitates breast development Alters carbohydrate, protein, and fat metabolism Facilitates fetal growth by altering maternal metabolism; acts as an insulin antagonist
Hyperplasia and increased vascularity of thyroid	Enlargement of thyroid Heat intolerance and fatigue
Increased BMR related to fetal metabolic activity	Depletion of maternal glucose stores leads to increased risk of maternal hypoglycemia. Increased production of insulin Increase in maternal resistance to insulin leads to increased risk of hyperglycemia.
Increased need for glucose due to developing fetus Increase in cortisol	

Sources: Blackburn (2007); Dillon (2007); Mattson & Smith (2004); Simpson & Creehan (2008).

Reproductive System

Maternal physiologic adaptations to pregnancy are most profound in the reproductive system. The uterus undergoes phenomenal growth, breasts prepare for lactation, the vagina changes to accomodate the birthing process (Fig. 4-3).

Breast

Breast changes begin early in pregnancy and continue throughout gestation and into the postpartum period. These changes are primarily influenced by increases in hormone levels and occur in preparation for lactation (see Table 4-2).

Uterus

The uterus is described in three parts:

- **Fundus** or upper portion
- **Isthmus** or lower segment
- **Cervix,** the lower part, or neck; the external part of the cervix interfaces with the vagina

Uterine changes over the course of pregnancy are profound (see Table 4-2).

- Before pregnancy, this elastic, muscular organ is the size and shape of a small pear, approximately 3 inches × 2 inches × 1 inch in its dimensions.

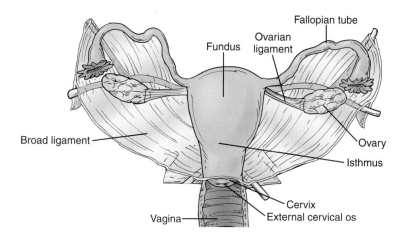

Figure 4-3   Reproductive system.

■ By mid-pregnancy, the uterine fundus reaches the level of the umbilicus abdominally.

■ Toward the end of pregnancy, the enlarged uterus, containing a full-term fetus, fills the abdominal cavity and has altered the placement of the lungs and rib cage in addition to the abdominal organs (Fig. 4-4).

■ The uterine wall progressively thins as the uterus expands to accommodate the developing fetus.

Vagina

The vagina is a muscular canal. As pregnancy progresses, various changes take place in the vasculature and tone of structures (see Table 4-2):

■ An increase of vascularity due to the expanded circulatory needs

■ An increase of vaginal discharge (**leukorrhea**) which is in response to the estrogen-induced hypertrophy of the vaginal glands

■ Relaxation of the vaginal wall and perineal body which allows stretching of tissues to accommodate the birthing process.

■ Acid pH of the vagina which inhibits growth of bacteria, but allows overgrowth of *Candida albicans*. This places the pregnant woman at risk for candidiasis (yeast infection).

Ovaries

The corpus luteum, which normally degenerates after ovulation when pregnancy does not occur, is maintained during the first trimester by high levels of human chorionic gonadotropin (hCG). At the beginning of pregnancy, the corpus luteum of pregnancy produces progesterone and some estrogen in order to maintain the uterine lining, referred to as the **endometrium**, to allow for implantation and establishment of the pregnancy. There is subsequently no shedding of the endometrium that would result in menstruation. Follicle maturation and release are inhibited by hormones of pregnancy and ovulation ceases.

Cardiovascular System

The cardiovascular system undergoes significant adaptations in pregnancy to support the maintenance and development of the pregnancy while meeting maternal physiological needs. Changes are seen in the hemodynamic, anatomical, and hematological areas (see Table 4-2). Hemodynamic changes include:

■ Blood volume increases by 1,500 mL or by 40% to 50%. This is referred to as hypervolemia of pregnancy.

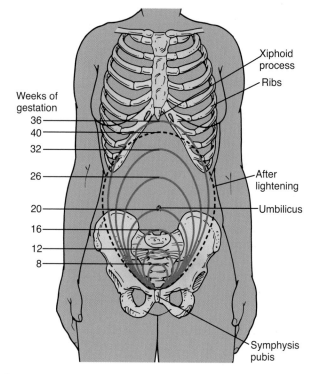

Figure 4-4   Uterine heights by weeks of gestation with anatomical landmarks.

■ Blood volume increases to support uteroplacental demands and maintenance of pregnancy.

■ Plasma and red blood cell (RBC) volume increase in response to increased uteroplacental and renal perfusion needs.

■ Cardiac output increases 30% to 50% with an increase in heart rate of 15 to 20 beats per minute (bpm; 20% increase).

■ Enlarging uterus can compress the inferior vena cava (Critical Component: Supine Hypotensive Syndrome).

■ The hemodynamic changes are also a protective mechanism for the inevitable intrapartum blood loss.

Anatomical changes include:

■ The heart enlarges slightly as a result of hypervolemia and increased cardiac output.

■ The heart shifts upward and laterally as the growing uterus displaces the diaphragm (Fig. 4-5).

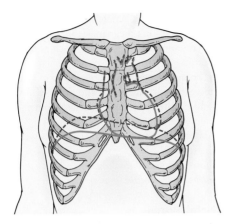

Figure 4-5 Term uterus and fetus indicating displacement of heart and lungs and indicates pregnancy changes.

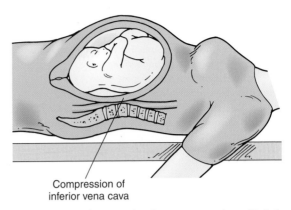

Compression of
inferior vena cava

Figure 4-6 Supine hypotension from compression of inferior vena cava.

Hematological changes include:

■ The RBC count increases 30% and RBC volume increases 17% to 33% in response to increased oxygen requirements of pregnancy.
■ Blood volume expansion leads to physiological anemia of pregnancy.
  ■ *Physiological anemia of pregnancy, also referred to as pseudoanemia of pregnancy, is due to hemodilution. The increase in plasma volume is relatively larger than the increase in RBCs and results in decreased hemoglobin and hematocrit values.*
■ Iron-deficiency anemia, defined as hemoglobin of less than 11.0 g/dL and hematocrit less than 33%.
  ■ *Maternal iron stores are insufficient to meet the demands for iron in fetal development.*
■ The white blood cell (WBC) count increases, with values up to 15,000 mm³ in the absence of infection
  ■ *The increase is hormonally induced and similar to elevations seen in physiological stress such as exercise.*
■ Hypercoagulation occurs during pregnancy to decrease the risk of postpartum hemorrhage. These changes place the woman at increased risk for thrombosis and coagulopathies.
  ■ *Plasma fibrin increase of 40%*
  ■ *Fibrinogen increase of 50%*
  ■ *Coagulation inhibiting factors decrease.*

CRITICAL COMPONENT

Supine Hypotensive Syndrome

Supine hypotensive syndrome is a hypotensive condition resulting from a woman lying on her back in mid to late pregnancy (Fig. 4-6). In a supine position, the enlarged uterus compresses the inferior vena cava, leading to a significant drop in cardiac output and blood pressure, and resulting in the woman feeling dizzy and faint. Pregnant women should be advised to lie on their side and rise slowly when in a supine position to decrease the risk of a hypotensive event.

Respiratory System

Throughout the course of pregnancy, the respiratory system adapts in response to physiological and anatomical demands related to fetal growth and development as well as maternal metabolic needs (see Table 4-2). Pulmonary function is not compromised in a normal pregnancy.

Physiological changes that occur to accommodate the additional requirements for oxygen delivery and carbon dioxide removal in mother and fetus during pregnancy.

Physiological changes include:

■ Tidal volume increase
■ Slight respiratory alkalosis
  ■ *Decrease in P_{CO_2} leads to an increase in pH (more alkaline) and decrease in bicarbonate*
  ■ *This change promotes transport of carbon dioxide away from the fetus.*

Increases in estrogen, progesterone, and prostaglandins cause vascular engorgement and smooth muscle relaxation resulting in edema and tissue congestion, which can lead to:

■ Nasal and sinus congestion
■ Epistaxis (nosebleeds)

Anatomical changes include:

■ Diaphragm is displaced upward.
■ There is a shift from abdominal to thoracic breathing as the pregnancy progresses (see Fig. 4-5).
■ Increase in chest circumference of 6 cm with an increase in the costal angle of greater than 90 degrees.
■ These anatomical changes may contribute to the physiological dyspnea that is common during pregnancy.

Renal System

The kidneys undergo change during pregnancy as they adapt to perform their basic functions of regulating fluid and electrolyte balance, eliminating metabolic waste products, and helping to regulate blood pressure (see Table 4-2).

Physiological changes include:

■ Renal plasma flow increases.
■ Glomerular filtration rate (GFR) increases.
■ Renal tubular reabsorption increases.
■ Proteinuria and glucosuria can normally occur in small amounts related to tubal reabsorption threshold of protein and glucose being exceeded due to increased volume.
  ■ *Even though a small amount can be normal, it is important to assess and monitor for pathology.*

■ Shift in fluid and electrolyte balance
  ■ *The need for increase fluid and electrolytes results in alteration of regulating mechanisms including the renin–angiotensin–aldosterone system and antidiuretic hormone.*
■ Positional variation in renal function
  ■ *In the supine and upright maternal position, blood pools in the lower body, causing a decrease in cardiac output, GFR, and urine output; also causing excess sodium and fluid retention.*
  ■ *A left lateral recumbent maternal position can:*
    ■ Maximize cardiac output, renal plasma volume, and urine output
    ■ Stabilize fluid and electrolyte balance
    ■ Minimize dependent edema
    ■ Maintain optimal blood pressure

These changes support the increased circulatory and metabolic demands of the pregnancy because the renal system secretes both maternal and fetal waste products.
Anatomical changes include:

■ Renal pelvis dilation with increased renal plasma flow
■ Ureter alterations
  ■ *Become elongated, tortuous, and dilated*
■ Bladder alterations
  ■ *Bladder capacity increases and bladder tone decreases related to progesterone effect on smooth muscle of the bladder causing relaxation and stretching.*
■ Urinary stasis
  ■ *Progesterone reduces the tone of renal structures, allowing for pooling of urine.*
  ■ *Stasis promotes bacterial growth and increases the woman's risk for urinary tract infections and pyelonephritis.*
■ Hyperemia of bladder and urethra related to increased vascularity that results in pelvic congestion; edematous mucus is easily traumatized.
■ Most women experience urinary symptoms of frequency, urgency, and nocturia beginning early in pregnancy and continuing to varying degrees throughout the pregnancy. These symptoms are primarily a result of the systemic hormonal changes of pregnancy and may also be attributed to anatomical changes in the renal system and other body system changes during pregnancy, but are not generally indicative of infection.

Gastrointestinal System

The gastrointestinal (GI) system adapts in its anatomy and physiology during pregnancy in support of maternal and fetal nutritional requirements (see Table 4-2). The adaptations are related to hormonal influences as well as the impact of the enlarging uterus on the GI system as pregnancy progresses.
Alterations in nutritional patterns commonly seen in pregnancy include:

■ Some degree of nausea and vomiting in early pregnancy
■ Increase in appetite and intake, cravings for specific foods, avoidance of specific foods

Anatomical and physiological changes include:

■ Uterine enlargement displaces the stomach, liver, and intestines as the pregnancy progresses.
■ By the end of pregnancy, the appendix is situated high and to the right along the costal margin.

■ The GI tract experiences a general relaxation and slowing of its digestive processes during pregnancy, contributing to many of the common discomforts of pregnancy such as heartburn and constipation.
■ Gallstones: Progesterone-induced relaxation of smooth muscle results in distention of gallbladder and slows emptying of bile; bile stasis and elevated levels of cholesterol contribute to formation of gallstones.
■ Pruritus: Abdominal pruritus may be an early sign of cholestasis.
■ Ptyalism: Increase in saliva
■ Bleeding gums and periodontal disease
  ■ *Increased vascularity of the gums can result in gingivitis.*

Musculoskeletal System

Significant adaptation occurs in the musculoskeletal system as a result of pregnancy (see Table 4-2). Hormonal shifts are responsible for many of these changes. Mechanical factors attributable to the growing uterus also contribute to musculoskeletal adaptation.
Anatomical and physiological changes include:

■ Altered posture and center of gravity related to distention of the abdomen by the expanding uterus and reduced abdominal tone that shifts the center of gravity forward.
  ■ *A shift in the center of gravity places the woman at higher risk for falls.*
■ Altered gait ("pregnant waddle"): Hormonal influences of progesterone and relaxin soften joints and increase joint mobility.
■ **Lordosis:** Abnormal anterior curvature of the lumbar spine. The body compensates for the shift in center of gravity by developing an increased curvature of the spine.
■ Joint discomfort: Hormonal influences of progesterone and relaxin soften cartilage and connective tissue, leading to joint instability.
■ Round ligament spasm: Estrogen and relaxin increase elasticity and relaxation of ligaments and abdominal distention stretches round ligaments causing spasm and pain.
■ **Diastasis recti:** This is the separation of the rectus abdominis muscle in the midline caused by the abdominal distention. It is a benign condition that can occur in the third trimester.
■ The impact of all of the musculoskeletal adaptations in pregnancy resulting in numerous common discomforts of pregnancy can sometimes be reduced if the woman maintains a normal body weight and exercises regularly prior to and throughout her pregnancy.

Integumentary System

The integumentary system includes the skin and related structures such as hair, nails, and glands. Hormonal influences are primary factors in integumentary system adaptations during pregnancy, with mechanical factors associated with the enlarging uterus playing a lesser role in changes associated with this body system (see Table 4-2).
Anatomical and physiological changes include:

■ Hyperpigmentation: Estrogen and progesterone stimulate increased melanin deposition of light brown to dark brown pigmentation.
  ■ *Linea nigra: Darkened line in midline of abdomen (Fig. 4-7)*
  ■ *Melasma (chloasma), also referred to as mask of pregnancy, is a brownish pigmentation of the skin over the cheeks, nose, and*

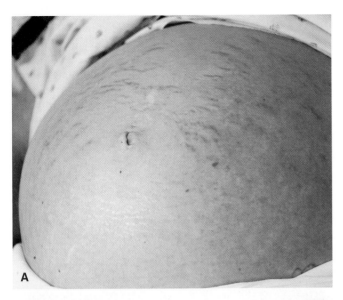

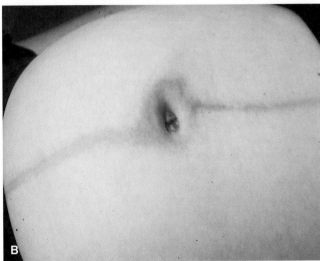

Figure 4-7   Pregnant abdomen with striae (*A*) and linea nigra (*B*).

forehead. This occurs in 50% of 70% of pregnant women and is more common in darker skinned woman. It usually occurs after the 16th week of pregnancy.
- **Striae** (stretch marks): Stretching of skin due to growth of breast, hips, abdomen, and buttock plus the effects of estrogen, relaxin, and adrenocorticoids may result in tearing of subcutaneous connective tissue/collagen (see Fig. 4-7).
- Varicosities, spider nevi, and palmer erythema: Vascular changes related to hormonally induced increased elasticity of vessels and increased venous pressure from enlarged uterus.
- Hot flashes and facial flushing: Caused by increased blood supply to skin, increase in basal metabolic rate, progesterone-induced increased body temperature, and vasomotor instability.
- Oily skin and acne: Effects of increase in androgens.
- Sweating: Thermoregulation process at the level of skin increased in response to increases in thyroid activity, basal metabolic rate (BMR), metabolic activity of fetus, and increase maternal body weight.

- Although none of these integumentary system adaptations is seen universally, each alteration is seen commonly, is not of pathological significance, and typically resolves or regresses significantly after pregnancy.

Endocrine System

Endocrine system adaptations are essential for maintaining the stability of both the woman and her pregnancy and for promoting fetal growth and development. Endocrine glands mediate the many metabolic process adaptations in pregnancy. There are general endocrine system alterations as a result of pregnancy as well as pregnancy-specific endocrine adaptations related to the placenta that develop once conception has occurred (see Table 4-2).

General Physiological Changes

Significant alterations in pituitary, adrenal, thyroid, parathyroid, and pancreatic functioning occur in pregnancy. For example, the hormonal production activity and size of the thyroid gland increase during pregnancy in support of maternal and fetal physiological needs and there is an increase in pancreatic activity during pregnancy to meet both maternal and fetal needs related to carbohydrate metabolism.

Pregnancy-Specific Hormones

The hormones of pregnancy are responsible for most of the physiological adaptations and physical changes seen throughout the entire pregnancy. The placental hormones are initially produced by the corpus luteum of pregnancy. Once implantation occurs, the fertilized ovum and chorionic villi produce hCG.

- The function of the high hCG level in early pregnancy is to maintain the corpus luteum and its production of progesterone and, to a lesser extent, estrogen until the placenta develops and takes over this function.
- After the development of a functioning placenta, the placenta produces most of the hormones of pregnancy including estrogen, progesterone, human placental lactogen (hPL), and relaxin.
- Each of these hormones plays a role in the physiology of pregnancy, resulting in specific alterations in nearly all body systems, as described in this chapter, to support maternal physiological needs, maintenance and progression of the pregnancy, and fetal growth and development (see Table 4-2).

Immune System

Every aspect of the body's very complicated immune system undergoes adaptation during pregnancy in order to maintain a tenuous balance between preservation of maternal–fetal well-being through normal immune responses on the one hand, and the necessary alterations of the maternal immune system required for maintenance of the pregnancy on the other. This adaptive process involves the maternal immune system becoming tolerant of the "foreign" fetal system so that the fetus is not rejected, and further, so that the fetus is protected from infection. Immune function changes in pregnancy are far-reaching and beyond the scope of this chapter. This is also a relatively new body of science that is not fully understood.

ANTEPARTAL NURSING CARE: PHYSIOLOGY-BASED NURSING ASSESSMENT AND NURSING ACTIONS

Prenatal Assessment

The **prenatal period** is the entire time period during which a woman is pregnant through the birth of the baby. It is a time of transition in the life of a family as they prepare for the birth of a child. This time period affords an opportunity for positive change in all aspects of health and health maintenance behaviors. During ongoing interactions, the nurse places emphasis on health education and health promotion involving the woman in her care. The holistic view of health inherent in nursing care for the childbearing woman and her family contribute to a unique situation in which the antepartal patient has ready access to health information, support, and guidance to help her achieve the healthiest possible pregnancy. The impact of this **prenatal care** (health care related to pregnancy) and the possibility for positive change it engenders can extend well beyond the antepartal period into the life of the new family. Prenatal nursing care and interventions also contribute to the woman's and family's ability to make informed choices about the health care of the entire family throughout the childbearing cycle, choices based on an integration of information provided by the nurse with the family's personal values, preferences, and beliefs. **Family-centered maternity care** is a model of obstetrical care based on a view of pregnancy and childbirth as a normal life event, a life transition that is not primarily medical but rather developmental.

■ The initial prenatal visit parallels a preconception health care visit (see Table 4-1). It also includes information about the health and health history of the father of the baby (age, blood type and Rh status, current health status and history of any chronic or past medical problems, genetic history, occupation, lifestyle factors impacting health, and his involvement in the woman's life and with her pregnancy).

■ The focus of patient education and anticipatory guidance shifts toward pregnancy-related health concerns, but the basic components of the visit as well as the emphasis on health maintenance and health promotion remain the same. Prenatal visits also include specific assessment of the pregnancy and fetal status. Some of these components are uniform across all prenatal visits and others are specific to one or more trimesters of the pregnancy.

■ Subsequent prenatal visits are more abbreviated than the initial visit, with nursing care and interventions focused on current pregnancy status and patient needs, always with an emphasis on patient education and anticipatory guidance (Table 4-3).

■ The standard accepted frequency of prenatal care visits in a low-risk population in the United States results in approximately 14 to 16 prenatal visits per pregnancy. However, available evidence suggests that a schedule with reduced frequency of prenatal visits for this population is not associated with an increase in adverse maternal or perinatal outcomes and may be associated with increased levels of patient satisfaction. In spite of this evidence, the routine remains unchanged for the present (Villar, Carrolli, Khan-Neelofer, Piaggio, & Gulmezoglo, 2007; Walker, McCully, & Vest, 2001).

■ The efficacy of the current model for individual prenatal care visits has been questioned as well (Evidence-Based Practice: Centering Pregnancy).

Evidence-Based Practice: Centering Pregnancy

The generally accepted model of individual prenatal care currently in use in the United States lacks a scientific basis; there is also some question as to its effectiveness in meeting public health objectives in care provision to a healthy population (Walker & Rising, 2004). An innovative group model of prenatal care delivery, Centering Pregnancy, is designed to promote individual responsibility for health in pregnancy; provide appropriate prenatal assessment and risk screening; and provide education, social support, and a sense of community, all in a cost-effective and efficient manner. The existing, preliminary evidence for Centering Pregnancy supports it as a viable model for delivery of care for a low-risk population, although more research is needed. In the pilot study, perinatal outcomes were comparable to the traditional care control group and women reported satisfaction with their care, with 96% of the Centering Pregnancy participants preferring this alternative model to a traditional model of prenatal care (Rising, 1998). Subsequent research has shown positive benefits including higher birth weights in a low socioeconomic status population (Ickovics et al., 2003); fewer missed prenatal appointments, preterm births, and low birth weight babies, and increased rates of breastfeeding in an adolescent population (Grady & Bloom, 2004); and increased knowledge about pregnancy in the Centering Pregnancy group compared to the traditional care group (Baldwin, 2006).

Rising developed the Centering Pregnancy program as a pilot project. The program begins with an initial comprehensive prenatal visit in the traditional format. Subsequent visits are group-based with between 8 and 12 other women of similar gestational age. A reduced number of prenatal visits are scheduled between the initial visit and the postpartum follow-up compared with traditional care. Facilitation of the sessions is consistent and led by a professional skilled in group process, typically a nurse-midwife. Partners and support people are included in the group. The women are participatory in their care—obtaining their weight and blood pressure, testing their urine, and documenting results in their charts. Each session includes a brief individual assessment on the periphery of the group space for each woman, allowing for assessment of the pregnancy and discussion of individual progress and/or concerns. There are two discussion and education segments to each session, including topics related to health maintenance and promotion, pregnancy, childbirth, and parenting (Rising, 1998).

Advantages of the Centering Pregnancy model of care include: focus on the normalcy of pregnancy, increased time with the care provider during the pregnancy, a perceived benefit for both the care provider and the pregnant woman; efficiency for the care provider in providing important prenatal education content; development of social connections between group members; social support for participants in managing the normal challenges of pregnancy; and validation of the woman's experience of pregnancy by a peer group. Studies are ongoing and more research is needed to evaluate the benefit of Centering Pregnancy as a safe, effective, and satisfying model of health care delivery for a low-risk prenatal population.

(Baldwin, 2006; Grady & Bloom, 2004; Ickovics et al., 2003; Rising, 1998; Walker & Rising, 2004)

TABLE 4–3 PRENATAL CARE: CONTENT AND TIMING OF ROUTINE PRENATAL VISITS

	HISTORY AND PHYSICAL ASSESSMENT	LABORATORY/DIAGNOSTIC STUDIES IN NORMAL PREGNANCY (RECOMMENDED TIMING)
First Trimester		

Initial visit	Comprehensive health and risk assessment (see Table 4-1)
	Current pregnancy history
	Complete physical and pelvic examination
	Determine EDD
	Nutrition assessment including 24-hour diet recall
	Psychosocial assessment (see Chapter 5)
	Assessment for intimate partner violence
		Blood type and Rh factor
		Antibody screen
		Complete blood count (CBC) including:
		  Hemoglobin
		  Hematocrit
		  White blood cell count (WBC)
		  Platelet count
		  RPR, VDRL (syphilis serology)
		  HIV screen and hepatitis B screen
		  (surface antigen)
		Genetic screening based on
		  family history, racial/ethnic
		  background (e.g., sickle cell
		  disease, Tay-Sachs)
		Rubella titer
		PPD (tuberculosis screen)
		Urinalysis
		Urine culture and sensitivity
		Pap smear
		Gonorrhea and *Chlamydia* cultures
		Ultrasound

Return visit (4 weeks after initial visit)	Chart review Interval history Focused physical assessment: Vital signs, urine, weight, fundal height Clinical pelvimetry	
Second Trimester		
Return visits (Every 4 weeks)	Chart review Interval history Focused physical assessment: Vital signs, urine dipstick for glucose, albumin, ketones, weight, fundal height, FHR, fetal movement, Leopold maneuver, edema Pelvic exam or sterile vaginal examination if indicated Confirm established due date.	Triple screen or quad screen Ultrasound Screening for gestational diabetes Hemoglobin and hematocrit Antibody screen Administration of RhoGAM if Rh-negative with a negative antibody screen
Third Trimester		
RETURN VISITS (Every 2 weeks until 36 weeks, then weekly until 40 weeks; typically twice weekly after 40 weeks)	Chart review Interval history Focused physical assessment: Vital signs, urine dipstick for glucose, albumin, ketones, weight, fundal height, FHR, fetal movement, Leopold maneuver, edema Pelvic exam or sterile vaginal examination if indicated Nutrition follow up	Group B *Streptococcus* screening: ■ Culture at 35–37 weeks of gestation ■ A quarter to a third of all women are colonized with Group B *Streptococcus* bacteria (GBS) in the lower GI or urogenital tract (typically asymptomatic) ■ Vaginal and rectal swabs to determine presence of GBS bacterial colonization before the onset of labor in order to anticipate treatment during labor for a positive culture as recommended by the CDC (2002)

Continued

	HISTORY AND PHYSICAL ASSESSMENT	LABORATORY/DIAGNOSTIC STUDIES IN NORMAL PREGNANCY (RECOMMENDED TIMING)
TABLE 4–3 PRENATAL CARE: CONTENT AND TIMING OF ROUTINE PRENATAL VISITS—CON'TD		
Third Trimester		
		■ GBS infection in a newborn, either early-onset (first week of life) or late onset (after first week of life), can be invasive and severe, with potential long-term neurological sequelae
		■ Treatment with IV antibiotics in labor recommended for positive screening results; unknown screening results; risk factors of PTL, prolonged rupture of membranes, or maternal temperature over 100.4°F (38°C); history of infant with invasive GBS disease (no screening needed); and history of GBS in urine (no screening needed)
		■ Treatment not indicated for planned cesarean birth without labor or rupture of membranes, regardless of screening results (CDC, 2002)
		Additional screening testing:
		■ CBC
		■ Repeat GC, *Chlamydia*, RPR, HIV, HbSAg (if indicated), antibody screen if Rh negative
		■ 1-hour glucose challenge test 24–28 weeks

Goals of Prenatal Care

■ Maintenance of maternal fetal health
■ Accurate determination of gestational age
■ Ongoing assessment of risk status and implementation of risk-appropriate intervention
■ Build rapport with the childbearing family
■ Referrals to appropriate resources

Nursing Actions

■ Provide for comfort and privacy.
■ Use therapeutic communication techniques during the interview and conversation.
■ Demonstrate sensitivity toward the patient related to the personal nature of the interview and conversation.
■ Obtain the woman's identifying information (initial prenatal visit).
■ Obtain a complete health history (initial prenatal visit) or an interval history (subsequent visits) (see Tables 4-1 and 4-3).
■ Conduct a Review of Systems (initial prenatal visit).
■ Obtain blood pressure, temperature, pulse, respirations, height (initial prenatal visit), weight, and body mass index (BMI; initial prenatal visit).
■ Assess urine specimen for protein, glucose, and ketones.

■ Assess for absence or presence of edema.
■ Provide anticipatory guidance for the patient before and during the physical examination (initial prenatal visit and subsequent visits when indicated).
■ Assist with physical and pelvic examination as needed (initial prenatal visit and subsequent visits when indicated).
■ Assist with obtaining specimens for laboratory or diagnostic studies as ordered (initial prenatal visit and subsequent visits when indicated).
■ Provide teaching about procedures as needed (initial prenatal visit and subsequent visits when indicated).
■ Provide anticipatory guidance related to the plan of care and appropriate follow-up, including how and when to contact care provider with warning signs or symptoms (see Critical Component Boxes).
■ Provide teaching appropriate for the woman, her family, and her gestational age.
■ Assess the woman's understanding of the teaching provided.
■ Allow time for the woman to ask questions.
■ Document, according to agency protocol, all findings, interventions, and education provided.
■ Assess for intimate partner violence (Critical Component: Intimate Partner Violence).

CRITICAL COMPONENT

Intimate Partner Violence (Abuse)

Intimate partner violence (IPV) against women consists of actual or threatened physical or sexual violence and psychological and emotional abuse. IVP crosses all ethnic, racial, religious, ethnic, and socioeconomic levels. Pregnancy does not protect women from abuse. Homicide is the most likely cause of death in pregnant or recently pregnant women, and a significant portion of those homicides are committed by their intimate partners (Association of Women's Health, Obstetrics and Neonatal Nursing [AWHONN], 2007). Based on the Abuse Assessment Screen, 16% or one in six pregnant women reported physical or sexual abuse during pregnancy (McFarlane, Parker, & Moran, 2007) seriously impacting maternal and fetal health and infant birth weight. Men who abuse pregnant women jeopardize the safety of the woman and infant. Pregnancy is often the only time a woman may come into frequent contact with a health provider. Research has documented that three simple screening tools can reliably identify abused women. Those questions are:

Within the last year have you been hit, slapped, kicked, or otherwise physically hurt by someone?

Since you have been pregnant have you been hit, slapped, kicked, or otherwise physically hurt by someone?

Within the last year, has anyone forced you to have sexual activities?

Assessment for abuse during pregnancy with education, advocacy, and referral to community resources should be standard for all pregnancy women. AWHONN advocates for universal screening for domestic violence for all pregnant women and recommends the ABC's of patient care to guide nurses caring for victims of abuse (AWHONN, 2007).

Learn and practice the ABCs of Patient Care:

A: Alone. Reassure the woman that she is not alone, that there have been others in her position before, and that help is available.

B: Belief. Articulate your belief in the victim—that you know the abuse is not her fault and that no one deserves to be hurt or mistreated.

C: Confidentiality. Ensure the confidentiality of the information that is being provided and explain the implication of mandatory reporting laws, where applicable.

D: Documentation. Descriptive documentation with photographs, taken with the woman's permission, and a verbatim account from the patient's perspective is helpful to accurately capture and record the nature and extent of injuries.

E: Education. Education about community resources can be life-saving. Know where you can refer a woman for help and have information about local shelters readily available. Also ask if she know how to obtain a restraining order.

S: Safety. One of the most dangerous times for women is the point at which they decide to leave. Tell the woman to call 911 if she is in imminent danger, and to consider alerting neighbors to call the police if they hear and/or see signs of conflict.

(AWHONN, 2007; Campbell & Furniss, 2002; McFarlane, Parker, & Moran, 2007)

Prenatal Assessment Terminology

A set of terms is used to describe obstetrical history and to define a woman's obstetrical status. An important shorthand system for explaining a woman's obstetrical history uses the terms *gravida* and *para* in describing numbers of pregnancies and births.

■ **G/P** is a two-digit system to denote pregnancy and births

■ **Gravida** refers to the number of times a woman has been pregnant. This is without reference to how many fetuses there were with each pregnancy or when the pregnancy ended. It is simply how many times a woman has been pregnant, including a current pregnancy.

■ **Para** refers to any birth that occurred after 20 weeks' gestation, regardless of whether or not the baby was born alive and also without reference to number of fetuses. A pregnancy that ends before the end of 20 weeks' gestation is considered an abortion, whether it is spontaneous (miscarriage) or induced (elective or therapeutic).

■ **GTPAL** is a more comprehensive system for notation of obstetrical history. This system goes further and designates numbers of term infants, preterm infants, abortions, and living children using the acronym **TPAL** as follows: **T** = number of *term* infants born (after 37 weeks' gestation), **P** = number of *preterm* infants born (between 20 weeks' gestation and 37 weeks' gestation), **A** = number of pregnancies ending before 20 weeks' gestation, either spontaneous or induced (*abortion*), and **L** = the number of children currently *living*.

■ **Nulligravida** is a woman who has never been pregnant or given birth.

■ **Primigravida** is a woman who has been pregnant for the first time.

■ **Multigravida** is someone who is pregnant for at least the second time.

In a clinical setting, these terms are sometimes used incorrectly by convention. For example, a woman who is pregnant with her first baby is frequently referred to as a "primip" meaning primipara when she has, in fact, not given birth yet.

First Trimester

It is best to begin prenatal care in the first trimester. Current reports from the National Center for Health Statistics indicate that 84% of women receive prenatal care in the first trimester; however, almost 4% of women receive late or no prenatal care (Martin, Hamilton, Menacker, Sutton, & Mathews, 2007). The proportion of women beginning prenatal care in the first trimester has risen 11% since 1990 and the percentage of women receiving late or no prenatal care has declined 6% (Martin et al., 2007).

Components of Initial Prenatal Assessment (see Table 4-3)

■ History of current pregnancy:
  ■ *First day of last normal menstrual period (LNMP) and degree of certainty about the date*
  ■ *Regularity, frequency, and length of menstrual cycles*
  ■ *Recent use or cessation of contraception*
  ■ *Woman's knowledge of conception date*
  ■ *Signs and symptoms of pregnancy*
  ■ *Whether the pregnancy was intended*
  ■ *The woman's response to being pregnant*
■ Obstetrical history, detail about all previous pregnancies:
  ■ *TPAL*
  ■ *Whether abortions, if any, were spontaneous or induced*
  ■ *Dates of pregnancies*
  ■ *Length of gestation*
  ■ *Type of birth experiences (e.g., induced or spontaneous labors, vaginal or cesarean births, use of forceps or vacuum-assist, type of pain management)*
  ■ *Complications with pregnancy, or labor and birth*
  ■ *Neonatal outcomes including Apgar scores, birth weight, neonatal complications, feeding method, health and development since birth*

Complications with Pregnancy or Labor and Birth

Neonatal outcomes including Apgar scores, birth weight, neonatal complications, feeding method, health and development since birth

- Physical and pelvic examinations:
  - *The bimanual component of the pelvic examination enables the examiner to palpate internally the dimensions of the enlarging uterus. This information assists with dating the pregnancy, either confirming an LMP-based EDD or providing information in the absence of a certain LMP. In the absence of a certain LMP or with conflicting data about gestational age, a decision may be made to perform an ultrasound examination of the pregnancy in order to determine an EDD. It is important to determine an accurate EDD as early as possible in a pregnancy because numerous decisions related to timing of interventions and management of pregnancy are based on gestational age as determined by the EDD.*
  - *Clinical pelvimetry (measurement of the dimensions of the bony pelvis through palpation during an internal pelvic examination) may be performed during the initial pelvic examination. Its purpose is to identify any variations in pelvic structure that might inhibit or preclude a fetus passing through the bony pelvis during a vaginal birth.*
- Assessment of uterine growth:
  - *Uterine growth after 10 to 12 weeks' gestation is assessed by measuring the height of the fundus with the use of a centimeter measuring tape. The zero point of the tape is placed on the symphysis pubis and the tape is then extended to the top of the fundus. The measurement should approximately equal the number of weeks pregnant. Instruct the woman to empty her bladder before the measurement because a full bladder can displace the uterus.*
  - *Maternal position and examiner uniformity are variables that render this evaluation somewhat imprecise, but it is useful as a gross measure of progressive fetal growth as well as to help identify a pregnancy that is growing outside the optimal or normal range, either too large or too small for its gestational age. This serves as a screening tool for fetal growth.*
- Assessment of fetal heart tones:
  - *Fetal heart tones are auscultated with an ultrasound Doppler in the first trimester, usually between about 10 and 12 weeks' gestation. The normal fetal heart rate (FHR) baseline is between 110 bpm up to 160 bpm.*
- Comprehensive laboratory and diagnostic studies:
  - *Laboratory studies are ordered or obtained at the initial prenatal visit to establish baseline values for follow-up and comparison as the pregnancy progresses (see Table 4–3).*
  - *Ultrasound might be performed to confirm intrauterine pregnancy, viability, and gestational age.*

Patient Education and Anticipatory Guidance

- General information about physical changes (see Table 4-2)
- General information about fetal development: By the end of the first trimester the fetus is 3 inches in length, weighs 1 to 2 ounces, all organ systems are present, the head is large, and the heartbeat is audible with Doppler.
- Warning/danger signs that need to be reported to the care provider (Critical Component: Warning/Danger Signs of the First Trimester)
- General health maintenance/health promotion information:
  - *Avoid exposure to tobacco, alcohol, recreational drugs.*
  - *Avoid exposure to environment hazards with teratogenic effects.*
  - *Obtain input from the care provider before using medications, complementary and alternative medicine (CAM), and nutritional supplements.*
  - *Use safety behaviors (e.g., seat belt, sunscreen).*
  - *Recognize the need for additional rest.*
  - *Maintain daily hygiene.*
  - *Decrease the risk for urinary tract infections (UTI) and vaginal infections by wiping from front to back, wearing cotton underwear, maintaining adequate hydration, voiding after intercourse, and not douching.*
  - *Maintain good oral hygiene: Gentle brushing of teeth and floss; continue routine preventative dental care.*
  - *Exercise 30 minutes each day: Avoid risk for trauma to abdomen, avoid overheating, and maintain adequate hydration while exercising.*
  - *Establish daily Kegel exercises routine to maintain pelvic floor muscle strength and decrease risk of urinary incontinence and uterine prolapse.*
  - *Travel is safe in low-risk pregnancy: Need to stop more frequently to stretch and walk to decrease risk of thrombophlebitis; take prenatal record.*
  - *Use coping strategies for stress such as relaxation and meditation.*
  - *Communicate with partner regarding changes in sexual responses: Sexual responses/desires change throughout pregnancy. Couples need to talk openly about these changes and explore different sexual positions that accommodate the changes of pregnancy.*
    - Relief measures for normal discomforts in early pregnancy are discussed based on patient need (Table 4-4).

CRITICAL COMPONENT

Warning/Danger Signs of the First Trimester

- Abdominal cramping or pain: Possible threatened abortion, UTI, appendicitis
- Vaginal spotting or bleeding: Possible threatened abortion
- Absence of fetal heart tone: Possible missed abortion
- Dysuria, frequency, urgency: Possible UTI
- Fever, chills: Infection
- Prolonged nausea and vomiting: Hyperemesis gravidarum; increased risk of dehydration

---

Nutritional Assessment and Education

- Obtain a 24-hour diet recall.
- Encourage the woman to eat a variety of unprocessed foods from all food groups including lean protein sources, fresh fruits, whole grains, and "good" fats (Table 4-5 and Fig. 4-8).
- Encourage the woman to drink 8 to 10 glasses of fluid per day.
- Both excessive and inadequate weight gain in pregnancy are associated with poor perinatal outcomes.
- Recommend weight gain of less than 5 pounds during the first trimester (see Boxes 4-1 and 4-2 for weight gain recommendations and USDA MyPyramid food guidelines).

During the initial prenatal visit, the woman learns the frequency of follow-up visits and what to expect from her prenatal visits as the pregnancy progresses (see Table 4-3). If the patient is seen for her initial prenatal visit early in the first trimester, she may have more than one visit during that trimester. Subsequent visits are similar to those described for the second trimester. If the woman presents late for prenatal care and is in her second or third trimester at her initial prenatal visit, the nurse may need to modify typical patient education content to meet the current needs of the patient and her family.

At every prenatal care encounter, it is imperative that the nurse provides a relaxed environment for the woman and her family, one in which the childbearing family feels comfortable asking questions and sharing personal details about their lives related to the health of the woman, her fetus, and the developing family.

TABLE 4–4   SELF-CARE/RELIEF MEASURES FOR PHYSICAL CHANGES AND COMMON DISCOMFORTS OF PREGNANCY

BODY SYSTEM	PHYSICAL CHANGES AND COMMON DISCOMFORTS OF PREGNANCY (COMMON TIMING)	NURSING ACTIONS FOR PATIENT EDUCATION FOR SELF-CARE AND RELIEF MEASURES
GENERALIZED OR MULTISYSTEM	Fatigue (first and third trimesters)	Reassure the woman of the normalcy of her response. Encourage the woman to plan for extra rest during the day and at night; focus on "work" of growing a healthy baby. Enlist support and assistance from friends and family. Encourage the woman to eat an optimal diet with adequate caloric intake and iron-rich foods and iron supplementation if anemic
	Insomnia (throughout pregnancy)	Instruct the woman to implement sleep hygiene measures (regular bedtime, relaxing or low-key activities pre-bedtime). Encourage the woman to create a comfortable sleep environment (body pillow, additional pillows). Teach breathing exercises and relaxation techniques/measures [progressive relaxation, effleurage (a massage technique using a very light touch of the fingers in two repetitive circular patterns over the gravid abdomen), warm bath or warm beverage pre-bedtime] Evaluate caffeine use.
	Emotional lability (throughout pregnancy)	Reassure the woman of the normalcy of response. Encourage adequate rest and optimal nutrition. Encourage communication with partner/significant support people. Refer to pregnancy support group.
REPRODUCTIVE Breasts	Tenderness, enlargement, upper back pain (throughout pregnancy; tenderness mostly in the first trimester)	Encourage the woman to wear a well-fitting, supportive bra. Instruct woman in correct use of good body mechanics.
Uterus	Braxton-Hicks contractions (mid-pregnancy onward)	Reassure the woman that occasional contractions are normal. Instruct the woman to call her provider if contractions become regular and persist before 37 weeks. Ensure adequate fluid intake. Recommend a maternity girdle for uterus support.
Cervix/vagina	Increased secretions Yeast infections (throughout pregnancy)	Encourage daily bathing. Recommend cotton underwear. Recommend wearing panty liner, changing pad frequently. Instruct the woman to avoid douching using feminine hygiene sprays.
	Dyspareunia (throughout pregnancy)	Reassure the woman/couple of normalcy of response, provide information. Suggest alternative positions for sexual intercourse and alternative sexual activity to sexual intercourse.
CARDIOVASCULAR	Supine hypotension (mid-pregnancy onward)	Instruct the woman to avoid supine position from mid-pregnancy onward
	Anemia (throughout pregnancy; more common in late second trimester)	Encourage the woman to include iron-rich foods in daily dietary intake and take iron supplementation

Continued

TABLE 4–4   SELF-CARE/RELIEF MEASURES FOR PHYSICAL CHANGES AND COMMON DISCOMFORTS OF PREGNANCY—CONT'D

BODY SYSTEM	PHYSICAL CHANGES AND COMMON DISCOMFORTS OF PREGNANCY (COMMON TIMING)	NURSING ACTIONS FOR PATIENT EDUCATION FOR SELF-CARE AND RELIEF MEASURES
	Dependent edema (lower extremities and/or vulva) (late pregnancy)	Instruct the woman to: ■ Wear loose clothing ■ Use a maternity girdle (abdominal support), which may help reduce venous pressure in pelvis/lower extremities and enhance circulation ■ Avoid prolonged standing or sitting; dorsiflex feet periodically when standing or sitting ■ Elevate legs when sitting ■ Position on side when lying down
	Varicosities (later pregnancy)	Instruct woman in all measures for dependent edema (see above) Suggest the woman wear support hose (put on before rising in the morning, before legs have been in dependent position) Instruct the woman to lie on her back with legs propped against a wall in an approximately 45-degree angle to spine periodically throughout the day Instruct the woman to avoid crossing legs when sitting.
RESPIRATORY	Hyperventilation and dyspnea (throughout pregnancy; may worsen in later pregnancy)	Reassure the woman of the normalcy of her response and provide information. Instruct the woman to slow down respiration rate and depth when hyperventilating Encourage good posture. Instruct the woman to stand and stretch, taking a deep breath, periodically throughout the day; stretch and take a deep breath periodically throughout the night. Suggest sleeping semi-sitting with additional pillows for support.
	Nasal and sinus congestion/ Epistaxis (throughout pregnancy)	Suggest the woman try a cool-air humidifier. Instruct the woman to avoid use of decongestants and nasal sprays and instead to use normal saline drops.
RENAL	Frequency and urgency/nocturia (may be throughout pregnancy; most common in first and third trimesters)	Reassure the woman of normalcy of response. Encourage the woman to empty her bladder frequently. Stress the importance of maintaining adequate hydration, reducing fluid intake only near bedtime. Encourage Kegel exercises; wear perineal pad if needed.
GASTROINTESTINAL	Nausea and/or vomiting (first trimester and sometimes into the second trimester)	Reassure the woman of normalcy and self-limiting nature of response. Suggest eating small, frequent meals. Avoid strong odors and causative factors (e.g., spicy foods, greasy foods, large meals). Encourage women to experiment with alleviating factors (e.g., crackers or dry toast before rising or whenever nauseous, avoiding fluid intake with meals, sweet beverages, carbonated beverages). Suggest vitamin B6, 25 mg by mouth three times daily or ginger, 350 mg by mouth three times daily (Smith, Crowther, Willson, Hotham, & McMillian, 2004).
	Bleeding gums (throughout pregnancy)	Encourage the woman to maintain good oral hygiene (brush gently with soft toothbrush, daily flossing). Maintain optimal nutrition.

TABLE 4–4   SELF-CARE/RELIEF MEASURES FOR PHYSICAL CHANGES AND COMMON DISCOMFORTS OF PREGNANCY—CONT'D

BODY SYSTEM	PHYSICAL CHANGES AND COMMON DISCOMFORTS OF PREGNANCY (COMMON TIMING)	NURSING ACTIONS FOR PATIENT EDUCATION FOR SELF-CARE AND RELIEF MEASURES
	Increase or sense of increase in salivation (mostly first trimester if associated with nausea)	Suggest use of gum or hard candy or use astringent mouth wash.
	Flatulence (throughout pregnancy)	Encourage the woman to: ■ Maintain regular bowel habits ■ Engage in regular exercise ■ Avoid gas-producing foods ■ Chew food slowly and thoroughly ■ Use the knee–chest position during periods of discomfort
	Heartburn (later pregnancy)	Suggest ■ Small, frequent meals ■ Maintain good posture ■ Maintain adequate fluid intake, but avoid fluid intake with meals ■ Avoid fatty or fried foods ■ Remain upright for 30–45 minutes after eating
	Constipation (throughout pregnancy) (see Concept Map)	Encourage the woman to ■ Maintain adequate fluid intake ■ Engage in regular exercise ■ Increase fiber in diet ■ Maintain regular bowel habits ■ Maintain good posture and body mechanics
	Hemorrhoids (later pregnancy)	Avoid constipation (see above) Instruct the woman to avoid bearing down with bowel movements Instruct the woman in comfort measures (e.g., ice packs, warm baths or sitz baths, witch hazel compresses) Elevate the hips and lower extremities during rest periods throughout the day. Gently reinsert into the rectum while doing Kegel exercises.
	Severe pruritus (itching) (later pregnancy)	Suggestions for maintaining skin comfort (e.g., lotions, oatmeal baths, non-binding clothing)
MUSCULOSKELETAL	Low back pain/joint discomfort/difficulty walking (later pregnancy)	Instruct the woman to: ■ Utilize proper body mechanics (e.g., stoop using knees vs. bend for lifting) ■ Maintain good posture ■ Do pelvic rock/pelvic tilt exercises ■ Wear supportive shoes with low heels ■ Apply warmth or ice to painful area ■ Use of maternity girdle ■ Use massage ■ Use relaxation techniques ■ Sleep on a firm mattress with pillows for additional support of extremities, abdomen, and back

Continued

	PHYSICAL CHANGES AND COMMON	
BODY SYSTEM	DISCOMFORTS OF PREGNANCY (COMMON TIMING)	NURSING ACTIONS FOR PATIENT EDUCATION FOR SELF-CARE AND RELIEF MEASURES

TABLE 4–4   SELF-CARE/RELIEF MEASURES FOR PHYSICAL CHANGES AND COMMON DISCOMFORTS OF PREGNANCY—CONT'D

BODY SYSTEM	PHYSICAL CHANGES AND COMMON DISCOMFORTS OF PREGNANCY (COMMON TIMING)	NURSING ACTIONS FOR PATIENT EDUCATION FOR SELF-CARE AND RELIEF MEASURES
	Diastasis recti (later pregnancy)	Instruct the woman to do gentle abdominal strengthening exercises (e.g., tiny abdominal crunches, may cross arms over abdomen to opposite sides for splinting, no sit-ups). Teach proper technique for sitting up from lying down (i.e., roll to side, lift torso up using arms until in sitting position)
	Round ligament spasm (pain) (late second and third trimester)	Instruct the woman to: ■ Lie on side and flex knees up to abdomen ■ Bend toward pain ■ Do pelvic tilt/pelvic rock exercises ■ Use warm baths or compresses ■ Use side-lying in exaggerated Sim's position with pillows for additional support of abdomen and in between legs ■ Use of a maternity belt
	Leg cramps (throughout pregnancy)	Instruct the woman to: ■ Dorsiflex foot to stretch calf muscle ■ Warm baths or compresses to the affected area ■ Change position slowly ■ Massage the affected area ■ Regular exercise and muscle conditioning
INTEGUMENTARY	Striae (stretch marks) (later pregnancy)	Reassure the woman that there is no method to prevent them. Suggest maintaining skin comfort (e.g., lotions, oatmeal baths, non-binding clothing). Good weight control
	Hot flushes, hot and cold sensations (throughout pregnancy)	Suggest that the woman: ■ Dress in layers ■ Wear loose clothing ■ Maintain adequate fluid intake

Second Trimester

Subsequent or return prenatal visits begin with a chart review from the previous visit(s) and an interval history. This history includes information about the pregnancy since the previous prenatal visit (see Table 4-3).

Components of Second-Trimester Prenatal Assessments

- Focused physical assessment
- Vital signs
  - *Vital signs within normal limits; slight decrease in blood pressure toward end of second trimester*
- Weight
  - *Average weight gain of 0.5 to 1 lb./week*
- Urine dipstick for glucose, albumin, and ketones
  - *Mild proteinuria and glucosuria are normal.*
- Fundal height measurement (Fig. 4-9)
  - *Fundal height should equal weeks of gestation.*

- FHR
  - *Able to auscultate FHR with Doppler*
- Fetal movement
  - *Quickening occurs around 18 weeks' gestation.*
- Leopold maneuver
  - *Examiner able to palpate fetal parts*
- Presence of edema
  - *Slight lower body edema is normal due to decreased venous return.*
  - *Upper body edema, especially of the face, is abnormal and needs further evaluation.*
- Confirm established due date:
  - *Assess for **quickening** (when the woman feels her baby move for the first time). This usually occurs between 18 and 20 weeks' gestation, but sometimes as early as 16 weeks' gestation in a multigravida and occasionally as late as 22 weeks' gestation in some primigravidas.*
  - *Use of ultrasound to estimate gestational age by measuring fetus.*

TABLE 4–5   PRENATAL NUTRITION RECOMMENDATIONS

General Recommendations:

1. Eat foods high in iron—heme iron from meats, iron-rich plant foods, or iron-fortified foods.
2. Eat foods high in folate and add a folic acid supplement daily (preconception and through first trimester).
3. Eat a variety of foods in a balanced pattern across and within all food groups. Focus on fruits and vegetables.
4. Choose foods with highest nutrient value and limit saturated fats, trans fats, cholesterol, and added sugar and salt.
5. Add an additional 300 kcal/day to pre-pregnant calorie needs in the second and third trimesters, and monitor for appropriate weight gain.
6. Drink at least 8–10 (8-ounce) glasses of fluid daily (primarily water).
7. To prevent food-borne illnesses: Thoroughly cook meat, poultry, fish and shellfish, and eggs to prevent food-borne illnesses; reheat leftover foods and ready-to-eat foods; avoid raw sprouts and thoroughly wash all fruits and vegetables; avoid unpasteurized dairy products and soft cheeses.
8. Fat intake guidelines: Limit saturated fats and cholesterol, eliminate trans fatty acids; fat intake = 20%–35% of total calories; good sources include fish, nuts, and vegetable oils.

Food Groups	
FRUITS	2 cups Avoid raw, unpasteurized juices
VEGETABLES	2 1/2 cups, 3 cups second and third trimesters Vegetables with dark, rich colors contain more nutrients. Avoid raw sprouts.
LOW-FAT OR NONFAT DAIRY PRODUCTS	3 servings (1 1/2-ounces of cheese, 1 cup milk or yogurt) Avoid raw, unpasteurized products. Avoid soft cheeses.
MEATS, POULTRY, FISH, EGGS, DRY BEANS, NUTS NOTE: It is possible to meet recommendations for food group needs as a vegetarian. Vegan, lacto-, and lacto-ovo-vegetarians need to carefully monitor: intake of micronutrients, especially vitamin B12, calcium, iron, and zinc; and adequate intake of macronutrients and calories)	3 (2-ounce) servings Select lean and low-fat sources. Limit fish and shellfish to 12 ounces/week and avoid large fish with high mercury content—swordfish, shark, tilefish, king mackerel. Reheat leftovers and ready-to-eat foods. May reheat or avoid deli meats (but risk is low).
GRAINS	6 (1-ounce) servings, 7 ounces second trimester, 8 ounces third trimester Select whole-grain products for at least half of the servings.

Based on current recommendations for total energy needs (kilocalories) during pregnancy and the Dietary Guidelines for Americans 2005 document from which the new individualized Food Pyramid is derived (Kaiser & Allen, 2002; U.S. Department of Health and Human Services, 2005).

■ Laboratory and diagnostic studies:
  ■ *Triple screen or quad screen at 15 to 20 weeks' gestation (Chapter 6): Screens for neural tube defect and trisomy 21 screening test are not diagnostic. Amniocentesis is done if screening tests are positive.*
  ■ *Ultrasound around 20 weeks' gestation to confirm EDD and scan fetal anatomy*
  ■ *Screening for gestational diabetes: 1–hour glucose challenge test recommended between 24 and 28 weeks*
  ■ *Hemoglobin and hematocrit to identify anemia and the need for iron supplement. This is the time in pregnancy when the hemoglobin and hematocrit are likely to be at their lowest, so the result provides the care provider with valuable information for management of late pregnancy.*
  ■ *Antibody screen for Rh-negative women*
■ Administer RhoGAM.
  ■ *RhoGAM is administered to Rh-negative women with negative antibody screen results. This is administered at 28 weeks' gestation to help prevent isoimmunization and the resulting risk of hemolytic disease in fetuses in subsequent pregnancies (Medication Box).*

Medication

Rho (D) Immune Globulin (RhoGAM)

■ Indication: Administered to Rh-negative women prophylactically at 28 weeks' gestation to prevent isoimmunization from potential exposure to Rh-positive fetal blood during the normal course of pregnancy. Also administered with likely exposure to Rh-positive blood, such as with pregnancy loss, amniocentesis, or abdominal trauma.

■ Specific mechanism of action: Prevents production of anti-Rho (D) antibodies in Rho (D) negative women exposed to Rho (D) positive blood. Prevention of antibody response and hemolytic diseases of the newborn (erythroblastosis fetalis) in future pregnancies of women who have conceived an Rho (D)-positive fetus.

■ Adverse reactions: Pain at IM site; fever.

■ Route/dosage: 1 vial standard dose (300 mcg) IM at 28 weeks' gestation

(Data from Deglin & Vallerand, 2009)

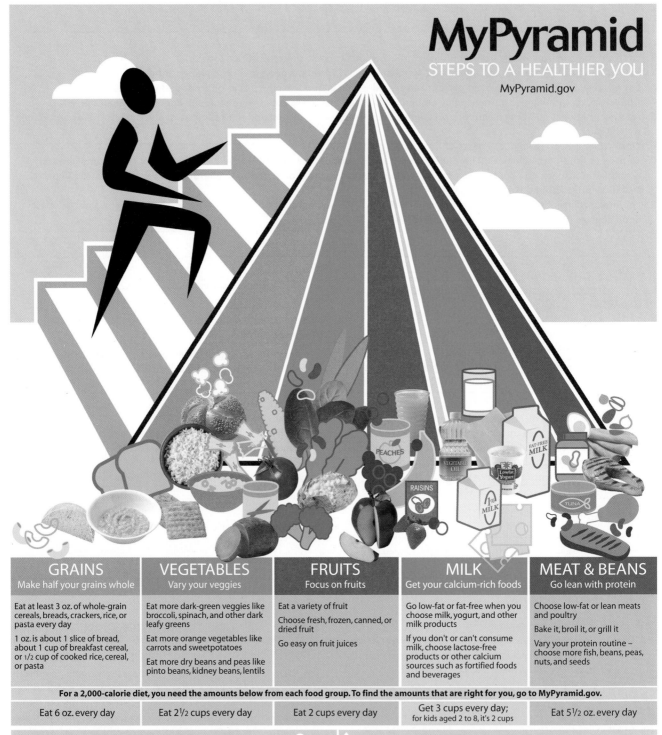

MyPyramid
STEPS TO A HEALTHIER YOU
MyPyramid.gov

GRAINS	VEGETABLES	FRUITS	MILK	MEAT & BEANS
Make half your grains whole	Vary your veggies	Focus on fruits	Get your calcium-rich foods	Go lean with protein
Eat at least 3 oz. of whole-grain cereals, breads, crackers, rice, or pasta every day	Eat more dark-green veggies like broccoli, spinach, and other dark leafy greens	Eat a variety of fruit	Go low-fat or fat-free when you choose milk, yogurt, and other milk products	Choose low-fat or lean meats and poultry
1 oz. is about 1 slice of bread, about 1 cup of breakfast cereal, or 1/2 cup of cooked rice, cereal, or pasta	Eat more orange vegetables like carrots and sweetpotatoes Eat more dry beans and peas like pinto beans, kidney beans, lentils	Choose fresh, frozen, canned, or dried fruit Go easy on fruit juices	If you don't or can't consume milk, choose lactose-free products or other calcium sources such as fortified foods and beverages	Bake it, broil it, or grill it Vary your protein routine – choose more fish, beans, peas, nuts, and seeds

For a 2,000-calorie diet, you need the amounts below from each food group. To find the amounts that are right for you, go to MyPyramid.gov.

Eat 6 oz. every day	Eat 2½ cups every day	Eat 2 cups every day	Get 3 cups every day; for kids aged 2 to 8, it's 2 cups	Eat 5½ oz. every day

Find your balance between food and physical activity

- Be sure to stay within your daily calorie needs.
- Be physically active for at least 30 minutes most days of the week.
- About 60 minutes a day of physical activity may be needed to prevent weight gain.
- For sustaining weight loss, at least 60 to 90 minutes a day of physical activity may be required.
- Children and teenagers should be physically active for 60 minutes every day, or most days.

Know the limits on fats, sugars, and salt (sodium)

- Make most of your fat sources from fish, nuts, and vegetable oils.
- Limit solid fats like butter, margarine, shortening, and lard, as well as foods that contain these.
- Check the Nutrition Facts label to keep saturated fats, *trans* fats, and sodium low.
- Choose food and beverages low in added sugars. Added sugars contribute calories with few, if any, nutrients.

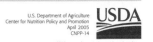

U.S. Department of Agriculture
Center for Nutrition Policy and Promotion
April 2005
CNPP-14

Figure 4-8   USDA MyPyramid Nonpregnant Food Guidelines.

BOX 4–1 PRE-PREGNANCY WEIGHT AND PRENATAL WEIGHT GAIN RECOMMENDATIONS

The impact of pre-pregnancy weight and gestational weight gain on perinatal outcomes is significant and is directly related to infant birth weight, morbidity and mortality. The recommendations for maternal weight gain in pregnancy are individualized based on pre-pregnancy weight and BMI as follows:

- Underweight (BMI <19.8): 28–40 lbs.
- Average weight (BMI 19.8–26.0): 25–35 lbs.
- Overweight (BMI 26.1–29.0): 15–25 lbs.
- Obese (BMI >29.0): 15 lbs.

This set of recommendations remains in current use despite a significant shift in the weight characteristics of the childbearing population (Institute of Medicine, 1990). The recommendations were developed in response to concern over inadequate maternal nutrition and weight gain resulting in low birth weight infants. More recently, the Committee on the Impact of Pregnancy Weight on Maternal and Child Health, National Research Council (2007) through the Institute of Medicine issued a report summarizing the research and identifying emerging themes for future research.

Since the 1990 IOM recommendations, pre-pregnancy weight and BMI as well as gestational weight gain have increased nationally. The current concern lies with the emerging issue of obesity and excessive weight gain in pregnancy and its impact on maternal and child health in both the short-term and the long-term. The current evidence suggests that inadequate weight gain and/or an underweight pre-pregnancy weight increase risk for poor fetal growth and low birth weight. At the other end of the spectrum, excessive weight gain and/or an overweight or obese pre-pregnancy weight increase the risk for poor maternal and neonatal outcomes and may have far-reaching implications for long-term health and development of chronic disease.

Suggestions from the 2007 Committee report included possible modification of the 1990 IOM recommendations and additional research in all related areas to create a body of evidence-based information that can be used to develop recommendations regarding weight gain in pregnancy in order to achieve optimal maternal and child health outcomes.

Source: Committee on the Impact of Pregnancy Weight on Maternal and Child Health, National Research Council (2007).

BOX 4–2 USDA MYPYRAMID FOOD GUIDELINES

Provide food groups info (the color coded lists of food groups with examples, what constitutes a serving, how much to eat of each group daily) and a small version of the new pyramid (with steps on the side to indicate physical activity) (Fig. 4-8).

Source: U.S. Department of Health and Human Services (2005).

- *Leaking of amniotic fluid*
- *Increased vaginal discharge*
- *Vaginal spotting or bleeding*
- Signs and symptoms of hypertensive disorders
  - *Severe headache that does not respond to usual relief measures*
  - *Visual changes*
  - *Facial or generalized edema*
- Information about the benefits and risks of procedures and tests with goal of enabling the woman to make informed decisions about what procedures she will choose based on her knowledge of the available options coupled with her and her family's values and beliefs.

CRITICAL COMPONENT

Warning/Danger Signs of the Second Trimester

- Abdominal or pelvic pain indicates possible PTL, UTI, pyelonephritis, appendicitis.
- Absence of fetal movement once the woman is feeling daily movement indicates possible fetal death.
- Prolonged nausea and vomiting indicates possible hyperemesis gravidarum; at risk for dehydration.
- Fever and chills indicates possible infection.
- Dysuria, frequency, and urgency indicate possible UTI.
- Vaginal bleeding indicates possible infection, friable cervix due to pregnancy changes, placenta previa, abruptio placenta, PTL.

Patient Education and Anticipatory Guidance

- Information on physical changes during the second trimester
- Information on fetal development during the second trimester
  - *At 20 weeks' gestation, the fetus is 8 inches long, weighs 1 pound, is relatively long and skinny.*
- General health maintenance/health promotion topics
- Relief measures for normal discomforts commonly experienced during the second trimester (see Table 4-4)
- Warning/danger signs that need to be reported to care provider (Critical Component: Warning/Danger Signs of the Second Trimester)
- Signs and symptoms of preterm labor (PTL)
  - *Rhythmic lower abdominal cramping or pain*
  - *Low backache*
  - *Pelvic pressure*

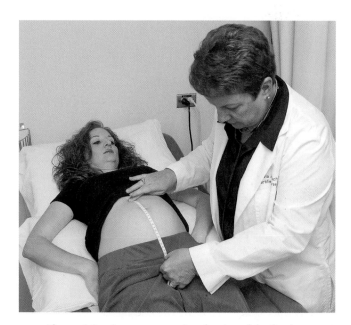

Figure 4-9 A nurse measuring the size of the fundus.

Third Trimester

The focused assessment includes all aspects of the second trimester assessment and may also include a pelvic examination to identify cervical change, depending on weeks of gestation and maternal symptoms. Assessment of pregnancy in the third trimester becomes more frequent and involved than in previous return visits as the pregnancy advances and the fetus nears term (see Table 4-3).

Components of Third Trimester Assessments

- Chart review
- Interval history
- Focused assessment (e.g., fundal height)
- Assessment of fetal well-being
  - *Auscultation of FHR (Fig. 4-10)*
  - *Record woman's assessment of "kick counts"*
    - Daily **fetal movement count (kick counts)** is a maternal assessment of fetal movement by counting fetal movements in a period of time to identify potentially hypoxic fetuses. Maternal perception of fetal movement was one of the earliest tests of fetal well being and remains an essential assessment of fetal health. The pregnant woman is instructed to palpate the abdomen and track fetal movements daily by tracking fetal movements for 1 or 2 hours.
    - In the 2-hour approach, maternal perception of 10 distinct fetal movements within 2 hours is considered reassuring; once movement is achieved counts can be discontinued for the day.
    - In the 1-hour approach, the count is considered reassuring if it equals or exceeds the established baseline, in general 4 movements in 1 hour is reassuring.
    - Decreased fetal activity should be reported to the provider and is an indication for further fetal assessment, such as a non stress test or biophysical profile. If there is reduction in fetal movement, further evaluation of the fetus is indicated.
- Pelvic examination to identify cervical change, depending on weeks of gestation and maternal symptoms

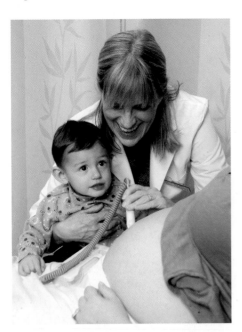

Figure 4-10: A nurse-midwife listening to fetal heart tone with a pregnant mom and her toddler.

- **Leopold's maneuvers** (palpation of the abdomen) to identify the position of the fetus in utero (Chapter 8)
- Nutritional follow-up
- Screening for Group B *Streptococcus*
  - *A quarter to a third of all women are colonized with Group B* Streptococcus *(GBS) in the lower gastrointestinal or urogenital tract (typically asymptomatic)*
  - *Culture at 35 to 37 weeks' gestation*
  - *Vaginal and rectal swabs to determine presence of GBS bacterial colonization before the onset of labor in order to anticipate treatment during labor for a positive culture as recommended by the CDC (2002)*
  - *GBS infection in a newborn, either early-onset (first week of life) or late onset (after first week of life), can be invasive and severe, with potential long-term neurological sequelae.*
  - *Treatment with IV antibiotics in labor recommended for positive screening results; unknown screening results; risk factors of PTL, prolonged rupture of membranes, or maternal temperature greater than 100.4°F (38°C); history of infant with invasive GBS disease (no screening needed); and history of GBS in urine (no screening needed)*
  - *Treatment not indicated for planned cesarean birth without labor or rupture of membranes, regardless of screening results (CDC, 2002)*
- Laboratory tests and screening
  - *1-hour glucose test at 24 to 28 weeks' gestation*
  - *CBC*
  - *Repeat gonorrhea culture (GC), Chlamydia, rapid plasma reagin (RPR), human immunodeficiency virus (HIV), and hepatitis B surface antigen (HbSAg) tests as indicated*

Patient Education and Anticipatory Guidance

- Information about physical changes during the third trimester

---

CRITICAL COMPONENT

Warning/Danger Signs of the Third Trimester

- Abdominal or pelvic pain (PTL, UTI, pyelonephritis, appendicitis)
- Decreased or absent fetal movement
- Prolonged nausea and vomiting (dehydration, hyperemesis gravidarum)
- Fever, chills (infection)
- Dysuria, frequency, urgency (UTI)
- Vaginal bleeding (infection, friable cervix due to pregnancy changes or pathology, placenta previa, placenta abruptio, PTL)
- Signs/symptoms of PTL: Rhythmic lower abdominal cramping or pain, low backache, pelvic pressure, leaking of amniotic fluid, increased vaginal discharge,
- Vaginal spotting or bleeding
- Signs/symptoms of hypertensive disorders:
  Severe headache that does not respond to usual relief measures
  Visual changes
  Facial or generalized edema
- Nausea and vomiting
- Absence of fetal movement
- Absence of fetal heart tones

- Information about fetal growth during the third trimester
  - *At term fetus is about 17 to 20 inches in length, weighs between 6 to 8 pounds, increased deposits of subcutaneous fat, has established sleep and activity cycles*
- Self-care measures
- General health maintenance/health promotion topics
- Relief measures for normal discomforts commonly experienced during the third trimester (see Table 4-4).
- Warning/danger signs that need to be reported to care provider (Critical Component: Warning/Danger Signs of the Third Trimester)
- Travel is usually limited in the last month.
- Discussion of preparation for labor and birth
  - *Attend childbirth classes.*
  - *Discuss the method of labor pain management.*
  - *Develop birth plan; list preferences for routine procedures*
- Signs of impending labor
- Discussion of true versus false labor
- Instruction on when to contact the doctor or midwife
- Instructions on when to go to the birthing unit
- Discussion on parenting and infant care
  - *Attend parenting classes*
  - *Select the method of infant feeding*
  - *Select the infant health care provider*
  - *Preparation of siblings*

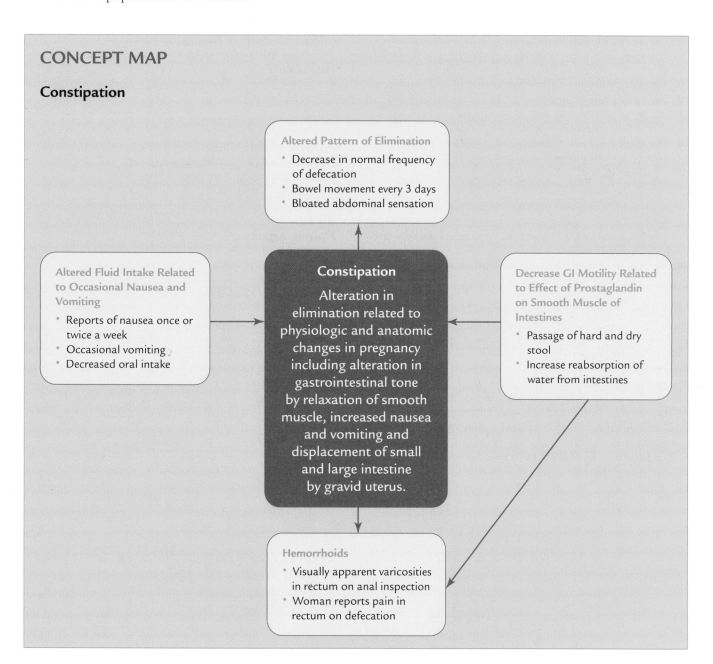

CONCEPT MAP

Constipation

Altered Pattern of Elimination
- Decrease in normal frequency of defecation
- Bowel movement every 3 days
- Bloated abdominal sensation

Altered Fluid Intake Related to Occasional Nausea and Vomiting
- Reports of nausea once or twice a week
- Occasional vomiting
- Decreased oral intake

Constipation
Alteration in elimination related to physiologic and anatomic changes in pregnancy including alteration in gastrointestinal tone by relaxation of smooth muscle, increased nausea and vomiting and displacement of small and large intestine by gravid uterus.

Decrease GI Motility Related to Effect of Prostaglandin on Smooth Muscle of Intestines
- Passage of hard and dry stool
- Increase reabsorption of water from intestines

Hemorrhoids
- Visually apparent varicosities in rectum on anal inspection
- Woman reports pain in rectum on defecation

Problem No. 1: Altered pattern of elimination
Goal: Resumption of typical bowel patterns
Outcome: Patient will resume her normal bowel patterns.

Nursing Actions

1. Assess prior bowel patterns before pregnancy including frequency, consistency, shape, and color.
2. Auscultate bowel sounds.
3. Assess prior experiences with constipation.
4. Explore prior successful strategies for constipation.
5. Explain contributing factors to constipation in pregnancy.
6. Teaching strategies for dealing with constipation including diet, exercise, and adequate fluid intake.
7. Encourage high-fiber foods and fresh fruits and vegetables.
8. Encourage dietary experimentation to evaluate what works for her.
9. Establish regular time for bowel movement.
10. Discuss rationale for strategies.
11. Explore with the woman and discuss with the care provider use of stool softener and/or bulk laxative.
12. Encourage the patient to discuss concerns about constipation by asking open-end questions

Problem No. 2: Altered fluid intake related to nausea and vomiting
Goal: Normal fluid intake
Outcome: Normal fluid intake and decreased nausea and vomiting

Nursing Actions

1. Assess factors that increase nausea and vomiting.
2. Suggest small frequent meals.
3. Decrease fluid intake with meals.
4. Avoid high-fat and spicy food.
5. Explore contributing factors to nausea in pregnancy.
6. Teach strategies for dealing with nausea in pregnancy.
7. Encourage the woman to experiment with strategies to alleviate nausea
8. Suggest vitamin B_6 or ginger to decrease nausea.

Problem 3: Decreased gastric motility
Goal: Increased motility
Outcome: Patient has normal bowel movement.

Nursing Actions

1. Provide dietary information to increase fiber and roughage in diet.
2. Review high fiber foods, for example, pears, apples, prunes, kiwis and dried fruits.
3. Bran cereal in the morning and instruct woman to check labels for at least 4-5 grams per serving of fiber.
4. Discuss strategies to increase fluid intake
5. Drink warm liquid upon rising.
6. Encourage exercise to promote peristalsis.
7. Reinforce relationship of diet, exercise, and fluid intake on constipation.

Problem 4: Discomfort with defecation because of hemorrhoids
Goal: Decreased pain with bowel movement
Outcome: Patient will have decreased pain and maintain adequate bowel function.

Nursing Actions

1. Reinforce strategies to avoid constipation.
2. Encourage the woman to not avoid defecation.
3. Discuss care of hemorrhoids including TUCKS pads and hemorrhoid creams.
4. Discuss use of stool softeners.
5. Instruct the woman to avoid straining on evacuation.
6. Recommend that the woman support a foot on a foot stool to facilitate bowel evacuation.
7. Reinforce relationship of diet, exercise, and fluid intake on constipation.

TYING IT ALL TOGETHER

As a nurse in an antenatal clinic you are part of an interdisciplinary team that is caring for Margarite Sanchez during her pregnancy. Margarite is a 28-year-old G3 P1 Hispanic woman here for her first prenatal care appointment. By her LMP she is 8 weeks' gestation. Margarite reports some spotting at 2 weeks ago that prompted her to do a home pregnancy test that was positive. The spotting has stopped. She tells you that she is very tired throughout the day, has some nausea in the morning and breast tenderness. She is happy to be pregnant but a bit surprised.

Outline the aspects of your initial assessment.

Outline for Margarite what laboratory tests are done during this first prenatal visit and rationale for the tests.

Detail the prenatal education and anticipatory guidance appropriate to the first trimester of pregnancy.

What teaching would you do for Margarite's discomforts of pregnancy?

Discuss nursing diagnosis, nursing activities and expected outcomes related to this woman.

At 18 weeks' gestation Margarite comes to the clinic for a prenatal visit. She states she thinks she felt her baby move last week and that the pregnancy now feels real to her. She states she feels "Great! The nausea and fatigue are gone". She is concerned she is not eating enough protein as she has little interest in red meat, but eats beans and rice at dinner. She remembers discussing with you at her first visit some screening tests for problems with the baby but now is unsure how they are done and what they are for.

Outline for Margarite nutritional needs during pregnancy highlighting protein requirements.

Outline for Margarite the screening tests that are done in the second trimester and what they are for.

Detail the prenatal education and anticipatory guidance appropriate to the second trimester of pregnancy.

Discuss nursing diagnosis, nursing activities, and expected outcomes related to this woman.

Margarite comes to your clinic for a prenatal visit and is now 34 weeks' gestation. She states she feels well but has some swelling in her legs at the end of the day, has a backache at the end of the day and difficulty getting comfortable to fall asleep, she is having difficulty sleeping as she gets up to go to the bathroom two or three times a night.

She remembers from her first pregnancy some things she should be aware of that indicate a problem at the end of pregnancy but is not sure what they are.

Detail the prenatal education and anticipatory guidance appropriate to the third trimester of pregnancy.

What teaching would you do for Margarite's discomforts of pregnancy?

Discuss nursing diagnosis, nursing activities, and expected outcomes specific to Margarite.

■ ■ ■ Review Questions ■ ■ ■

1. The appropriate recommended weight gain during pregnancy with a woman with a normal BMI:
   A. 10–15 lbs.
   B. 6–20 lbs.
   C. 21–25 lbs.
   D. 25–35 lbs.

2. The purpose of preconception care is to:
   A. Prevent unwanted pregnancies
   B. Improve perinatal outcomes
   C. Facilitate desired pregnancy
   D. Screen for sexually transmitted diseases

3. Presumptive signs of pregnancy are:
   A. All the objective signs of pregnancy
   B. Those perceived by the healthcare provider
   C. Physiological changes perceived by the woman herself
   D. Those attributed to the fetus.

4. Physiological changes in pregnancy:
   A. Involve primarily reproductive organs
   B. Are protective of the woman and/or fetus
   C. Are most profound in the first trimester
   D. Primarily impact the musculoskeletal system

5. Intimate partner violence:
   A. Consists of physical abuse
   B. Decreases during pregnancy
   C. Crosses all ethnic, racial, religious, and socioeconomic levels
   D. Primarily impacts maternal health

6. RhoGAM would be administered during pregnancy at 28 weeks' gestation to women with the following:
   A. Blood type O+
   B. Blood type A+
   C. Blood type O–
   D. Blood type AB

7. Blood volume increases during pregnancy by:
   A. 500 mL
   B. 1,000 mL
   C. 1,500 mL
   D. 2,000 mL

8. A woman presents for prenatal care at 10 weeks' gestation reporting nausea and vomiting. Self-care and relief measures include:
   A. Suggest a high protein diet
   B. Suggest avoiding eating early in the day
   C. Suggest increasing fluid intake
   D. Suggest small, frequent meals

References

Association for Women's Health, Obstetric and Neonatal Nurses (AWHONN). (2007). *Universal screening for domestic violence.* Washington, DC: Author.

Baldwin, K. A. (2006). Comparison of selected outcomes of centering pregnancy versus traditional prenatal care. *Journal of Midwifery & Women's Health, 51*(4), 266–272.

Blackburn, S. T. (2007). *Maternal, fetal, & neonatal physiology: A clinical perspective* (3rd ed.). St. Louis, MO: W. B. Saunders.

Campbell, J., & Furniss, K. (2002). *Violence against women: Identification, screening and management of intimate partner violence.* Washington, DC: Association of Women's Health, Obstetric, and Neonatal Nurses.

Centers for Disease Control and Prevention (CDC). (1992). Recommendations for the use of folic acid to reduce the number of cases of spina bifida and other neural tube defects. *MMWR Recommendations and Reports, 41*(RR-14); 001.

Centers for Disease Control and Prevention (CDC). (2002). Prevention of perinatal group B streptococcal disease: Revised guidelines from CDC. *MMWR Recommendations and Reports, 51*(RR-11); 1–22.

Centers for Disease Control and Prevention (2006). Recommendations to Improve Preconception Health and Health Care—United States. *MMWR Recommendations and Reports, 55*(RR-6); 1–23.

Committee on the Impact of Pregnancy Weight on Maternal and Child Health, National Research Council. (2007). *Influence of pregnancy weight on maternal and child health: Workshop report.* Washington, DC: The National Academies Press.

Deglin, J., & Vallerand, A. (2009). *Davis's drug guide for nurses* (11th ed.). Philadelphia: F. A. Davis.

Dillon, P. (2007). *Nursing health assessment.* Philadelphia: F. A. Davis.

Grady, M. A., & Bloom, K. C. (2004). Pregnancy outcomes of adolescents enrolled in a Centering Pregnancy program. *Journal of Midwifery & Women's Health, 49*(5), 412–420.

Ickovics, J. R., Kershaw, T. S., Westdahl, C., Rising, S. S., Klima, C., Reynolds, H., & Magriples, U. (2003). Group prenatal care and preterm birth weight: Results from a matched cohort study at public clinics. *Obstetrics & Gynecology, 102*(5), Part 1, 1051–1057.

Institute of Medicine. (1990). *Nutrition during pregnancy.* Washington, DC: National Academies Press.

Kaiser, L., & Allen, L. (2002). Position of the American Dietetic Association: Nutrition and lifestyle for a healthy pregnancy outcome. *Journal of the American Dietetic Association, 102*(10), 1479–1490.

Mattson, S., & Smith, J. (2004). *Core curriculum for maternal-newborn nursing* (3rd ed). St. Louis, MO: Elsevier.

Martin, J. A., Hamilton, B. E., Menacker, F., Sutton, P., & Mathews, T. (2007). *Preliminary births for 2004: Infant and maternal health.* Hyattsville, MD: National Center for Health Statistics.

McFarlane, J., Parker, B., & Moran, B. (2007). *Abuse during pregnancy: A protocol for prevention and intervention* (3rd ed.). White Plains, NY: March of Dimes.

McFarlane, J., Parker, B., & Soekin, K. (1996). Abuse during pregnancy: Associations with maternal health and infant birth weight. *Nursing Research, 45,* 37–42.

National Center for Health Statistics. (2006). *Births: Final data for 2004.* Hyattsville, MD: Author.

Rising, S. S. (1998). Centering pregnancy: An interdisciplinary model of empowerment. *Journal of Nurse-Midwifery, 43*(1), 46–54.

Simpson, K., & Creehan, P. (2008). *Perinatal nursing.* Philadelphia: Lippincott Williams & Wilkins.

Smith, C., Crowther, C., Willson, K., Hotham, N., & McMillian, V. (2004). A randomized controlled trial of ginger to treat nausea and vomiting in pregnancy. *Obstetrics & Gynecology, 103*(4), 639–645.

U.S. Department of Health and Human Services. (2005). *Dietary guidelines for Americans 2005.* Retrieved from www.healthierus.gov/dietaryguidelines (Accessed May 24, 2007).

Villar, J., Carroli, G., Khan-Neelofur, D., Piaggio, G., & Gulmezoglu, M. (2007). Patterns of routine antenatal care for low-risk pregnancy. *Cochrane Database of Systematic Reviews,* Volume 2, 2007. Oxford: Update Software.

Walker, D. S., McCully, L., & Vest, V. (2001). Evidence-based prenatal care visits: When less is more. *Journal of Midwifery & Women's Health, 46*(3), 146–151.

Walker, D. S., & Rising, S. S. (2004/2005). Revolutionizing prenatal care: New evidence-based prenatal care delivery models. *Journal of the New York State Nurses Association,* Fall/Winter, 18–21.

Psycho–Social–Cultural Aspects of the Antepartum Period

5

OBJECTIVES

On completion of this chapter, students will be able to:
- ☐ Describe expected emotional changes of the pregnant woman and appropriate nursing responses to these changes.
- ☐ Identify the major developmental tasks of pregnancy as they relate to maternal, paternal, and family adaptation.
- ☐ Identify critical variables that influence adaptation to pregnancy, including age, parity, social and cultural factors.
- ☐ Identify nursing assessments and interventions that promote positive psycho–social–cultural adaptations for the pregnant woman and her family.
- ☐ Analyze critical factors in preparing for birth, including choosing a provider and birth setting and creating a birth plan.
- ☐ Identify key components of childbirth preparation education for expectant families.
- ☐ Analyze and critique current evidence-based research in the area of psycho–social–cultural adaptation to pregnancy.

Nursing Diagnosis
- ☐ At risk for anxiety and fear related to:
  - ☐ Unknown processes of pregnancy
  - ☐ Changes in roles related to pregnancy
  - ☐ Changes in family dynamics
  - ☐ Changes in body image
- ☐ Knowledge deficit related to pregnancy changes
- ☐ At risk for impaired adjustment related to role changes in pregnancy
- ☐ At risk for interrupted family processes related to developmental stressors of pregnancy
- ☐ At risk for impaired communication related to cultural differences between family and health care providers
- ☐ At risk for ineffective coping related to inadequate social support during pregnancy

Nursing Outcomes
- ☐ The pregnant woman and her family will:
  - ☐ Be able to communicate effectively with health care providers
  - ☐ Verbalize decreased anxiety
  - ☐ Verbalize appropriate family dynamics
  - ☐ Report increasing acceptance of changes in body image
  - ☐ Seek clarification of information about pregnancy and birth
  - ☐ Demonstrate knowledge regarding expected changes of pregnancy
  - ☐ Develop a realistic birth plan
  - ☐ Exhibit acceptance of roles as mother and father
  - ☐ Identify appropriate support systems
  - ☐ Receive positive and effective social support
  - ☐ Express satisfaction with adherence to traditional beliefs and practices of their culture

---

MATERNAL ADAPTATION TO PREGNANCY

The news of pregnancy confers profound and irrevocable changes in a woman's life and the lives of those around her. With this news, the woman begins her journey toward becoming a mother. Less visible than the physical adaptations of pregnancy, but just as profound, the pregnant woman's psychological adaptations and development of her identity as a mother are crucial aspects of the childbearing cycle. Psychological, cultural, and social factors all significantly influence this process. Psychosocial support for the pregnant woman and her family is a distinct and major nursing responsibility during the antepartal period. This chapter presents the changes a woman and her family must navigate to achieve a positive adaptation to pregnancy. Factors influencing these changes are also described.

Want to reinforce your reading? Need to review for a test? Listen to this chapter on your accompanying CD.

Pregnancy provides the time for the woman to prepare for the labor and birth experience, complete the tasks of pregnancy, and take on the role of mother. Motherhood, an irrevocable change in a woman's life, progressively becomes part of a woman's total identity (Koniak-Griffin, Logsdon, Hines, & Turner, 2006; Mercer, 1995, 2004). Becoming a mother has been noted to occur on a long continuum, with the psychological groundwork laid during the course of each woman's individual experience during pregnancy. The pregnant woman is able to use the 9 months of pregnancy to restructure her psychological and cognitive self toward motherhood. Nursing care is based on an understanding of the maternal tasks of pregnancy and variables that influence maternal adaptation.

Maternal Tasks of Pregnancy

Maternal tasks of pregnancy were first identified in the psychoanalytic literature (Bibring, Dwyer, Huntington, & Valenstein, 1961), then further explored and outlined by classic maternity nurse researchers Reva Rubin, Ramona Mercer and Regina Lederman.

Rubin's research has provided a framework and core knowledge base from which researchers and clinicians have worked. Rubin identified significant maternal tasks women undergo during the course of pregnancy on their journey toward motherhood (1975, 1984):

■ Ensuring a safe passage for herself and her child refers to the mother's knowledge and care-seeking behaviors to ensure that both she and the newborn emerge from pregnancy healthy.
■ Ensuring social acceptance of the child by significant others refers to the woman engaging her social network in the pregnancy.
■ Attaching or "binding-in" to the child refers to the development of maternal–fetal attachment.
■ Giving of oneself to the demands of being a mother refers to the mother's willingness and efforts to make personal sacrifices for the child.

Building on Rubin's work, Regina Lederman (1996) identified seven dimensions of maternal role development.

■ Acceptance of pregnancy
   ■ *This task focuses on the woman's adaptive responses to the changes that occur related to pregnancy growth and development (Lederman, 1996). These responses include:*
      ■ Responding to mood changes
      ■ Responding to ambivalent feelings
      ■ Responding to nausea, fatigue, and other physical discomforts of the early months of pregnancy
      ■ Responding to financial concerns
      ■ Responding to increased dependency needs
   ■ *Expected findings:*
      ■ Desired and/or acceptance of pregnancy (Critical Component: Ambivalent Feelings Toward Pregnancy)
      ■ Predominantly happy feelings during pregnancy
      ■ Little physical discomfort or a high tolerance for the discomfort
      ■ Acceptance of body changes
      ■ Minimal ambivalent feelings and conflict regarding pregnancy by the end of her pregnancy
      ■ A dislike of being pregnant but feels love for the unborn child

CRITICAL COMPONENT

Ambivalent Feelings Toward Pregnancy

It is common for women to experience ambivalent feelings toward pregnancy during the first trimester. These feelings decrease as pregnancy progresses. Ambivalent feelings toward pregnancy that continues into the third trimester may indicate unresolved conflict. When evaluating ambivalence it is important to assess:

■ The reason for the ambivalence
■ The intensity of the ambivalence

(Lederman, 1996; Mercer, 1995)

■ Identification with the motherhood role
   ■ *Accomplishment of this task is influenced by the woman's acceptance of pregnancy and the relationship the woman has with her own mother. Women who have accepted their pregnancy and who have a positive relationship with their own mothers have an easier time accomplishing this task (Lederman, 1996).*
   ■ *Accomplishment of this task is also influenced by the woman's degree of fears about labor related to helplessness, pain, loss of control, and loss of self-esteem (Lederman, 1996).*
   ■ *Vivid dreams are common during pregnancy, which allows the woman to envision herself as a mother in various situations. A woman often rehearses or pictures herself in her new role in different scenarios (Rubin, 1975; Sorensen & Schuelke, 1999).*
   ■ *The motherhood role is strengthened as the woman attaches to her fetus. Events that facilitate fetal attachment are:*
      ■ Hearing the fetal heart beat
      ■ Seeing the fetus move during an ultrasound examination
      ■ Feeling the fetus kick or move
   ■ *Fetal attachment influences the woman's sense of her child and her sense of being competent as a mother.*
   ■ *Expected findings:*
      ■ The woman moves from viewing herself as a woman-without-child to a woman-with-child.
      ■ Anticipates changes motherhood will bring to her life
      ■ Seeks company of other pregnant women
      ■ Highly motivated to assume the motherhood role
      ■ Actively prepares for the motherhood role
■ Relationship to her mother
   ■ *Four components important to the woman's relationship with her own mother are:*
      ■ Availability of the woman's mother to her in the past and in the present
      ■ The mother's reaction to her daughter's pregnancy
      ■ The mother's relationship to her daughter
      ■ The mother's willingness to reminisce with her daughter about her own childbirth and childrearing experiences
   ■ *Unresolved mother–daughter conflicts reemerge and confront the woman during pregnancy (Lederman, 1996).*
   ■ *Expected findings:*
      ■ The woman's mother was available to her in the past and continues to be available during the pregnancy (Fig. 5-1).
      ■ The woman's mother is accepting of the pregnancy, respects her autonomy, and acknowledges her daughter becoming a mother.
      ■ The woman's mother relates to her daughter as an adult versus as a child.

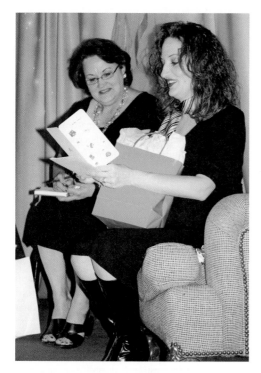

Figure 5-1   Pregnant woman and her mother participating in baby shower.

■ The woman's mother reminisces about her own childbearing and childrearing experiences.

■ Reordering relationship with her husband or partner

■ *Pregnancy has a dramatic effect on the couple's relationship. Some couples view pregnancy and childbirth as a growth experience and as an expression of deep commitment to their bond, while others view it as an added stressor to a relationship already in conflict.*

■ *The partner's support during pregnancy enhances the woman's feelings of well-being during pregnancy and is associated with earlier and continuous prenatal care (Lederman, 1996).*

■ *Assessment of the relationship between the couple includes:*

■ The partner's concern for the woman's needs during pregnancy

■ The woman's concerns for her partner's needs during pregnancy

■ The varying desires for sexual activity among pregnant women

■ The effect pregnancy has on the relationship (e.g., does it bring them closer together or cause conflict?)

■ The partner's adjustment to his or her new role

■ *Expected findings:*

■ The partner is understanding and supportive of the woman.

■ The partner is thoughtful and "pampers" the woman during pregnancy.

■ The partner is involved in the pregnancy.

■ The woman perceives that her partner is supportive.

■ The woman is concerned about her partner's needs of making emotional adjustments to the pregnancy and new role. Women in relationships with established open communication about sexuality are likely to have less difficulty with changes in sexual activity.

■ Couples indicate that they are growing closer to each other during pregnancy.

■ The partner is happy and excited about the pregnancy and prepares for the new role.

■ Preparation for labor

■ *Preparation for labor means preparation for the physiological processes of labor as well as the psychological processes of separating from the fetus and becoming a mother to the child.*

■ *Preparation for labor and birth occur by taking classes, reading, fantasizing, and dreaming about labor and birth (Lederman, 1996).*

■ *The degree of preparation for labor and birth has an effect on the woman's level of anxiety and fear. The more prepared a woman feels, the lower the level of anxiety and fear.*

■ *Feeling loved and valued and having her child accepted by her partner are two major contributors to positive adaptation (Cannella, 2006; Kroelinger & Oths, 2000; Orr, 2004).*

■ *Expected findings:*

■ The woman attends childbirth classes and reads books about labor and birth.

■ The woman mentally rehearses (fantasizes) the labor and birthing process.

■ The woman has dreams about labor and birth.

■ The woman develops realistic expectations of labor and birth.

■ The pregnant woman may engage in a flurry of activities, known as "nesting behavior," wherein she is hurrying to prepare for the newborn's arrival (Driscoll, 2001; Lederman, 1996).

■ Prenatal fear of loss of control in labor

■ *Loss of control includes two factors (Lederman, 1996):*

■ Loss of control over the body

■ Loss of control over emotions

■ *The degree of fear is related to:*

■ The woman's degree of trust with the medical and nursing staff, her partner, and other support persons

■ The woman's attitude regarding the use of medication and anesthesia for labor pain management

■ *Expected findings:*

■ The woman perceives individual attention from medical staff.

■ Woman perceives that she is being treated as an adult and her questions and concerns are addressed by the medical staff.

■ The woman perceives that the nursing staff is compassionate, understanding, and available.

■ The woman perceives that she is being supported by her partner and family/friends.

■ The woman has realistic expectations regarding management of labor pain and these expectations are met.

■ Prenatal fear of loss of self-esteem in labor

■ *Some women have fears that they will lose self-esteem in labor and "fail" during labor (Lederman, 1996).*

■ *When a woman feels a threat to her self-esteem it is important to assess the following areas (Lederman, 1996).*

■ The source of the threat

■ The response to the threat

■ The intensity of the reaction to the threat

■ *Behaviors that reflect self esteem are:*

■ Tolerance of self

■ Value of self and assertiveness

■ Body image and appearance

Expected findings:

- Able to develop realistic expectations of self during labor and birth and an awareness of risks and potential complications
- Able to identify and respect her own feelings
- Able to assert herself in acquiring information needed to make decisions
- Able to recognize own needs and limitations
- Able to adjust to the unexpected and unknown
- Able to recover from threats quickly

As the woman prepares to experience labor, give birth, and take on the maternal role, the process of maternal adaptation to pregnancy is completed. With the dominating physical discomforts of the third trimester, most women become impatient for labor to begin. There is relief and excitement about going into labor. The mother is ready and eager to deliver and hold her baby. She has prepared for her future as a mother (Rubin, 1984).

Nursing Actions

- During the antepartal period, the nurse can take on a variety of roles: teacher, counselor, clinician, resource person, role model (Critical Component: Nursing Actions that Facilitate Adaptation to Pregnancy).

- Nursing actions should be focused on health promotion, individualized care, and prevention of individual and family crises (Driscoll, 2001; Mattson & Smith, 2004; May & Mahlmeister, 1994).

Variables that Influence Maternal Adaptation

The ability of the woman to adapt to the maternal role is influenced by a variety of factors, including parity, maternal age, sexual orientation, single parenting, multiple pregnancies (twins, triples), socioeconomic factors, and abuse.

Parity

- Multigravidas may have the benefit of experience, but it should not be assumed that they need less help than a first-time mother. They know more of what to expect in terms of pain during labor, postpartum adaptation, and the many added responsibilities of motherhood, but they may need time to process and develop strategies for integrating a new member into the family.
- Pregnancy tasks may be more complex. Giving adequate attention to all of her children and supporting sibling adaptation are unique challenges faced by the multigravida. She may spend a

---

CRITICAL COMPONENT

Nursing Actions that Facilitate Adaptation to Pregnancy

First Trimester	Begin psychosocial assessment at initial contact; assess the woman's response to pregnancy; assess stressors in woman's life.
	Promote pregnancy and birth as a family experience; encourage family and partner participation in prenatal visits; encourage questions from partner and family members about the pregnancy.
	Assess learning needs.
	Offer anticipatory guidance regarding normal developmental stressors of pregnancy, such as ambivalence during early pregnancy, feelings of vulnerability, mood changes, and active dream/fantasy life.
	Assess for increased anxieties and fear; if anxieties seem greater than normal refer to mental health care provider.
	Listen, validate, provide reassurance, teach expected emotional changes to decrease anxiety, educate the partner and family members; stress normalcy of feelings.
	If appropriate, discuss common phases through which expectant fathers/partners progress through pregnancy; be aware of phases of paternal adaptation when counseling parents about expected changes of pregnancy; provide anticipatory guidance regarding potential communication conflicts.
Second Trimester	Encourage verbalization regarding possible grief process during pregnancy related to body image changes, loss of previous lifestyle, changing relationships with family and friends.
	Provide anticipatory guidance regarding normal changes and concerns
	Discuss normal changes in sexual activity
	Encourage "tuning in" to fetal movements; discuss the fetus' ability to hear and respond to interaction and maternal movement.
	Reinforce to partners and family importance of giving the expectant mother extra support; offer specific examples of ways to help (helping her eat well, helping with heavy work, giving extra attention).
Third Trimester	Encourage attendance at childbirth classes.
	Discuss preparations for birth, parenthood; explore expectations of labor
	Assess the partner's interest in a labor coach role and reassure as needed; stress that help in labor will be available; and if appropriate encourage the presence of a second support person.
	Refer to appropriate educational materials on parenthood.
	Encourage discussions of plans and expectations with the partner.
	Provide anticipatory guidance regarding normal changes and concerns
	Give anticipatory guidance regarding the realities of infant care, breastfeeding, etc.
	Plan for appropriate referrals to accommodate psychosocial complications; coordinate with social workers, nutritionist, and community agencies.
	Help the expectant mother identify and use support systems.

(Driscoll, 2001; Mattson, 2004; May, 1994; Simpson, 2008)

great deal of time working out a new relationship with the first child, and grieve for the loss of their special relationship. She also has to consider the financial issues associated with feeding, clothing, and providing for another child while at the same time maintaining a relationship with her partner and continuing her career, whether inside or outside the home (Jordan, 1989).

Maternal Age

■ Adolescent mothers

■ *The major developmental task of adolescence is to form and become comfortable with a sense of self. Pregnancy presents a challenge for teenagers who, as expectant parents, must cope with the conflicting developmental tasks of pregnancy and adolescence at the same time.*

■ *Adolescents who have an unintended pregnancy face a number of challenges, including abandonment by their partners, increased adverse pregnancy outcomes, and inability to complete school education, which may ultimately limit their future social and economic opportunities (Ehiri, Meremikwu, & Meremikwu, 2005).*

■ *Achieving a maternal identity is very difficult for an adolescent who is in the throes of evolving her own identity as an adult capable of psychosocial independence from her family. Although she may achieve the maternal role, research indicates that she functions at a lower level of competence than do older women (Mercer, 2004).*

■ *The younger she is, the more difficulties the adolescent woman has with body image changes, acknowledging the pregnancy, seeking health care, and planning for the changes that pregnancy and parenting will bring. Delayed entry into prenatal care is common. There is also a higher rate of abuse among pregnant adolescents (Montgomery, 2003; Spear, 2004; Spear & Lock, 2003).*

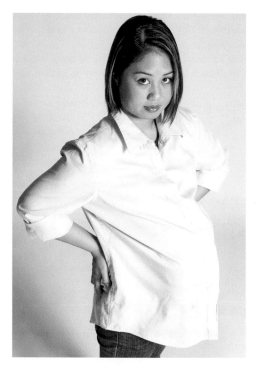

Figure 5-2   Pregnant adolescent. (Photo courtesy of Randi Willis and Gwen Ortiz.)

■ *Successful adaptation to pregnancy and parenthood may greatly depend on the age of the adolescent (Fig. 5-2).*

■ Early adolescence can be defined as the period between 11 and 15 years. Adolescents in this phase of life are self-centered and oriented toward the present. There is a greater likelihood that pregnancy at this age is a result of abuse or coercion. Moving into the maternal role is a difficult challenge for this age group. Grandmothers play a significant role in caring for the infant as well as providing guidance to their daughters regarding mothering skills (Mercer, 1995; Montgomery, 2003; Sadler & Clemmens, 2004).

■ Middle adolescence is defined as the period between 14 and 16 years. During this time, the adolescent is more capable of abstract thinking and understanding consequences of current behaviors.

■ Late adolescence is defined as the period of time between 17 and 20 years. The older pregnant adolescent is more likely to be a capable and active participant in health care decisions (Montgomery, 2003).

■ *Comprehensive and community-based health care programs for adolescents have been shown to be effective in improving outcomes for the teen mother and her infant. Examples include programs that have been implemented in schools, clinics, community agencies, or home visitation programs.*

■ Higher levels of support and higher self-esteem are associated with a more positive adaptation to mothering for adolescents (Breedlove, 2005; Kirby, 1999; Logsdon, Gagne, Hughes, Patterson, & Rakestraw, 2005; Philliber, Brooks, Lehere, Oakley, & Waggoner, 2003).

■ Older mothers

■ *In North America, increasing numbers of women have delayed childbearing until after the age of 30 to 35. The majority of women in this age group deliver at term without adverse outcomes. Even with good prenatal care, there is an increased incidence of adverse perinatal outcomes.*

■ *Chronic diseases that are more common in women older than 35 may affect the pregnancy.*

■ *Evidence indicates that older mothers are also more likely to have miscarriages, fetal chromosomal abnormalities, low birth weight infants, premature births, and multiple births. In women older than 40, the risk increases for placenta previa, placenta abruption, caesarean, deliveries, and gestational diabetes (Cleary-Goldman et al., 2005; Joseph et al., 2005).*

■ *The more mature woman is better equipped psychosocially to assume the maternal role. She also might have increased difficulty with the changing roles in her life, experiencing heightened ambivalence. She might have difficulty balancing a career with the physical and psychological demands of pregnancy. The sometimes unpredictable nature of pregnancy, labor, and life with a newborn may challenge a woman who may have developed a predictable life over which she has much control (Carolan, 2005; Dobrzykowski & Stern, 2003; Schardt, 2005).*

■ *Older mothers are more commonly from a higher socioeconomic background and have a greater number of years of education. They are more established in a career, their relationships, and their lifestyles.*

■ *Pregnancy is often chosen and planned. Often it culminates after infertility treatments and the use of reproductive technologies such as in vitro fertilization (IVF) or gamete intrafallopian transfer (GIFT).*

■ *Pregnant women in this age group are highly motivated to seek information about childbirth and parenting from books, friends, and electronic resources.*

Lesbian Mothers

■ Little research has been conducted on the process of maternal adaptation to pregnancy among lesbian women. The lesbian woman faces unique obstacles and challenges in today's health care environment such as homophobic attitudes from some health care professionals.

■ Lesbian women may be more likely to lack social support, particularly from their families of origin. They may be exposed to additional stress due to homophobic attitudes.

■ Finding supportive health care providers with whom they are comfortable disclosing sexual orientation is an important need identified by lesbian women. The role of the woman's partner and legal considerations of the growing family will also affect the lesbian experience of pregnancy (McManus, Hunter, & Renn, 2006; Ross, 2005).

■ Lesbian mothers most commonly plan their pregnancies, conceiving through donor insemination. Many lesbian couples participate in a relatively equal division of child care (Fig. 5-3). These factors can combine to help decrease the stress a lesbian mother might experience and act as protection from perinatal depression (Ross, 2005).

■ Nursing assessments of lesbian women should be adapted accordingly. Nurses need to strive toward the use of inclusive language and avoid making assumptions about a woman's sexual orientation without further information.

Single Parenting

■ The literature reports a higher degree of stress for pregnant single women (e.g., greater anxiety; less tangible, reliable support from family and friends).

■ Single mothers may live at or below the poverty level, facing greater financial challenges, resulting in a higher risk of depression.

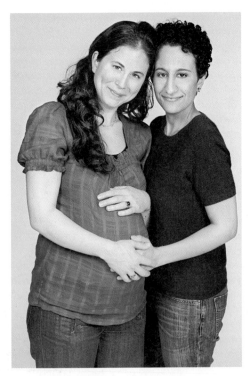

Figure 5-3 Lesbian pregnant couple. (Photo courtesy of Gwen Ortiz and Randi Willis.)

■ Single women engage in the maternal tasks of pregnancy and face more complex tasks and a variety of challenges. With the initial news, the decision must be made whether or not to proceed with the pregnancy.
  ■ *Telling family may cause concern.*
  ■ *Issues regarding legal guardianship in the event she is incapacitated must be considered.*
  ■ *Putting the father's name on the birth certificate is another decision she must make.*

■ The reasons surrounding the pregnancy and the presence or absence of strong support persons can significantly influence her adaptation. Initial assessments are crucial for providing appropriate care:
  ■ *Is the woman single by choice?*
  ■ *Is she a single mother by accident (i.e., death of partner after conception, separation, divorce)?*
  ■ *Did she become pregnant by a casual acquaintance?*

Multifetal Pregnancy

■ A multiple pregnancy (twins, triples, etc.) places added psychosocial stressors on the family unit. The diagnosis shocks many expectant parents, and they may need additional support and education to help them cope with the changes they face. The increased risk for adverse outcomes results in increased fears and anxieties for the pregnant woman.

■ If the woman is found to be carrying more than three fetuses, the parents may receive counseling regarding selective reduction of the pregnancies to reduce the incidence of premature birth and allow the remaining fetuses to grow to term gestation.
  ■ *This situation poses an ethical dilemma and emotional strain for many parents, particularly if they have been attempting to achieve pregnancy for a lengthy time (Begley, 2000; Collopy, 2004; Damato, 2003; Maifeld et al., 2003).*

Socioeconomic Factors

■ The resources of the family to meet the needs for food, shelter, and health care play a crucial role in how a family responds to pregnancy.

■ Financial barriers have been identified as the most important factor contributing to maternal inability to receive adequate prenatal care.

■ The nature of immigrant women's work must also be carefully assessed.
  ■ *Low-income service-oriented work is typical of immigrant populations, and these groups are often marginalized. This puts additional demands on the woman and access to health care may be constrained (Meleis, 2003).*

The Abused Woman

■ Pregnancy can often be a trigger for beginning or increased abuse, or intimate partner violence (see Chapters 4 and 7).

■ Pregnancy offers a unique opportunity for health care providers to recognize abuse and to intervene appropriately.

■ Screen all pregnant women for abuse.

Nursing Actions

■ Assess adaptation to pregnancy at every prenatal visit. Early assessment and intervention may prevent or greatly reduce later problems for the pregnant woman and her family.

■ Identify areas of concern, validate major issues, and make suggestions for possible changes.

■ Refer to the appropriate member of the health care team.
■ Establish a trusting relationship, as women may be reluctant to share information until one has been formed (e.g., questions asked at the first prenatal visit bear repeating with ongoing prenatal care).
■ Use psychosocial health assessment screening tools.
  ■ *A variety of screening tools can be used to assess adaptation to pregnancy and to identify risk factors. Psychosocial assessment reported in the literature ranges from a few questions asked by the health care provider to questionnaires and risk screening tools focusing on a specific area such as depression or abuse (Beck, 2002; Carroll et al., 2005; Midmer, Carroll, Bryanton, & Stewart, 2002; Priest, Austin & Sullivan, 2006; Spietz & Kelly, 2003).*
  ■ *The Antenatal Psychosocial Health Assessment (ALPHA) form, developed in Ontario, Canada has been demonstrated to be a useful evidence-based prenatal tool that can identify women who would benefit from additional support and intervention (Box 5-1) (Carroll et al., 2005; Midmer et al., 2002).*

PATERNAL ADAPTATION DURING PREGNANCY

The news of a pregnancy has a profound effect on the man. Men have fears, questions, and concerns regarding the pregnancy, his partner, and his transition to fatherhood. Each man brings to pregnancy a unique history with which he begins his own experience of becoming a father. Some men relish the role and look forward to actively nurturing a child. Others may be more detached or even hostile to the idea of fatherhood.

Changing cultural and professional attitudes have encouraged fathers' participation in the pregnancy and birth experience.

■ Some fathers respond well to this expectation, wishing to explore every aspect of pregnancy, childbirth, and parenting (May, 1980).
■ Others are more task-oriented and view themselves as managers. They may direct the woman's diet and rest periods and act as coaches during childbirth but remain detached from the emotional aspects of the experience (May, 1980).
■ Some men are more comfortable as observers and prefer not to participate (May, 1980).

BOX 5–1 ANTENATAL PSYCHOSOCIAL HEALTH ASSESSMENT (ALPHA)

Assess the following areas:
■ Social support
■ Recent stressful life events
■ Couple's relationship
■ Onset of prenatal care
■ Plans for prenatal education
■ Feelings toward pregnancy after 20 weeks
■ Relationship with parents in childhood
■ Self-esteem
■ History or psychiatric/emotional problems
■ Depression in this pregnancy
■ Alcohol/drug use
■ Family violence

Source: Carroll, Reid, Biringer, Midmer, Glazier, Wilson, et al. (2005).

■ In some cultures men view pregnancy and childbirth as "women's work" and may be removed from the experience completely (Buist, Morse, & Durkin, 2003; Finnbogadottir, Svalenius, & Persson, 2003).

Effect of Pregnancy on Fathers

■ Concerns about the well-being of his partner are heightened.
■ Worries may be present about whether he and his partner will be good parents.
■ Increased emphasis on his role as provider causes a reevaluation of lifestyle and job or career status.
  ■ *There may be anxiety about providing financial stability for his growing family.*
■ Changes in relationships and roles may challenge expectant fathers, creating the potential for distancing from their partners.
■ The man may struggle at times to feel like he is relevant in the pregnancy related to the focus of prenatal care being on the woman and the growing fetus (Jordan, 1990).
■ Some men are without models to assist them in taking on the role of an active and involved parent (Jordan, 1990).
■ Abuse may begin or escalate with the news of pregnancy. Extramarital affairs may occur.

Developmental Tasks

There is evidence that paternal adaptation involves unique developmental tasks for fathers (Table 5-1). May's classic research (1982) on men identified three phases that fathers experience as the pregnancy progresses:

■ The announcement phase
■ The moratorium phase
■ The focusing phase

These experiences unfold concurrently but in a distinctly different manner than the pregnant woman's adaptive experience.

Nursing Actions

■ Explore the man's response to news of pregnancy.
■ Reassure that ambivalence is common in the early months of pregnancy.
■ Encourage attendance in childbirth classes (i.e., provide resources for classes, discuss advantages of attending classes).
■ Encourage the man to negotiate his role in labor with his partner.
■ Explore his attitudes and expectations of pregnancy, childbirth, and parenting (Critical Component: Nursing Actions that Facilitate Adaptation to Pregnancy)

Couvade Syndrome

■ **Couvade syndrome** is a condition in which men may experience pregnancy symptoms and discomforts similar to those of their pregnant partner.
■ Ritual couvade has been reported as a custom in many societies in which the father takes to his bed as if he himself has suffered the pains of labor, cares for the child, or submits himself to fasting, purification, or various taboos (Murphy, 1992).
■ More current versions of couvade involve the partners of the pregnant woman experiencing pregnancy-like symptoms such as nausea, weight gain, or abdominal pains.

TABLE 5–1   PATERNAL ADAPTATION TO PREGNANCY

ANNOUNCEMENT PHASE	Begins when the news of the pregnancy is revealed. It may last from a few hours to several weeks. Men react to the news of pregnancy with joy, distress, or a combination of emotions, depending on whether the pregnancy is planned or unwanted. It is very common during this phase for men to feel ambivalence. The main developmental task is to accept the biological fact of pregnancy. Men will begin to attempt to take on the expectant father role.
MORATORIUM PHASE	During this phase, many men appear to put conscious thought of the pregnancy aside for some time, even as their partners are undergoing dramatic physical and emotional changes right before their eyes. This can cause potential conflict when women attempt to communicate with their partners about the pregnancy. Sexual adaptation will be necessary; men may fear hurting the fetus during intercourse. Feelings of rivalry may surface as the fetus grows larger and the woman becomes more preoccupied with her own thoughts of impending motherhood. Men's main developmental task during this phase is to accept the pregnancy. This includes accepting the changing body and emotional state of his partner, as well as accepting the reality of the fetus, especially when fetal movement is felt.
FOCUSING PHASE	The focusing phase begins in the last trimester. Men will be actively involved in the pregnancy and relationship with the child. Men begin to think of themselves as fathers. Men participate in planning for labor and delivery, and the newborn. Men's main developmental task is to negotiate with their partner the role they will play in labor and to prepare for parenthood.

Source: May (1982).

Both ritual couvade and the more current versions of couvade have been reported in the literature (Buist et al., 2003; Draper, 2003; Murphy, 1992).

SEXUALITY IN PREGNANCY

Sexuality in pregnancy occurs on a wide continuum of responses for women. Some women feel more beautiful and desirable with advancing pregnancy and others unattractive and ungainly. The sexual relationship can be significantly affected during pregnancy. Physical, emotional and interactional factors all play a part in the womans and her partners sexual reponse during pregnancy.

- The desire for sexual activity varies among pregnant women. Sexual desire can vary even in the same woman at different times during the pregnancy.
  - *During the first trimester, fatigue, nausea, and breast tenderness may affect sexual desire.*
  - *During the second trimester, there may be an increase in desire as a result of increased sense of well-being and the pelvic congestion associated with this time in pregnancy.*
  - *During the third trimester, sexual interest may once again decrease as the enlarging abdomen creates feelings of awkwardness and bulkiness.*
- Women in relationships with established open communication about sexuality are likely to have less difficulty with changes in sexual activity.
- It may be necessary for a couple to modify intercourse positions for the pregnant woman's comfort.
  - *The side-by-side, woman-above, and rear-entry positions are generally more comfortable than the man-above positions.*
- Nonsexual expression of affection is important.

- Common concerns related to sexual activity include:
  - *Fears about hurting the fetus during intercourse or causing permanent anomalies as a result of sexual activity.*
  - *Fear the birth process will drastically change the woman's genitals.*
- Changes in body shape and body image can influence both partners' desire for sexual expression.

Nursing Actions

- Discuss fears and concerns related to sexual activity.
- Encourage communication between partners and discuss possible changes with couples.
  - *Encourage the couple to verbalize fears and to ask questions.*
  - *Use humor and encourage the couple to use humor to relieve anxiety or embarrassment.*
- Advise pregnant women that there are no contraindications to intercourse or masturbation to orgasm provided the woman's membranes are intact, there is no vaginal bleeding, and she has no current problems or history of premature labor (Crooks & Baur, 2007).
- Review sexual positions to increase comfort for couple with advancing pregnancy.
- Discuss alternative forms of sexual expression.

FAMILY ADAPTATION DURING PREGNANCY

The family is the basic structural unit of the community and constitutes one of society's most important institutions. It is a key target for perinatal assessment and intervention. This primary social group assumes major responsibility for the introduction and socialization of children, and forms a potent network of support for its members.

■ The family has traditionally been defined as the fundamental social group in society typically consisting of one or two parents and their children (Friedman, Bowden, & Jones, 2003).

■ The structure of families varies widely among and within cultures. Social scientists now commonly recognize that families exist in a variety of forms, and that during the course of their lives, children may indeed belong to several different family groups.

An understanding of the different family structures and the life cycle of the family and the related developmental tasks can assist the nurse in the development of nursing care during pregnancy.

Changing Structures of the Family

The U.S. census data indicate major shifts in the configuration of families over the past several decades. A woman's family is the primary support during the childbearing year and has a direct influence on her emotional and physical health. It is essential that the nurse identify the woman's definition of family and provide care on that basis.

Nurses must support all types of families. The variety of family configurations includes (Friedman et al., 2003):

■ The nuclear family: A father, mother, and child living together but apart from both sets of grandparents

■ The extended family: Three generations, including married brothers and sisters and their families

■ The single-parent family: Divorced, never married, separated, or widowed man or woman and at least one child

■ Three-generational families: Any combination of first, second, and third generation members living within a household

■ Dyad family: Couple living alone without children

■ Stepparent family: One or both spouses have been divorced or widowed and have remarried into a family with at least one child

■ Blended or reconstituted family: A combination of two families with children from one or both families and sometimes children of the newly married couple

■ Cohabiting family: An unmarried couple living together

■ Gay or lesbian family: A homosexual couple living together with or without children; children may be adopted, from previous relationships, or conceived via artificial insemination

■ Adoptive family: Single persons or couples who have at least one child who is not biologically related to them and to whom they have legally become parents

Eight Stages in the Life Cycle of a Family

Family theorists have identified eight stages in the life cycle of a family that provide a framework for nurses caring for childbearing families (Duvall, 1985; Friedman, et al, 2003):

■ Beginning families
■ Childbearing families
■ Families with preschool children
■ Families with school-aged children
■ Families with teenagers
■ Families launching young adults
■ Middle-aged parents
■ Family in retirement

Each of these stages has developmental tasks that the family needs to accomplish to successfully move to the next stage.

Developmental Tasks

■ The events of pregnancy and childbirth are considered a developmental (maturational) crisis in the life of a family (i.e., those changes associated with normal growth and development).

■ All family members are significantly affected.
  ■ *Previous life patterns may be disturbed and there may be a sense of disorganization.*

■ Certain developmental tasks have been identified which a family must face and master to successfully incorporate a new member into the family unit and allow the family to be ready for further growth and development. The developmental tasks for the childbearing family are:
  ■ *Acquiring knowledge and plans for the specific needs of pregnancy, childbirth, and early parenthood*
  ■ *Preparing to provide for the physical care of the newborn*
  ■ *Adapting financial patterns to meet increasing needs*
  ■ *Realigning tasks and responsibilities*
  ■ *Adjusting patterns of sexual expression to accommodate pregnancy*
  ■ *Expanding communication to meet emotional needs. Reorienting of relationships with relatives*
  ■ *Adapting relationships with friends and community to take account of the realities of pregnancy and the anticipated newborn*

The accomplishment of these tasks during pregnancy lays the groundwork for later adaptation required when the newborn is added to the family unit (Duvall, 1985; Friedman et al., 2003).

Nursing Actions

■ Assess knowledge related to pregnancy, childbirth, and early parenting.

■ Assess progress in developmental tasks of pregnancy.

■ Explore patterns of communications related to emotional needs, responsibilities, and new roles.

■ Include the entire family; assessments and interventions must be considered in a family-centered perspective (Barron, 2001).

■ Provide education and guidance related to pregnancy, childbirth, and early parenting (see Critical Component: Nursing Actions that Facilitate Adaptation to Pregnancy).

GRANDPARENT ADAPTATION

■ Grandparents are often the first family members to be told about the pregnancy. They must make complex adjustments to the news. When it is their first grandchild, most grandparents are delighted. A first pregnancy is also undeniable evidence that they are growing older, and some may respond negatively, indicating that they are not ready to be grandparents.

■ New parents recognize that the tie to the future represented by the fetus is of special significance to grandparents.

■ Grandparents provide a unique sense of family history to expectant parents that may not be available elsewhere. They can be a valuable resource and can strengthen family systems by widening the circle of support and nurturance.

■ Grandparents may be called upon to help with the care and upbringing of the newborn, particularly in the case of adolescent pregnancies. The demands of helping to raise their grandchild may create added stressors in their lives that they may not have anticipated. Community and home-based multigenerational parent support interventions may address some of these concerns (McBride & Shore, 2001; Sadler & Clemmens, 2004).

Nursing Actions

■ Assess the grandparents' response to pregnancy.

■ Explore grandparents as a resource during pregnancy and early parenting.

SIBLING ADAPTATION

Sharing the spotlight with a new brother or sister can be a major crisis for a child. The older child often experiences a sense of loss or feels jealous at being "replaced" by the new sibling. During pregnancy, areas of change that impact siblings the most involve maternal appearance, parental behavior, and changes in the home environment such as sleeping arrangements.

■ Sibling adaptation is greatly influenced by the child's age and developmental level and the attitude of the parents.

   ■ *Children younger than 2 years of age are usually unaware of the pregnancy, and do not understand explanations about the future arrival of the newborn.*

   ■ *Children from 2 to 4 years of age may respond to the obvious changes in their mother's body, but may not remember from month to month why the changes are occurring. This age group is particularly sensitive to disruptions of the physical environment. If the parents plan to change the sibling's sleeping arrangements to accommodate the new baby, these arrangements should be implemented well in advance of the birth. Children still sleeping in a crib should be moved to a bed at least 2 months before the baby is due.*

   ■ *Children ages 4 to 5 often enjoy listening to the fetal heartbeat and may show interest in the development of the fetus. As pregnancy progresses, they may resent the changes in their mother's body that interfere with her ability to lift and hold them, or engage in physical play.*

   ■ *School-age children ages 6 to 12 are usually enthusiastic and keenly interested in the details of pregnancy and birth. They have many questions and are eager to learn. They often plan elaborate welcomes for the newborn and want to be able to help when their new sibling comes home (Fortier, Carson, Will, & Shubkagel, 1991).*

   ■ *Adolescent responses to pregnancy vary according to their developmental status. They may be uncomfortable with the obvious evidence of their parents' sexuality, or be embarrassed by the changes in their mother's appearance. They may be fascinated and repelled by the birth process all at once. Older adolescents may be somewhat indifferent to the changes associated with pregnancy, but also may respond in a more adult fashion by offering support and help.*

■ Expectant parents should make a special effort to prepare and include the older child as much as their developmental age allows. Preparation must be carried out at the child's level of understanding and readiness to learn (Box 5-2).

■ Some children may express interest in being present at the birth. If siblings are to attend the birth, they should participate in a class that prepares them for the event. During the labor and birth, a familiar person who has no other role should be available to explain what is taking place and to comfort or remove them if the situation becomes overwhelming.

Nursing Actions

■ Explore with parents strategies for sibling preparation (see Box 5-2).

■ Discuss strategies to facilitate sibling adaptation based on the child's age and development.

BOX 5–2   TIPS FOR SIBLING PREPARATION

Pregnancy
■ Take the child on a prenatal visit. Let the child listen to the fetal heartbeat and feel the baby move.
■ Take the child to the homes of friends who have babies to given him or her an opportunity to see firsthand what babies are like.
■ Take the child on a tour of the hospital or birthing center. Enroll in a sibling preparation class.

After the Birth
■ Encourage parents to be sensitive to the changes the sibling is experiencing, that jealousy and a sense of loss are normal feelings at this time.
■ Plan for high-quality, uninterrupted time with the older child.
■ Encourage older children to participate in care of their sibling (e.g., bringing a diaper, singing to the baby, sitting with mom during infant feeding times).
■ Teach parents to be watchful when the older child is with the newborn; natural expressions of sibling jealousy may involve rough handling, slapping or hitting, throwing toys, etc.
■ Reassure parents that regressive behaviors in the very young child may be a normal part of sibling adjustment (e.g., return to diapers, wanting to breastfeed or take a bottle, tantrums) and with consistent attention and patience the behaviors will decrease.
■ Praise the child for acting age appropriately; show the child how and where to touch the baby.
■ Encourage sibling visitation while in the hospital; call older children on the phone; have visitors greet the older child before focusing on the newborn.
■ Give a gift to the new sibling from the newborn; let the sibling select a gift for the baby before delivery to bring to the newborn after the birth.

■ Facilitate discussion of the birth plan if parents want the children present during the sibling's birth.

MATERNAL MALADAPTATION TO PREGNANCY

Mental health issues during pregnancy can create problems for the pregnant woman across several dimensions. Difficulty with taking on the maternal role, making the necessary transitions to parenthood, and mourning losses associated with the time before pregnancy are all potential areas of concern. Prenatal depression, maternal stress, and maternal anxiety may have an impact on not only the course of the woman's pregnancy, labor, and birth experience, but also the actual physiology and birth outcome of the developing fetus (Giurgescu, Penckofer, Maurer, & Bryant, 2006; Grussu, 2005; May, 1994; Orr, 2004).

Signs of possible maladaptation:

■ Strong, intense resistance to pregnancy
■ Disabling physical symptoms
■ Quickening experienced as unpleasant; avoidance of maternity clothes
■ Denial of any need to change in couple relationship
■ Total avoidance of sexual contact with partner

- Avoidance of weight gain; strong distress about changing pregnant body
- Denial of fears about childbirth
- Unrealistic expectations about birth
- Lack of preparation for infant

During ongoing assessment of adaptation to pregnancy and the potential for maladaptation to pregnancy, it is essential to assess the pregnant woman's mood, anxiety, and emotional states. During ongoing assessment of mood, anxiety, and emotional status, consider three aspects: frequency, duration, and intensity of woman's response to pregnancy (Simpson & Creehan, 2008). If a woman is having difficulty functioning in her daily life and having difficulty coping, referral to mental health services is necessary. Collaborating with colleagues and referrals to other health professionals is essential to ensure good care.

Nursing Actions

- Assess the woman's mood, anxiety, and emotional state.
- Assess the woman's support system and coping mechanisms.
- Discuss expectations about pregnancy, childbirth, and parenting.
- Make appropriate referrals to other health professionals when needed.

PSYCHOSOCIAL ADAPTATION TO PREGNANCY COMPLICATIONS

The majority of the time, pregnancy progresses with few problems and results in generally positive outcomes. With the diagnosis of pregnancy complications, normal concerns and anxieties of pregnancy are exacerbated even more. Uncertainty of fetal outcome can interfere with maternal and paternal attachment.

- Response to pregnancy complication depends on:
  - *Pregnancy condition*
  - *Perceived threat to mother or fetus*
  - *Coping skills*
  - *Available support*
- Disequilibrium, feelings of powerlessness, increased anxiety and fear, and a sense of loss are all responses to the news of a pregnancy complication.
- The pregnant woman may distance herself emotionally from the fetus as she faces varying levels of uncertainty about the pregnancy, impacting attachment (Gilbert, 2007).
- Events such as antepartal hospitalization or activity restrictions may contribute to a greater incidence of depression in the pregnant woman.
- The risk of crisis for the pregnant woman and her family clearly increases due to an unpredictable or uncertain pregnancy outcome (Durham, 1998).
- How a woman and her family respond to this additional stress is crucial in determining whether a crisis will develop.
  - *Realistic perception of the event, adequate situational support, and positive coping mechanisms are all factors that help a woman maintain her equilibrium and avoid crisis.*
  - *Poor self-esteem, lack of confidence in the mothering role, and an inability to communicate concerns to health care providers and close family members are all factors that increase the risk of crisis.*

Nursing Actions

When caring for a pregnant woman with complications, the first priority is to reestablish and maintain physiological stability. However, nurses must also be able to intervene to promote psychosocial adaptation to the news of pregnancy complications (Giurgescu et al., 2006; May, 1994; Mattson & Smith, 2004). (See Concept Map: Maternal Adaptation to Pregnancy Complication.)

The following actions can assist to reduce or limit the detrimental effects of complications on individual or family functioning:

- Provide frequent and clear explanations about the problem, planned interventions, and therapy.
- Assess and encourage the use of the woman's support systems.
- Support individual adaptive coping mechanisms.
- Make appropriate referrals when additional assistance is needed.

SOCIAL SUPPORT DURING PREGNANCY

Social support refers to that support given by someone with whom the expectant mother has a personal relationship. It involves the primary groups of most importance to the individual woman (material, emotional, informational, and comparison support).

- Material support, or instrumental support, consists of practical help such as assistance with chores, meals, and managing finances.
- Emotional support involves support that gives affection, approval, encouragement, and feelings of togetherness.
- Informational support consists of sharing information and helping women investigate new sources of information.
- Comparison support consists of help given by someone in a similar situation. Their shared information is useful and credible because they are experiencing or have experienced the same events in their lives.

Social support is not generally considered professional support, although professionals can provide supportive actions such as counseling, teaching, role modeling, or problem solving. When expectant mothers have no other means of support, some community programs will employ paraprofessionals to visit expectant mothers, providing education and social support. Programs that capitalize on the skills of experienced mothers living in the communities may be less expensive and more culturally sensitive than purely hospital-based programs led by teams of health care professionals. Post-delivery follow-up programs offering home-based social support may also have important benefits for socially disadvantaged mothers and children (Cannella, 2006; Dawley & Beam, 2005; Logsdon, 2000; Logsdon et al., 2005).

Social Support Research

- The predominant sources of support for the pregnant woman are her spouse or partner and her mother. A high-quality relationship with one's partner has a positive effect on physical and emotional well being (Logsdon, 2000).
- Research from several disciplines provides evidence for the importance of social support for the pregnant woman's health, positive adaptation to pregnancy, and the prevention of pregnancy complications. It is a naturally occurring resource that can prevent health problems and complications and promote health. Receiving adequate help from others enhances self-esteem and feelings of being in control (Evidence-Based Practice: Measurable Outcomes of Social Support Interventions). Women who have little support during pregnancy are more likely to begin prenatal care late and experience depression during pregnancy and postpartum (Beeber & Canuso, 2005; Giurgescu et al., 2006; Logsdon, 2000; Logsdon et al., 2005; Mercer, 1995; Orr, 2004; Tilden, 1983).
- Social support benefits the expectant mother the most when it matches the pregnant woman's expectations ("perceived social

support"). It is important that the woman identify and clarify her expectations and needs for support. Perceived support expectations that do not materialize for the pregnant woman can lead to increased distress and problems with adaptation to pregnancy (Nichols & Humenick, 2000).

■ Pregnant women frequently need social support that differs from that which they receive. Nurses can advise the pregnant woman how best to use her existing support networks or how to expand her support network so her needs are met. Nurses have the opportunity and responsibility to help women explore potential sources of support such as childbirth education classes, church, work, or school. High-risk populations including adolescents, women with pregnancy complications, and low-income women may need particular direction from nurses in obtaining adequate support (Beeber & Canuso, 2005; Logsdon et al., 2005).

■ A woman's cultural background influences the amount of social support received and who provides this support. Women in cultures that value individualism, self-sufficiency, and independence may have more difficulty receiving social support than women from a culture who values interdependence and collectivism (Meleis, 2003).

■ Recent immigrants face many challenges in obtaining needed social support. The disruption of lifelong attachments can cause anxieties and a sense of disorientation. Language barriers and socioeconomic struggles are additional stressors facing immigrant women, creating a higher risk for depression (Zelkowitz et al., 2004). Their families, experiencing the same difficulties, may not be able to provide sufficient support. Further research is needed in the area of examining the impact of culture on social support.

Assessing Social Support

Assessing social support is a crucial component of prenatal care. The following areas of assessment should be addressed when planning care:

■ Who is available to help provide support? Who is available to provide each type of support (material, emotional, informational, and comparison)? Is the support adequate in each category?

■ With whom does the pregnant woman have the strongest relationships and what type of support is provided by these individuals?

■ Is there conflict in relationships with support providers?

■ Is there potential for improvement of the woman's support network? Should members who provide more stress than support be deleted? Should new members be added?

■ Who are the people living with the pregnant woman?

■ Who assists with household chores?

■ Who assists with child care and parenting activities?

■ Who does the pregnant woman turn to when problems occur or during a crisis?

Nursing Actions

Because there is good evidence that social support improves pregnancy outcomes, the nurse has a role in providing support to women (Lodgson, 2000).

■ Provide opportunities for the woman to ask for support, and rehearse with her appropriate language to use in asking for support.

■ Invite key support providers to attend prenatal and postpartum visits.

■ Facilitate supportive functioning and interactions within the family.

■ Encourage the pregnant woman to interact with other pregnant or postpartum women she knows.

■ Suggest church, health clubs, work, and/or school as sites to meet women with similar interests and concerns.

■ Provide information regarding community resources.

Evidence-Based Practice: Measurable Outcomes of Social Support Interventions

■ Attachment to infant and improved interactions with infant
■ Compliance with health care regimen
■ Improved functional status
■ Improved coping
■ Improved birth outcomes (e.g., fewer low birth weight infants)
■ Increased incidence of breastfeeding
■ Reduced physical symptoms
■ Reduced loneliness
■ Satisfaction with support
■ Satisfaction with intimate relationships

Adapted from Logdson, C. (2000). Social support for pregnant and postpartum women. Washington, DC: Association of Women's Health, Obstetric and Neonatal Nurses.

CHILDBEARING AND CULTURE

Statistics of U.S. Population

Estimates indicate that by the year 2050, more than 50% of the U.S. population will be made up of ethnic minorities (Martin, Hamilton, Sutton, Ventura, Menacker, & Kimeyer, 2006). From a global perspective, the movement of immigrants, refugees, and their families worldwide has resulted in increasingly diverse populations. With such dramatic population shifts, it is critical that nurses develop skills to provide quality care to culturally divergent groups. Expectations of nursing practice will increasingly demand sensitivity to the cultural needs of families and competence in providing care.

Behavioral Practices

Every culture has a set of behaviors, beliefs, and practices that influence women and their families profoundly during childbearing.

■ Preventing harm to the fetus and ensuring a safe and easy birth are common themes through various cultures.

■ Common themes influencing labor and delivery include general attitudes toward birth, preferred positions, methods of pain management, and the role of family members and the health care provider.

■ The postpartum period is generally considered to be a time of increased vulnerability for both mothers and babies, influencing care of the new mother as well as infant care practices related to bathing, swaddling, feeding, umbilical cord care, and circumcision (Lauderdale, 2007; Mattson & Smith, 2004).

■ Pregnancy and childbirth may elicit certain customs, beliefs, and behaviors during pregnancy about acceptable and unacceptable practices that have implications for planning nursing care and interventions. Take all of these beliefs and behaviors into consideration when assessing and promoting adaptation to pregnancy (Box 5-3).

BOX 5–3 CULTURAL PRESCRIPTIONS, RESTRICTIONS, AND TABOOS

Prescriptive Beliefs

- Remain active during pregnancy to aid the baby's circulation (Crow Indian).
- Remain happy to bring the baby joy and good fortune (Navajo, Mexican, Japanese).
- Drink chamomile tea to ensure an effective labor (Hispanic).
- Soup with ginseng root is a good general strength tonic (Asian).
- Pregnancy cravings need to be satisfied or the baby will be born with a birthmark (Hispanic).
- Sleeping flat on your back protects the fetus from harm (Mexican).
- Attach a safety pin to an undergarment protects the fetus from cleft lip or palate (Hispanic).

Restrictive Beliefs

- Do not have your picture taken because it might cause still-birth (African American).
- Avoid sexual intercourse during the third trimester because it will cause respiratory distress in the newborn (Southeast Asian).
- Coldness in any form may cause arthritis or other chronic illness (Korean).
- Avoid seeing an eclipse of the moon because it will result in a cleft lip or palate (Hispanic).
- Do not reach over your head or the cord will wrap around the baby's neck (African American, White, Hispanic, Asian).

Taboos

- Avoid funerals and visits from widows or women who have lost children because they will bring bad fortune to the baby (Asian).
- Avoid hot and spicy foods as they can cause overexcitement for the pregnant woman (Hindu).
- An early baby shower will invite the evil eye (mal ojo) and should be avoided (Hispanic, Arab).
- Avoid praising the newborn; it will call the attention of the gods to the vulnerable infant (Asian).

Source: Lauderdale (2007).

- ***Prescriptive behavior*** *is an expected behavior of the pregnant woman during the childbearing period.*
- ***Restrictive behavior*** *describes activities during the childbearing period that are limited for the pregnant woman.*
- ***Taboos*** *are cultural restrictions believed to have serious supernatural consequences.*

Throughout the childbearing cycle, cultural background provides a framework within which each woman and her family can think, make decisions, and act (Callister, 2001a; Lauderdale, 2007).

Barriers to Culturally Competent Care

Mainstream models of obstetric care as practiced in North America can present a strange and confusing picture to many women from different ethnic backgrounds. With the predominant culture's emphasis on formal prenatal care, technology, hospital deliveries, and a bureaucratic health care system, conflict with traditional cultures can be inevitable. Immigrant and ethnic minority women may have experienced vastly different models of care in their home country, town, reservation, or family of origin. Health care decisions may be influenced by the elderly members of the family (e.g., grandmothers have historically played an influential role in women's health care) (Meleis, 2003).

If pregnancy is considered a normal and healthy event, prenatal care may be delayed. Fear or modesty may prevent other women from seeking care. Barriers to seeking cultural competent care include:

- Protocols, a strange environment, and health care providers who speak only English all create barriers that confuse and intimidate. The American way of birth may seem as foreign to people outside the United States as non-American ways do to U.S. health professionals (Meleis, 2003).
- Nurses' attitudes can also create barriers to culturally competent care. **Ethnocentrism,** the belief that the customs and values of the dominant culture are preferred or superior in some way, create obstacles that can make culturally sensitive care challenging to implement. The challenges are compounded by the fact that only 12% of registered nurses come from racial or ethnic minority backgrounds (US Department of Heath and Human Services, 2004).
- In recent years, nurses have attempted to incorporate individual beliefs and cultural practices into health care to raise the quality of care and improve outcomes. Mandates from professional health care accrediting bodies have also signaled a nationwide commitment to providing sensitive and competent cultural care:
    - *The Joint Commission has mandated a plan of patient care that includes cultural and spiritual assessments and interventions (www.jointcommission.org; Andrews & Boyle, 2007).*
    - *The American Association of Colleges of Nursing (AACN) has stated that "nursing graduates should have the knowledge and skills to provide holistic care that addresses the needs of diverse populations" (Callister, 2001a).*
    - *Cultural competence is addressed explicitly in the DHHS Healthy People 2010 focus area of health communications, stating that cultural sensitivity is necessary for effective communication with individuals and the public to stimulate systems change and to influence health behavior (Callister, 2001a).*

Cultural Groups in the United States

- The U.S. Census Bureau identifies five major cultural groups in the United States: African American/blacks, American Indian/Alaska Native, Asian American/Pacific Islander, Hispanic/Latino, and white/Caucasian. The Arab-American and Jewish populations together comprise another 2% to 3% of the total population (Callister, 2001a; Kridi, 2002; Semenic, Callister & Feldman, 2004).
- All nursing care is given within the context of many cultures (that of the patient, nurse, health care system, and the larger culture of the society). The following descriptions of various populations must be reviewed within a context of diversity within each group. Many women follow only some or few of the typical customs of their cultural groups. A holistic approach to care provides the most effective outcomes (Meleis, 2003).

African American/Blacks

- 12.9% of the population
- Ethnic origins include Africa and the Caribbean Islands, including West Indies, Dominican Republic, Haiti, and Jamaica; languages spoken may include French, Spanish, African dialects, and various regional forms of English.

- Strong religious commitment
- 51% single-parent families with female head of household, extensive networks of extended families
- Infant mortality rates twice those of the overall population
- Becoming a mother at young age accepted
- Comfortable with touch, physical contact, and emotional sharing
- Pregnancy considered a state of wellness and often a reason for delay in seeking prenatal care
- Use of pica (eating nonedible substances)
- Beliefs: Having a picture taken during pregnancy will cause stillbirth; reaching up will cause the cord to strangle the baby
- Low-income populations may fear public clinics or hospitals (Andrews & Boyle, 2007; Purnell & Paulanka, 2008; St. Hill, 2003).

Arab American

- 0.5% to 1% of the population
- Ethnic origins include Saudi Arabia, Yemen, Iran, Iraq, Jordan, Syria, Egypt, and Lebanon
- Religious traditions: Muslim and Christian
- Western medicine generally highly valued, although recent immigrants do not usually engage in preventive medicine and may not seek prenatal care; medical care seen as unnecessary unless there are complications
- Sons highly valued as a source of economic security
- Pregnant women seek most knowledge from female relatives
- Excessive planning seen as defying God's will and risking bringing the "evil eye" to mother or baby
- Special attention given to nutrition for the pregnant woman (e.g., Muslim pregnant women exempted from daily fasting during holy month of Ramadan)
- Muslim dietary laws prohibit pork and alcoholic beverage
- Labor and birth strictly female; husband's participation is not expected
- Very vocal and expressive of emotions during labor
- Expected to remain in bed or stay at home for 40 days after birth
- Breastfeeding expected (Kridi, 2002)

Asian American

- 4% of population
- Ethnic origins include China, Japan, Korea, the Philippines, Vietnam, Cambodia and Laos, as well as the Indian subcontinent and the Pacific Islands, with a great diversity of languages and dialects.
- Philosophical traditions of Buddhism, Hinduism, and Christianity. Pregnancy seen as natural process; childbearing a family-centered event
- Belief in the polarity of yin/yang as major life force: Health requires a balance between cold (yin) and heat (yang).
- Pregnancy considered a "hot" condition that is depleted during birth; balance must be restored after delivery by avoidance of "cold" foods (fruits and beverages), staying indoors, avoiding baths and showers for 30 days, wearing more clothing.
- Breastfeeding may be delayed because colostrum thought to be harmful.
- May omit prenatal vitamins during pregnancy as they are considered "hot" medications.
- Avoid public displays of affection

- Traditional therapies often used concurrently with Western medicine (Callister, 2001b; Purnell & Paulanka, 2008)

Caucasian/European American

- 81% of population (dominant culture)
- Ethnic origins include Europe and North Africa and parts of the Middle East.
- Pregnancy viewed as a condition that requires medical attention to ensure health
- Emphasis on early prenatal care, participation in childbirth education, father participation
- Technology driven, with written sources of information valued
- May encounter "premium birth/baby syndrome": Middle-class couples expecting to have a small family will do everything in their power to ensure a good outcome.
- May disdain those who fail to eliminate unhealthy practices, such as smoking.
- May lead to intense self-doubt and guilt if expectations for a "good birth" and a healthy newborn are not met. This may be true even if the outcome was not preventable (Callister, 2001b; May, 1994).

Hispanic

- 10.2% of the population, most rapidly growing ethnic group in United States
- Ethnic origins include Mexico, Puerto Rico, Cuba, Spain, and South or Central America.
- Assimilation is minimal, with strongly held cultural beliefs and behaviors; Catholic church strong influence
- Strong family relationships and loyalty valued over individual choice; motherhood highly esteemed
- Early marriage is more common than in general population; childbearing is seen as the duty of a married woman.
- The man is the unquestioned head of the family; "machismo" a predominant cultural expectation for men (strong, in control, and the providers for their families).
- Very modest; may be unacceptable and frightening to have pelvic exam by male health care provider
- Pregnancy is a delicate and perilous time for the fetus; the goal is to maintain a state of equilibrium and harmony between natural and supernatural forces of the world.
- Female relatives active in pregnancy support
- Strong cultural preference for sons
- Elderly well respected
- Beliefs: "*Mal ojo*" (evil eye): A fixed stare will result in illness and "susto": folk illness that occurs if pregnant woman attends a funeral; avoid milk because it causes large babies and a difficult birth; unsatisfied food cravings will cause a birthmark
- Folk medicine (*curanderismo*) frequently used (Callister, 2001b; Harley & Eskenazi, 2006; Jiminez, 1995)

Jewish

- 1.8% of U.S. population; 40% of world Jewish population lives in United States
- Extent of religious observance is highly variable among Jews of differing degrees of orthodoxy and assimilation.
- Birth and childrearing are central to the Orthodox Jewish culture.
- Some women feel moral responsibility to bring "just one more child" into the world because of the destruction of their ancestors during the Holocaust.

- Circumcision performed on all male children on the eighth day of life by a mohel (skilled circumcisionist)
- Orthodox dietary laws prohibit pork, predatory fowl, shellfish, blood by ingestion, and the mixing of dairy and meat dishes at the same meal; foods should be kosher (i.e., properly preserved and animals ritually slaughtered)
- Ritual cleansing bath 7 days after cessation of any blood flow (menses or postpartum lochia)
- Strong relationship between health status and spiritual well-being (Callister, 2001b; Semenic et al., 2004)

Native American

- 0.9% of the population, high unemployment, poverty, lack of education compared to general population
- Ethnic origins include American Indian, Eskimo, and Aleut
- Higher unemployment, poverty, lack of education compared to general population
- Greater pregnancy risks related to diabetes, alcohol use, and smoking
- Strong spiritual foundation with holistic focus on "Mother Earth"
- Traditional stories, songs, and dances highly valued, respect for ancestors and elders
- May avoid eye contact and limit touch
- Pregnancy considered special time during which actions and thoughts should be as positive as possible
- Prenatal care may be delayed.
- Umbilical cord may be saved after delivery due to a belief in its spiritual significance (Callister, 2001b; Roberts, 2003).

Culturally Competent Nursing Practice

- Nurses have an obligation to provide to patients and their families effective, understandable, and respectful care in a manner that is compatible with their cultural beliefs, practices and preferred language.
- It may be unrealistic for any individual nurse to be familiar with every cultural variation. However, if the nurse is willing to maintain an open attitude and a sensitivity to differences, the chances of providing culturally competent care increase greatly (Fuller, 2003).
- Nurses must be able to differentiate among beliefs and practices that are harmful, benign, and health promoting. When considering a cultural practice, three crucial questions present themselves to the nurse:
  - *Is the practice safe?*
  - *Is it feasible?*
  - *Is it important to the woman?*
- Nurses need to keep in mind that few cultural customs related to pregnancy are dangerous; although they might cause a woman to limit her activity and her exposure to some aspects of life, they are rarely harmful to her or her fetus (see Box 5-3).
- Nurses need to be careful to avoid **cultural stereotyping**, or making sweeping generalizations about women based on their ethnicity. Because of the complex dimensions of culture, simplistic assumptions should be avoided.
  - *Cultural practices or beliefs may not apply to all individuals, and a great deal of diversity is found among women of any ethnic group. Educational background, family heritage, social class, economic factors, work/occupational experience, urban/rural origin, length of time in the United States (or place of migration), and a variety of individual characteristics or choices such as sexual orientation,*

disability, and strength of ethnic identity all influence how women experience health and illness (Machado, 2001; Meleis, 2003).
  - *Socioeconomic factors may be blended with culturally influenced patterns of behavior. Variations that appear to be cultural may actually be a reflection of socioeconomic conditions in which many minority groups live. This arises in part because ethnic minorities tend to be poorer than European Americans, are overrepresented among the very poor, and have fewer opportunities for education and upward mobility. The economic gap accentuates differences and soon the assumption is made that observed differences are cultural in origin (May, 1994).*

Cultural Assessment

When considering cultural aspects of care for expectant families answer a variety of questions (Andrews & Boyle, 2007):

- What is the woman's predominant culture? To what degree does the client identify with the cultural group?
- What language does the client speak at home? What are the styles of nonverbal communication?
- How does the women's culture influence her beliefs about pregnancy and childbirth? Is pregnancy considered a state of illness or health? Are there particular attitudes toward age at the time of pregnancy? Marriage? Who would be an acceptable father or partner? What is considered acceptable in terms of pregnancy frequency?
- Are there cultural prescriptions, restrictions, or taboos related to certain activities, dietary practices, or expressions of emotion? What does the pregnant woman consider to be normal practice during pregnancy, birth, postpartum?
- How does the culture interpret and respond to experiences of pain?
- How is modesty expressed by men and women?
- Are there culturally defined expectations about male–female relationships?
- What is the client's educational background? Does it affect her knowledge level concerning the health care delivery system, teaching/learning, written material given?
- How does the client relate to persons outside her cultural group? Does she prefer a caregiver with the same cultural background?
- What is the role of religious beliefs related to pregnancy and childbirth?

Nursing Actions

With the increasingly diverse patient population it is imperative nurses provide culturally sensitive care. Culturally sensitive health care does not require professionals to become experts in cultural differences in health practices; however, it is important that professionals acknowledge belief and value systems different from their own, and consider these differences when delivering care to childbearing women and their families (Box 5-4). Nursing actions that facilitate culturally appropriate care are (Callister, 2001a, 2001b; Leininger, 1991; Purnell & Paulanka, 2008; Willis, 1999):

- Enhance communication.
  - *Greet respectfully.*
  - *Establish rapport.*
  - *Demonstrate empathy and interest.*
  - *Listen actively.*
- Emphasize the woman's strengths; consider each woman's individuality regarding how they conform to traditional values and norms.

BOX 5–4   ACHIEVING CULTURAL COMPETENCE

Strategies for Achieving Cultural Competence
- Maintain an open attitude.
- Recognize yourself as a part of the diversity in society and acknowledge your own belief system.
- Be aware of your own biases and assumptions, and that you are most likely carrying cultural, racial, or ethnic "baggage."
- Confront your own issues about genetically determined attributes.
- Avoid preconceptions and cultural stereotyping.
- Talk to another person about mainstream society's definitions and images of white, black, brown, red, and yellow.
- Acknowledge the power you have to use professional privilege positively or negatively.
- Recall your commitment to "individualized care," "respect," and "professionalism."
- Identify whom the client calls "family."
- Include notes on cultural preferences and family strengths and resources as part of all intake and ongoing assessments and nursing care plans.
- Use the cultural wisdom (beliefs, values, customs, and habits) of the client to shape his or her participation in health practices and care plans.
- Seek out culture-friendly teaching and assessment tools.
- Review the literature to generate a culture database.
- Read literature from other cultures.
- Discourage negativism and discrimination on the unit.
- Participate in professional development/continuing education programs that address cultural competence.
- Recognize that all care is given within the context of many cultures.
- Develop linguistic skills related to your patient population.
- Learn to use nonverbal communication in an appropriate way.
- Learn about the communication patterns of various cultures.

Sources: Willis (1999); Simpson, Creehan, & Association of Women's Health, Obstetrics and Neonatal Nursing (2008).

- If proposed practices are not harmful, allow them to continue.
- If proposed practices are harmful, attempt to alter behaviors to include more beneficial ones.
- Accommodate cultural practices as appropriate.
- Identify who the client calls "family."
- Determine who family decision makers are and include them.
- Provide an interpreter when necessary.
  - *Use language assistance devises.*
  - *Many agencies use "translator telephones" to ensure that patients receive professionally accurate and confidential translation services.*
- Recognize that a patient agreeing and nodding "yes" to the nurse's instruction or questions may not always guarantee comprehension.
- Use nonverbal communication and visual aids in an appropriate way.
- When providing patient education, include family and elicit support from the established caretakers in the family (i.e., grandmother, aunt, etc.).
- Demonstrate how scientific and folk practices can be combined to provide optimal care.

PLANNING FOR BIRTH

Planning and preparing for childbirth requires many decisions by the woman and her family during pregnancy (i.e., choosing a provider, choosing a place of birth, planning for the birth, and preparing for labor through education). These choices affect how the woman approaches her pregnancy, and can contribute significantly to a positive adaptation.

Choosing a Provider

One of the first decisions a woman makes is who will be her care provider during her pregnancy and childbirth. This important decision also influences where her birth will take place.

Physicians

- Obstetricians and family practice physicians attend approximately 91% of births in the United States. Most physicians manage birth in a hospital setting.
- Care often includes pharmacological and medical management of problems as well as use of technological procedures.
- They see both low- and high-risk patients.

Midwives

- The focus of midwifery is on noninterventionist care, with an emphasis on the normalcy of the birth process.
- Most births are managed in hospital settings or alternative birth centers; a small number may be managed in a home setting.
- In many countries, midwives are the primary providers of care for healthy pregnant women, and physicians are consulted when medical or surgical intervention is required (Kennedy & Shannon, 2004).
- Nurse-midwives are registered nurses with advance training in care of obstetric patients. They provide care for about 10% of births in the United States and Canada, usually seeing low-risk patients. Nurse-midwives practice with physicians or independently with a contracted health care provider agency for physician backup.
- Lay midwives, or independent midwives, are nonprofessional caregivers. Their training varies greatly, from being self-taught to having formal training. They manage about 1% of the births in the United States and Canada, with the majority taking place in the home setting.
- Direct entry midwives are trained in midwifery schools or universities as a profession distinct from nursing. Increasing numbers of midwives in the United Kingdom and Ireland fall into this category.
- Given the variations in midwifery training and knowledge, pregnant women considering midwifery care may need education and information regarding the experience and credentials of the midwife providing their care in order to make informed decisions (Box 5-5).

Choosing a Place of Birth

Hospitals

- In the United States, approximately 99% of all births take place in hospital settings.
- Hospital maternity services can vary greatly, from traditional labor and delivery rooms with separate newborn and postpartum units, to in-hospital birth centers.

BOX 5–5   PROFESSIONAL POSITION STATEMENT: AWHONN POSITION STATEMENT ON MIDWIFERY

AWHONN supports the practice of the certified nurse-midwife as a primary care provider who is prepared to independently manage most aspects of women's health care. The certified nurse-midwife's practice should include appropriate professional consultation, collaboration, and referral as indicated by the health status of the patient and applicable state and federal laws.

Background
AWHONN identifies a wide range of disparate educational requirements and certification standards in the United States that fall under the umbrella category of midwifery. The following titles are attributed to midwives without prior nursing credentials who are not graduates of ACNM-accredited programs: direct entry, lay, licensed, or professional. Direct entry midwives cover the spectrum from the doctorally prepared European midwife to the self-taught, beginning practitioner.

The wide range of what is actually meant by the designation, "midwife," can easily confuse consumers, health care institutions, and legislators. Definitions of various certification levels are:

- CNM: Certified Nurse-Midwife (administered by ACNM)
- CM: Certified Midwife (administered by ACNM)
- CPM: Certified Professional Midwife [administered by NARM (North American Registry of Midwives)]. Also referred to as *direct entry, lay,* or *licensed midwife.*
- Midwives with a state license or permit (administered on a state-by-state basis). Also referred to as *direct entry, lay,* or *licensed midwife.*
- Midwives without formal credentials (no administrative oversight). Also referred to as *direct entry* or *lay midwife.*

Individual state-by-state laws govern the practice of midwifery in the United States. Certified nurse-midwives and certified midwives often practice in collaboration and consultation with other health care professionals to provide primary, gynecological, and maternity care to women in the context of the larger health care system. Certified nurse-midwives may have prescriptive privileges, admitting privileges to hospitals, and may own and/or manage freestanding practices. The scope of practice for a direct entry, or lay, midwife who is not ACC-accredited is typically limited to the practice of home birth or birth center options for women, but varies according to state-by-state regulations.

Association of Women's Health, Obstetric and Neonatal Nurses (AWHONN). (2000b). Policy position statement: Midwifery. *Washington, DC: Author.*

- Labor, delivery, and recovery rooms (LDRs) may be available in which the expectant mother is admitted, labors, gives birth, and spends the first several hours of recovery.
- In labor, delivery, recovery, and postpartum units (LDRPs), the mother remains in the same room for her entire hospital stay.

Birth Centers

- Free-standing birth centers are usually built in locations separate from the hospital but may be located nearby in case transfer of the woman or newborn is needed.
- Only women at low risk for complications are included in care.

- Birth centers are usually staffed by nurse-midwives or physicians who also have privileges at the local hospital.
- They offer homelike accommodations, with emergency equipment available but stored out of view.

Home Births

- Home births are popular in European countries such as Sweden and the Netherlands.
- In developing countries, home birth may be a necessity due to the lack of hospitals or adequate birthing facilities. In North America, home births account for fewer than 1% of births.
- Home births allow the expectant family to be in control of the experience, and the mother may be more relaxed than in the hospital environment. It may be less expensive, and there may be decreased risk of serious infection.
- Many physicians and nurses believe home birth exposes the mother and fetus to unnecessary danger. Consequently they are not widely accepted by the North American medical community, making it difficult for a woman to find a qualified health care provider willing to give prenatal care and attend the birth.
- There is agreement that if home birth is the woman's choice, the following criteria will promote a safe home birth experience:
  - *The woman must be comfortable with her decision.*
  - *The woman should be in good health. Home birth is not appropriate for a high-risk pregnancy.*
  - *A hospital should be no more than a 10- to 15-minute drive.*
  - *The woman should be attended by a well-trained physician or midwife with adequate medical supplies and resuscitation equipment.*

The Birth Plan

- A birth plan is a tool by which parents can explore their childbirth options and choose those that are most important to them. A written birth plan can help women clarify their desires and expectations and communicate those desires with their care providers (Lothian, 2006).
- Birth plans typically emphasize specific requests for labor and immediate post-delivery care. Some involve expectations surrounding postpartum and newborn care as well.
- The birth plan document can be inserted into the woman's prenatal record or hospital chart as a way of communicating with care providers.

The Doula

- The word "doula" comes from ancient Greek and means "woman's servant" (International Childbirth Education Association, 1999).
- A doula is a trained individual who provides support to women and their partners during labor, birth, and postpartum, but not clinical care.
- Continuous support by a trained doula during labor has been associated with shorter labors, decreased need for analgesics, decreased need for many forms of medical interventions, and increased maternal satisfaction (Campbell, Lake, Falk, & Backstrand, 2006; Pascali-Bonaro & Kroeger, 2004; Sauls, 2002; Scott, Berkowitz, & Klaus, 1999; Yogev, 2004).

Childbirth Education

- The roots of prenatal education began in the early 1900s with classes in maternal hygiene, nutrition, and baby care taught by the American Red Cross in New York City.

- Childbirth education as we know it today developed as a consumer response to the increasing medical control and technological management of normal labor and birth during the 1950s and 1960s in Europe and North America.
- Early proponents of childbirth education such as Lamaze, Bradley, and Dick-Read focused primarily on the prevention of pain in childbirth. Methods of "natural childbirth" (Dick-Read), "psychoprophylaxis" (Lamaze), and "husband coached childbirth" (Bradley) attained great popularity among middle-class groups.
- Since that time, the distinctions between the schools of prepared childbirth have faded, and many childbirth educators present an eclectic approach to labor techniques (Nichols & Humenick, 2000). The content of childbirth education classes has also greatly expanded, assisting women and their families to make informed decisions about pregnancy and birth based on knowledge of their options and choices.
- Specialized classes have been developed to meet the needs of specific groups as well (e.g., classes for breastfeeding, sibling preparation, early pregnancy, refresher, or prenatal/postpartum exercise). Programs have been developed for adolescents, mothers expecting twins, and mothers older than age 35. Nurses and childbirth educators have played an important role in the development of these innovative education programs (Enkin et al., 2000).
- Professional organizations including ICEA, Lamaze International, and AWHONN have all published position papers that delineate expectations of basic components of prenatal education (AWHONN, 2000a). Through the development of position papers as well as teacher training and certification programs, these organizations have ensured that childbirth educators have a sound knowledge base and specific competencies. Leaders of these organizations have demonstrated the further influence of this specialty by successfully convincing committee members of the *Healthy People 2010* program to include in their list of objectives one that is committed to "increasing the proportion of pregnant women who attend a formal series of prepared childbirth classes" (Nichols & Humenick, 2000).
- Childbirth education is to promote the competence of expectant parents in meeting the challenges of childbirth and early parenting. The focus is on promoting healthy pregnancy and birth outcomes and facilitating a positive transition to parenting.

Class content typically includes the physical and emotional aspects of pregnancy, childbirth and early parenting, coping skills, and labor support techniques. Values clarification and informed decision making are emphasized, as well as the promotion of wellness behaviors. Pregnant women are encouraged to identify their own unique goals for childbirth, balancing these aims within the existing health care system and their own personal situation, and moving toward their fulfillment (Box 5-6) (Nichols & Humenick, 2000).

- Childbirth classes remain a popular and well established component of care during the childbearing year. As the body of research on childbirth and childbirth education increases and as more childbirth educators use research findings as a basis for their teaching, evidence-based practice will be enhanced (Evidence-Based Practice: Effectiveness of Antenatal Education).
- In addition to attending classes, there are books, pamphlets, magazines, and videos aimed at childbearing women and their families. The Internet is a widely used resource for information and advice (Box 5-7).

BOX 5–6 PERINATAL EDUCATION: SAMPLE CONTENT OF A 6-WEEK CHILDBIRTH PREPARATION SERIES

Week 1
- Introductions
- Overview of childbirth education: Rationale and pain theory
- Physical and emotional changes of pregnancy; fetal development
- Nutrition, exercise, and self-care during pregnancy
- Introduction to breathing and relaxation techniques

Week 2
- Signs of labor
- Stages and phases of labor and delivery
- Labor support techniques; the role of the support person in labor
- Practice of breathing and relaxation techniques

Week 3
- Labor review, incorporating labor support techniques and nonpharmacological comfort strategies
- Birth options and birth plans: Developing advocacy skills
- Pharmacological interventions
- Practice of breathing and relaxation techniques
- Hospital tour

Week 4
- Variations of labor: back labor, prodromal labor, precipitous labor
- Cesarean delivery
- Medical procedures (IV's, episiotomy, assisted delivery, EFM, Pitocin, epidurals)
- Practice of relaxation and breathing techniques

Week 5
- Review of labor; practice of relaxation and breathing techniques
- Newborn care
- Breastfeeding

Week 6
- Postpartum and transition to parenthood
- Community resources for new parents

Box 5–7 INTERNET RESOURCES FOR EXPECTANT FAMILIES

- Babycenter: www.babycenter.com
- Childbirth Connection: www.childbirthconnection.org
- Doulas of North America: www.dona.org
- Healthy Mothers, Healthy Babies Coalition: www.hmhb.org
- ICEA (International Childbirth Education Association): www.icea.org
- La Leche League: www.lalecheleague.org
- Lamaze International: www.lamaze.org
- March of Dimes: www.marchofdimes.com

- Nurses need to be aware of these potentially powerful influences on the health-related decisions of childbearing women and their families. The quality of information and advice varies widely, from excellent to inaccurate and potentially dangerous.

Evidence-Based Practice: Effectiveness of Antenatal Education

Gagnon, A. (2006). Individual or group antenatal education for childbirth/parenthood (Cochrane Review). In *The Cochrane Library*, Issue 4, 2006, Oxford: Update Software.

A great deal of research has attempted to assess the effectiveness of antenatal education in preparing women for pregnancy, birth, and childcare. Researchers have attempted to link attendance at childbirth classes with a variety of outcomes, including shorter labors, higher Apgar scores, decreased incidence of Cesarean sections, decreased anxiety, breastfeeding success, pain management, maternal satisfaction, infant care competencies, and teaching methods. The majority of the evidence has been inconclusive. Difficulties with sample size, poorly designed methodologies, and lack of funding have persistently hindered the creation of an evidence-based body of knowledge. More research is needed to determine the effects and benefits of childbirth education in a variety of populations and programs.

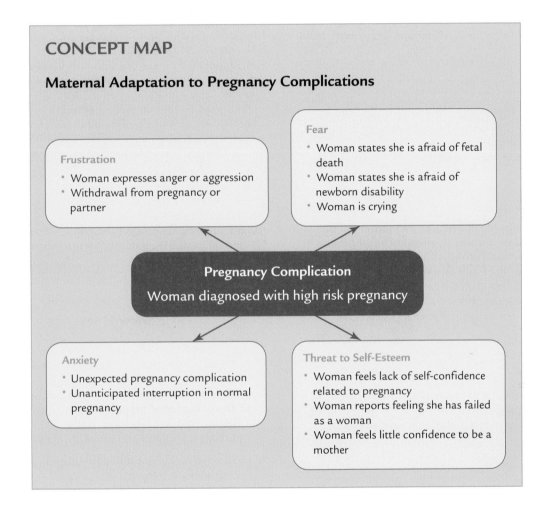

CONCEPT MAP

Maternal Adaptation to Pregnancy Complications

Frustration
- Woman expresses anger or aggression
- Withdrawal from pregnancy or partner

Fear
- Woman states she is afraid of fetal death
- Woman states she is afraid of newborn disability
- Woman is crying

Pregnancy Complication
Woman diagnosed with high risk pregnancy

Anxiety
- Unexpected pregnancy complication
- Unanticipated interruption in normal pregnancy

Threat to Self-Esteem
- Woman feels lack of self-confidence related to pregnancy
- Woman reports feeling she has failed as a woman
- Woman feels little confidence to be a mother

Problem No. 1: Fear related to uncertain fetal outcome
Goal: Decreased fear
Outcome: Patient will express decreased fear related to uncertain fetal outcome.

Nursing Actions

1. Provide time for the patient and family to express their concerns regarding fetal outcome.

2. Encourage the woman to vent apprehension, uncertainty, anger, fear, and/or worry.
3. Discuss prior pregnancy outcomes if applicable.
4. Explain pregnancy complication, management, and reason for each treatment.
5. Help the woman to obtain needed social support.
6. Refer the family to community or hospital resources such as social worker, case manager, or chaplain services as needed
7. Provide contact information for the woman and family as issues arise.

Problem No. 2: Impaired self-esteem related to pregnancy compli-
cation
Goal: Improved self-esteem
Outcome: Patient will express improved self-esteem

Nursing Actions

1. Encourage verbalization of feelings.
2. Practice active listening.
3. Provide emotional support.
4. Encourage the patient to participate in decision making.
5. Make needed referrals to social services and mental health
specialists.

Problem 3: Anxiety related to unexpected pregnancy complication
Goal: Decreased anxiety
Outcome: Patient verbalizes that she feels less anxious

Nursing Actions

1. Be calm and reassuring in interactions with patient and family.
2. Explain all information repeatedly related to complication.
3. Provide autonomy and choices.
4. Encourage patient and family to verbalize their feelings regarding diagnosis by asking open-end questions.
5. Explore past coping strategies.
6. Explore with the woman spiritual practices and beliefs.

Problem 4: Frustration related to pregnancy complication
Goal: Positive pregnancy adaptation
Outcome: Patient demonstrates adaptation to pregnancy.

Nursing Actions

1. Allow the woman to express her feelings related to loss of normal
pregnancy.
2. Allow the woman to express her feelings related to not having a
normal birth.
3. Allow the woman to express her feelings related to uncertainty of
fetal outcome.
4. Provide choices related to management when possible.

TYING IT ALL TOGETHER

As a nurse in an antenatal clinic you are part of an interdisciplinary team that is caring for Margarite Sanchez during her
pregnancy. Margarite is 10 weeks pregnant and is a 28-year-old
G3 P1 Hispanic woman. She began prenatal care at
8 weeks gestation visit. She works in a day care center. She has
a 2-year-old son. José, her husband, has not accompanied her
to her second prenatal appointment as he is in his busy season
at work in landscaping. Margarite reports they are pleased
about the pregnancy although planned to wait another year or
two before attempting another pregnancy. Margarite was seen
for some spotting at 6 weeks' gestation that has resolved.
Marguerite tells you has she has been irritable and short tem-
pered with her husband and son, particularly at the end of the
day when she feels exhausted. She states she is relieved the
spotting stopped but is not sure she feels ready to be a mother
of two children. Her mother lives 4 blocks away and they speak
on the phone daily and see each other several times a week. She
is very involved in her parish and the women in her church study
group all know she is pregnant and are all certain this is a girl.

Detail the aspects of your psychosocial assessment at 10 weeks gestation.
Discuss the rationale for the assessment.
Discuss the nursing diagnosis, nursing activities and expected outcomes
related to this problem.
Discuss the importance of the pregnant woman's mother during pregnancy.
Suggest two interventions that could help to prepare Margarite's 2-year-
old son during the pregnancy.

■ ■ ■   Review Questions   ■ ■ ■

1. Signs of possible maladaptation to pregnancy include:
   A. Denial of fears about childbirth and unrealistic expectations
      about birth
   B. Excessive maternal weight gain and limiting physical activity
   C. Denial of physical symptoms of pregnancy and emotional
      lability
   D. Changes in couple's interactions and sexual activity

2. Nursing interventions that facilitate adaptation to pregnancy in
   the first trimester focus on:
   A. Physiological changes in pregnancy
   B. Promoting pregnancy and birth as a family experience
   C. Readiness for parenting
   D. Partners role during labor and birth

3. Ambivalent feelings toward pregnancy in the third trimester
   may indicate:
   A. Normal expected finding
   B. Unresolved conflict
   C. Depression
   D. Unwanted pregnancy

4. Prescriptive behavior is:
   A. Behavior during childbearing period that is limited for preg-
      nant women
   B. Expected behavior for pregnant women
   C. Behavior that is restricted for pregnant women that has
      supernatural consequences
   D. Unacceptable practices that have implications for pregnant
      women

5. Measurable outcomes of social support interventions during pregnancy include:
   A. Improved coping and functional status
   B. Improves relationship with mother
   C. Reduced stress
   D. Reduced depression

6. When conducting a psychosocial assessment it is important to determine the ____, ____, and ____ of mood or emotional disturbances.
   A. Anxiety, depression, level
   B. Coping, support, distress
   C. Frequency, duration, intensity
   D. Acceptance, avoidance, character

References

Andrews, M., & Boyle, J. (2007). *Transcultural concepts in nursing care* (5th ed.). Philadelphia: Lippincott, Williams & Wilkins.

Association of Women's Health, Obstetric and Neonatal Nurses, AWHONN. (2000a). *Nurse providers of perinatal education: Competencies and program guide.* Washington, DC: Author.

Association of Women's Health, Obstetric and Neonatal Nurses (AWHONN). (2000b). *Policy position statement: Midwifery.* Washington, DC: Author.

Barron, M. (2001). Prenatal risk assessment. In K. Simpson & P. Creehan (Eds.), *AWHONN Perinatal Nursing* (2nd ed., pp.125–160). Philadelphia: Lippincott Williams & Wilkins.

Beck, C. (2002). Revision of the Postpartum Depression Predictors Inventory. *Journal of Obstetric, Gynecologic, and Neonatal Nursing, 31* (4), 394–402.

Beeber, L., & Canuso, R. (2005). Strengthening social support for the low income mother: Five critical questions and a guide for intervention. *Journal of Obstetric, Gynecologic, and Neonatal Nursing, 34*(6), 769–776.

Begley, A. (2000). Preparation for practice in the new millennium: A discussion of the moral implications of multifetal pregnancy reduction. *Nursing Ethics, 7*(2), 99–112.

Bibring, G., Dwyer, T., Huntington, D., & Valenstein, D. (1961). A study of the psychological processes in pregnancy and of the early mother-child relationships. *Psychoanalytic Study of the Child, 16*(9), 9–24.

Breedlove, G. (2005). Perceptions of social support from pregnant and parenting teens using community-based doulas. *Journal of Perinatal Education, 14*(3), 15–22.

Buist, A., Morse, C., & Durkin, S. (2003). Men's adjustment to fatherhood: Implications for obstetrical health care. *Journal of Obstetric, Gynecologic, and Neonatal Nursing, 32*(2), 172–180.

Callister, L. (2001a). Culturally competent care of women and newborns: Knowledge, attitude, and skills. *Journal of Obstetric, Gynecologic, and Neonatal Nursing, 30*(2), 209–215.

Callister, L. (2001b). Integrating cultural beliefs and practices into the care of childbearing women. In K. Simpson & P. Creehan (Eds.), *AWHONN perinatal nursing* (2nd ed., pp. 68–94). Philadelphia: Lippincott Williams & Wilkins.

Campbell, D., Lake, M., Falk, M., & Backstrand, J. (2006). A randomized trial of continuous support in labor by a lay doula. *Journal of Obstetric, Gynecologic, and Neonatal Nursing, 35*(4), 456–464.

Cannella, B. (2006). Mediators of the relationship between social support and positive health practices in pregnant women. *Nursing Research, 55*(6), 437–445.

Carolan, M. (2005). "Doing it properly": The experience of first time mothering over 35 years. *Health Care for Women International, 26*(9), 764–787.

Carroll, J., Reid, A., Biringer, A., Midmer, D., Glazier, R., Wilson, L., et al. (2005). Effectiveness of the Antenatal Psychosocial Health Assessment (ALPHA) form in detecting psychosocial concerns: A randomized controlled trial. *CMAJ: Canadian Medical Association Journal, 173*(3), 253–259.

Cleary-Goldman, J., Malone, F., Vidaver, J., Ball, R., Nyberg, D., Comstock, C., et al. (2005). Impact of maternal age on obstetric outcome. *Obstetrics and Gynecology, 105*(5, Part 1), 983–990.

Collopy, K. (2004). "I couldn't think that far": Infertile women's decision making about multifetal reduction. *Research in Nursing and Health, 27*(2), 75–86.

Crooks, R., & Baur, K. (2007). *Our sexuality* (10th ed.). Menlo Park, CA: Benjamin Cummings.

Damato, E. (2003). Predictors of prenatal attachment in mothers of twins. *Journal of Obstetric, Gynecologic, and Neonatal Nursing, 33*(4), 436–445.

Dawley, K., & Beam, R. (2005). "My nurse taught me how to have a healthy baby and be a good mother:" Nurse home visiting with pregnant women 1888 to 2005. *Nursing Clinics of North America, 40,* 803–815.

Dobrzykowski, T., & Stern, P. (2003). Out of sync: A generation of first-time mothers over 30. *Health Care for Women International, 24*(3), 242–253.

Draper, J. (2003). Blurring, moving and broken boundaries: Men's encounters with the pregnant body. *Sociology of Health and Illness, 25*(7), 743–767.

Driscoll, J. (2001). Psychosocial adaptation to pregnancy and postpartum. In K. Simpson & P. Creehan (Eds.), *AWHONN perinatal nursing* (2nd ed., pp. 115–124). Philadelphia: Lippincott Williams & Wilkins.

Durham, R. (1998). Strategies women engage in when analyzing preterm labor at home. *Journal of Perinatology, 18*, 61–69.

Duvall, E. (1985). *Marriage and family development.* New York: Harper & Row.

Ehiri, J., Meremikwu, A., & Meremikwu, M. (2005). Interventions for preventing unintended pregnancies among adolescents. (Protocol) *Cochrane Database of Systematic Reviews* 2. Art. No.: CD005215. DOI: 10.1002/14651858.CD005215.

Enkin, M., Keirse, M., Neilson, J., Crowther, C., Duley, L., Hodnett, E., & Hofmeyr, J. (2000). *A guide to effective care in pregnancy and childbirth* (3rd ed.). Oxford, UK: Oxford University Press.

Finnbogadottir, H., Svalenius, E., & Persson, E. (2003). Expectant first-time fathers' experiences of pregnancy. *Midwifery, 19*(2), 96–105.

Fortier, J., Carson, V., Will, S., & Shubkagel, B. (1991). Adjustment to a newborn: Sibling preparation makes a difference. *Journal of Obstetric, Gynecologic, and Neonatal Nursing, 20*(4), 73–78.

Friedman, M., Bowden, V., & Jones, E. (2003). *Family nursing: Research, theory, and practice* (5th ed.). Upper Saddle River, NJ: Prentice-Hall.

Fuller, J. (2003). Intercultural health care as reflective negotiated practice. *Western Journal of Nursing Research, 25*(7), 781–797.

Gagnon, A. (2006). Individual or group antenatal education for childbirth/parenthood (Cochrane Review). In *The Cochrane Library*, Issue 4, 2006, Oxford: Update Software.

Gilbert, E. (2007). *Manual of high risk pregnancy and delivery* (4th ed.). St. Louis, MO: C. V. Mosby.

Giurgescu, C., Penckofer, S., Maurer, M., & Bryant, F. (2006). Impact of uncertainty, social support, and prenatal coping on the psychological well-being of high risk pregnant women. *Nursing Research, 55*(5), 356–365.

Grussu, P. (2005). Profile of mood states and parental attitudes in motherhood: comparing women with planned and unplanned pregnancies. *Birth: Issues in Perinatal Care, 32*(2), 107–114.

Harley, K., & Eskenazi, B. (2006). Time in the United States, social support and health behaviors during pregnancy among women of Mexican descent. *Social Science & Medicine, 62*(12), 3048–3061.

International Childbirth Education Association (ICEA). (1999). Position paper: The role and scope of the doula. *International Journal of Childbirth Education, 14*(1), 38–45.

Jordan, P. (1989). Support behaviors identified as helpful and desired by second time parents over the perinatal period. *Maternal Child Nursing Journal, 18*(2), 133–145.

Jordan, P. (1990). Laboring for relevance: Expectant and new fatherhood. *Nursing Research, 39*(6), 11–15.

Joseph, K., Allen, A., Dodds, L., Turner, L., Scott, H., & Liston, R. (2005). The perinatal effects of delayed childbearing. *Obstetrics and Gynecology, 105*(6), 1410–1418.

Kennedy, H., & Shannon, M. (2004). Keeping birth normal: Research findings on midwifery care during childbirth. *Journal of Obstetric, Gynecologic, and Neonatal Nursing, 33*(5), 554–560.

Kirby, D. (1999). Reflections on two decades of research on teen sexual behavior and pregnancy. *Journal of School Health, 69*(3), 89–94.

Koniak-Griffin, D., Logsdon, C., Hines-Martin, V., & Turner, C. (2006). Contemporary mothering in a diverse society. *Journal of Obstetric, Gynecologic, and Neonatal Nursing, 35*(5), 671–678.

Kridi, S. (2002). Health beliefs and practices among Arab women. *MCN: The American Journal of Maternal Child Nursing, 27*(3), 178–182.

Kroelinger, C., & Oths, K. (2000). Partner support and pregnancy wantedness. *Birth: Issues in Perinatal Care, 27*(2), 112–119.

Lauderdale, J. (2007). Transcultural perspectives in childbearing. In M. Andrews & J. Boyle, *Transcultural concepts in nursing care* (5th ed.). Philadelphia: Lippincott, Williams & Wilkins.

Lederman, R. (1996). *Psychosocial adaptation in pregnancy* (2nd ed.). New York: Springer.

Leininger, M. (Ed). (1991). *Culture care diversity & universality: A theory of nursing.* New York: National League for Nursing Press.

Logdson, C. (2000). *Social support for pregnant and postpartum women.* Washington DC: Association of Women's Health, Obstetric and Neonatal Nurses.

Logsdon, C., Gagne, P., Hughes, T., Patterson, J., & Rakestraw, V. (2005). Social support during adolescent pregnancy: Piecing together a quilt. *Journal of Obstetric, Gynecologic, & Neonatal Nursing, 34*(5), 606–614.

Lothian, J. (2006). Birth plans: The good, the bad, and the future. *Journal of Obstetric, Gynecologic, & Neonatal Nursing, 35*(2), 295–303.

Machado, G. (2001). Cultural sensitivity and stereotypes. *Journal of Multicultural Nursing and Health, 7*(2), 13–15.

Maifeld, M., Hahn, S., Titler, M., Marita, G., & Mullen, M. (2003). Decision making regarding multifetal reduction. *Journal of Obstetric, Gynecologic, & Neonatal Nursing, 32*(3), 357–369.

Martin, J. A., Hamilton, B. E., Sutton, P. D., Ventura, S., Menacker, F., & Kimeyer, S. (2006). Births: Final data for 2004. *National Vital Statistics Reports, 55*(1), Hyattsville, MD: National Center for Health Statistics.

Mattson, S., & Smith, J. (Eds.). (2004). *Core curriculum for maternal newborn nursing* (3rd ed.). St. Louis, MO: Elsevier Saunders.

May, K. (1980). A typology of detachment/involvement styles adopted by first-time expectant fathers. *Western Journal of Nursing Research, 2*, 443–453.

May, K. (1982). Three phases of father involvement in pregnancy. *Nursing Research, 31*(6), 337–342.

May, K. (1994). Impact of maternal activity restriction on the expectant father. *Journal of Obstetric, Gynecologic, & Neonatal Nursing, 23*, 246–251.

May, K., & Mahlmeister, L. (1994). *Maternal & neonatal nursing, family centered care.* Philadelphia: Lippincott Williams & Wilkins.

McBride, A., & Shore, C. (2001). Women as mothers and grandmothers. *Annual Review of Nursing Research, 19*, 63–85.

McManus, A., Hunter, L., & Renn, H. (2006). Lesbian experiences and needs during childbirth: Guidance for health care providers. *Journal of Obstetric, Gynecologic, & Neonatal Nursing, 35*(1), 13–23.

Meleis, A. (2003). Theoretical consideration of health care for immigrant and minority women. In P. St. Hill, J. Lipson, & A. Meleis (Eds.), *Caring for women crossculturally.* Philadelphia: F. A. Davis.

Mercer, R. (1995). *Becoming a mother.* New York: Springer.

Mercer, R. (2004). Becoming a mother versus maternal role attainment. *Journal of Nursing Scholarship, 36*(3), 226–233.

Midmer, D., Carroll, J., Bryanton, J., & Stewart, D. (2002). From research to application: The development of an antenatal psychosocial health assessment tool. *Canadian Journal of Public Health, 93*(4), 291–296.

Montgomery, K. (2003). Nursing care for pregnant adolescents. *Journal of Obstetric, Gynecologic, and Neonatal Nursing, 32*(2), 249–256.

Murphy, R. (1992). Couvade: The pregnant male. *Journal of Perinatal Education, 1*(2), 13–18.

Nichols, F., & Humenick, S. (2000). *Childbirth education, practice, research and theory* (2nd ed.). Philadelphia: W. B. Saunders.

Orr, S. (2004). Social support and pregnancy outcome: A review of the literature. *Clinical Obstetrics & Gynecology, 47*(4), 842–855.

Pascali-Bonaro, D., & Kroeger, M. (2004). Continuous female companionship during childbirth: A crucial resource in times of stress or calm. *Journal of Midwifery & Women's Health, 49*(4), 19–27.

Philliber, S., Brooks, L., Lehrer, L., Oakley, M., & Waggoner, S. (2003). Outcomes of teen parenting programs in New Mexico. *Adolescence, 38*(151), 535–553.

Price, S., Lake, M., Breene, G., Carson, G., Quinn, C., & O'Connor, T. (2007). The spiritual experience of high-risk pregnancy. *Journal of Obstetric, Gynecologic & Neonatal Nursing, 36*(1), 63–69.

Priest, S., Austin, M., & Sullivan, E. (2006). Antenatal psychosocial screening for prevention of antenatal and postnatal anxiety and depression (Protocol). In *The Cochrane Library,* Issue 1, 2006. Oxford: Update Software.

Purnell, L., & Paulanka, B. (2008). *Guide to culturally competent health care* (3rd ed). Philadelphia: F. A. Davis.

Roberts, S. (2003). Native American health: Examining our commitment to Indian health services. *AWHONN Lifelines, 7*(3), 244–250.

Ross, L. (2005). Perinatal mental health in lesbian mothers: A review of potential risk and protective factors. *Women & Health, 41*(3), 113–128.

Rubin, R. (1975). Maternal tasks in pregnancy. *Maternal-Child Nursing Journal, 4*(3), 143–153.

Rubin, R. (1984). *Maternal identity and the maternal experience.* New York: Springer.

Sadler, L., & Clemmens, D. (2004). Ambivalent grandmothers raising teen daughters and their babies. *Journal of Family Nursing, 10*(2), 211–231.

Sauls, D. (2002). Effects of labor support on mothers, babies, and birth outcomes. *Journal of Obstetric, Gynecologic, and Neonatal Nursing, 31*(6), 733–741.

Schardt, D. (2005). Delayed childbearing: Underestimated psychological implications. *International Journal of Childbirth Education, 20*(3), 34–37.

Scott, K., Berkowitz, G., & Klaus, M. (1999). A comparison of intermittent and continuous support during labor: A meta-analysis. *American Journal of Obstetrics and Gynecology, 180*(5), 1054–1059.

Semenic, S., Callister, L., & Feldman, P. (2004). Giving birth: The voices of orthodox Jewish women living in Canada. *Journal of Obstetric, Gynecologic, and Neonatal Nursing, 33*(1), 80–87.

Simpson, K., Creehan, P., and Association of Women's Health, Obstetrics and Neonatal Nursing (AWHONN). (2008). *Perinatal nursing* (3rd ed.). Philadelphia: Lippincott Williams & Wilkins.

Spear, H. (2004). Personal narratives of adolescent mothers-to-be: Contraception, decision making and future expectations. *Public Health Nursing, 21*(4), 338–346.

Spear, H., & Lock, S. (2003). Qualitative research on adolescent pregnancy: A descriptive review and analysis. *Journal of Pediatric Nursing, 18*(6), 397–408.

Spietz, A., & Kelly, J. (2003). The importance of maternal mental health during pregnancy: Theory, practice and intervention. *Public Health Nursing, 19*(3), 153–155.

St. Hill, P. (2003). African Americans. In P. St. Hill, J. Lipson, & A. Meleis (Eds.), *Caring for women crossculturally.* Philadelphia: F. A. Davis.

Tilden, V. (1983). The relation of life stress and social support to emotional disequilibrium during pregnancy. *Research in Nursing and Health, 6*, 167–174.

U.S. Department of Health and Human Services, Health Resources and Services Administration (2004). *The registered nurse population: Findings from the National Sample Survey of Registered Nurses.* Washington, DC: Author.

Willis, W. (1999). Culturally competent nursing care during the perinatal period. *Journal of Perinatal and Neonatal Nursing, 13*(3), 45–59.

Yogev, S. (2004). Support in labour: A literature review. *Midwifery Digest, 14*(4), 486–492.

Zelkowitz, P., Schinazi, J., Katofsky, L., Saucier, J., Valenzuela, M., Westreich, R., & Dayan, J. (2004). Factors associated with depression in pregnant immigrant women. *Transcultural Psychiatry, 41*(4), 445–464.

Antepartal Tests

Nursing Diagnosis
- Knowledge deficit related to antenatal tests
- Anxiety related to antenatal tests
- Risk of fetal injury or death related invasive antenatal tests

Nursing Outcomes
- The pregnant woman and her family will verbalize understanding of antenatal tests.
- If complications occur, they will be identified promptly and appropriate nursing interventions will be initiated.

INTRODUCTION

This chapter presents various antenatal tests offered to pregnant women. The focus of the chapter is on tests for at risk and/or high-risk pregnancies. Common maternal conditions indicating need for antenatal tests are presented in Table 6-1. The purpose, indication, basic procedure, interpretation, advantages, risks, and nursing responsibilities are outlined. Specifics on procedures are not detailed as they may vary from institution to institution. Routine tests performed during pregnancy are presented in Chapter 4. Antenatal tests are often performed as outpatient procedures, such as ultrasound, amniocentesis, and non-stress tests. Antenatal tests may also be performed during an antenatal hospitalization for a high-risk pregnancy. The nurse's role and responsibility related to antenatal tests may vary based on the inpatient or outpatient setting. Nursing care may be provided before, during, and/or after a procedure.

ASSESSMENT FOR RISK FACTORS

The nurse needs to assess for factors that place the woman and/or her fetus at risk for adverse outcomes:

- **Biophysical factors** originate from the mother or fetus and impact the development or function of the mother or fetus. They include genetic, nutritional, medical, and obstetric issues (see Table 6-1).
- **Psychosocial factors** are maternal behaviors or lifestyles that have a negative effect on the mother or fetus. Examples include smoking, caffeine use, alcohol/drug use, and psychological status.
- **Sociodemographic factors** are variables that pertain to the woman and her family and place the mother and the fetus at increased risk. Examples include access to prenatal care, age, parity, marital status, income, and ethnicity.
- **Environmental factors** are hazards in the workplace or the general environment that impact pregnancy outcomes. Various environmental substances can affect fetal development. Examples include exposure to chemicals, radiation, and pollutants.

The underlying mechanism for how some risk factors impact pregnancy outcomes is not fully understood. Many risk factors appear to have a combined or cumulative effect. Identification of risk factors for poor perinatal outcomes is essential to minimize maternal and neonatal morbidity and mortality. Risk factors are described in more detail in Chapters 7, 10, 14, and 17 as they relate specifically to pregnancy, labor, the postpartum period, and the neonate.

THE NURSE'S ROLE IN ANTEPARTAL TESTING

The nurse's role during antepartal testing varies based on the specific test. In general, it includes providing information and emotional support and comfort to women undergoing antenatal tests and their families. Many women having antenatal tests are at high risk for fetal and maternal complications and are anxious and vulnerable. In some instances, the nurse assists or performs the antenatal test, but in most instances this requires advanced competencies (i.e., ultrasound).

To provide appropriate support to families, nurses need to understand:

- The variety of tests available during pregnancy
- The indications for the test/procedure
- The interpretation of findings
- The nursing care associated with the test/procedure
- The physical and psychological benefits, limitations, and implications of the test/procedure (Simpson & Creehan, 2001)

TABLE 6–1	COMMON MATERNAL CONDITIONS INDICATING NEED FOR ANTENATAL TESTS
PREEXISTING MEDICAL CONDITIONS	Hypertensive disorders Renal disease Autoimmune disease Type 1 diabetes
PREGNANCY-RELATED CONDITIONS	Pregnancy-related hypertension Decreased fetal movement Hydramnios Intrauterine growth restriction Multiple gestation Post-term pregnancy Previous unexplained fetal demise Isoimmunization Fetal anomalies

Nursing Actions for Women Undergoing Antenatal Testing

■ Provide information regarding the test.
  ■ *Explain how the test/procedure is performed.*
  ■ *Explain what the woman can expect during the test/procedure.*
  ■ *Explain what the test measures.*
■ Provide comfort.
  ■ *Assist woman into a comfortable position.*
  ■ *Preserve the woman's modesty by closing doors and exposing only the portions of her body necessary for the test/procedure.*
■ Reassure the woman and her partner.
  ■ *Address the woman's and her partner's concerns regarding the test/procedure such as type of discomfort or pain she may experience and effects on her and/or her unborn child.*
  ■ *If she prefers, encourage the woman's significant others to be with her during procedures.*

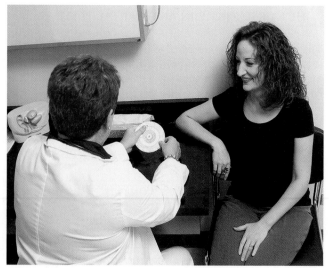

Figure 6-1   Nurse counseling a pregnant woman.

■ Provide psychological support to woman and her partner (Fig. 6-1).
  ■ *Incorporate understanding of cultural and social issues.*
  ■ *Remain with the woman and her partner during the test/procedure.*
  ■ *Assess for anxiety and provide care to reduce the level of anxiety.*
  ■ *Allow woman to express feelings related to high-risk pregnancy.*
■ Document the woman's response and the results of tests.
■ Report results of tests to care providers.
■ Schedule appropriate follow-up.
■ Reinforce information given by the woman's provider regarding the results of the tests and need for further testing, treatment, or referral.

CRITICAL COMPONENT

Antepartal Screening and Diagnostic Tests

Screening Test

A screening test is a test designed to identify those who are not affected by a disease or abnormality. Some screening tests are offered to all pregnant women and include multiple marker screening and ultrasound. Other screening tests are reserved for high-risk pregnancies to provide information on fetal status and well-being. If the results of screening tests indicate an abnormality, further testing is indicated. Screening tests include:

■ Amniotic fluid index
■ Biophysical profile
■ Contraction stress test
■ Daily fetal movement count
■ Multiple marker screening: Alpha–fetoprotein screening, triple marker, and quad marker
■ Non-stress test
■ Ultrasonography
■ Umbilical artery Doppler flow
■ Vibroacoustic stimulation

Diagnostic Tests

Diagnostic tests help to identify a particular disease or provide information which aids in the making of a diagnosis. Most fetal diagnostic tests are reserved for high-risk pregnancies where there is increased risk to fetus for developmental or physical problems. Diagnostic tests include:

■ Amniocentesis
■ Chorionic villi sampling
■ Magnetic resonance imaging
■ Percutaneous umbilical blood sampling
■ Ultrasonography

BIOPHYSICAL ASSESSMENT

Since the 1970s, the fetus has become more accessible with the refinement of new technology such as ultrasound. Fetal physiological parameters that can now be assessed include fetal movement, urine production, and observing fetal structures and blood flow. Tests used in biophysical assessment of the fetus are ultrasonography, umbilical artery Doppler flow, and magnetic resonance imaging (MRI).

Ultrasonography

Ultrasonography is the use of high-frequency sound waves to produce an image of an organ or tissue. It is the most common diagnostic test during pregnancy (Simpson & Creehan, 2001) and its use varies based on trimester (Table 6-2). Ultrasonography is commonly used to obtain vital information:

- Gestational age
- Fetal growth
- Fetal anatomy
- Placental abnormalities and location
- Fetal activity
- Amount of amniotic fluid
- Visual assistance for some invasive procedures such as amniocentesis.

Procedures

- Transvaginal ultrasound
  - *Is generally performed in the first trimester.*
  - *The woman is in a lithotomy position.*
  - *A sterile covered probe/transducer is inserted into the vagina.*
- Abdominal ultrasound (Fig. 6-2)
  - *A full bladder is necessary to elevate the uterus out of the pelvis for better visualization when abdominal ultrasound is performed during the first half of pregnancy.*
  - *The woman is in a supine position.*
  - *Transmission gel and transducer are placed on the maternal abdomen.*
  - *The transducer is moved over the maternal abdomen to create an image of the structure being evaluated.*

Interpretation

- Post-procedure interpretation is typically done by a practitioner such as a radiologist, obstetrician, or nurse-midwife.
- Ultrasound for gestational age is determined through measurements of fetal–crown rump length, biparietal diameter, and femur length. It is most accurate when performed before 20 weeks' gestation (American Academy of Pediatrics & the American College of Obstetricians and Gynecologists [AAP & ACOG], 2002).
- Normal findings for the fetus are appropriate age, size, viability, position, and functional capacities.
- Normal findings for the placenta are expected size, normal position and structure, and adequate volume of amniotic fluid.
- Nurses can perform limited obstetrical ultrasound (Box 6-1).

Advantages

- Noninvasive
- Provides information on fetal structures and status

BOX 6–1   AWHONN STANDARD OF CARE

Limited Obstetric Ultrasound

Components of a limited obstetric ultrasound are:

- Assessing the number of fetuses
- Assessing for the presence or absence of fetal cardiac activity
- Assessing fetal presentation
- Assessing placental location
- Assessing amniotic fluid

The Association of Women's Health, Obstetric, and Neonatal Nurses (AWHONN) has developed guidelines for the didactic and clinical preparation for nurses who perform limited obstetric ultrasound. A minimum of 12 hours of didactic content is recommended in the following four areas: (1) ultrasound physics and instrumentation; (2) patient education; (3) nursing accountability; and (4) OB content (AWHONN, 1998). According to one study, nurses obtained competence in limited OB ultrasound after completing 12 hours of didactic training with a clinical practicum of 6 to 9 hours and approximately 15 ultrasound scans (Stringer, Miesnik, Brown, Menei, & Macones, 2003).

Currently there are no certification requirements for nurses performing limited ultrasound. Appropriate institutional policies, didactic and clinical education, and evaluation components are needed to ensure competence for nurses to perform limited ultrasound.

Sources: AWHONN (1998); Menihan (2000); Stringer, Miesnik, Brown, Menei, & Macones (2003).

Risks

- None, but controversy exists on the use of routine ultrasound for low-risk pregnant women as there is no evidence it improves outcomes.

Nursing Actions

- Explain the procedure to the woman and her family.
- Assess for latex allergies with transvaginal ultrasound.
- Inform the woman that a sterile sheathed probe is used for transvaginal ultrasound and is inserted into the vagina.

TABLE 6–2   INDICATIONS FOR ULTRASOUND BY TRIMESTER OF PREGNANCY

FIRST TRIMESTER	SECOND TRIMESTER	THIRD TRIMESTER
Confirm the pregnancy.	Confirm the due date.	Confirm gestational age.
Confirm fetal viability (detecting fetal cardiac activity).	Confirm fetal viability.	Confirm fetal viability.
Detect multiple gestation (number and size of gestational sacs).	Confirm fetal number, position, gestational age.	Detect placental abruption, previa, or maturity.
Visualization during chorionic villus sampling.	Confirm placental location.	Detect fetal position, congenital anomalies, IUGR.
Measure gestational age.	Detect fetal anomalies (best after 18 weeks) or intrauterine growth restriction (IUGR)	Assess biophysical profile (BPP).
Evaluate uterine structures.	Visualize for amniocentesis.	Assess amniotic fluid volume (AFI).
Detect missed abortion, tubal, or ectopic pregnancy.	Evaluate uterine and cervical structures.	Perform Doppler flow studies.
Evaluate vaginal bleeding.	Evaluate vaginal bleeding.	Visualize for diagnostic tests and external version.
		Evaluate vaginal bleeding.

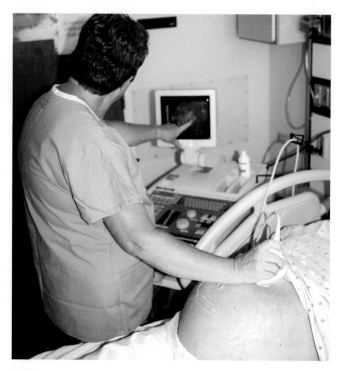

Figure 6-2 Nurse explains ultrasound to a pregnant woman having an ultrasound test.

■ Provide comfort measures to the woman during the procedure such as a pillow under her head and a warm blanket above and below her abdomen.
■ Be sensitive to cultural and social as well as modesty issues.
■ Provide emotional support.
■ Schedule appropriate follow-up.

Umbilical Artery Doppler Flow

Umbilical artery Doppler flow studies assess the rate and volume of blood flow through placenta and umbilical cord vessels using ultrasound. This is a noninvasive, screening technique used to assess resistance to blood flow in the placenta. It is commonly used in combination with other diagnostic tests to assess fetal status in intrauterine growth restricted (IUGR) fetuses.

Procedure

■ The woman is assisted into a supine position.
■ Transmission gel and transducer are placed on the woman's abdomen.
■ Images are obtained of blood flow in the umbilical artery.

Interpretation

■ The directed blood flow within the umbilical arteries is calculated using the difference between systolic and diastolic flow (Gilbert & Harmon, 2003).
■ As peripheral resistance increases, diastolic flow decreases and the systolic/diastolic increases. Reversed end-diastolic flow can be seen with severe cases of intrauterine growth restriction (AAP & ACOG, 2002).
■ Umbilical artery Doppler is considered abnormal if the systolic/diastolic (S/D) ratio is above the 95th percentile for gestational age, or a ratio above 3.0, or the end-diastolic flow is absent or reversed (Cunningham et al., 2005).

Advantages

■ Noninvasive
■ Assesses placental perfusion

Risks

■ None

Nursing Actions

■ Explain the procedure to the woman and her family.
■ Address questions and concerns.
■ Provide comfort measures.
■ Provide emotional support.
■ Schedule appropriate follow-up.

Magnetic Resonance Imaging

Magnetic resonance imaging (MRI) is a diagnostic radiologic evaluation of tissue and organs from multiple planes. During pregnancy, it is used to visualize maternal and/or fetal structures for detailed imaging when screening tests indicate possible abnormalities. It is most commonly performed for suspected brain abnormality.

Procedure

■ The woman is instructed to remove all metallic objects before the test.
■ The woman is placed in a supine position with left lateral tilt on the MRI table.
■ The woman's abdominal area is scanned.

Interpretation

■ Interpretation of the study is done by a radiologist.

Advantages

■ Provides very detailed images of fetal anatomy; particularly useful for brain abnormalities and complex abnormalities.

Risks

■ No known harmful effects

Nursing Actions

■ Nurses are involved in the pre- and post-procedure.
■ Explain the procedure to the woman and her family.
■ Address questions and concerns.

BIOCHEMICAL ASSESSMENT

Biochemical assessment involves biological examination and chemical determination. Procedures used to obtain biochemical specimens include amniocentesis, chorionic villi sampling, percutaneous blood sampling, and maternal assays. More than 15% of pregnancies are at sufficient risk to warrant invasive testing (Queenan, Hobbins, & Spong, 2005).

Amniocentesis

Amniocentesis is a diagnostic procedure in which a needle is inserted through the maternal abdominal wall into the uterine cavity to obtain amniotic fluid. It is commonly performed for genetic testing (at 14–20 weeks' gestation), assessment of fetal lung maturity, and assessment of hemolytic disease in fetus or for intrauterine infection.

Risk factors for fetal genetic disorders include advanced maternal age (older than 35 years of age), history of genetic disorders, positive screening test such as a positive alpha-fetoprotein, and known or suspected hemolytic disease in the fetus

Procedure

■ A needle is inserted transabdominally into the uterine cavity using ultrasonography to guide placement (Fig. 6-3).
■ Amniotic fluid is obtained.

Interpretation

■ Results of chromosomal studies is available within 2 weeks.
■ Elevated bilirubin levels indicate fetal hemolytic disease.
■ A positive culture indicates infection.
■ If the purpose of the test is to determine fetal lung maturity, lecithin/sphingomyelin (L/S) ratio, phosphatidyl glycerol (PG), lamellar body count (LBC), results are interpreted as follows:
    ■ *L:S ratio >2:1 indicates fetal lung maturity*
    ■ *L:S ratio <2:1 indicates fetal lung immaturity in increased risk of respiratory distress syndrome*
    ■ *Positive PG indicates fetal lung maturity*
    ■ *Negative PG indicates immature fetal lungs*
    ■ *Lamellar bodies are indicative of fetal lung maturity*

Advantages

■ Examines fetal chromosomes for genetic disorders.
■ Direct examination of biochemical specimens.

Risks

■ Less than 1% fetal loss rate after 15 weeks' gestation; increases to 2% to 5% earlier in gestation (AAP & ACOG, 2002).

Nursing Actions

■ Review the procedure with the woman and assure her that precautions are followed during the procedure with ultrasound visualization of fetus to avoid fetal or placental injury (Leeuwen, Kranpitz, & Smith, 2006).
■ Explain that during needle aspiration discomfort will be minimized with the use of a local anesthetic.
■ Explain that a full bladder may be required for ultrasound visualization if the woman is less than 20 weeks' gestation.

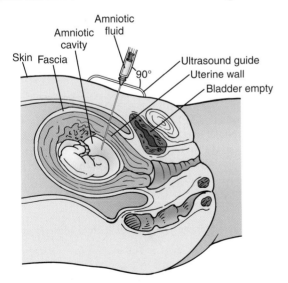

Figure 6-3 Amniocentesis procedure.

■ Instruct the woman in breathing and relaxation techniques she can use during the procedure.
■ Provide comfort measures.
■ Provide emotional support.
■ Recognize anxiety related to test results.
■ Label specimens.
■ Assess fetal and maternal well-being post-procedure.
■ Instruct the woman to report abdominal pain or cramping, leaking of fluid, bleeding, decreased fetal movement, fever, or chills to the care provider.
■ Administer Rh$_o$(D) immune globulin (RhoGAM) to Rh-negative women post-procedure as per order to prevent antibody formation in the Rh-negative women.

Chorionic Villus Sampling

Chorionic villus sampling (CVS) is aspiration of a small amount of placental tissue (chorion) for chromosomal, metabolic, or DNA testing. This test is used for chromosomal analysis between 10 and 12 weeks' gestation to detect fetal abnormalities caused by genetic disorders. It tests for metabolic disorders such as cystic fibrosis but does not test for neural tube defects (NTDs).

Procedure

■ The woman is in a supine position.
■ A catheter is inserted transvaginally through the cervix using ultrasonography to guide placement (sometimes through the maternal abdomen).
■ A small sample of chorionic (placental) tissue is removed.
■ The villi are harvested and cultured for chromosomal analysis and processed for DNA and enzymatic analysis as indicated (Fig. 6-4).

Interpretation

■ Results of chromosomal studies are available within 2 weeks.
■ Detailed information is provided on specific chromosomal abnormality detected.

Advantages

■ Can be performed earlier than amniocentesis, but is not recommended before 10 weeks (AAP & ACOG, 2002).
■ Examination of fetal chromosomes.

Risks

■ There is a 7% fetal loss rate due to bleeding, infection, and rupture of membranes.
■ 10% of women experience some bleeding after the procedure.

Nursing Actions

■ Review the procedure with the woman and her family.
■ Instruct the woman in breathing and relaxation techniques she can use during the procedure.
■ Assist the woman into the proper position.
    ■ *Lithotomy for transvaginal aspiration*
    ■ *Supine for transabdominal aspiration*
■ Provide comfort measures.
■ Provide emotional support.
■ Recognize anxiety related to test results.
■ Label specimens.
■ Assess fetal and maternal well-being post-procedure.
■ Instruct the woman to report abdominal pain or cramping, leaking of fluid, bleeding, fever, or chills to the care provider.

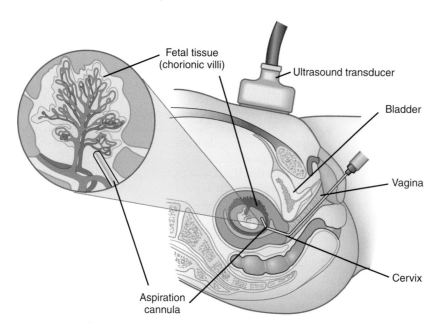

Figure 6-4 Chorionic villi sampling procedure.

■ Administer RhoGAM to Rh-negative women post-procedure as per order to prevent antibody formation in Rh-negative women.

Percutaneous Umbilical Blood Sampling

Percutaneous umbilical blood sampling (PUBS), or cordocentesis, is the removal of fetal blood from the umbilical cord for fetal blood sampling. The blood is used to test for metabolic and hematological disorders, fetal infection, and fetal karyotyping. It can also be used for fetal therapies such as red blood cell and platelet transfusions.

Procedure

■ A needle is inserted into the umbilical vein and a small sample of fetal blood is aspirated (Fig. 6-5).
■ Ultrasound is used to guide the needle.

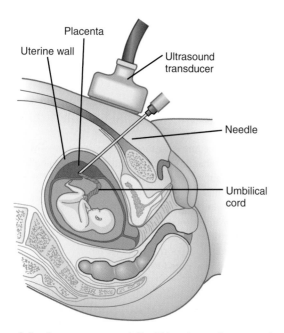

Figure 6-5 Percutaneous umbilical blood sampling procedure.

Interpretation

■ Interpretation of studies is based on the indication for the procedure.

Advantages

■ Direct examination of fetal blood sample

Risks

■ Complications are similar to those for amniocentesis and include cord vessel bleeding, maternal–fetal hemorrhage, and fetal bradycardia.
■ The overall procedure-related fetal death rate is 1.4% (Cunningham et al., 2005).

Nursing Actions

■ Nurses may be involved in the pre- and post-procedure.
■ Explain the procedure to the woman and her family.
■ Address questions and concerns.
■ Assess fetal well-being post-procedure.

MATERNAL ASSAYS

Alpha-Fetoprotein/α_1-Fetoprotein/Maternal Serum Alpha-Fetoprotein

Alpha-fetoprotein (AFP) is a glycoprotein produced in the fetal liver, gastrointestinal tract, and yolk sac in early gestation. Assessing for the levels of AFP in the maternal blood is a screening tool for certain developmental defects in the fetus such as fetal NTDs and ventral abdominal wall defects.

Procedure

■ Maternal blood is drawn and analyzed at 16 to 18 weeks' gestation.

Interpretation

■ Increased levels are associated with defects such as NTDs, anencephaly, omphalocele, and gastroschisis.
■ Decreased levels are associated with trisomy 21 (Down syndrome).

■ Abnormal findings require additional testing such as amniocentesis or ultrasonography.

Advantages

■ 80% to 85% of all open NTDs and open abdominal wall defects and 90% of anencephalies can be detected early in pregnancy (AAP & ACOG, 2002).

Risks

■ There is a high false-positive rate (meaning the test results indicate an abnormality in a normal fetus) that can result in increased anxiety for woman and her family related to identification of a potential defect as they wait for results of additional testing.

Nursing Actions

■ Educate the woman about the screening test.
■ Support the woman and her family, particularly if results are abnormal.
■ Assist in scheduling diagnostic testing when results are abnormal.
■ Provide information on support groups if a NTD occurs.

Multiple Marker Screen

Triple marker screening combines all three chemical markers—AFP, human chorionic gonadotropin (hCG) and estriol levels—with maternal age to detect some trisomies and NTDs. It is sometimes used as an alternative to amniocentesis. **Quad screen** adds inhibin-A to the triple marker screen to increase detection of trisomy 21 to 80% (Queenan, Hobbins, & Spong, 2005).

Procedure

■ Maternal blood is drawn by the laboratory at 15 to 16 weeks of gestation.

Interpretation

■ Low levels of maternal serum alpha-fetoprotein (MSAFP) and unconjugated estriol levels suggest an abnormality.
■ hCG and inhibin-A levels are twice as high in pregnancies with trisomy 21.
■ Decreased estriol levels are an indicator of NTDs.

Advantages

■ 60% to 80% of cases of Down syndrome can be identified.
■ 85% to 90% of open NTDs are detected.

Risks

■ None

Nursing Actions

■ Educate the woman about the test.
■ Provide emotional support for the woman and her family.
■ Assist in scheduling additional testing if needed.
■ Provide information on support groups if a NTD occurs.

TESTS OF FETAL STATUS AND WELL-BEING

The assessment of fetal status is a key component of perinatal care. A variety of methods are available for ongoing assessment of fetal well-being during pregnancy (AWHONN, 2008):

■ Daily fetal movement count (kick counts)
■ Non-stress test (NST)

■ Contraction stress test (CST)
■ Amniotic fluid index (AFI)
■ Biophysical profile (BPP)

The goal of fetal testing is to reduce the number of preventable stillbirths. The purpose of antenatal testing is to validate fetal well-being or identify fetal hypoxemia and to intervene before permanent injury or death occurs (AWHONN, 2008). In most clinical situations a normal test result indicates that intrauterine fetal death is highly unlikely in the next 7 days (AAP & ACOG, 2002).

Daily Fetal Movement Count

Daily fetal movement count (kick counts) is a maternal assessment of fetal movement by counting fetal movements in a period of time to identify potentially hypoxic fetuses. Maternal perception of fetal movement was one of the earliest and easiest tests of fetal well-being and remains an essential assessment of fetal health. Fetal activity is diminished in the compromised fetus and cessation of fetal movement has been documented preceding fetal demise (AWHONN, 2008). Kick counts have been proposed as a primary method of fetal surveillance for all pregnancies after 28 weeks' gestation.

Procedure

■ The pregnant woman is instructed to palpate her abdomen and track fetal movements daily for 1 or 2 hours.

Interpretation

■ In the 2-hour approach, maternal perception of 10 distinct fetal movements within 2 hours is considered reassuring; once movement is achieved, counts can be discontinued for the day.
■ In the 1-hour approach, the count is considered reassuring if it equals or exceeds the established baseline; in general 4 movements in 1 hour is reassuring.
■ Reports of decreased fetal movement should be reported to the provider and is an indication for further fetal assessment such as a non-stress test or biophysical profile.

Advantages

■ Done by pregnant women
■ Inexpensive, reassuring, and relatively easily taught to pregnant women

Risks

■ None

Nursing Actions

■ Teach the woman how to do kick counts and provide a means to record them (Fig. 6-6).
■ If fetal movement is decreased, the woman should be instructed to have something to eat, rest, and focus on fetal movement for 1 hour. Four movements in one hour is considered reassuring.
■ Instruct the woman to report decreased fetal movement below normal as decreasing fetal movements are an indication for further assessment by care providers.

Non-Stress Test

The **non-stress tests (NST)** is a screening tool that uses electronic fetal monitoring (EFM) to assess fetal well-being (Fig. 6-7). The heart rate of a physiologically normal fetus with adequate oxygenation and intact autonomic nervous system accelerates in response to movement (AWHONN, 2008). The NST records accelerations in

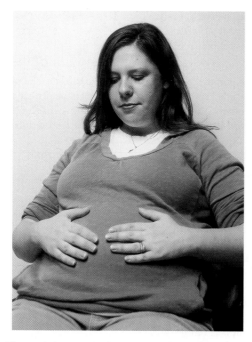

Figure 6-6   A pregnant woman doing kick counts.

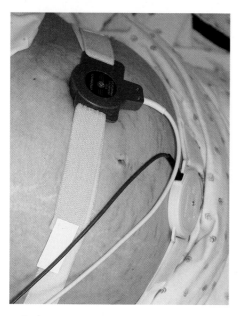

Figure 6-7   Monitoring for a non-stress test.

the fetal heart rate (FHR) in relation to fetal activity. It is the most widely accepted method of evaluating fetal status, particularly for high-risk pregnant women with complications such as hypertension, diabetes, and placental abnormalities.

Procedure

- The FHR is monitored with the external FHR transducer until reactive (up to 40 minutes).
- Monitor FHR and fetal activity for 20 to 30 minutes (placement of EFM and interpretation of EFM are described in Chapter 9).

Interpretation

- The NST is considered reactive when the FHR increases 15 beats above baseline for 15 seconds twice in 20 minutes.
- In fetuses less than 32 weeks' gestation two accelerations peaking at least 10 bpm above baseline and lasting 10 seconds in a 20-minute period is reactive (AWHONN, 2008).
- Nonreactive NST is one without sufficient FHR accelerations in 40 minutes and should be followed up with further testing such as a BPP (AAP & ACOG, 2002).

Advantages

- Noninvasive, easily performed, and reliable indicator of fetal well-being

Risks

- None

Nursing Actions

- Explain the procedure to the woman and her family.
- Provide comfort measures.
- Provide emotional support.
- Interpret FHR and accelerations; report results to the care provider.
- Schedule appropriate follow-up; the typical interval for testing is biweekly.

Vibroacoustic Stimulation

Vibroacoustic stimulation (VAS) is a screening tool that uses auditory stimulation (using an artificial larynx) to assess fetal well-being with EFM when NST is nonreactive.

Procedure

- VAS is conducted by activating an artificial larynx on the maternal abdomen near the fetal head for 1 second. This can be repeated at 1-minute intervals up to 3 times.

Interpretation

- The NST using VAS is considered reactive when the FHR increases 15 beats above baseline for 15 seconds twice in 20 minutes.

Advantages

- Using VAS to stimulate the fetus has reduced the incidence of nonreactive NSTs and reduced the time required to conduct NSTs.

Risks

- No adverse effects reported

Nursing Actions

- Explain the procedure to the woman and her family.
- Provide comfort measures.
- Provide emotional support.
- Interpret FHR and accelerations and conduct VAS appropriately.
- Schedule appropriate follow-up.

Contraction Stress Test

The **contraction stress test (CST)** is a screening tool to assess fetal well-being with EFM in women with nonreactive NST at term gestation. The purpose of the CST is to identify a fetus that is at risk for compromise through observation of the fetal response to intermittent reduction in utero placental blood flow associated with stimulated uterine contractions (UCs) (AWHONN, 2008).

Procedure

- Monitor FHR and fetal activity for 20 minutes.
- If no spontaneous UCs, stimulate UCs with oxytocin via IV until 3 UCs in 10 to 20 minutes lasting 40 seconds occur (placement of EFM and interpretation of EFM are described in Chapter 9).

Interpretation

- The CST is considered negative or normal when there are no significant variable decelerations or no late decelerations.
- The CST is positive where there are late decelerations of FHR with 50% of UCs; this requires further testing such as BPP.
- The CST is equivocal or suspicious when there are intermittent late or variable decelerations.

Advantages

- Negative CSTs are associated with good fetal outcomes.

Risks

- CST has a high false-positive rate which can result in unnecessary intervention.
- Cannot be used with women who have a contraindication for uterine activity.

Nursing Actions

- Explain the procedure to the woman and her family.
- Provide comfort measures.
- Provide emotional support.
- Correctly interpret FHR and contractions.
- Safely administer oxytocin (i.e., avoid uterine tachysystole).
- Recognize adverse effects of oxytocin.
- Schedule appropriate follow-up.

Amniotic Fluid Index

The **amniotic fluid index (AFI)** is a screening tool that measures the volume of amniotic fluid with ultrasound to assess fetal well-being and placental function. The amniotic fluid level is based on fetal urine production which is the predominate source of amniotic fluid and is directly dependent on renal perfusion (Queenan, Hobbins, & Spong, 2005). In prolonged fetal hypoxemia, blood is shunted away from fetal kidneys to other vital organs. Persistent decreased blood flow to the fetal kidneys results in reduction of amniotic fluid production and oligohydramnios. In conjunction with NST, AFI is a strong indicator of fetal status, as it is accurate in detecting fetal hypoxia.

Procedure

- Measurement of pockets of amniotic fluid in four quadrants of the uterine cavity via ultrasound.

Interpretation

- Average measurement in pregnancy is 8 to 24 cm (Cunningham et al., 2005).
- Abnormal AFI is below 5 cm. An AFI ≤ 5 cm is indicative of **oligohydramnios**. Oligohydramnios is associated with increased prenatal mortality.

- An AFI above 24 cm **(polyhydramnios)** may indicate a fetal malformation such as NTDs, obstruction of fetal gastrointestinal tract, or fetal hydrops.

Advantages

- AFI is a reflection of placental function and perfusion to the fetus as well as overall fetal condition.

Risks

- None

Nursing Actions

- Explain the procedure to the woman and her family.
- Provide comfort measures.
- Provide emotional support.
- Schedule appropriate follow-up.
- Special training in obstetric ultrasound is required for evaluation of amniotic fluid volume (see Box 6-1).

Biophysical Profile

The **biophysical profile (BPP/BPA)** is an ultrasound assessment of fetal status along with an NST. It involves evaluation of fetal status through ultrasound observation of various fetal reflex activities that are central nervous system (CNS) controlled and sensitive to fetal hypoxia. If fetal oxygen consumption is reduced, the immediate fetal response is reduction of activity regulated by the CNS. The BPP includes assessment of fetal breathing movement, gross body movement, fetal tone, amniotic fluid volume, and heart rate reactivity. The BPP provides improved prognostic information because physiological parameters associated with chronic and acute hypoxia are evaluated. It is indicated in pregnancies involving increased risk of fetal hypoxia and placental insufficiency such as maternal diabetes and hypertension.

Some controversy exists related to this test as a recent Cochrane review concluded that available evidence from randomized clinical trials provides no support for the use of BPP as a test of fetal well-being in high-risk pregnancies (Alfirevic & Neilson, 2006).

Procedure

- BPP consists of a NST with the addition of 30 minutes of ultrasound observation for four indicators: fetal breathing movements, fetal movement, fetal tone, and measurement of amniotic fluid.
  - *Assess fetal breathing movements: One or more episodes of rhythmic breathing movements of 30 seconds or move within 30 minutes is expected.*
  - *Assess fetal movement: Three or more discrete body or limb movements in 30 minutes are expected.*
  - *Assess fetal tone: One or more fetal extremity extension with return to fetal flexion or opening and closing of the hand is expected.*
  - *Assess amniotic fluid volume: A pocket of amniotic fluid that measures at least 2 cm in two planes perpendicular to each other is expected.*

Interpretation

- A score of 2 (present) or 0 (absent) is assigned to each of the five components.
- A score of 8 or 10 is reassuring.
- A score of 6 is equivocal and may indicate the need for delivery depending on gestational age.

■ A score of 4 or less is non-reassuring and warrants further evaluation and consideration for delivery (AAP & ACOG, 2002).

■ Fetal activity decreases or stops to reduce energy and oxygen consumption as fetal hypoxemia worsens. Decreased activity occurs in reverse order of normal development.

■ Fetal activities that appear earliest in pregnancy (tone and movement) are usually the last to cease and activities that are the last to develop are usually the first to be diminished (FHR variability).

Advantages

■ Lower false-positive rate

Risks

■ None

Nursing Actions

■ Explain the procedure to the woman and her family.
■ Provide comfort measures.
■ Provide emotional support.
■ Special training in obstetric ultrasound is required for interpretation of ultrasound components of the test (see Box 6-1).
■ Schedule appropriate follow–up; the typical interval for testing is 1 week but for specific pregnancy complications may be biweekly.

Modified Biophysical Profile

The **modified BPP** combines an NST with an AFI as an indicator of short-term fetal well-being and AFI as an indicator of long-term placental function to evaluate fetal well-being. It is indicated in high-risk pregnancy related to maternal conditions or pregnancy-related conditions (see Table 6-1).

Procedure

■ A modified BPP combines the use of an NST with an AFI.

Interpretation

■ A modified BPP is considered normal when the NST is reactive and the AFI is greater than 5 cm. An AFI less than or equal to 5 is indicative of oligohydramnios. Oligohydramnios is associated with increased perinatal mortality and decreased amniotic fluid may be a reflection of acute or chronic fetal asphyxia (Feinstein, Torgesen, & Atterbury, 2003).

Advantages

■ Less time to complete
■ Predictive of fetal well-being

Risks

■ None

Nursing Actions

■ Explain the procedure to the woman and her family.
■ Provide comfort measures.
■ Provide emotional support.
■ Special training in ultrasound is required for interpretation of amniotic fluid volume (see Box 6-1).
■ Schedule appropriate follow-up; the typical interval for testing is 1 week, but for specific pregnancy complications may be biweekly.

■ ■ ■ Review Questions ■ ■ ■

1. Assessment for risk factors includes:
   A. Cultural factors
   B. Medical and obstetrical issues
   C. Religion

2. The nurse's role in antepartal testing includes:
   A. Interpreting results
   B. Obtaining consent
   C. Explaining how and why test is performed
   D. Referring the woman's question to a physician

3. Screening tests are designed to:
   A. Be offered to all pregnant women
   B. Identify those not affected by a disease
   C. Identify a particular disease
   D. Make a specific diagnosis

4. Amniocentesis done after 15 weeks is associated with a fetal death rate of:
   A. Less than 1%
   B. Less than 5%
   C. Greater than 1%
   D. Approximately 5%

5. Daily fetal movement counts are done:
   A. Only in high-risk pregnancies
   B. By care providers during prenatal visits
   C. As soon as the pregnancy is confirmed.
   D. To identify potentially hypoxic fetuses

References

Alfirevic, Z., & Neilson, J. (2006). Biophysical profile for fetal assessment in high risk pregnancies. (Cochrane review). Cochrane Library, Issue 1, 2006. Oxford: Update Software.

American Academy of Pediatrics and the American College of Obstetricians and Gynecologists (2002). *Guidelines for perinatal care* (5th ed.). Washington, DC: Author.

Association of Women's Health, Obstetric, and Neonatal Nurses (AWHONN). (1998). *Clinical Competencies and education guide: Limited ultrasound examinations in obstetrics and gynecology/infertility settings* (2nd ed.). Washington, DC: Author.

Association of Women's Health, Obstetric, and Neonatal Nurses (AWHONN). (2008). *Fetal heart rate monitoring: Principles and practice* (4th ed.). Washington, DC: Author.

Cunningham, F., Leveno, K., Bloom, S., Hauth, J., Gilstrap, L., & Wenstrom, K. (2005). *Williams obstetrics* (22nd ed.). New York: McGraw-Hill.

Feinstein, N., Torgersen, K., & Atterbury, J. (2003). *AWHONN's fetal heart monitoring principles and practices* (3rd ed.). Washington, DC: Association of Women's Health, Obstetric and Neonatal Nurses.

Gilbert, E., & Harmon, J. (2003). *Manual of high risk pregnancy and delivery.* St. Louis, MO: C. V. Mosby.

Leeuwen, A., Kranpitz, T., & Smith, L. (2006). *Davis's comprehensive handbook of laboratory and diagnostic tests with nursing implications. Philadelphia:* F. A. Davis.

Menihan, A. (2000). Limited ultrasound examinations in nursing practice. *Journal of Obstetric, Gynecologic and Neonatal Nursing, 29*(3), 325–330.

Queenan, J., Hobbins, J., & Spong, C. (2005). *Protocols in high risk pregnancies.* Malden, MA: Blackwell.

Simpson, K., & Creehan, P., & Association of Women's Health, Obstetrics and Neonatal Nursing. (2001). *Perinatal nursing.* Philadelphia: Lippincott.

Stringer, M., Miesnik, S., Brown, L., Menei, L., & Macones, G. (2003). Limited obstetric ultrasound examinations: Competency and cost. *Journal of Obstetric, Gynecologic and Neonatal Nursing, 32*(3), 307–312.

High-Risk Antepartum Nursing Care

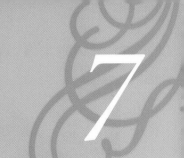

OBJECTIVES

On completion of this chapter, the student will be able to:

- ☐ Define key terms.
- ☐ Describe the primary complications of pregnancy and the related nursing and medical care.
- ☐ Demonstrate understanding of knowledge related to preexisting medical complications of pregnancy and related management.
- ☐ Identify potential antenatal complications for the woman, the fetus and the newborn.
- ☐ Describe the key aspects of discharge teaching for women with antenatal complications.

Nursing Diagnosis

- Risk of maternal injury related to pregnancy complications
- Risk of maternal injury related to preexisting medical conditions
- Risk of fetal injury related to complications of pregnancy

Nursing Outcomes

- The woman will understand management of a high-risk pregnancy condition and warning signs.
- The woman will give birth without serious complications.
- The woman will give birth to a healthy infant without complications.

INTRODUCTION

This chapter presents information on key complications that can occur during pregnancy and on preexisting medical conditions that have the potential to be exacerbated by pregnancy. An overview of each complication is presented including underlying pathophysiology, risk factors, risks posed to the woman and fetus, and typical medical management and nursing actions.

The nature of perinatal nursing is unpredictable, and pregnancy complications can arise abruptly, resulting in rapid deterioration of maternal and fetal status. It is imperative that nurses understand the underlying physiological mechanisms of pregnancy, the impact of complications on maternal and fetal well-being, and current interventions to optimize maternal and fetal outcomes.

GESTATIONAL COMPLICATIONS

Although most pregnant women experience a normal pregnancy, various complications can develop during pregnancy that affect maternal and fetal well-being. When women experience pregnancy complications, astute assessment, rapid intervention, and a team approach are essential to optimize maternal and neonatal outcomes. In this section, complications related to pregnancy are presented along with the physiological and pathological basis for the most common complications of pregnancy. Nursing care and appropriate management are discussed.

Preterm Labor and Birth

Premature labor (PTL) is the onset of labor before 37 weeks' gestation. **Preterm birth (PTB)** refers to gestational age at birth of less than 37 weeks. A **preterm/premature infant** is born after 20 weeks and before 37 completed weeks of gestation (Fig. 7-1).

More specific classifications of prematurity include (Peristats, 2008):

- **Late preterm infant:** An infant born between 34 and 36 weeks of gestation
- **Moderately preterm infant:** An infant born between 32 and 36 completed weeks of gestation
- **Very preterm infant:** An infant born before 32 completed weeks of gestation
- **Low birth weight infant (LBW):** An infant who weighs less than 2,500 grams at delivery, regardless of gestational age; Among low birth weight infants, two thirds are preterm.
- **Very low birth weight infant:** An infant who weighs less than 1,500 grams at birth
- **Extremely low birth weight infant:** An infant who weighs less than 1,000 grams at birth

During the last 20 years, the preterm birth rate has increased more than 28%, from 9.6% in 1983 to 11.0% in 1993 to 12.3% in 2003 and now 12.7% (March of Dimes, 2006a; Martin et al., 2006). Prematurity is the number one cause of neonatal mortality and the number two cause of infant mortality in the United States. Data from 2006 indicate hospital charges for premature infants that year

Want to reinforce your reading? Need to review for a test? Listen to this chapter on your accompanying CD.

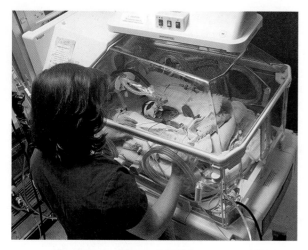

Figure 7-1 Premature infant in the NICU.

totaled more than $18 billion in immediate costs of neonatal intensive care and the morbidity associated with prematurity such as respiratory distress syndrome, intraventricular hemorrhages, and necrotizing enterocolitis (March of Dimes, 2006b). Long-term sequelae for preterm infants include cerebral palsy, sensory deficits, and special health care and learning needs. Long-term costs include not only health care costs but also special education costs for learning problems, costs of developmental services and health care costs for long-term sequelae associated with prematurity. The goals of *Healthy People 2010* and the March of Dimes are to reduce the preterm birth rate to 7.6% (March of Dimes, 2006a).

Pathophysiological Pathways of Preterm Labor

The specific causes of spontaneous preterm labor and delivery are largely unknown. Preterm labor is characterized as a series of complex interactions of factors. No single factor acts alone but multiple factors interact to initiate a cascade of events that result in preterm labor and birth (Simpson & Creehan, 2008). The pathways to preterm birth are thought to be multicausal and contributing factors include (March of Dimes, 2006a) (Fig. 7-2):

■ Inflammation and infection contribute 40%.
  ■ *Inflammatory cytokines or bacterial endotoxins can stimulate prostaglandin release.*
■ Activation of fetal hypothalamic–pituitary adrenal (HPA) axis from maternal–fetal stress or physiological initiators contributes 30%.

■ Decidual hemorrhage/abruption contributes 20%.
■ Uterine overdistension contributes 10%.
  ■ *Prostaglandin can be produced, stimulating the uterus to contract when overdistended.*
■ Psychosocial factors are also hypothesized to contribute to a stress response that results in uterine contractions (UCs).

Because we do not know what triggers normal labor at term, it is difficult to know what causes preterm labor. Extensive research has been conducted over the past three decades to predict which women are at risk to deliver preterm so that intensive interventions can be implemented to prevent prematurity. The risk factors predict only about half the women who will deliver preterm.

Risk Factors for Preterm Labor and Birth

Fifty percent of women who deliver preterm have no risk factors. Seventy percent of women who are at risk for preterm delivery go on to deliver at term. Research indicates it is a complex interplay of multiple risk factors (Peristats, 2008). Significant racial disparities remain largely unexplained (Creasy, Resnik, & Iams, 2004).

Common risk factors include (Freda, Patterson, & Wieczorek, 2004):

■ Multiple gestation (50% of twins delivered preterm, ≥90% higher multiples delivered preterm)
■ Prior preterm birth (single most important factor)
■ Uterine/cervical abnormalities, diethylstilbestrol (DES) exposure
■ Infection, especially genitourinary infections and periodontal disease
■ Premature rupture of membranes
■ Stress
■ Domestic violence
■ Vaginal bleeding
■ Lack of social support
■ Inadequate nutrition
■ Age younger than 17 or older than 35 years old
■ Smoking, alcohol, and illicit drug use
■ Late or no prenatal care
■ Low socioeconomic status
■ Ancestry and ethnicity
  ■ *Preterm birth rates are highest for African American infants.*
■ Chronic health problems such as hypertension, diabetes, or clotting disorders
■ Working long hours, long periods of standing

Most preterm births (75%) are a result of preterm labor and/or preterm premature rupture of membrane (PPROM) and related

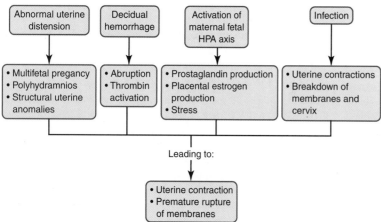

Figure 7-2 Pathophysiological pathway to preterm labor.

diagnoses (Creasy, Resnik, & Iams, 2004). However, 25% of preterm births are clinically indicated for complications (intentional preterm birth) that place the woman or fetus at risk such as preeclampsia or intrauterine growth restriction.

Risks for the Woman Related to Preterm Labor and Birth

■ Complications related to bedrest and treatment with tocolytics

Risks for the Fetus Related to Preterm Labor and Birth

■ Complications of prematurity (see Chapter 17)

Assessment Findings

■ Persistent uterine contractions (Critical Component: Diagnosis of Preterm Labor)
■ Dilated to 1 cm or greater or 80% effaced
■ Positive biochemical marker
   ■ *Fetal fibronectin (fFN) is a protein detected via immunoassay; a positive test is greater than 50 ng/mL. A negative fFN has a high negative predictive value (up to 95%) that the woman will not deliver in 7 to 14 days. It has a poor positive predictive value (25%–40%), which limits its ability to predict women who will deliver preterm (Simpson & Creehan, 2008). In other words, fFN is better at predicting who will not deliver preterm than who will deliver preterm.*

CRITICAL COMPONENT

Diagnosis of Preterm Labor

The diagnosis of preterm labor is made when the follow criteria are met:

■ Gestational age of >20 weeks and <37 weeks
■ Documented regular uterine contractions (UCs) ≥6/hour. *and* at least one of the following:
■ Rupture of membranes (ROM)
■ Cervical change: Cervix ≥1 cm dilated or 80% effaced (criteria for cervical dilation varies)

Medical Management

Current interventions to stop preterm labor have not been proven to be effective. The cornerstones of management of preterm labor are still administration of medications to stop uterine contractions and bed rest. Typically management is focused on delaying delivery for several days (optimal is 72 hours) to give glucocorticoids (corticosteroids) time to facilitate fetal lung maturity. Medical management includes:

■ **Tocolytic drugs** are medications that are used to suppress uterine contractions in preterm labor. These agents have drawbacks and potential serious adverse effects (Table 7-1). A review of evidence on tocolytic therapy revealed a small improvement in pregnancy prolongation and that extended use has little or no value (Berkman et al., 2003). Current management now is focused on delaying delivery for several days to give corticosteroids time to work and to treat Group B *Streptococcus* infections. Using tocolytic drugs to delay delivery for a few days is well documented. However, their impact on decreasing prematurity is yet unproved (Creasy, Resnik, & Iams, 2004). Terbutaline pump therapy has not been shown to decrease the risk of preterm birth by prolonging pregnancy (Nanda, Cook, Gallo, & Grimes, 2002).
■ **Bed rest** is a widely used first step in the treatment of preterm labor, but there is no evidence to support or refute its use at home

or in the hospital to prevent preterm birth. Current evidence based on systematic reviews of research on bed rest during pregnancy highlight potential adverse effects on the woman and her family (Maloni, 1993, 1998; Sosa, Althabe, Belizán, & Bergel, 2004):
   ■ *Muscle atrophy*
   ■ *Cardiovascular deconditioning*
   ■ *Maternal weight loss*
   ■ *Stress for the woman and her family*
■ **Intravenous hydration** is a common strategy to reduce preterm uterine contractions because it increases vascular volume and may help to decrease contractions. It should be used with caution due to the potential for pulmonary edema when tocolytic agents are used.
■ **Antibiotics** are commonly used to treat genital urinary infections but prophylactic antibiotic treatment is not recommended (Creasy, Resnik, & Iams, 2004).
■ **Corticosteroid therapy**, with antenatal steroids, are currently recommended to women at risk of preterm birth (Medication Box: Corticosteroids). Betamethasone is one antenatal steroid given to women to accelerate fetal lung maturity, thereby decreasing the severity of respiratory distress syndrome and other complications of prematurity in the neonate. Treatment with antenatal corticosteroids reduces the risk of neonatal respiratory distress syndrome, cerebroventricular hemorrhage, necrotizing enterocolitis, and infectious morbidity in the neonate when used between 24 and 34 weeks' gestation (Roberts & Dalziel, 2006).
■ If UCs decrease to fewer than five per hour, then women are often transferred to less acute antenatal units for further observations for several days. If they remain stable they may be discharged to home undelivered. Discharge instructions typically include bedrest or activity restriction, self-monitoring of uterine activity, and signs and symptoms of preterm labor, and may include oral tocolytics or use of terbutaline pump therapy.
■ Contraindications to treating preterm labor include:
   ■ *Active hemorrhage*
   ■ *Severe maternal disease*
   ■ *Fetal compromise*
   ■ *Chorioamnionitis*
   ■ *Fetal death*

Medication

Corticosteroids
Betamethasone/Dexamethasone

■ Indication: Given to women at 24 and 34 weeks' gestation with signs of preterm labor or at risk to deliver preterm
■ Action: Stimulate the production of more mature surfactant in the fetal lungs to prevent respiratory distress syndrome in premature infants
■ Adverse reactions: None
■ Route and dose:
   Betamethasone 12 mg IM every 24 hours × 2 doses
   Dexamethasone 6 mg IM every 12 hours × 2 doses

(Data from Deglin & Vallerand, 2009)

Nursing Actions

Nurses can provide expertise in directing patient care, stabilizing the woman and fetus, counseling, coordinating care, and providing patient teaching (Grey, 2006; March of Dimes, 2006b). Immediate care, including assessment and stabilization, occurs in labor and

TABLE 7–1   COMMON TOCOLYTIC DRUGS

DRUG	PHARMACOLOGY AND ACTION	DOSAGE AND ADMINISTRATION	MATERNAL EFFECTS	FETAL EFFECTS	NURSING CONSIDERATIONS
MAGNESIUM SULFATE (MgSO₄)	Depresses myometrium contractility, relaxes smooth muscle of the uterus. It has not been proven to have either short- or long-term effectiveness as a tocolytic agent.	Administered continuous IV infusion via a pump, Initial loading dose of 4–6 grams in 20 minutes, then 2 g/hr. Therapeutic level at 5–8 mg/dL in maternal serum levels, or as tolerated by the patient.	Flushing, drowsiness, headache, lethargy, nausea and vomiting. Respiratory depression can occur with serum levels above 9 mg/dL.	No demonstrable effect on the neonate	Monitor FHR and UCs. Monitor serum magnesium levels. Signs and symptoms of maternal toxicity include: ■ Absent DTRs, respiratory rate < 14 breaths/min, severe hypotension and muscle relaxation, decreased level of consciousness ■ Assess lungs for signs and symptoms of pulmonary edema. Check I&O for fluid overload or output of <30 mL/hr. For details of care of the woman and Magnesium Sulfate see Critical Component box Care of the Woman on Magnesium Sulfate page 116.
PROSTAGLANDIN SYNTHESIS INHIBITORS Indomethacin Naproxen Fenoprofen	Depresses synthesis of prostaglandins Effective in delaying delivery 48+ hours; because of fetal side effects generally used short term and before 32 weeks	Indomethacin 50 mg orally loading dose, then 25–50 mg orally every 6 hours	GI upset; serious side effects are uncommon.	Serious fetal side effects include constriction of the patent ductus arteriosis, neonatal pulmonary hypertension, oligohydramniosis, and intraventricular hemorrhages.	Monitor FHR and UCs. Treat nausea and heartburn.

CALCIUM CHANNEL BLOCKERS Nifedipine Nicardipine	Inhibits smooth muscle contractions of uterus by blocking calcium availability for muscle contraction As effective or superior as other agents in delaying delivery 48–72 hours	10–20 mg PO every 4–6 hours	Flushing, headache, nausea, transient tachycardia and hypotension	Limited clinical evidence on fetal effects, may decrease uteroplacental blood flow.	Monitor FHR and UCs. Monitor maternal blood pressure and heart rate and may hold dose for blood pressure <90/50 or heart rate >120
BETA-ADRENERGIC AGONISTS Ritodrine Terbutaline	Beta 2 adrenergic effects to suppress uterine activity Can delay delivery for 3 days Given IV or SQ Oral use of drugs has not demonstrated any improvement in preterm birth or preterm labor.	Terbutaline IV/SQ IV maximum dose 0.08 mg/min SQ; 0.25 mg every 3–4 hours Ritodrine IV maximum dose .350 mg/min	Highest rates of serious maternal side effects including tachycardia, cardiac arrhythmia, myocardial ischemia and pulmonary edema, elevation in maternal glucose, hypokalemia	Mild fetal tachycardia, conflicting reports on incidence of IVH	Monitor FHR and UCs. Monitor I&O for fluid overload. Auscultate lungs for pulmonary edema. Monitor maternal HR and may hold dose for heart rate >120. Monitor blood glucose. Life-threatening complications are pulmonary edema, myocardial failure, and fluid overload. Contraindicated in women with cardiac disease.

Sources: Gilbert (2007); Deglin & Vallerand (2007); Simpson & Creehan (2008).

delivery. If uterine activity decreases, generally to fewer than 5 UCs/hr, and there is no further cervical change, women are often moved to a less intensive care setting than a labor and delivery unit. Once moved to an antenatal high-risk unit they are often observed for several days and if stable discharged to home undelivered.

Immediate care:

- Review the prenatal record for risk factors and establish gestational age through history and ultrasound (ultrasound early in pregnancy is more reliable for gestational age).
- Assess the woman and fetus for signs and symptoms of:
  - *Vaginal and urinary infection*
  - *Rupture of membranes*
    - A sterile speculum exam may be performed to assess for ferning of the amniotic fluid
  - *Vaginal bleeding or vaginal discharge*
  - *Dehydration*
- Assess fetal heart rate (FHR) and uterine contractions.
  - *Report fetal tachycardia or increased uterine contractions to the health care provider.*
- Obtain vaginal and urine cultures as per orders.
- Obtain fFN as per orders.
  - *This should be obtained before the sterile vaginal exam.*
- Maintain strict input and output (I&O).
- Provide oral or IV hydration.
  - *May restrict total intake to 3,000 mL/24 hr if on tocolytics*
- Administer tocolytic agents as per orders.
  - *Monitor for adverse reactions (see Table 7-1).*
- Administer glucocorticoids (betamethasone) as per orders.
- Position the patient on her side to increase uteroplacental perfusion and decrease pressure on the maternal inferior vena cava.
- Assess vital signs per protocol for tocolytic administered.
  - *Report to the provider blood pressure greater than 140/90 mm Hg or less than 90/50 mm Hg; heart rate greater than 120; temperature greater than 100.4°F (38°C).*
- Auscultate lungs for evidence of pulmonary edema.
- Assess cervical status with a sterile vaginal exam unless contraindicated by ROM or bleeding (may be done by the health care provider to minimize multiple exams); cervical ultrasound may be done (cervical length of less than 30 mm is clinically significant).
- Notify the care provider of findings.

Continuing care once stable:

- Provide emotional support to the woman by providing opportunities to discuss her feelings. Women often feel guilt that they caused the preterm labor and are concerned for the infant's health and have anxiety and sadness over loss of "normal" newborn and normal pregnancy labor and delivery (Critical Component: Nursing Actions to Promote Adaptation to Pregnancy Complications).
- Facilitate a clear understanding of the treatment plan and the woman's and family's involvement in clinical decision-making.
- Facilitate consultations with the neonatal staff regarding neonatal survival rates, the anticipated care of the newborn, treatments, complications, and possible long-term disabilities. The family may be taken on a tour of NICU.
- Monitor the woman's response to treatment including FHR baseline and variability and uterine contractions, maternal vital signs, woman's response to tocolytics, increase in vaginal discharge or ROM.
- Assessment of women on tocolytics is based on tocolytic used and is detailed in Table 7-1, but generally includes monitoring of blood pressure and pulse and auscultation of lungs for pulmonary edema. Watch for:

- *Shortness of breath, chest tightness or discomfort, cough, oxygen saturation less than 95%, increased respiratory and heart rates*
- *Changes in behavior such as apprehension, anxiety, or restlessness*
- Encourage a side-lying position to enhance placental perfusion.
- Evaluate laboratory reports such as urine and cervical cultures.
  - *White blood cell (WBC) counts are elevated in women who have received corticosteroids, therefore, elevated WBCs are not indicative of infection.*
- Provide ongoing reassurance and explanations to the woman and her family.
- Explain the purpose and side effects of the medication.
- Set short-term goals such as completion of a gestational week or milestones.
- Facilitate family interactions and visiting by having flexible visiting policies.
- Facilitate a clear understanding of the treatment plan and the woman's involvement in clinical decision making.
- Assist with passive limb exercises for women on bedrest to decrease muscle deterioration.
- Assist with hygiene and self-care based on orders for activity.
- Provide diversional activities that interest the woman.

CRITICAL COMPONENT

Nursing Activities to Promote Adaptation to Pregnancy Complications

Pregnancy complications represent a threat to both the woman's and fetus's health and to the emotional well-being of the family. Assessment of emotional status and coping of the entire family is necessary to provide comprehensive care. Implementing individualized plan of care will facilitate the family's transition during an often unexpected and frightening experience (Gilbert, 2007).

Some general nursing actions include:

- Provide time for the woman and family to express their concerns, which may include apprehension, fear, anger, and frustration.
- Explain high-risk conditions, procedures, diagnostic tests, and treatment plan in layman's terms.
  - Provide ongoing updates.
  - Clarify misconceptions.
- Facilitate referrals related to the condition which may include social services and chaplain services.
- Practice active listening.
- Encourage the woman and her family to participate in decision making and care.

Discharge Plan

All plans should be decided with the woman's and family's strengths, needs, and goals in mind and with their participation (March of Dimes, 2006b) (Fig. 7-3). Discharge teaching should include:

- Warning signs and how and when to call the provider (Box 7-1)
- A clear understanding of the treatment plan including use of tocolytics and bedrest/activity restriction (Box 7-2)

Programs have demonstrated some improvement in outcomes with nurse phone or home care follow-up (Freda, Patterson, & Wieczorek, 2004; Gilbert, 2007). Typically women treated for preterm labor are sent home without follow-up at home except weekly prenatal visits. Topics that should be discussed include (Durham, 1998; Maloni, 1998):

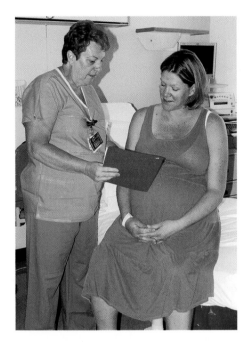

Figure 7-3 Nurse doing discharge teaching with high-risk pregnant woman in the hospital.

BOX 7–1 WARNING SIGNS OF PRETERM LABOR

Call you doctor or midwife or the hospital for any of the following:

- Your bag of waters breaks.
- Your baby stops moving.
- You have more than _____ contractions in an hour.
- You have a low backache, menstrual like cramps, pelvic pressure, or intestinal cramps with or without diarrhea.
- You have increased discharge from your vagina.
- You have a fever higher than 100.4°F (38°C).
- You feel "something is not right."

MD or midwife number is _____
Hospital labor and delivery number is _____

- Effects of activity restriction on the woman and family including emotional distress (Evidence-Based Practice: Cochrane Review on Social Support during at-risk Pregnancy)
- Maternal anxiety about the health of the woman and fetus
- Childcare difficulties when on bed rest and plan for at home
- Financial and career difficulties
- Physical activity restrictions may include restricted sexual activity.

Preterm Premature Rupture of Membranes/Chorioamnionitis

Premature rupture of membranes is defined as rupture of the chorioamniotic membranes before the onset of labor. **Preterm premature rupture of membranes (PPROM)** is rupture of membranes with a premature gestation (<37 weeks). Adding to the confusion is **prolonged rupture of membranes** which is greater than 24 hours (PROM). This section focuses on those women that have rupture of membranes preterm (PPROM), as it accounts for approximately

BOX 7–2 HOME CARE INSTRUCTIONS FOR PRETERM LABOR

Baby movements and contractions	Lie on your side for 1 hour and count the number of times your baby moves. If your baby does not move ___ times call your doctor or midwife. While lying on your sides, place your fingertips on your abdomen and feel for tightening. If you have more than ____ contractions in 1 hour call your doctor or midwife.
Activity restrictions	Indicate restrictions on physical activity and be specific.
Sexual relations	Indicate restrictions on sexual relations.
Diet	Small meals and snacks may be easier to tolerate and be sure to include foods high in fiber, calcium, and iron.
Fluids	Drink at least eight 8-ounce glasses of fluid a day including water, milk, and juices.
Medication schedule	Per discharge orders with teaching related to specific medications May include: tocolytic, prenatal vitamin (PNV), iron sulfate, stool softeners

30% of premature births. Bacterial infections are thought to weaken the membranes leading to rupture. Once the membranes rupture, labor usually begins within 24 hours.

Risk Factors for PPROM

- Previous PPROM
- Previous preterm delivery
- Bleeding during pregnancy
- Multiple gestation (up to 15% in twins, up to 20% in triplets)
- Sexually transmitted diseases (STDs)
- Cigarette smoking

(Queenan, Hobbins, & Spong, 2005)

Risks for the Woman

- Maternal infection (i.e., chorioamnionitis)
- Preterm labor and birth
- Increased rates of cesarean birth

Risks for the Newborn

- Fetal or neonatal sepsis
  - *The earlier the fetal gestation at ROM, the greater the risk for infection*
  - *The membranes serve as a protective barrier that separates the sterile fetus and fluid from the bacteria-laden vaginal canal*
- Preterm delivery and complications of prematurity
- Hypoxia or asphyxia because of umbilical cord compression due to decreased fluid
- Fetal deformities if PPROM before 26 weeks' gestation

Assessment Findings

- Confirmed premature gestational age by prenatal history and ultrasound
- Confirmed rupture of membranes with speculum exam and positive ferning test
- Oligohydramniosis on ultrasound

Evidence-Based Practice: Cochrane Review on Social Support during at-risk Pregnancy

Hodnett E. D., & Fredericks, S. (2003). Support during pregnancy for women at increased risk of low birth weight babies. *Cochrane Database of Systematic Reviews* 2003, Issue 3. Art. No.: CD000198. DOI: 10.1002/14651858.CD000198.

Studies consistently show a relationship between social disadvantage and low birth weight. Many countries have programs offering special assistance to women thought to be at risk for giving birth to a low birth weight infant. These programs may include advice and counseling (about nutrition, rest, stress management, alcohol and recreational drug use), tangible assistance (e.g., transportation to clinic appointments, help with household responsibilities), and emotional support. The programs may be delivered by multidisciplinary teams of health professionals, by specially trained lay workers, or by a combination of lay and professional workers.

This Cochrane Review evaluated the effects of programs offering additional social support for pregnant women who are believed to be at risk for giving birth to preterm or low birth weight babies.

Randomized trials of interventions offering additional support during at-risk pregnancy by either a professional (social worker, midwife, or nurse) or specially trained lay person, compared to routine care were evaluated. Additional support was defined as some form of emotional support (e.g., counseling, reassurance, sympathetic listening) and information or advice or both, either in home visits or during clinic appointments, and could include tangible assistance (e.g., transportation to clinic appointments, assistance with the care of other children at home).

Main Results:

Eighteen trials, involving 12,658 women, were included. The trials were generally of good to excellent quality, although three used an allocation method likely to introduce bias. Programs offering additional social support for at-risk pregnant women were not associated with improvements in any perinatal outcomes, but there was a reduction in the likelihood of caesarean birth. Some improvements in immediate maternal psychosocial outcomes were found in individual trials.

Authors' Conclusions:

Pregnant women need the support of caring family members, friends, and health professionals. Although programs that offer additional support during pregnancy are unlikely to prevent the pregnancy from resulting in a low birth weight or preterm baby, they may be helpful in reducing the likelihood of cesarean birth.

Medical Management

Medical treatment is aimed at balancing the risks of prematurity and the risks of infections. In the woman with PPROM, management is aimed at prolonging gestation for the woman that is not in labor, not infected, and not experiencing fetal compromise.

■ Monitor for infection, labor, and fetal compromise.
■ Assess for fetal lung maturity with LS ratio/phosphatidyl glycerol (PG).
■ Administer prophylactic antibiotic therapy to reduce maternal and fetal infections.

■ The use of tocolytics is controversial, as is the use of corticosteroids to accelerate lung maturity but they appear to improve outcomes when used before 32 weeks' gestation and in conjunction with prophylactic antibiotic therapy (Creasy, Resnik, & Iams, 2004).

Nursing Actions

■ Assess FHR and uterine contractions.
■ Assess for signs of infection including:
  ■ *Maternal and/or fetal tachycardia*
  ■ *Maternal fever 100.4°F (38°C) or greater*
  ■ *Uterine tenderness*
  ■ *Malodorous fluid or vaginal discharge*
■ Monitor for labor and for fetal compromise.
■ Provide antenatal testing including non-stress tests (NSTs) and biophysical profiles (BPPs).
■ See Critical Component Box: Nursing Activities to Promote Adaptation to Pregnancy Complications

Incompetent Cervix

Incompetent cervix is a mechanical defect in the cervix that results in painless cervical dilation and ballooning of the membranes into the vagina followed by expulsion of a premature fetus during the second trimester (Cunningham et al., 2005). When undiagnosed, it can result in repeated second trimester abortions.

The cause of cervical incompetence is unclear but it is associated with previous cervical trauma such as cervical dilation or cauterization and diethylstilbestrol (DES) exposure in utero. Cervical incompetence frequently results in multiple second trimester abortions without contractions.

Risks to the Woman

■ Repeated second trimester losses (e.g., spontaneous abortions)
■ Preterm delivery
■ Rupture of membranes/infection

Risk to the Newborn

■ Preterm birth

Assessment Findings

■ Shortened cervical length or funneling of the cervix
■ Obstetrical history of second trimester cervical dilation or fetal losses
■ Live fetus and intact membranes

Medical Management

■ Obtain transcervical ultrasound to evaluate cervix for cervical length and funneling.
■ Treatment of incompetent cervix is **cerclage,** which is a type of purse string suture placed cervically to reinforce a weak cervix (Fig. 7-4).
  ■ *Cerclage may be placed prophylactically before cervical dilation, generally between 12 and 16 weeks of gestation or emergently after the cervix has dilated, up to about 24 weeks of gestation (Cunningham et al., 2005).*
■ Administer antibiotics or tocolytics as needed.
■ Remove sutures if membranes rupture, infection occurs, or labor develops.

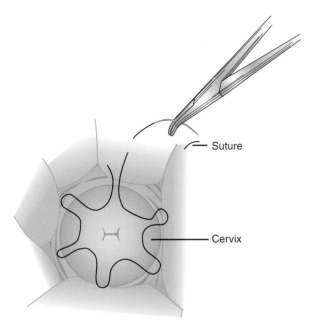

Figure 7-4 Cerclage.

Postoperative Nursing Actions

■ Provide emotional support.
■ Monitor for uterine activity with palpation.
■ Monitor for vaginal bleeding and leaking of fluid/rupture of membranes.
■ Monitor for infection.
  ■ *Maternal fever*
  ■ *Uterine tenderness*
■ Administer tocolytics to suppress uterine activity as per orders.

Multiple Gestations

Multiple gestation pregnancies are pregnancies with more than one fetus. They are more common now because of the use of ovulation-stimulating drugs and assisted reproductive technology (ART). Approximately one third of twins are monozygotic (from one egg) and two thirds are dizygotic (from two eggs).

■ **Monozygotic twins** are from one zygote that divides in the first week of gestation. They are genetically identical and similar in appearance and always have the same gender.
■ **Dizygotic twins** result from fertilization of two eggs. Dizygotic twins may be the same or differing genders.
■ There are two principal placental types, monochorionic (one chorion) and dichorionic (two chorions). About 20% of twins are monochorionic. Monoamniotic twins are the least common (1%) and results in an amniotic sac containing both twins. Because they share the same sac, monoamniotic twins have a fetal mortality rate of 50% to 60% due to entangling of umbilical cords (Creasy, Resnik, & Iams, 2004) (Fig. 7-5).

Although multiple gestations are only about 3% of births in the United States they contribute disproportionately to maternal, fetal, and neonatal morbidity and mortality (Simpson & Creehan, 2008). Risks for both the fetus and the woman increase with increased number of fetuses (Creasy, Resnik, & Iams, 2004).

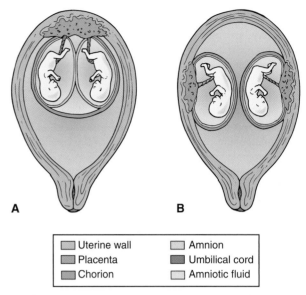

Uterine wall	Amnion
Placenta	Umbilical cord
Chorion	Amniotic fluid

Figure 7-5 *A.* Monozygotic twins. *B.* Dizygotic twins.

Risks for the Woman

■ Compared with women with twins, women with triplets or higher order multiples (HOM) are at even higher risk of pregnancy related morbidities and mortality (Simpson & Creehan, 2008).
■ Preterm labor and delivery rate is 50% or greater related to overdistension of the uterus.
■ Premature prolonged rupture of membranes related to overdistension of the uterus, occurs with up to 15% in twins and up to 20% in triplets.
■ Hypertensive disorders and preeclampsia, which tend to develop earlier and be more severe, are related to enlarged placenta.
■ Gestational diabetes often occurs due to physiological changes related to supporting multiple fetuses.
■ Antepartum hemorrhage, abruptio placenta, placenta previa
■ Anemia related to dilutional anemia.
■ Pulmonary edema related to increase cardiac workload
■ Cesarean birth

Risks for the Fetus

■ Increase in fetal morbidity and mortality due to sharing uterine space and placental circulation
  ■ *Increased perinatal mortality (threefold higher than in singleton pregnancy).*
  ■ *Intrauterine fetal death of one fetus after 20 weeks' gestation increases the risks to the surviving fetus(es).*
■ Increase of preterm delivery (50% higher in twins and >90% higher in multiples) (i.e., triplets or higher).
■ Increase of low birth weight neonates (20% higher than singleton)
■ Increase of intrauterine growth restriction (IUGR) and discordant growth (weight of one fetus differs significantly than others, usually ≥ 25%) related to placental insufficiency (Simpson & Creehan, 2008)
  ■ *Discordant growth and twin-to-twin transfusions from sharing a placenta occurs*
  ■ **Twin-to-twin transfusion** *due to an imbalance in blood flow through the vasculature of the placenta, leading to overperfusion of one twin and underperfusion of the co-twin*
■ Increase of congenital, chromosomal, and genetic defects

Assessment Findings

Nearly every maternal system is affected by the physiological changes that occur in multiple gestations. These changes are greater in multiple pregnancies than in singleton pregnancies (Simpson & Creehan, 2008).

■ Ultrasound confirmation of multiple gestation
■ Fundal height and size greater than dates and palpation of excessive number of fetal parts during Leopold's maneuver
■ Elevation of human chorionic gonadotropin (hCG) and alpha-fetoprotein
■ Increased cardiac output and plasma volume, which increases the risk of pulmonary edema
■ Increased dyspnea and shortness of breath
■ Increased plasma volume 50% to 100% (results in dilutional anemia)
■ Increased iron-deficiency anemia
■ Increased uterine size which leads to increased susceptibility to uterine hypotensive syndrome and PTL and PPROM
■ Increased nausea and vomiting
■ Increased lower back and ligament pain
■ Increased dermatosis

Antepartal Medical Management

A woman pregnant with multiple fetuses needs ongoing, frequent surveillance of the pregnancy because of the increased rates of complications, including:

■ Ultrasound for discordant fetal growth and IUGR, as well as placental sites, dividing membranes, congenital anomalies, and gender
■ Genetic testing for anomalies
■ Monitor for preterm labor.
■ Monitor for maternal anemia.
■ Fetal surveillance including NST, BPP
■ Monitor for hypertension and preeclampsia.
■ Monitor for hydramnios.
■ Monitor for antepartal hemorrhage.
■ Monitor for intrauterine fetal demise.
■ Nutritional consult
■ Consultation with perinatologist if complications occur

Intrapartum Medical Management

■ Ultrasound to confirm placental location and fetal positions
■ Continuous electronic fetal monitoring (EFM) of all fetuses
■ Cesarean birth access should be immediately available, including anesthesia, obstetricians, circulating nurse, and scrub personnel
■ Agents for hemorrhagic management available, including medications and blood products
■ The neonatal team available should be sufficient for all infants.
■ Birth mode varies with fetal presentations, maternal, and fetal health, and preference of the mother and the clinician and can be:
    ■ *Vaginal birth for both infants*
    ■ *Cesarean birth for both*
    ■ *Combined vaginal and cesarean birth if first fetus is born vaginally and second fetus needs to be delivery by cesarean birth for malpresentation or non-reassuring fetal status*
■ Triplets and higher multiples are delivered by cesarean birth.

Nursing Actions

■ Assess for the following possible complications:
    ■ *Preterm labor, however, uterine contractions as preterm labor can be more difficult to identify in women pregnant with multiple*

gestations because of more discomfort, stretching, and pressure with multiple fetuses, and overdistension of the uterus results in more uterine irritability (Gilbert, 2007).
    ■ *Hypertension or preeclampsia*
    ■ *Antepartal hemorrhage*
■ Conduct antepartal surveillance including NST, amniotic fluid index (AFI), and BPP.
■ Provide emotional support to the woman and family. The woman and her family often experience an increase of stress related to fear of pregnancy loss, high-risk pregnancy and potential complications during pregnancy and delivery, and anxiety related to caring for more than one infant.
■ Provide information to the woman and her family regarding signs and symptoms of preterm labor, preeclampsia, and other possible complications related to multiple gestations.
■ Facilitate nutritional consult. The woman has an increased need for iron, calcium, and magnesium to support growth of multiple fetuses.
■ Discuss the plan of care for delivery. Cesarean birth is often recommended for multiples.
■ Facilitate referrals such as perinatologist, neonatologist, and social worker.

Hyperemesis Gravidarum

Hyperemesis gravidarum is vomiting during pregnancy that is so severe it leads to dehydration, electrolyte and acid–base imbalance, and starvation ketosis. It appears to be related to rising chorionic gonadotropin and/or estrogen levels. Other factors may include a psychological component related to ambivalence about the pregnancy, but this is controversial. Regardless of the cause, a woman experiencing hyperemesis presents in the clinical situation severely dehydrated and physically and emotionally debilitated, sometimes in need of hospitalization to manage profound and prolonged nausea and vomiting (Gilbert, 2007; Queenan, Hobbins, & Spong, 2005).

Assessment Findings

■ Vomiting that may be prolonged, frequent, and severe
■ Weight loss, acetonuria, and ketosis
■ Signs and symptoms of dehydration including;
    ■ *Dry mucous membranes*
    ■ *Poor skin turgor*
    ■ *Malaise*
    ■ *Low blood pressure*

Medical Management

■ Vitamin B_6 and antiemetics for treatment of nausea and vomiting
■ IV hydration for fluid, electrolytes, and vitamin replacement
■ Laboratory studies to monitor kidney and liver function

Nursing Actions

■ Assess factors that contribute to nausea and vomiting.
■ Reduce or eliminate factors that contribute to nausea and vomiting such as eliminating odors.
■ Provide emotional support.
■ Provide comfort measures such as good oral hygiene.
■ Provide IV hydration, electrolytes, and antiemetics as per orders.
■ Check weight daily.
■ Monitor I&O and specific gravity of urine to monitor hydration.
■ Monitor nausea and vomiting.

- Monitor laboratory values for fluid and electrolyte imbalances.
- Ensure that the woman remains NPO until vomiting is controlled, then slowly advance the diet as tolerated.
- Facilitate nutritional and dietary consult.
- Determine the woman's food preferences and provide them.
- Minimizing fluid intake with meals can decrease nausea and vomiting.

DIABETES

Diabetes mellitus is a chronic metabolic disease characterized by hyperglycemia as a result of limited or no insulin production. Diabetes is characterized into two categories:

- **Type 1 diabetes** is a result of autoimmunity of beta cells of the pancreas resulting in absolute insulin deficiency and is managed with insulin.
- **Type 2 diabetes** is characterized by insulin resistance and inadequate insulin production. This is the most prevalent form of diabetes, and the rates are increasing as it is linked to increased rates of obesity. It is typically controlled with diet, exercise, and oral glycemic agents. Oral hypoglycemic agents are not recommended for use during pregnancy in type 2 diabetic women (Simpson & Creehan, 2008).

Diabetes in Pregnancy

For many of the complications of pregnancy, and particularly for diabetes, medical management is continually under investigation and recommendations for treatment are changing. This chapter provides a general discussion of diabetes in pregnancy, then considers pregestational diabetes, followed by a discussion of gestational diabetes. Many of the same principles apply in the approach to both conditions. Diabetes in pregnancy is categorized into two groups:

- Pregestational diabetes (either type 1 or 2 diabetes)
- Gestational diabetes mellitus (GDM), diabetes that begins during pregnancy

Some of the normal physiological changes in pregnancy present challenges for managing diabetes in pregnancy. The physiological changes that accompany pregnancy produce a state of insulin resistance. To spare glucose for the developing fetus the placenta produces several hormones that antagonize insulin:

- Human placental lactogen
- Progesterone
- Growth hormone
- Corticotropin-releasing hormone

These hormones shift the primary energy sources to ketones and free fatty acids.

Most pregnant women maintain a normal glucose level in pregnancy despite increasing insulin resistance by producing increased insulin. Whether preexisting or gestational diabetes, the risk of the perinatal morbidity and mortality for the woman and neonate are significant.

For preexisting or gestational diabetes the treatment goals are the same and management strategies are similar:

- Maintain euglycemia control.
- Minimize complications.
- Prevent prematurity.

Overall, diabetes in pregnancy is a complex health problem that requires a multidisciplinary approach to facilitate a healthy outcome for both the woman and her baby. Care for women with diabetes should begin before conception and for GDM at the time of diagnosis. The goal of preconception care is to maintain the lowest possible glycosylated hemoglobin (HbA1C) without episodes of hypoglycemia and the care should include (Kendrick, 2004):

- Assessment and education regarding current diabetes self-management skills
- Exploration of strategies to improve adherence to treatment regimen
- Involvement of the woman and her family in the treatment regimen (essential in improving adherence to treatment regimen)
- Establishment of mutual goals for glycemic controls and self monitoring

Pregestational Diabetes

Women with preexisting pregestational diabetes have a fivefold increase in the incidence of major fetal anomalies of the heart and central nervous system (CNS). The precise mechanism for teratogenesis in diabetic women is not well understood but is believed to be related to hyperglycemia and deficiencies in membrane lipids and prostaglandin pathways.

Risks for the Woman

- Hypoglycemia
- Diabetic ketoacidosis (DKA, 1%)
- Hypertensive disorders and preeclampsia (10%–15% risk)
- Preterm labor (25% risk)
- Spontaneous abortion (30+% risk)
- Polyhydramnios/oligohydramnios: Polyhydramnios related to fetal anomalies and fetal hyperglycemia (20% risk). Oligohydramnios related to decreased placental perfusion.
- Cesarean delivery
- Exacerbation of chronic diabetes-related conditions such as: retinopathy, nephropathy, neuropathy
- Infection related to hyperglycemia (80% risk)
- Induction of labor

Risks for the Newborn

- Hypoglycemia related to fetal hyperinsulinemia
- Hypocalcemia and hypomagnesemia
- Intrauterine growth restriction related to maternal vasculopathy and decreased maternal perfusion
- Asphyxia related to fetal hyperglycemia and hyperinsulinemia
- Respiratory distress syndrome related to delayed fetal lung maturity
- Polycythemia (hematocrit <65%) related to increased fetal erythropoietin
- Hyperbilirubinemia related to polycythemia and red blood cell (RBC) breakdown
- Prematurity because of maternal complications
- Congenital defects including cardiac, skeletal, neurological, genitourinary, and gastrointestinal related to maternal hyperglycemia during organogenesis (first 6–8 weeks of pregnancy) (up to 12% risk)
- Cardiomyopathy related to maternal hyperglycemia
- Macrosomia related to fetal hyperinsulinemia
- Birth injury related to macrosomia
- Stillbirth in poorly controlled maternal diabetes

Assessment Findings

- Pregestational diabetes, history type 1 or type 2 diabetes
- Abnormal of blood glucose levels
- Woman may have abnormal blood glucose levels.

Self-Management

Comprehensive self-management of diabetes is complex yet essential for successful pregnancy outcomes:

■ Self-monitoring of blood glucose (SMBG) 4 to 8 times per day in pregnancy is the most important parameter for determining metabolic control. Table 7-2 indicates glycemic goals for pregnancy.
■ Self-monitoring of urine ketone. This is done by testing the first void specimen for ketones. Moderate to large amounts of ketones is an indication of inadequate food intake. Moderate to large amounts of ketone should be reported to care provider.
■ Record keeping of blood glucose levels, food intake, insulin, and activity need to be maintained for appropriate management of treatment regimen (Fig. 7-6).
■ Exercise is beneficial for glycemia control and overall well-being. Generally exercise three times a week for at least 20 minutes is recommended, but some contraindications such as hypertension and preeclampsia do exist.

Medical Nutritional Therapy

Medical nutritional therapy (MNT) is a cornerstone of diabetes management for all diabetic women and the goal is to provide adequate nutrition, prevent diabetic ketoacidosis, and promote euglycemia. MNT needs to be individualized and continually adjusted based on blood glucose values and insulin regimen and the woman's lifestyle. A registered dietician should meet with the woman regularly to assess and reevaluate the nutritional needs of the woman.

Medical Management

Preconception care for women with preexisting diabetes is key to a successful pregnancy and decreasing risks to the woman and her fetus. Achieving euglycemic control for 1 to 2 months is recommended, achieving a HbA1C less than 6.1%. Pregnancies complicated by preexisting diabetes are managed by a multidisciplinary team including a perinatologist, diabetes nurse educator, and dietician. Screening at diagnosis of pregnancy may include kidney, heart, and thyroid function and ophthalmic exams. Additional diagnostic testing is typically done related to the fetus including regular ultrasound examinations, intensive prenatal care schedule, and antenatal testing. The insulin needs of type 1 diabetic women increase such that by the end of pregnancy insulin requirements may be two to three times that of pre-pregnancy levels and may require three or four injections per day of Humulin insulin.

TABLE 7–2	GLYCEMIC GOALS FOR PREGNANCY COMPLICATED BY DIABETES	
TIMING	WHOLE BLOOD GLUCOSE (MG/DL)	PLASMA GLUCOSE (MG/DL)
Fasting	<95	<105
Premeal	<105	<115
1-hour postprandial	<140	<155
2-hour postprandial	<120	<130

Source: American Diabetes Association (ADA) (2004).

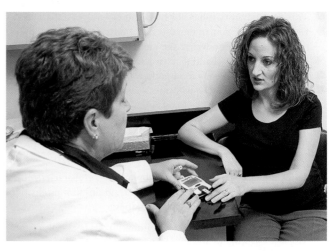

Figure 7-6   Blood glucose levels need to checked regularly for any woman who has diabetes at any time during pregnancy.

Delivery Issues

Timing of delivery is a tremendous challenge in pregnancies complicated by diabetes. At term, the risk of stillbirth increases, as does that of macrosomia. In contrast, intervention may place the woman at risk for prolonged labor and operative deliveries. Thus it is necessary for care providers to determine the pregnancies that should be allowed to go into spontaneous labor and those in need of labor induction. Most guidelines state that diabetes in pregnancy is not an automatic indication for scheduled cesarean delivery (Cunningham et al., 2005).

Complicating the issue of when and how to deliver is the fact that infants of diabetic women (IDM) have delayed pulmonary lung maturity and are at risk for respiratory distress syndrome (RDS). These risks seem to be related to glycemic control (Griffith & Conway, 2004).

The following are general recommendations for intrapartal care:

■ Evaluate fetal lung maturity by checking if amniotic fluid is positive for phosphatidylglycerol, to try to avert RDS in the newborn who is less than 38 weeks' gestation. The lecithin/sphingomyelin (L/S) ratio is not a specific indicator for fetal lung maturity in diabetic women.
■ Maintain plasma glucose levels at 70 to 110 mg/dL during labor.
■ Administer intravenous insulin when necessary to achieve desired glucose levels.

Nursing Actions

Extensive teaching is needed for women with diabetes in pregnancy. For type 1 diabetic pregnant women, this means learning about the effects pregnancy has on the management of diabetes and the adjustments required to the prior diabetic management regimen. The pregnancy represents new stressors and challenges for diabetic women and their families. Women may feel vulnerable and anxious related to their health and that of their fetus.

■ Provide information on:
 ■ *Physiological changes in pregnancy and the impact on diabetes*
 ■ *Changes in insulin requirements during pregnancy with advancing gestation*
■ Assist the woman in arranging for dietary counseling with a dietician.
 ■ *Dietary counseling should include the woman's preferences and pregnancy requirements.*

■ Review self-monitoring of blood glucose, dietary intake, and activity.

■ Emphasize the importance of record keeping of dietary intake, glucose, and activity.

   ■ *Instruct the woman to bring records to prenatal appointments to be reviewed by the primary health care provider.*

■ Review signs and symptoms, and treatment of hypoglycemia (blood glucose <70 mg/dL) including:

   ■ *Diaphoresis, tachycardia, shakiness, cold, clammy skin, blurred vision, extreme fatigue, mental confusion and irritability, somnolence, and pallor (Simpson & Creehan, 2008)*

   ■ *Ingest 10 to 15 g of carbohydrate for blood glucose of 60 mg/dL to raise blood glucose by 30 to 40 mg/dL in 30 minutes*

■ Review signs and symptoms, and treatment of hyperglycemia based on the individualized treatment plan.

■ Review signs and symptoms of diabetic ketoacidosis including:

   ■ *Abdominal pain, nausea and vomiting, polyuria, polydipsia, fruity breath, leg cramps, altered mental status, and rapid respirations (Simpson & Creehan, 2008).*

   ■ *Care for women admitted to the hospital in diabetic ketoacidosis during pregnancy should be provided by nurses with experience in intensive care and obstetrics and the goals of care include fluid resuscitation, restoring electrolyte imbalance, reduction of hyperglycemia, and treatment of underlying cause such as infection (Kendrick, 2004).*

■ Provide information on when and how to call the care provider:

   ■ *Glucose levels greater than 200 mg/dL, moderate ketones in urine, persistent nausea and vomiting, decreased fetal movement, and other indicators based on individualized plan of care (Simpson & Creehan, 2008).*

■ Provide information on management of nausea, vomiting, and illness:

   ■ *The glucose level should be checked every 1 to 2 hours, urine ketones checked every 4 hours; insulin should still be given with vomiting (Simpson & Creehan, 2008).*

■ Provide an expected plan of prenatal care, antenatal tests, and fetal surveillance.

■ Provide an expected plan for labor and delivery.

■ Assist the woman in arranging to meet with a diabetic nurse educator:

   ■ *Ideally women are referred to a diabetic nurse educator to help them to learn self-care management of diabetes and to facilitate regulation of diabetes in pregnancy.*

■ Emphasize that changes in the management plan may be necessary every few weeks due to the physiological changes of pregnancy.

■ Arrange for antenatal testing:

   ■ *Antenatal testing generally starts at 28 weeks' gestation and includes NST and BPP.*

Gestational Diabetes Mellitus

Gestational diabetes mellitus (GDM) is defined as any degree of glucose intolerance with the onset or first recognition in pregnancy (American Diabetes Association [ADA], 2004). This definition applies whether the GDM is controlled only with diet and exercise or with insulin as well. When medical nutrition therapy is inadequate to control glucose in GDM, insulin is required. Approximately 7% of pregnancies are complicated by GDM, resulting in more than 200,000 cases annually (ADA, 2004). Pregnancy is a condition characterized by progressive insulin resistance that begins mid-pregnancy

and progresses throughout the gestation. Two main contributors to insulin resistance are:

■ Increased maternal adiposity

■ Insulin desensitizing hormones produced by the placenta

The placenta produces human chorionic somatomammotropin (HCS), cortisol, estrogen, and progesterone. HCS stimulates pancreatic secretion of insulin in the fetus and reduces peripheral uptake of glucose in the woman. It has been proposed that, as the placenta increases in size with increasing gestation, so does the production of these hormones, leading to a progressive insulin-resistant state. Women with deficient insulin secretory capacity develop GDM. Because maternal insulin does not cross the placenta, the fetus is exposed to maternal hyperglycemia and in response the fetus produces more insulin, which promotes growth and subsequent macrosomia.

The American Association of Obstetricians and Gynecologists recommends routine screening for all pregnant women at 24 to 28 weeks of gestation, with a non-fasting 1-hour 50-gram oral glucose tolerance test. A positive test is a result of 130 mg/dL or 140 mg/dL depending on the criteria used (Griffith & Conway, 2004). For women who test positive, a 3-hour glucose tolerance test is done after the woman ingests a 100-gram glucose load; plasma glucose levels are drawn at 1, 2, and 3 hours post glucose load. If two or more glucose levels are above these thresholds, a diagnosis of GDM is made: fasting 95 mg/dL, 1-hour 180 mg/dL, 2-hour 155 mg/dL, and 3-hour 140 mg/dL (Griffith & Conway, 2004). Less stringent criteria have been proposed and may be used.

Risks for the Woman

■ Hypoglycemia and DKA

■ Development of nongestational diabetes

Risks for the Newborn

■ See risks with preexisting diabetes.

■ Risks of GDM for newborns are similar to risks with pregestational diabetes, except they are not at risk for congenital anomalies.

■ Macrosomia is the most common morbidity (15%–45%) (Perkins, Dunn, & Jagasia, 2007).

   ■ *Macrosomia places the fetus at risk for birth trauma such as brachial plexus injury.*

■ Hypoglycemia during the first few hours post-birth

■ The magnitude of fetal–neonatal complications is proportional to the severity of maternal hyperglycemia.

Assessment Findings

■ Abnormal glucose screening results

Medical Management

■ GDM may be managed by care providers with consultation and referral as appropriate.

■ For most women with GDM, the condition is controlled with diet and exercise.

■ 40% of women with GDM may need to be managed with insulin.

■ Women with GDM need to be monitored for type 2 diabetes after the birth. About one third of women will have recurrent GDM in subsequent pregnancies (Griffith & Conway, 2004).

Nursing Actions

For women diagnosed during pregnancy with GDM this means learning many complex skills and management strategies to maintain a healthy pregnancy. Nursing actions include:

■ Teach the woman to test glucose 4 times a day, one fasting and three 2-hour postprandial checks/day (suggested glucose control is maintaining fasting glucoses less than 95 before meals, greater than 140 at 1 hour after meals, and less than 120 at 2 hours after meals) (Perkins et al., 2007) (see Table 7-2).

■ Teach the woman to monitor fasting ketonuria levels in the morning.

■ Teach proper self-administration of insulin (site selection, insulin onset, peak, duration, administration). For the gestational diabetic, consider that it may be the first insulin administration time related to the pregnancy. Unlike women with preexisting diabetes, this can create a tremendous change in lifestyle. Successful self-administration of insulin requires patience, support and encouragement, and reassurance by the nurse educator (Kendrick, 2004).

■ Teach the woman signs and symptoms and treatment for hypoglycemia and hyperglycemia and diabetic ketoacidosis outlined above.

HYPERTENSIVE DISORDERS OF PREGNANCY

Hypertension is identified as systolic pressure 140 mm Hg or greater and diastolic pressure 90 mm Hg or greater. Hypertensive disorders of pregnancy have a 6% to 8% occurrence rate are the most common complication of pregnancy and are the second leading cause of maternal death and contribute to neonatal morbidity and mortality (Cunningham et al., 2005; National High Blood Pressure Education Working Group [NHBPEP], 2000).

Hypertensive disorders are classified into four categories by NHBPEP:

■ **Chronic hypertension**: Hypertension before conception or before the 20th week of gestation; may put the woman at high risk for developing preeclampsia.

■ **Preeclampsia–eclampsia**: Preeclampsia, a systemic disease with hypertension accompanied by proteinuria after the 20th week of gestation; eclampsia, a convulsive stage of the disease. Ten percent of all first pregnancies are affected by preeclampsia–eclampsia (Gibson, Carson, & Letterie, 2007).

■ **Preeclampsia superimposed on chronic hypertension:** Hypertensive women who develop new-onset proteinuria; proteinuria before the 20th week gestation; or sudden uncontrolled hypertension. Up to 25% of women with chronic hypertension develop preeclampsia (Gibson, Carson, & Letterie, 2007).

■ **Gestational hypertension:** High blood pressure detected for the first time after mid-pregnancy, without proteinuria. The diagnosis is made postpartum and it is relatively benign without underlying physiological changes in the woman. In the United States, gestational hypertension develops in 5% to 6% of all pregnancies (Gibson, Carson, & Letterie, 2007).

Preeclampsia

Preeclampsia is a disease of pregnancy that ranges from mild to severe and is hypertension accompanied by underlying systemic pathology that can have severe maternal and fetal impact.

Evidence-Based Practice: Cochrane Review: Antenatal Day Care Units versus Hospital Admission for Women with Complicated Pregnancy

Kröner, C., Turnbull, D., & Wilkinson, C. Antenatal day care units versus hospital admission for women with complicated pregnancy. Cochrane Database of Systematic Reviews 2001, Issue 4. Art.No.:CD001803. DOI:10.1002/14651858. CD001803.

The use of antenatal day care units is widely recognized internationally as an alternative for inpatient care for women with pregnancy complications. Antenatal day care units allow women with pregnancy complications to spend part or most of a day at an outpatient setting cared for by nurses and midwives with physician and perinatologist consults receiving complication-based antenatal testing and assessments and interventions.

The objective of this Cochrane Review was to assess the clinical safety, plus maternal, perinatal, and psychosocial consequences for the women and cost-effectiveness of this type of care. Randomized trials comparing antenatal day care with inpatient hospitalization for women with pregnancy complications were reviewed.

Main Results

One trial involving 54 women with a variety of pregnancy-related complications was included for this review. This trial was of average quality methodologically. It was found that day care assessment for nonproteinuria hypertension can reduce inpatient stay (difference in mean stay: 4.0 days; 95% confidence interval (CI): 2.1–5.9 days). In addition, a significant increase in the rate of induction of labor in the control group was found (4.9 times more likely: 95% CI: 1.6–13.8). The other clinical outcomes did not show a statistically significant difference between the control and intervention group. No other significant differences were observed. This means that women were able to be cared for safely without hospitalization in antenatal day care units.

Admission to day care for nonproteinuria hypertension reduces the amount of time spent in the hospital and the proportion of women induced for labor. However, one trial of 54 women is not sufficient to draw sound conclusions. Additional studies are needed to provide more solid evidence to confirm the advantages of antenatal day care units.

Summary

Some evidence exists that admission to antenatal day care units may help reduce the length of time spent in the hospital for women with a complicated pregnancy. Complications during pregnancy include high blood pressure, excessive vomiting, preterm labor, and heavy bleeding (hemorrhage). Admission to the hospital is necessary but disruptive to the mother and her family. Sometimes this care can be given without the need for an overnight stay in hospital. Day care units can provide a more relaxed atmosphere and better access for families, while still providing high-quality medical and midwifery care. The review of trials found some evidence that inpatient stay and the rate of induced labor was reduced by admission to antenatal day care units, but more research is needed. These findings may suggest a strategy to reduce hospitalizations for complications during pregnancy in the United States that extends beyond brief antenatal testing appointments done in the United States.

■ The incidence of preeclampsia complicating pregnancy is 5% to 8% (Martin et al., 2006).

■ Despite extensive research, there is no consensus as to the cause of preeclampsia.

■ The only cure for preeclampsia–eclampsia is delivery of the neonate and placenta.

To understand the pathophysiological mechanisms of preeclampsia, it is important to review the normal physiological changes of pregnancy. Normal pregnancy is a vasodilated state in which peripheral vascular resistance decreases 25%. Diastolic blood pressure drops 10 mm Hg at mid-pregnancy and gradually returns to pre-pregnant levels at term. There is a 50% rise in total blood volume by the end of the second trimester and cardiac output increases 30% to 50%. Increased renal blood flow leads to an increased glomerular filtration rate.

Pathophysiology of Preeclampsia

Preeclampsia is best described as a pregnancy-specific syndrome of reduced organ perfusion secondary to vasospasm and endothelial activation (Cunningham et al., 2005; Mignini, Villar, & Khalid, 2006). Blood pressure in preeclampsia is characterized by an increase in peripheral resistance. Preeclampsia is more than just hypertension, it is a systemic disorder with both maternal and fetal implications and manifestations (Peters & Flack, 2004).

In normotensive pregnancies, the spiral arteries of the uterus are remodeled by invasion of endovascular trophoblast cells, of the placenta, which allows them to widen to accommodate a 10-fold increase in blood flow. In a preeclamptic woman, this remodeling is incomplete and the spiral arteries remain thick walled, resulting in suboptimal placental perfusion. Uteroplacental perfusion can be diminished 50% before the onset of symptoms. It is believed that the resulting ischemia leads to endothelial cell dysfunction, resulting in multiorgan endothelial cell damage and dysfunction. This triggers generalized vasospasm with consequential poor tissue perfusion to all organs, resulting in increased peripheral resistance which manifests in elevated blood pressure (Cunningham et al., 2005; Gilbert, 2007; Peters & Flack, 2004). The criteria for diagnosis of preeclampsia and preeclampsia superimposed on chronic hypertension are presented in the Critical Component that follows (Criteria for Diagnosis of Preeclampsia-Eclampsia and Preeclampsia Superimposed on Chronic Hypertension).

The physiological changes that predispose women to preeclampsia also have an effect on other organs/systems such as the hepatic system, renal system, coagulation system, central nervous system, eyes, fluid and electrolytes, and pulmonary system (Fig. 7-7).

■ In preeclampsia there is an increase in microvascular fat deposition within the liver, which is postulated as one cause of epigastric pain. Liver damage may be mild or may progress to HELLP syndrome (**H**emolysis, **E**levated **L**iver enzymes, and **L**ow **P**latelets). Hepatic involvement can lead to periportal hemorrhagic necrosis in the liver which can cause a subcapsular hematoma, which can result in right upper quadrant pain or epigastric pain and may signal worsening preeclampsia (NHBPEP, 2000).

■ In 70% of preeclamptic patients, glomerular endothelial damage, fibrin deposition, and resulting ischemia reduce renal plasma flow and glomerular filtration rate (NHBPEP, 2000). Protein is excreted in the urine. Uric acid, creatinine, and calcium clearance are decreased and oliguria develops as the condition worsens. Oliguria is a sign of severe preeclampsia and kidney damage.

■ The coagulation system is activated in preeclampsia and thrombocytopenia occurs, possibly due to increased platelet aggregation and deposition at sites of endothelial damage, activating the

---

CRITICAL COMPONENT

Criteria for Diagnosis of Preeclampsia–Eclampsia and Preecclamsia Superimposed on Chronic Hypertension

Preeclampsia–Eclampsia

■ Diagnosed after the 20th week of pregnancy.

■ Blood pressure is >140 mm Hg systolic or >90 mm Hg diastolic with proteinuria (measurement of 3.0 g [300 mg/dL] or more of protein in a 24-hour urine collection period).

■ If proteinuria is absent, the diagnosis is suspected if headache, visual changes, abdominal pain, or laboratory abnormalities, specifically, low platelets or elevated levels of liver enzymes, are noted along with hypertension.

■ Eclampsia describes grand mal seizure in a preeclamptic woman.

Edema occurs in many normal pregnant women and therefore is no longer considered a clinical marker for preeclampsia.

Preeclampsia Superimposed on Chronic Hypertension

■ New-onset proteinuria or an abrupt increase in proteinuria

■ Increase in blood pressure that previously had been under control

■ Changes in laboratory values, specifically platelet count <100,000 cells/mm^3 and abnormal alanine transaminase (ALT) or aspartate aminotransferase (AST).

Because of poorer prognosis and difficulty in determining preeclampsia from an exacerbation of chronic hypertension, over diagnosis of preeclampsia is acceptable.

(Report of the National High Blood Pressure Education Program Working Group on High Blood Pressure in Pregnancy, 2000)

---

clotting cascade. A platelet count below 100,000 cells/mm^3 is an indication of severe preeclampsia (NHBPEP, 2000).

■ Endothelial damage to the brain results in fibrin deposition, edema, and cerebral hemorrhage which may lead to hyperreflexia and severe headaches and can progress to eclampsia (NHBPEP, 2000).

■ Retinal arterial spasms may cause blurring or double vision, photophobia, or scotoma (NHBPEP, 2000).

■ The leakage of serum protein into extracellular spaces and into urine, by way of damaged capillary walls, results in decreased serum albumin and tissue edema (NHBPEP, 2000).

■ Pulmonary edema is most commonly caused by volume overload related to left ventricular failure as the result of extremely high vascular resistance (Gilbert, 2007).

Risk Factors for Preeclampsia/Eclampsia

■ Nulliparity
■ Age younger than 19 or older than 35 years
■ Obesity
■ Multiple gestation
■ Family history of preeclampsia
■ Preexisting hypertension or renal disease
■ Previous preeclampsia or eclampsia
■ Diabetes mellitus

(Queenan, Hobbins, & Spong, 2005)

Risks for the Woman

■ Cerebral edema/hemorrhage/stroke
■ Disseminated intravascular coagulation (DIC)

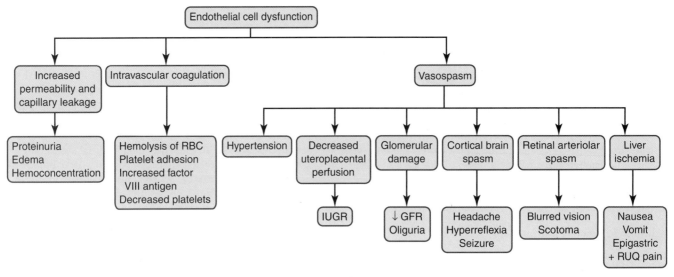

Figure 7-7 Pathophysiological changes of preeclampsia.

- Pulmonary edema
- Congestive heart failure
- Hepatic failure
- Renal failure
- Abruptio placenta

Risks for the Newborn

- Prematurity, delivery may be indicated preterm related to deterioration of maternal status
- Intrauterine growth restriction (IUGR) related to decrease uteroplacental perfusion
- Low birth weight
- Fetal intolerance to labor because of decrease placental perfusion
- Stillbirth

Assessment Findings

Accurate assessment is essential so that early recognition of worsening disease will allow for timely intervention that may improve maternal and neonatal outcome.

- Elevated blood pressure: Hypertension with systolic pressure 140 mm Hg or greater and diastolic pressure 90 mm Hg or greater.
- Proteinuria is 1+ or greater.
- Lab values may indicate elevations in liver function tests, diminished kidney function, and altered coagulopathies.

Medical Management

Once diagnosed, the woman and fetus should be monitored weekly for indications of worsening condition, as preeclampsia can be a progressive disease (Critical Component: Comparison of Assessment Findings Between Mild and Severe Preeclampsia). Women can also present with abrupt onset of the disease. Indications of worsening of the disease from mild to severe and severe preeclampsia are treated with hospitalization and evaluation. Antihypertensive drugs are used to control elevated blood pressure but because the only cure for preeclampsia is delivery, delivery is indicated in severe preeclampsia, even before term to protect the woman and fetus from severe sequelae. Care in labor and delivery includes use of magnesium sulfate to prevent seizures.

The primary goal in preeclampsia and preeclampsia superimposed on chronic hypertension is to control the woman's blood

CRITICAL COMPONENT

Comparison of Assessment Findings Between Mild and Severe Preeclampsia

Abnormality	Mild	Severe
Systolic blood pressure	140–160 mm Hg	>160 mm Hg
Diastolic blood pressure	<100 mm Hg	110 mm Hg or higher
Proteinuria	Trace to 1+	Persistent 2+ or more
Headache	Absent	Present
Visual disturbances	Absent	Present
Upper abdominal pain	Absent	Present
Oliguria	Absent	Present
Seizure (eclampsia)	Absent	May be present
Serum creatinine	Normal	Elevated
Thrombocytopenia	Absent	Present
Liver enzyme elevation	Minimal	Marked
Fetal growth restriction	Absent	Obvious
Pulmonary edema	Absent	May be present

Mild preeclampsia may progress rapidly to severe preeclampsia.

pressure and to prevent seizure activity and cerebral hemorrhage. Medical management includes:

- Magnesium sulfate, a central nervous system depressant, has been proven to help reduce seizure activity without documentation of long-term adverse effects to woman and fetus (Medication Box).
- Antihypertensive medications are used to control blood pressure (Box 7-3).
- Outpatient management for women with mild preeclampsia is an option if the woman can adhere to activity restriction, frequent office visits, and antenatal testing, and can monitor blood pressure (Evidence-Based Practice: Cochrane Review: Antenatal Day Care Units versus Hospital Admission for Women with Complicated Pregnancy).
- Delivery of the fetus and placenta is the only "cure" for preeclampsia. There are little data to suggest that any therapy

BOX 7–3   ANTIHYPERTENSIVE MEDICATIONS

First-line Drugs of Choice

Hydralazine (Apresoline, Neopreol) vasodilator: IV administration is used in severe preeclampsia; however, caution should be used to prevent rapid decreases in blood pressure. Rapid reduction in maternal blood pressure can decrease uteroplacental perfusion and decrease oxygen to fetus.

Methyldopa (Aldomet): Exact mechanism is unknown; may work on CNS. May take a few days for onset, so this drug is not a first choice in an acute situation. Research shows no long-term effects on fetus.

Labetalol (beta blocker): Slows the heart rate and decreases systemic vascular resistance. There is no significant research as to long-term effects on fetus.

Second-Line Drug

Nifedapine: Calcium channel blocker (Procardia) controls hypertension rapidly, increases cardiac index, and increases urinary output.

Sources: Deglin & Vallerand (2007); Gregg (2004); Sibai (2003).

alters the underlying pathophysiology. Therefore, all other interventions are designed to safeguard the mother while allowing time for fetal maturity. Although delivery cures preeclampsia, its effect is not immediate and women remain at risk of continuing problems, including eclampsia, as long as 5 days postpartum (Peters & Flack, 2004).

Nursing Actions

Accurate assessment is essential in that early recognition of worsening disease allows for timely intervention and may improve maternal and neonatal outcome.

■ Blood pressure should be measured with the woman seated and her arm at heart level, using an appropriate sized cuff (Fig. 7-8). Placing the woman in a left lateral recumbent position is no longer recommended to evaluate blood pressure as it gives an inaccurately low blood pressure reading (Cunningham et al., 2005; NHBPEP, 2000).

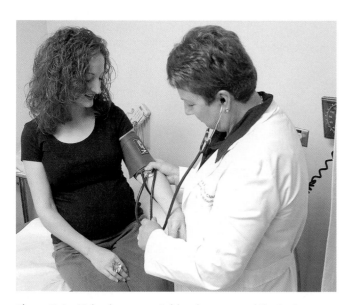

Figure 7-8   Take the woman's blood pressure while she is seated and with her arm at heart level.

BOX 7–4   ASSESSMENT OF DEEP TENDON REFLEXES

Physical Assessment	Grade
None elicited	0
Sluggish or dull	1
Active, normal	2
Brisk	3
Brisk with transient or sustained clonus	4
(Fig. 7.9)	

■ Administer antihypertensive as per orders (generally for blood pressure >160/110 mm Hg) (see Box 7-3).

■ Administer magnesium sulfate as per orders (Critical Component: Care of Woman on Magnesium Sulfate).

■ Assess for CNS changes including headache, visual changes; deep tendon reflexes (DTRs), and clonus (Box 7-4 and Fig. 7-9).

■ Auscultate lung sounds for clarity and monitor the respiratory rate.

■ Assess for signs and symptoms of pulmonary edema such as:

　■ *Shortness of breath, chest tightness or discomfort, cough, oxygen saturation less than 95%, increased respiratory and heart rates*

　■ *Changes in behavior such as apprehension, anxiety, or restlessness*

■ Assess for epigastric pain or right upper quadrant pain indicating liver involvement.

■ Assess weight daily and assess for edema to assess for fluid retention.

■ Check urine for proteinuria (may include 24-hour urine collection) and specific gravity.

■ Evaluate laboratory values including:

　■ *Elevations in serum creatinine (72 mg/dL)*

　■ *Hematocrit levels (>35)*

　■ *Low platelet count (100,000/mm³)*

　■ *Elevated liver enzymes (AST >41 units/L, ALT >30 units/L)*

■ Perform antenatal fetal testing and fetal heart rate monitoring (NST and BPP).

■ Check intake of adequate calories and protein.

■ Maintain accurate I&O to evaluate kidney function. Total fluid intake may be restricted to 2,000 mL/24 hr.

■ Provide a quiet environment to decrease CNS stimulation.

■ Maintain bedrest in the lateral recumbent position.

■ Provide information to the woman and her family. Education is key in helping with the understanding of the disease process and the plan of care.

■ Report deterioration in maternal or fetal status to provider.

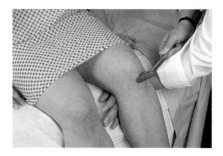

Figure 7-9   Assessing DTRs.

Medication

Intravenous Administration of Magnesium Sulfate

Continuous intravenous administration:

Loading dose: 4–6 g diluted in 100 mL of IV fluid administered over 15–20 minutes

Continuous infusion: 2 g/hr in 100 mL of IV fluid for maintenance

Laboratory evaluation: Measure serum magnesium level at 4–6 hours, after onset of treatment. Dosage should be adjusted to maintain a therapeutic level of 4–7 mEq/L

Duration: Intravenous infusion should continue for 24 hours post-delivery.

The antidote for magnesium toxicity is calcium gluconate or calcium chloride 5–10 mEq given IV slowly over 5–10 minutes.

(Magpie Trial Collaborative Group, 2002; Sibai, 2003)

Eclampsia

Eclampsia is the occurrence of seizure activity in the presence of preeclampsia (Gilbert, 2007). Eclampsia is thought to be triggered by one or more of the following:

- Cerebral vasospasm
- Cerebral hemorrhage
- Cerebral ischemia
- Cerebral edema

Warning signs of potential eclampsia include:

- Severe persistent headaches
- Epigastric pain
- Nausea and vomiting
- Hyperreflexia with clonus
- Restlessness

Care during a seizure includes:

- Remaining with the patient.
- Calling for help.
- Providing for patient safety by assessing airway and breathing.
  - *Lower the head of the bed and turn the woman's head to one side.*
  - *Anticipate the need for suctioning to decrease the risk of aspiration.*
- Preventing maternal injury.
  - *If possible, a padded tongue blade should be inserted to prevent tongue injury (using a tongue blade is still recommended by guidelines but not typically used in clinical practice).*
  - *Keep side rails up and padded if possible.*
- Recording the time, length, and type of seizure activity.
- Notifying the physician.

CRITICAL COMPONENT

Care of the Woman on Magnesium Sulfate

Potential Side Effects	Nursing Actions

Maternal:
  Nausea
  Flushing
  Diaphoresis
  Blurred vision
  Lethargy
  Hypocalcemia
  Depressed reflexes
  Respiratory depression-arrest
  Cardiac dysrhythmias
  Decreased platelet aggregation
  Circulatory collapse
	Assess vital signs before beginning infusion and every 5–15 minutes during loading dose, then every 30–60 minutes until the patient stabilizes. Frequency is then determined by the patient status.
	Assess DTRs every 2 hours.
	Monitor strict intake and output. Patients with oliguria or renal disease are at risk for toxic levels of magnesium.
	Monitor serum magnesium levels (therapeutic level is 5–7 mg/dL).
	Monitor for signs and symptoms of magnesium toxicity:
	
	■ Decreased reflexes could be a sign of pending respiratory depression
	■ Loss of DTRs
	■ Respiratory depression: respiratory rate < 14 breaths/min
	■ Oliguria, urine output <30 mL/hr
	■ Shortness of breath or respiratory rate <24
	■ Chest pain
	■ EKG changes
	■ If toxicity is suspected, discontinue the infusion and notify the health care provider. Respiration difficulty and cardiac arrest can occur with magnesium levels above 12 mEq/L.
	■ Keep calcium gluconate immediately available (1g IV).
	
	Maintain seizure precautions and keep resuscitation equipment nearby.
	Patients receiving IV labetalol for blood pressure control should have cardiac monitoring.
	Maintain continuous fetal heart rate monitoring

Fetal/neonatal:
  Fetal heart rate decreased variability
  Respiratory depression
  Hypotonia
  Decreased suck reflex
  Signs and symptoms of magnesium toxicity
	Monitor FHR
	Alert the neonatal team before delivery of use of magnesium sulfate in labor

(Mattson & Smith, 2004; Simpson, 2008)

After the seizure the following is done:

■ Rapidly assess maternal and fetal status.
■ Assess airway; suction if needed.
■ Administer supplemental oxygen: 10 L/min via mask.
■ Ensure IV access.
■ Administer magnesium sulfate per orders.
■ Provide a quiet environment.

HELLP Syndrome

HELLP syndrome (**H**emolysis, **E**levated **L**iver enzymes and **L**ow **P**latelets) is the acronym used to designate the variant changes in laboratory values that can occur as a complication of severe preeclampsia (Critical Component: Laboratory Values Indicative of HELLP Syndrome).

■ Hemolysis is a result of red blood cell destruction as they travel through constricted vessels.
■ Elevated liver enzymes result from decreased blood flow and damage to the liver.
■ Low platelets result from platelets aggregating at the site of damaged vascular endothelium causing platelet consumption and thrombocytopenia (Cunningham et al., 2005; Sibai, 2004).

Women with severe preeclampsia have an increased risk (7%–24%) of developing HELLP syndrome. HELLP may develop in women who do not present with the cardinal signs of severe preeclampsia. HELLP may appear at any time during the pregnancy in 70% of cases, and the immediate postpartum period accounts for 30% of cases (Queenan, Hobins, & Spong, 2005). The only definitive treatment is delivery. However, some women may experience worsening HELLP syndrome over the first 48-hour postpartum period. Women with only some of the laboratory changes are diagnosed with partial HELLP syndrome.

CRITICAL COMPONENT

Laboratory Values Indicative of HELLP Syndrome

Platelets	<100,000/mm³
Liver enzymes (AST, ALT)	Elevated AST: >70 units/L
	Elevated ALT: >50 units/L
Bilirubin (indirect)	Elevated: >1.2 mg/dL
LDH	Elevated: >600 units/L

(Mattson & Smith 2004).

Risks for the Woman

■ Abruptio placenta
■ Renal failure
■ Liver hematoma and possible rupture
■ Death

Risks for the Fetus

■ Preterm birth
■ Death

Assessment Findings

■ The woman may present with a complaint of general malaise, nausea, and right upper gastric pain.
■ The woman may have unexplained bruising, mucosal bleeding, petechiae, and bleeding from injection and IV sites.

■ Assessment findings are related to alternations in laboratory tests associated with changes in liver function and platelets (see Critical Component: Laboratory Values Indicative of HELLP Syndrome).

Medical Management

The only definitive cure for HELLP syndrome is immediate delivery of the fetus and placenta. Resolution of disease is generally in 48 hours postpartum. Medical management may include replacement of platelets.

Nursing Actions

■ Perform a thorough assessment of the woman related to the diagnosis of preeclampsia.
■ Evaluate laboratory tests.
■ Notify the physician immediately if HELLP syndrome is suspected or lab values deteriorate.
■ Administer platelets as per orders.
■ Provide the woman and the family with information regarding HELLP and its treatment.
■ Provide emotional support to the woman and her family, as the woman and family are at risk for increased levels of anxiety related to diagnosis.

(Mattson & Smith, 2004)

PLACENTAL ABNORMALITIES AND HEMORRHAGIC COMPLICATIONS

Major blood loss during pregnancy is a significant contributor to both maternal and fetal morbidity and mortality. Up to 1,000 mL/min of maternal blood flows through the placenta at term. Hemorrhage predisposes a woman to hypovolemia, anemia, infection, and premature birth. Significant maternal blood loss can result in decreased perfusion and oxygen to the fetus, resulting in progressive deterioration of fetal status and even death (Simpson & Creehan, 2008). Placental abnormalities and hemorrhagic complications of pregnancy are presented in this section.

Placenta Previa

The incidence of placenta previa is 1 in 300 deliveries (Cunningham et al., 2005). **Placenta previa** occurs when the placenta attaches to the lower uterine segment of the uterus, near or over the internal cervical os, instead of in the body or fundus of the uterus. Bleeding occurs due to placental separation from the internal cervical os or lower uterine segment and the inability of the uterus to contract at the vessel sites.

CRITICAL COMPONENT

Vaginal Bleeding

A sterile vaginal exam is contraindicated in all pregnant women with extensive vaginal bleeding until the source of bleeding is identified. If a vaginal exam is performed with a placenta previa, torrential vaginal bleeding could occur related to dislodging of the placenta from maternal tissues.

Maternal blood loss results in decreased oxygen-carrying capacity which directly impacts oxygen delivery to maternal organs and placental blood flow, thus decreasing oxygen to the fetus. Therefore, the management of placenta previa is dependent on maternal and fetal status. There are four classifications of placenta previa (Fig. 7-10; Cunningham et al., 2005):

- **Total placenta previa:** The placenta completely covers the internal cervical os.
- **Partial placenta previa:** The placenta partially covers the internal cervical os.
- **Marginal placenta previa:** The placenta is at the margin of the internal cervical os.
- **Low-lying placenta:** The placenta is implanted in the lower uterine segment in close proximity to the internal cervical os.

Risk Factors for Placenta Previa

- Endometrial scarring
  - *Previous placenta previa*
  - *Prior cesarean delivery*
  - *Abortion*
  - *Multiparity*
- Impeded endometrial vascularization
  - *Advance maternal age*
  - *Diabetes or hypertension*
  - *Cigarette smoking*
  - *Uterine anomalies/fibroids/endometritis*
- Increased placental mass
  - *Large placenta*
  - *Multiple gestation*

Risks for the Woman

- Hemorrhagic and hypovolemic shock related to excessive blood loss

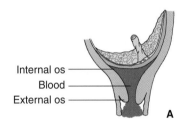

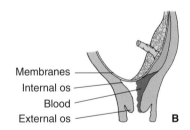

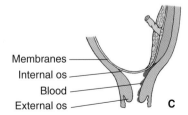

Figure 7-10 Classification of placenta previa. *A.* Total. *B.* Partial. *C.* Marginal/lowlying.

- Because of the large volume of maternal blood flow to the uteroplacental unit at term, unresolved bleeding can result in maternal exsanguinations in 10 minutes.
- Anemia
- Potential Rh sensitization as Rh-negative women can become sensitized during any antepartum bleeding episode.

Risks for the Newborn

- Disruption of uteroplacental blood flow can result in progressive deterioration of fetal status, and the degree of fetal compromise is related to the total volume of maternal blood loss fetal blood flow (Simpson & Creehan, 2008).
- Blood loss, hypoxia, anoxia, and death related to maternal hemorrhage may occur.
- Fetal anemia may develop due to maternal blood loss.
- Neonatal morbidity and mortality is related primarily to preterm birth.

Assessment Findings

- The classic presentation of a placenta previa is painless uterine bleeding.
- Bleeding usually occurs near the end of the second trimester or in the third trimester of pregnancy and initial bleeding episodes may be slight.
- The first episode of bleeding is rarely life threatening or a cause of hypovolemic shock.
- A vaginal exam is contraindicated (Critical Component: Vaginal Bleeding).

Emergency Medical Management

- Cesarean delivery is necessary when either maternal or fetal status is compromised as a result of extensive vaginal bleeding.
- Cesarean birth is necessary in practically all women with placenta previa because the placenta is at the cervix, and labor and cervical dilation results in placental hemorrhage (Cunningham et al., 2005).
- Vaginal delivery may be attempted with a low-lying placenta if one can proceed with an emergency cesarean birth if needed.
- Blood is transfused as needed.

Medical Management After Stabilization

When the maternal and fetal status is stable and bleeding is minimal, prolonging pregnancy and delaying delivery may be possible. This expectant management or conservative management is performed when the fetus is premature to allow for fetal lungs to mature. This typically includes close observation and hospitalization. If the woman and fetus remain stable and bleeding stops, discharge home may be considered with maternal bedrest, antenatal surveillance, and close proximity to the hospital.

Nursing Actions

Nursing actions are related to maternal fetal status and the amount of vaginal bleeding and include:

- Explain interventions, treatments, and procedure and plan of care.
- Inform the patient and family of maternal and fetal status.
- Reassure the patient and her family.
- Perform the initial assessment:
  - *Evaluation of color, character, and amount of vaginal bleeding*
  - *Arrangement for ultrasound to determine placental location*
  - *Determination of fetal gestational age and fetal lung maturity*

■ *Assessment of vital signs for increased pulse and respiratory rate and falling blood pressure every 5 to 15 minutes if active bleeding. The woman can have up to a 40% maternal blood loss before exhibiting hemorrhagic hemodynamic changes in the blood pressure and pulse.*
■ Monitor vaginal bleeding and uterine activity.
■ Ensure bedrest with bathroom privileges.
■ Maintain IV access with large-bore IV in case blood replacement therapy is needed.
■ Ensure availability of hold clot and blood components.
■ Assess FHR and UCs.
■ Give corticosteroids to accelerate fetal lung maturity, if indicated.
■ Monitor lab values including CBC, platelets, and clotting studies.
■ Notify the physician of any of the following:
 ■ *Onset or increase in vaginal bleeding*
 ■ *Blood pressure less than 90/60 mm Hg; pulse less than 60 or more than 120 bpm*
 ■ *Respirations less than 14 or more than 26 breaths/min*
 ■ *Temperature greater than 100.4°F (38°C)*
 ■ *Urine output less than 30 mL/hr*
 ■ *Saturated oxygen less than 95%*
 ■ *Decreased level of consciousness*
 ■ *Onset or increase in uterine activity*
 ■ *Non-reassuring fetal status*
■ Anticipate a cesarean birth.

Abruptio Placenta

An **abruptio placenta** is the separation of the placenta from its site of implantation after 20 weeks and before delivery. The separation may be partial or total and can be classified as grade 1, 2, or 3 (Gilbert, 2007). This is a uniquely dangerous condition for the woman and fetus because of its potentially serious complications. Bleeding into the decidua basalis results in hemorrhage and placental separation (Fig. 7-11 and Table 7-3).

Maternal and fetal status determines the management of the pregnancy. The classic signs and symptoms of abruption are:

■ Severe sudden onset of abdominal pain
■ Uterine contractions
■ Uterine tenderness
■ Vaginal bleeding (may or may not be present)
■ If separation is in the center of the placenta, then blood may be trapped between the placental and decidua, concealing the hemorrhage. A concealed hemorrhage occurs in about 10% of abruptions. This results in uterine tenderness and abdominal pain.

■ If the separation occurs at the edge of the placenta, then the blood usually escapes externally.

The fetal response to abruptio placenta depends on the volume of blood loss and the extent of uteroplacental insufficiency. Treatment depends on maternal and fetal status.

Risk Factors

■ Previous abruption increases the risk up to 15%.
■ Hypertensive disorders of pregnancy
■ Abdominal trauma
■ Cocaine, methamphetamine use, and/or cigarette smoking
■ Premature rupture of membranes
■ Uterine anomalies/fibroids

Risks for the Woman

■ Hemorrhagic shock
■ Disseminated intravascular coagulation (DIC)
■ Hypoxic damage to organs such as kidneys and liver
■ Postpartum hemorrhage

Risks for the Newborn

■ Preterm birth
■ Hypoxia, anoxia, neurological injury, and fetal death related to hemorrhage
■ Intrauterine growth restriction
■ 15% rate of neonatal death

Assessment Findings

■ Maternal assessment findings include (see Table 7-3):
 ■ *Hypovolemic shock, hypotension, oliguria, thready pulse, shallow/irregular respirations, pallor, anxiety*
 ■ *Vaginal bleeding (may be concealed hemorrhage)*
 ■ *Severe abdominal pain*
 ■ *Uterine contractions/tenderness/hypertonus/increasing uterine distension*
 ■ *Nausea and vomiting*
 ■ *Decreased renal output*
 ■ *Remember during pregnancy signs of shock are usually not until 25% to 30% of maternal blood loss has occurred.*
 ■ *Kleihauer–Betke test in maternal blood may be positive and indicate the presence of fetal red blood cells.*
■ Fetal assessment findings include (see Table 7-3):
 ■ *Tachycardia*
 ■ *Bradycardia*
 ■ *Loss or variability of FHR, late decelerations, decreasing baseline*

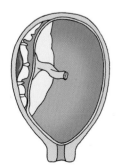
Mild Grade 1
(<15% placenta separates with concealed hemorrhage)

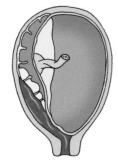
Moderate Grade 2
(up to 50% placenta separates with apparent hemorrhage)

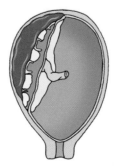
Severe Grade 3
(>50% placenta separates with concealed hemorrhage)

Figure 7-11 Three grades of abruption placentae.

TABLE 7–3   CLASSIFICATIONS OF MANAGEMENT OF ABRUPTIO PLACENTAE

	MILD: GRADE 1	MODERATE: GRADE 2	SEVERE: GRADE 3
DEFINITION	Less than one-sixth of placenta separates prematurely.	From one-sixth to one-half of placenta separates prematurely.	More than one-half of placenta separates prematurely.
SIGNS AND SYMPTOMS	Total blood loss <500 mL Dark vaginal bleeding (mild to moderate) Vague lower abdominal or back discomfort No uterine tenderness No uterine irritability	Total blood loss 1,000–1,500 mL 15%–30% of total blood volume Dark vaginal bleeding (mild to severe) Gradual or abrupt onset of abdominal pain Uterine tenderness present Uterine tone increased	Total blood loss >1,500 mL More than 30% of total blood volume Dark vaginal bleeding (moderate to severe) Usually abrupt onset of uterine pain described as tearing, knifelike, and continuous Uterus board like (hard)
MATERNAL EFFECTS	Vital signs normal	Mild shock Normal maternal blood pressure Maternal tachycardia Narrowed pulse pressure Orthostatic hypotension Tachypnea	Moderate-to-profound shock common Decreased maternal blood pressure Maternal tachycardia significant Narrowed pulse pressure Orthostatic hypotension severe Significant tachypnea
MATERNAL COMPLICATIONS	Normal fibrinogen of 450 mg/dL	Early signs of DIC common Fibrinogen 150–300 mg/dL	DIC usually develops unless condition is treated immediately Fibrinogen <150 mg/dL
FETAL/NEONATAL COMPLICATIONS	Normal FHR pattern	FHR shows non-reassuring signs of possible fetal compromise	FHR shows signs of fetal compromise and death can occur

Source: Gilbert (2007).

Emergency Medical Management

If abruption results in unstable maternal or fetal status, delivery by cesarean is indicated. Treatment includes:

- Monitoring maternal volume status
- Restoring blood loss
- Monitoring coagulation status
- Correcting coagulation defects

Medical Management after Stabilization

If the maternal status is stable and the fetus is immature, then expectant management would include:

- Hospitalization
- Close monitoring of maternal and fetal status including:
  - *FHR*
  - *Maternal bleeding*
  - *Uterine activity*
  - *Abdominal pain*
  - *Vaginal bleeding*
  - *Maternal laboratory and coagulation studies.*
- Corticosteroids may be given to accelerate fetal lung maturity

Nursing Actions

- Monitor vaginal bleeding (may be concealed hemorrhage).
- Assess abdominal pain.
- Palpate the uterus for contractions/tenderness/hypertonus/increasing uterine distension.
- Manage nausea and vomiting.
- Assess for decreased renal output.
- Monitor maternal cardiovascular status for hypotension and tachycardia.
- Maintain IV access with a large-bore needle.
- Administer oxygen at 8 to 10 L/min by mask.
- Assess FHR for baseline changes, variability and periodic changes indicative of an abnormal FHR.
- Monitor lab values including CBC and clotting studies.

■ Provide emotional support to the woman and her family.
■ Provide information to the woman and her family regarding treatment plan and status of their infant.

Placenta Accreta

Placenta accreta is an abnormality of implantation defined by degree of invasion into uterine wall of trophoblast of placenta:

■ **Placenta accrete:** Invasion of the trophoblast is beyond the normal boundary (80% of cases).
■ **Placenta increta:** Invasion of the trophoblast extends into uterine myometrium (15% of cases).
■ **Placenta percreta:** Invasion of the trophoblast extends into the uterine musculature and can adhere to other pelvic organs (5% of cases).

Placenta accreta can be diagnosed by ultrasound prenatally but typically is diagnosed after delivery when the placenta is retained. If the placenta does not separate readily, rapid surgical intervention is needed. Up to 90% of women lose more than 3,000 mL of blood operatively as a result of placenta accreta.

Risk Factors

■ Placenta accreta occurs in 5% to 10% of pregnancies with placenta previa.
■ Prevalence of placenta accreta increases if the woman has had a prior cesarean birth and has a placenta previa.
  ■ *A 10% to 25% increase with one prior cesarean birth*
  ■ *A 50% increase with two or more cesarean births*

Risks for the Woman

■ Postpartum hemorrhage
■ Hysterectomy when unable to remove placenta manually or with dilation and curettage (D & C)
■ 7% to 10% maternal mortality rate related to hemorrhage

Risks for the Newborn

■ Generally does not represent any increased risk to fetus or newborn

Assessment Findings

■ The placenta does not separate from the uterine wall after birth

Medical Management

■ Control hemorrhage and transfuse as needed.
■ Surgical intervention to remove the placenta
  ■ *D & C*
  ■ *Hysterectomy*

Nursing Actions

■ Control hemorrhage and anticipate surgical intervention and possible hysterectomy.
■ Monitor cardiovascular status for hypotensive shock.
■ Explain procedures.
■ Provide emotional support to the woman and her family.

Abortion

Abortion is the spontaneous or elective termination of pregnancy. Abortions are referred to as induced, elective, therapeutic, and spontaneous. **Induced abortion** is the medical or surgical termination of pregnancy before fetal viability. **Elective abortion** is termination of pregnancy before fetal viability at the request of the woman but not for reasons of impaired health of the mother or fetal disease. Termination of pregnancy is done transcervically through dilation of the cervix, then evacuation of the uterus mechanically by curettage, scraping of the contents, or vacuum. Legally induced abortions have an extremely low complication rate. Early medical abortion with medications such as mifepristone and misoprostol can be highly effective. **Therapeutic abortion** is termination of pregnancy for serious maternal medical indications or serious fetal anomalies. This section focuses on spontaneous abortion as it is associated with hemorrhage.

Spontaneous abortion (SAB) is abortion occurring without medical or mechanical means, also called **miscarriage**. Hemorrhage in the decidua basilis followed by necrosis of the tissue usually accompanies abortion. Approximately 10% to 30% of pregnancies end in spontaneous abortion. The majority (80%) occurs in the first 12 weeks of gestation and more than half of those are a result of chromosomal abnormalities (Cunningham et al., 2005). Early spontaneous abortions typically are related to an abnormality of the zygote, embryo, fetus, or at times the placenta.

Risk Factors for Spontaneous Abortion

■ Increased parity
■ Increased maternal and paternal age
■ Endocrine abnormalities such as diabetes or luteal phase defects
■ Drug use or environmental toxins
■ Immunological factors such as autoimmune diseases
■ Infections
■ Systemic disorders
■ Genetic factors
■ Uterine or cervical abnormalities

Assessment Findings for Spontaneous Abortion

■ Clinical manifestations and categories are listed in Table 7-4.
■ Uterine bleeding
■ Uterine contractions and cramping and pain
■ Ultrasound confirms diagnosis

Medical Management for Spontaneous Abortion

Medical management depends on classification and signs and symptoms and is presented in Table 7-4.

Nursing Actions Related to Spontaneous Abortion

■ Provide psychological support.
■ Monitor bleeding.
■ Follow agency guidelines and facilitate and support the family's decisions about disposition of the products of conception.
■ Discharge teaching related to self-care and warning signs including:
  ■ *Pelvic rest includes no tampons, douching, or intercourse for 6 weeks.*
  ■ *Monitoring for excessive bleeding and fever*
  ■ *Follow-up with care provider*

TABLE 7–4   CLASSIFICATION AND MANAGEMENT OF SPONTANEOUS ABORTIONS/ MISCARRIAGE

CLASSIFICATION	DEFINITION	MANIFESTATIONS	MEDICAL MANAGEMENT
THREATENED	Continuation of pregnancy is in doubt	Vaginal bleeding or spotting which may be associated with mild abdominal cramps Cervix closed Uterus soft, nontender, and enlarged appropriate to gestational age	Bedrest
INEVITABLE	Termination of pregnancy is in progress	Cervix dilated Membranes may be ruptured Vaginal bleeding Mild-to-painful uterine contractions	If bleeding, ROM, pain, or fever termination with D&C
INCOMPLETE	Fragments of products of conception are expelled and part is retained in uterus	Profuse bleeding because retained tissue parts interfere with myometrial contractions	D&C to evacuate uterus of products of conception
COMPLETE	Products of conception are totally expelled from uterus	Minimal vaginal bleeding	No intervention if minimal bleeding
MISSED	Embryo or fetus dies during first 20 weeks of gestation but is retained in uterus for 4 weeks or more afterward	Amenorrhea or intermittent vaginal bleeding, spotting, or brownish discharge No uterine growth No fetal movement felt Regression of breast changes	Evacuation of products of conception based on weeks of gestation
SEPTIC	Condition in which products of conception become infected during abortion process.	Foul-smelling vaginal discharge	Evacuation of products of conception based on weeks of gestation; antibiotics
RECURRENT	Condition in which two or more successive pregnancies have ended in spontaneous abortion		Treatment dependent on cause of spontaneous abortion

Source: Gilbert (2007).

Ectopic Pregnancy

An **ectopic pregnancy** develops as a result of the blastocyst implanting somewhere other than the endometrial lining of the uterus (Fig. 7-12). This is a nonviable pregnancy. The majority of ectopic pregnancies occur in the fallopian tube (>90%) but the fertilized ovum can also implant in the ovary, cervix, or abdominal cavity. Because the vast majority of ectopic pregnancies are tubal, the focus of this section is on tubular ectopic pregnancy. The incidence is increasing and not always reported, but accounts for 10% of maternal mortality (Cunningham et al.,

2005). Hemorrhage is the leading cause of death in women. The classic symptoms are:

■ Abdominal pain
■ Delayed menses
■ Vaginal bleeding or spotting 6 to 8 weeks after the last menstrual period

Risk Factors for Ectopic Pregnancy

■ Tubal corrective surgery
■ Tubal sterilization

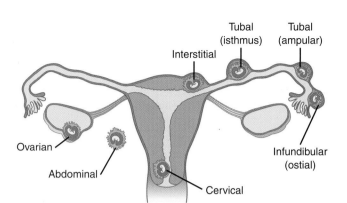

Figure 7-12 Sites for ectopic pregnancy.

- Previous ectopic pregnancies
- In utero diethylstilbestrol exposure
- Intrauterine device
- Pelvic inflammatory disease
- Assisted reproduction
- Previous ectopic pregnancies

Risks for the Woman

- Hemorrhage related to rupture of fallopian tube
- Decreased fertility related to removal of fallopian tube

Assessment Findings

- Signs and symptoms of ectopic pregnancy are often subtle or even absent
- Irregular vaginal spotting with dull, aching pelvic pain with or without signs of pregnancy
- Hemorrhage
- Positive pregnancy test
- Ultrasound confirmation of ectopic pregnancy

Assessment Findings Before Tubal Rupture

- Abdominal pain and tenderness
- Delayed menses
- Abnormal vaginal bleeding or spotting

Assessment Findings After Tubal Rupture

- Acute, severe lower abdominal pain and may have referred shoulder pain
- Faintness and dizziness
- Signs of shock (e.g., hypotension, tachycardia)

Medical Management

- Type of surgical management depends on the location and cause of the ectopic pregnancy, and extent of tissue involvement.
- Nonsurgical medical management of ectopic pregnancy may be indicated in hemodynamically unstable women. Methotrexate, a type of chemotherapy agent, will cause dissolution of the ectopic mass.

Nursing Actions

- Offer explanations and reassurance related to the plan of care.
- Provide support related to the pregnancy loss.
- Ensure stabilization of cardiovascular status.

Hydatiform Mole

A **hydatiform mole** is a benign proliferating growth of the trophoblast in which the chorionic villi develop into edematous, cystic, vascular transparent vesicles that hang in grapelike clusters without a viable fetus (Fig. 7-13). Hydatiform mole develops in 1 of 1,000 pregnancies in the United States and Europe (Cunningham et al., 2005). This is a nonviable pregnancy.

Risk Factors

- Maternal age younger than 15 or older than 45 years
- Previous molar pregnancy

Risks for the Woman

- Increased risk of choriocarcinoma

Assessment Findings

- Uterine bleeding from spotting to profuse hemorrhage
- Enlarged uterus
- Abdominal cramping and expulsion of vesicles
- Hyperemesis
- Absent fetal heart rate

Medical Management

- Immediate evacuation of the mole
- Follow-up of HCG levels for at least 6 months to detect trophoblastic neoplasia. After HCG levels fall to normal for 6 months, pregnancy can be considered.

Nursing Actions

- Offer emotional support related to pregnancy loss.
- Explain medical follow-up with regular HCG levels because of the risk of malignant trophoblastic disease and choriocarcinoma.

INFECTIONS

Infection is a common complication of pregnancy. The impact of infection on pregnancy is dependent on the infectious organism involved. Some infectious agents such as Trichomonas are easily treated and affect only the mother. Other infections such as rubella,

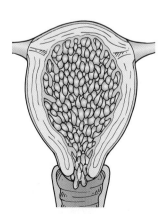

Figure 7-13 Hydatidiform mole.

can actively infect the fetus during pregnancy. Infections can be acquired by the fetus transplacentally, such as HIV; may ascend the birth canal; or can be acquired though contact at the time of a vaginal birth, such as herpes. In the following section, sexually transmitted diseases and TORCH infections are reviewed, highlighting maternal and fetal effects, treatment, and nursing implications.

Sexually Transmitted Diseases

Sexually transmitted diseases (STDs) remain a major public health challenge in the United States. The Centers for Disease Control and Prevention (CDC, 2005) estimates that 19 million new infections occur every year, almost half of them among young people ages 15 to 24 years. STDs affect women of every socioeconomic and educational level, age, race, and ethnicity.

In addition to the physical and psychological consequences, the costs of treating STDs are estimated at more than $14 billion annually (CDC, 2005). Women who are pregnant can become infected with the same STDs as women who are not pregnant. Pregnancy does not provide protection for the woman or the baby and consequences of an STD can be serious in pregnancy, even life-threatening for the woman and her baby. Intrauterine or perinatal transmitted STDs can have severely debilitating effects on women, their partners, and their fetuses. All women should be screened for STDs during their first prenatal visit. Table 7-5 shows the estimated number of women infected with specific STDs annually.

Risks for the Woman

■ STDs can cause pelvic inflammatory disease (Table 7-6).
■ Pelvic inflammatory disease (PID) can lead to infertility, chronic hepatitis, and cervical and other cancers.
■ STDs during pregnancy can lead to PTL, PROM and uterine infection.

Table 7-7 summarizes information on maternal effects and management of STDs (CDC, 2006).

TABLE 7–5	ESTIMATED INCIDENCES OF STDs IN PREGNANT WOMEN ANNUALLY
STD	**ESTIMATED NUMBER OF PREGNANT WOMEN**
Bacterial vaginosis	800,000
Herpes simplex	800,000
Chlamydia	200,000
Trichomoniasis	80,000
Gonorrhea	40,000
Hepatitis B	40,000
HIV	8,000
Syphilis	8,000

Source: Centers for Disease Control and Prevention (CDC). (2004).

Risks for the Fetus

■ STDs can pass to the fetus by crossing the placenta; some can be transmitted to the baby during delivery as the baby passes through the birth canal (see Table 7-7).
■ Harmful effects to babies include preterm birth, low birth weight, neonatal sepsis, and neurological damage.

Assessment Findings

■ Many STDs in women are "silent" without signs and symptoms, making routine screening for STDs during the first prenatal visit an important part of routine prenatal care.

Medical Management (see Table 7-7)

■ Provide routine screening of STDs and HIV at first prenatal visit.
■ Treat bacterial STDs with antibiotics.
■ Prescribe antiviral medications for viral STDs to reduce symptoms.

Nursing Actions (see Table 7-7)

■ Provide information on STDs.
■ Provide emotional support.
■ Instruct the woman on correct administration of medications and other treatments and importance of completing treatment.
■ Provide the partner with treatment as indicated.

TORCH Infections

TORCH is an acronym that stands for **T**oxoplasmosis, **O**ther (hepatitis B), **R**ubella, and **C**ytomegalovirus and **H**erpes simplex virus. TORCH infections are unique in their pathogenesis and have potentially devastating effects on the developing fetus (Table 7-8). Each disease is teratogenic to the developing fetus.

Risk Factors

The risk status for these infections varies based on route of transmission. Some are sexually transmitted diseases, such as herpes, others have various routes of transmission to woman (CDC, 2004b).

Risk for the Woman

■ Depends on the infectious agent (CDC, 2004b; see Table 7-8)

Risks for the Fetus

■ The usual route of transmission to the fetus is transplacentally (see Table 7-8).
■ Infections acquired in utero can result in intrauterine growth restriction, prematurity, chronic postnatal infection, and even death.

Assessment Findings

■ Maternal assessment findings vary with the organism (see Table 7-8).

Medical Management

■ Medical management varies based on the organism, trimester of exposure, and clinical evidence of neonatal sequelae (see Table 7-8).

Nursing Actions

■ Nursing considerations vary with the organism (see Table 7-8).

TABLE 7–6   PELVIC INFLAMMATORY DISEASE

PELVIC INFLAMMATORY DISEASE (PID)	Pelvic inflammatory disease is a general term that refers to an infection of the uterus, fallopian tubes, and other reproductive organs. It is a common and serious complication of STDs. Pregnant women with PID are at high risk for maternal morbidity and preterm delivery and should be hospitalized and treated with IV antibiotics.
INCIDENCE	An estimated more than 1 million women in the United States have an episode of acute PID.
CONSEQUENCES	Can lead to infertility, ectopic pregnancy, abscess formation and chronic pelvic pain. Scar tissue in fallopian tubes increase the occurrence of ectopic pregnancies. 100,000 women become infertile as a result of PID. 150 women per year die as a result of complications of PID.

SIGNS AND SYMPTOMS OF PID	Signs and symptoms vary from none to severe including:
	    Lower abdominal pain, fever, unusual vaginal discharge, painful urination, and irregular menstrual bleeding.
	    Vague symptoms may go unrecognized.

TREATMENT	PID can be cured with antibiotics, but treatment does not reverse damage to reproductive organs.

Source: Centers for Disease Control and Prevention (CDC). (2004).

*T*RAUMA DURING PREGNANCY

Trauma is the leading cause of maternal death during pregnancy and is more likely to cause maternal death than any other complication of pregnancy. The most common cause of maternal death by trauma is abdominal injury, resulting in hemorrhagic shock, and head injury. Injury to the pregnant woman can result from blunt or penetrating trauma. The most common cause of blunt injury is motor vehicle accidents. The most common cause of penetrating trauma is from gunshot wounds. Maternal outcome in trauma corresponds to the severity of the injury. Fetal outcome depends on injury and maternal physiological response (Mattson & Smith, 2004). Two catastrophic events can occur during pregnancy after blunt trauma to the abdomen:

- Abruptio placenta
- Uterine rupture

Extensive discussion of management and care during trauma in pregnancy is beyond the scope of this chapter but key elements of stabilization of the woman and the fetus and assessments are reviewed. Treatment priorities for injured pregnant women typically are directed as they would be for nonpregnant women. Some important considerations related to pregnancy are presented in the following section.

Assessment Findings

- Assessment findings are based on injury.
- If the fetus is viable, electronic fetal monitoring is the best indicator of the maternal and fetal condition (Mattson & Smith, 2004).
- Fetal well-being reflects maternal and fetal status and conversely fetal heart rate changes may indicate maternal deterioration such as hypoxia.

- Physiological changes in pregnancy might delay the usual vital sign changes of hypovolemia; blood loss of up to 1,500 mL can occur without a change in maternal vital sign changes.
- Uterine contractions more frequently than every 10 minutes may be an indication of placental abruption (Cunningham et al., 2005)

Medical Management

Admit all pregnant women with viable fetuses and with major injuries to the hospital for continuous fetal monitoring for 24 to 48 hours after stabilization, in particular for abdominal injuries because of the increased incidence of abruptio placenta.

Nursing Actions

- Treatment priorities for injured pregnant women typically are directed as they would be for nonpregnant women.
- Initial actions in trauma care are focused on maternal stabilization.
  - *Initiate ABCs: Airway, breathing and circulation.*
- Assess maternal vital signs.
- Assess FHR, fetal movement, and UCs.
  - *Continuous fetal monitoring*
- Complete focused assessment of the injured areas.
- Determine the mechanism of injury including intimate partner violence and physical abuse.
- Ensure that diagnostic procedures, which may include laboratory tests and diagnostic imaging are completed.
- Position the woman on her side to position the gravid uterus off the inferior vena cava.
- Provide emotional support to the woman and her family.
- Explain procedures and plan of care to the woman and her family.

TABLE 7-7   SUMMARY OF FETAL AND MATERNAL EFFECTS AND MANAGEMENT OF STDs

INFECTION	MATERNAL EFFECTS	FETAL EFFECTS	MANAGEMENT	NURSING ISSUES
CHLAMYDIA *CHLAMYDIA TRACHOMATIS*	Three-fourths of women have no symptoms, so it is known as a "silent" disease, may have burning on urination or abnormal vaginal discharge.	Contact at delivery may cause conjunctivitis and/or premature birth. The efficacy of ophthalmia neonatorum prophylaxis is unclear.	Antibiotics Amoxicillin Azithromycin Erythromycin	Can lead to PID. Treat all infected partners. Retest in 3 weeks.
GONORRHEA *NEISSERIA GONORRHOEAE*	Most women have no symptoms but may have burning on urination, increased purulent yellow-green vaginal discharge, or bleeding between periods. Rectal infection can cause anal itching, discharge, and bleeding. Can lead to PID.	Contact at birth. Ophthalmia neonatorum may cause sepsis and/or blindness. To prevent gonococcal ophthalmia neonatorum, a prophylactic antibiotic ointment should be instilled into the eyes of all newborns.	Antibiotics Cephalosporin	Can lead to PID Complete treatment
GROUP B STREPTOCOCCUS *STREPTOCOCCUS AGALACTIAE* (GBS)	Women are typically asymptomatic carriers. Symptoms can include abnormal vaginal discharge, urinary tract infections, chorioamnionitis	Transmission rates are low, 1–2%, but infection can result in invasive GBS with permanent neurological sequelae.	If GBS-positive at 35–37 weeks of gestation or GBS status unknown treat with antibiotics in labor to prevent neonatal transmission. Penicillin or ampicillin IV	GBS-positive women receive intrapartum antibiotic prophylaxis.
HEPATITIS B (HBV)	50% asymptomatic May have low-grade fever, anorexia, nausea and vomiting, fatigue, rashes. Chronic infection can lead to cirrhosis of the liver and liver cancer.	90% of infected infants have chronic infection Cirrhosis of the liver Liver cancer	No specific treatment	HBsAg-positive pregnant women should be reported to the state or local health department for timely and appropriate prophylaxis for their infants. Immunoprophylaxis of all newborns born to HBsAg-positive women. HBIG to neonate at delivery and hepatitis b vaccination series initiated.
HEPATITIS C RNA VIRUS (HCV)	80% of persons infected have no symptoms. Can lead to chronic liver disease, cirrhosis, and liver cancer.	Exposure transplacentally. Estimated 2%–7% transmission rate. Little research on treatment of children.	Ribavirin and interferon, but are contraindicated in pregnancy.	Breastfeeding is not contraindicated.

Organism	Description	Effects	Treatment	Notes
HUMAN PAPILLOMAVIRUS (HPV) Thirty or more types infect the genital area.	The majority of HPV infections are asymptomatic but can cause genital warts. Genital warts are flat, papular, or pedunculated growths on the genital mucosa.	Route of transmission unclear. Can cause respiratory papillomatosis.	Warts may be removed during pregnancy. Treatment reduces but does not eliminate HPV infection.	The presence of genital warts is not an indication for cesarean delivery.
SYPHILIS TREPONEMA PALLIDUM	Ulcer or chancre, then maculopapular rash advancing to CNS and multiorgan damage.	Transplacental transmission. Congenital syphilis may cause preterm birth, physical deformity, neurological complications, stillbirth, and/or neonatal death.	Penicillin	
TRICHOMONAS TRICHOMONAS VAGINALIS	Malodorous yellow-green vaginal discharge and vulvar irritation. Can lead to premature rupture of membrane and preterm labor.	Preterm delivery and low birth weight. Respiratory and genital infection.	Metronidazole	
CANDIDIASIS CANDIDA ALBICANS Not an STD	Results from a disturbance in vaginal flora. Pruritus, vaginal soreness, dyspareunia, abnormal vaginal discharge with a yeasty odor.		Topical azole therapies	
BACTERIAL VAGINOSIS A polymicrobial clinical syndrome Not an STD	50% of women are asymptomatic. A fishy odor and/or vaginal discharge. Can result in preterm labor and/or premature rupture of membranes.	Premature rupture of membranes, chorioamnionitis and/or preterm birth	Metronidazole or clindamycin	

Continued

TABLE 7-7　SUMMARY OF FETAL AND MATERNAL EFFECTS AND MANAGEMENT OF STDs—CONT'D

INFECTION	MATERNAL EFFECTS	FETAL EFFECTS	MANAGEMENT	NURSING ISSUES
Human immunodeficiency virus (HIV)	May be asymptomatic for years. HIV weakens the immune system. It may manifest as mononucleosis-like symptoms such as fever, fatigue, sore throat, and lymphadenopathy.	Early antiretroviral treatment has been shown to be effective in reducing maternal-fetal transmissions. Placental transmission but <2% transmission with maternal treatment with antiretroviral medications. 15%–25% transmission to fetus without maternal treatment. Antibody screening is not reliable during infancy because of maternally produced IgG antibodies to HIV are present up to 18 months.	Antiviral	Cesarean birth may be considered. Breastfeeding is contraindicated Case management follow-up for both the woman and her baby.

Source: CDC (2005, 2006).

TABLE 7–8   TORCH INFECTIONS

INFECTION	MATERNAL EFFECTS	FETAL EFFECTS	PREVENTION AND MANAGEMENT	NURSING ISSUES
TOXOPLASMOSIS *TOXOPLASMA GONDII* Single-celled protozoan parasite. Transplacental transmission	Most infections are asymptomatic but may cause fatigue, muscle pains, and lymphadenopathy.	Severity varies with gestational age and congenital infection. Can lead to spontaneous abortion, low birth weight, hepatosplenomegaly, icterous, anemia, and/or neurological disease. Incidence of congenital infection is low.	Avoid eating raw meat and contact with cat feces. Treatment with sulfadiazine or pyrimethamine after the first trimester	Teach women to avoid raw meat and cat feces. Almost 50% of adults have an antibody to this organism.
OTHER INFECTIONS HEPATITIS B Direct contact with blood or body fluid from infected person.	30%–50% of infected women are asymptomatic. Symptoms include low-grade fever, nausea, anorexia, jaundice, hepatomegaly, preterm labor, and preterm delivery.	1 in 1,000–8,000 infants have a 90% chance of becoming chronically infected, HBV carrier, and a 25% risk of developing significant liver disease.	Infant receives HBIG and hepatitis vaccine at delivery.	Universal screening recommended in pregnancy. HBV can be given in pregnancy.
RUBELLA (GERMAN MEASLES) Nasopharyngeal secretions Transplacental	Erythematous maculopapular rash, lymph node enlargement, slight fever, headache, malaise	Overall risk of congenital rubella syndrome is 20% for primary maternal infection in the first trimester with 50% if the woman is infected in the first 4 weeks of gestation. Anomalies include deafness, eye defects, CNS anomalies, and severe cardiac malformations.	Primary approach to rubella infection is immunization. If the woman is pregnant and not immune, she should not receive the vaccine until the postpartum period.	If the woman is not immune she should not receive the vaccine until the postpartum period and be counseled to not become pregnant for 3 months.
CYTOMEGALOVIRUS (CMV) Virus of herpes group Transmitted by droplet contact and transplacentally	Most infections are asymptomatic but symptoms may include mononucleosis-like syndrome.	Infection to fetus is most likely with primary maternal infection and timing of infection with first- and second-trimester exposure. May result in low birth weight, IUGR, hearing impairment microcephaly, and CNS abnormalities.	No treatment is available.	

Continued

TABLE 7–8   TORCH INFECTIONS—CONT'D

INFECTION	MATERNAL EFFECTS	FETAL EFFECTS	PREVENTION AND MANAGEMENT	NURSING ISSUES
HERPES SIMPLEX VIRUS (HSV) Chronic lifelong viral infection Contact at delivery and ascending infection	Painful genital lesions. Lesions may be on external or internal genitalia.	Transmission rate of 30%–50% among women who acquire genital herpes near time of delivery and is low (<1%) among women with recurrent genital herpes. Mortality of 50%–60% if neonatal exposure to active primary lesion is related to neurological complications of massive infection sepsis and neurological complications.	No cure available. Acyclovir to suppress outbreak of lesions.	Most common viral STD. Protect the neonate from exposure with cesarean delivery if active lesion.

Source: Queenan, Hobbins, & Spong (2005).

PREGESTATIONAL COMPLICATIONS

Women who enter pregnancy with a preexisting disease or chronic medical condition are at increased risk for complication and are considered high-risk. These high-risk pregnancies require extensive surveillance and collaboration of multiple disciplines to achieve an optimal pregnancy outcome. Women often experience fear and anxiety for their health and that of the fetus regarding the impact of the chronic disease on the pregnancy outcome. Any preexisting medical disease can complicate the pregnancy or be exacerbated during pregnancy. Increasing numbers of women with chronic diseases are achieving pregnancy. Nursing care is focused on decreasing complications and providing support and education to patients and families to facilitate their participation in their health care during pregnancy.

Women and their families should participate in decision-making and the plan of care to optimize outcomes for both the woman and the fetus. Maternal safety is the prime consideration in all pregnancies. The major preexisting medical complications that impact pregnancy are discussed in this chapter, although all of the possible preexisting medical conditions impacting pregnancy are beyond the scope of this chapter. When caring for women who have preexisting diseases, textbooks on high-risk pregnancy management and perinatal journals are the best sources of information.

Cardiovascular Disorders

Pregnancy complicated by cardiovascular disease is potentially dangerous to maternal and fetal well-being. The incidence of cardiac disease among pregnant women ranges from 0.5% to 2% and varies in form and severity (Gilbert, 2007). **Cardiac disease** during pregnancy may be categorized as congenital, acquired, rheumatic, or ischemic. Some of the normal cardiac changes during pregnancy can exacerbate cardiac disease during pregnancy, including:

- Increase in cardiac output that peaks at 28 to 32 weeks of gestation
- Plasma volume expansion by 45%
- Increase in RBC by 20%
- Increased cardiac output by 40%
- Increased heart rate by 15%
- Heart slightly enlarges and displaces upward and to the left anatomically.
- The weight of the gravid uterus can lie on the inferior vena cava causing compression and hypotension and decreasing cardiac output
- Increased estrogen leads to vasodilatation which lowers peripheral resistance and increases cardiac output.
- Autonomic nervous system influences are more prominent on blood pressure

Marked hemodynamic changes in pregnancy can have a profound effect on the pregnant woman with cardiac disease and may result in exceeding the functional capacity of the diseased heart, resulting in (Cunningham et al., 2005; Simpson & Creehan, 2008; Mattson & Smith, 2004):

- Pulmonary hypertension
- Pulmonary edema
- Congestive heart failure
- Maternal or fetal death

Extensive discussion of specific cardiac disorders and their management is beyond the scope of this text. Reference to texts that deal with management of high-risk pregnancy particularly during labor and

delivery is indicated when caring for women with underlying heart disease, but general principles are presented. The management of cardiac disease is related to the cardiac disorder that is present and the impact it has on cardiac function responsible for specific symptoms.

Risks for the Woman

- Maternal mortality with cardiac disorders ranges from 1% to 50% based on cardiac disorder.
- Maternal effects include severe pulmonary edema, systemic emboli, and congestive heart failure.

Risks for the Newborn

- Fetal effects are a result of decreased systemic circulation and/or decreased oxygenation.
- If maternal circulation is compromised because of decreased cardiac function, uterine blood flow is reduced, which can result in intrauterine growth restriction. Fetal oxygenation is impaired when maternal oxygenation is impaired.
- Fetal hypoxia can result in permanent CNS damage depending on length and severity of decreased oxygenation.
- Neonatal death secondary to maternal cardiac disease ranges from 3% to 50%.

Assessment Findings

- Diagnosis of cardiac disease is based on symptoms and diagnostic tests which may include ECG, echocardiogram, and lab tests.
- The usual signs of deteriorating cardiac function include:
  - *Dyspnea, severe enough to limit usual activity*
  - *Progressive orthopnea*
  - *Paroxysmal nocturnal dyspnea*
  - *Syncope during or after exertion*
  - *Chest pain with activity*
  - *Thromboembolitic changes*
  - *Palpations*
  - *Fluid retention*

Medical Management

- Medical management varies based on cardiac disease and should include collaboration between obstetricians, cardiologists, anesthesiologists, and other specialists as needed.
- Discuss with the woman estimations of maternal and fetal mortality, potential chronic morbidity, and interventions to minimize risk during pregnancy and delivery (Simpson & Creehan, 2008).
- Obtain laboratory test to evaluate renal function and profusion ofusion (electrolytes, serum creatinine, proteins, and uric acid).
- Invasive hemodynamic monitoring using pulmonary artery catheters, peripheral arterial catheters, or central venous pressure monitors may be necessary.
- Preterm delivery may be indicated for deteriorating maternal or fetal status.

Nursing Actions

- Review the woman's history related to cardiovascular disorder including previous therapies or surgery, current medications, and current functional classification of cardiac disease.
- Conduct a cardiovascular assessment (Simpson & Creehan, 2008) that includes:
  - *Auscultation of heart, lungs, and breath sounds*
  - *Identification of pathological edema*
  - *Evaluation of respiratory rate and rhythm*

- *Evaluation of cardiac rate and rhythm*
- *Body weight and weight gain*
- *Assessment of skin color, temperature, and turgor*
- *Capillary refill check*
- Additional noninvasive assessment may include:
  - *O₂ saturation via pulse oximeter*
  - *Arrhythmia assessment with 12-lead EKG*
  - *Electrocardiogram*
  - *Urinary output*
  - *Electronic fetal monitoring*
- Review laboratory results related to renal function and perfusion.
  - *Electrolytes, blood urea nitrogen (BUN), serum creatinine, proteins, uric acid*
- Provide information to the woman and her family regarding status of woman and fetus and plan of care.
  - *Antepartal testing including NSTs, BPPs, and ultrasounds*
  - *New medications may include anticoagulation therapy; therefore, women need to learn to give self-injections.*
- Assess FHR
- Provide emotional support to the woman and her family.

Anemia and Iron-Deficiency Anemia

Anemia complicates 15% to 25% of all pregnancies, and 80% of those anemias are a result of iron deficiency related to a diet low in iron content and insufficient iron stores. Pregnancy results in an intravascular volume expansion with the increase in plasma volume larger than the rise in RBCs resulting in the hemodilution of pregnancy; the net result is a physiological drop in hemoglobin and hematocrit values. Iron deficiency anemia during pregnancy is the consequence primarily of expansion of plasma volume without normal expansion of maternal hemoglobin mass (Cunningham et al., 2005). **Anemia** is present if the hemoglobin drops below 10 g/dL or the hematocrit falls below 30% (Mattson & Smith, 2004). Discussion of acquired and inherited anemias and hemoglobinopathies are beyond the scope of this chapter.

Risk Factors

- History of poor nutritional status or eating disorder
- Close spacing of pregnancies
- Multiple gestation
- Excessive bleeding
- Adolescence

Risks for the Woman

- Fatigue
- Reduced tolerance to activity

Risks for the Newborn

- Preterm birth
- Intrauterine growth restriction

Assessment Findings

- Pallor
- Fatigue, weakness, and malaise
- Reduced exercise tolerance and dyspnea
- Anorexia and/or pica
- Edema
- Hemoglobin below 10 g/dL
- Hematocrit below 30%

Medical Management

- Iron supplementation
  - *Supplement with 300 mg/day ferrous sulfate*

Nursing Actions

- Refer the woman to a dietician for nutritional counseling and reinforce dietary interventions.
- Advise that taking iron supplementation at bedtime and on an empty stomach may increase absorption and decrease gastrointestinal upset.
- Assess fatigue and develop interventions and a plan of care to deal with fatigue.

Pulmonary Disorders/Asthma

Normal physiological changes of pregnancy can cause a woman with a history of compromised respiratory function to decompensate. Pulmonary disease has become more prevalent in women of childbearing age. Pulmonary diseases can develop during pregnancy such as pneumonia or tocolytic induced pulmonary edema, whereas other conditions preexist. It is important to remember that some of the normal respiratory changes during pregnancy can exacerbate respiratory disease during pregnancy. Alteration in the immune system, and mechanical and anatomical changes have a cumulative effect to decrease tolerance to hypoxia and acute changes in pulmonary function (Simpson & Creehan, 2008). These include:

- Increased progesterone during pregnancy results in maternal hyperventilation and increase tidal volume.
- Changes in configuration of the thorax with advancing pregnancy decrease residual capacity and volume while oxygen consumption increases.
- Increased estrogen levels result in mucosal edema, hypersecretion, and capillary congestion.
- Respiratory physiology in normal pregnancy tends toward respiratory alkalosis.

Asthma is the most common form of lung disease that can impact pregnancy and complicates about 4% of pregnancies. **Asthma** is an irrevocable syndrome characterized by varying levels of airway obstruction, bronchial hyper responsiveness, and bronchial edema.

Diagnosis and management goals of asthma during pregnancy are the same as for nonpregnant women. People with asthma have airways that are hyperresponsive to allergens, viruses, air pollutants, exercise, and cold air. This hyperresponsiveness is manifested by bronchospasm, mucosal edema, and mucus plugging the airways. Goals of therapy include:

- Protection of the pulmonary system from irritants
- Prevention of pulmonary and inflammatory response to allergen exposure
- Relief of bronchospasm
- Resolution of airway inflammation to reduce airway hyperresponsiveness
- Improve pulmonary function

Risks for the Woman

- Pregnancy has varying effects on asthma with about one-third of pregnant women becoming worse, one-third improving, and one-third remaining the same (Gilbert, 2007).
- With aggressive management of asthma, pregnancy outcomes can be the same as for nonasthmatic pregnant women.

Risks for the Newborn

■ Hypoxia to the fetus is a major complication.
■ Preterm birth
■ Low birth weight

Assessment Findings

■ Signs and symptoms of asthma:
  ■ *Cough*
  ■ *Wheezing*
  ■ *Tightness in chest*
  ■ *Shortness of breath*
  ■ *Sputum production*
■ Signs and symptoms of hypoxia:
  ■ *Cyanosis*
  ■ *Lethargy*
  ■ *Agitation*
  ■ *Intercostal retractions*
  ■ *Respiratory rate greater than 30 breaths/min*

Medical Management

Asthma should be aggressively treated during pregnancy, as the benefits of asthma control far outweigh the risks of medication use. During pregnancy, monthly evaluation of pulmonary function and asthma history are conducted. Serial ultrasound for fetal growth and antepartal fetal testing is done for moderately or severely asthmatic women.

■ Medications commonly used for asthma management are considered safe during pregnancy and include bronchodilators, anti-inflammatory agents such as inhaled steroids, oral corticosteroids, allergy injections, and antihistamines.

Nursing Actions

■ Take a detailed history and assessment of respiratory status including pulmonary function and blood gases.
■ Assess for signs and symptoms including cough, wheezing, chest tightness, and sputum production.
■ Care for women with acute asthma exacerbations includes:
  ■ *Oxygen administration to maintain PaO_2 greater than 95%*
  ■ *Ongoing maternal pulse oximeter*
  ■ *Baseline arterial blood gases as per orders*
  ■ *Baseline pulmonary function tests performed to gather baseline data as per orders*
  ■ *Beta-agonist inhalation therapy as ordered*
■ Monitor maternal oxygen saturation (should be at 95% to oxygenate the fetus).
■ Assess fetal well-being and for signs of fetal hypoxia.
■ Evaluate pulmonary function test results and laboratory tests (i.e., arterial blood gases).
■ Explain the plan of care and goals.
■ Teach the woman to avoid allergens and triggers.
■ Teach the woman to monitor pulmonary function daily and her normal parameters.
■ Teach the woman the role of medications, correct use of medications, and adverse effects of medications.
■ Teach the woman to recognize signs and symptoms of worsening asthma and provide a treatment plan to manage exacerbations appropriately.
■ Discuss warning signs and symptoms to report to the provider, such as dyspnea, shortness of breath, chest tightness, or exacerbations of signs and symptoms beyond the woman's baseline asthma status.

Gastrointestinal Disorders

Cholelithiasis, presence of gall stones in the gall bladder, occurs in approximately 8% of pregnancies (Gilbert, 2007). Decreased muscle tone allows gall bladder distension and thickening of the bile and prolongs emptying time during pregnancy, increasing the risk of cholelithiasis.

Assessment Findings

■ Colicky abdominal pain presents in the right upper quadrant; anorexia, nausea, and vomiting; the woman may have a fever.
■ Gallstones are present on an ultrasound scan.

Medical Management

Cholelithiasis is typically treated with conservative management such as IV fluids, bowel rest, nasogastric suctioning, diet, and antibiotics. Increasingly, it is managed by surgical intervention with laparoscopic cholecystectomies (Cunningham et al., 2005). If gall bladder disease is nonacute, surgical intervention may be delayed until the postpartum period.

Nursing Actions

■ Manage pain, administering pain medication as needed.
■ Manage nausea and vomiting, minimizing environmental factors that cause nausea and vomiting such as odors.
■ Administer antiemetics as needed.
■ Provide comfort measures based on symptoms.
■ Explain procedures and plan of care including dietary restrictions.

SUBSTANCE ABUSE

The rate of substance abuse among childbearing women continues to increase (Gilbert, 2007). Approximately 15% of all pregnant women have a substance abuse problem (United States Department of Health and Human Services [USDHHS], 2008). Abusing any substance increases the risk of pregnancy and neonatal complications. Many pregnant women who use illicit drugs also use alcohol and tobacco, and it may be difficult to determine which complications are associated with which substance. Risks of specific complications vary based on substance used; however, general risks resulting from substance abuse for both the woman and fetus/newborn are presented. Pregnant women using illicit substances often fear legal consequences and may avoid seeking prenatal care. A nonjudgmental and factual approach with attention toward reducing risks offers the best approach for these complex pregnancies. Chemically dependent pregnant women may engage in other risky behaviors. A holistic, comprehensive approach to care that deals not only with the prenatal aspects of care, but also with the complex social and psychological contributing factors, is needed.

Smoking/Tobacco Use

At least 16% of women in the United States smoke during pregnancy (Martin et al., 2006; USDHHS, 2008). The physiological effects of smoking are a result of transient intrauterine hypoxemia. The more the woman smokes, the greater the risk (March of Dimes, 2008a). Cigarette smoke contains many chemicals, in particular nicotine and carbon monoxide, that cause adverse pregnancy outcomes, particularly low birth weight and prematurity.

■ Nicotine reduces uterine blood flow.
■ Carbon monoxide binds to hemoglobin, reducing the oxygen-carrying capacity of the blood (Creasy, Resnik, & Iams, 2004).

Alcohol

About 13% of pregnant women drink alcohol during pregnancy, and alcohol is the most common teratogen (Gilbert, 2007). When a pregnant woman drinks, alcohol passes swiftly to the fetus through the placenta. Because alcohol is processed more slowly in the fetus's liver, the alcohol level can be even higher and can remain elevated longer. Drinking alcohol during pregnancy can result in a wide range of physical and mental birth defects. The term fetal alcohol spectrum disorders (FASD) is used to describe the many problems associated with alcohol exposure prior to birth. Each year in the United States up to 40,000 infants are born with FASDs (March of Dimes, 2008b). Chapter 17 provides additional information on FASDs. The consensus is that no level of drinking alcohol is considered safe in pregnancy.

Illicit Drugs

An average of 5.2% of pregnant women use illicit drugs such as marijuana, cocaine, amphetamines, heroin and Ecstasy (USDHHS, 2008). The effect of the drug on placental function and fetal development depends on its nature.

For example, cocaine causes vasoconstriction that can impact the placenta and uterus, resulting in abruption of the placenta or preterm birth (Foley, 2002; March of Dimes, 2006c). Women who use illicit drugs are counseled to stop, except for heroin users, for whom methadone treatment is recommended to prevent stillbirth.

Risks for the Woman

■ Preterm labor
■ PPROM
■ Poor weight gain and nutritional status
■ Placental abnormalities (placenta previa, abruptio placenta)

Risks for the Newborn

■ Effects of maternal substance use on the neonate are detailed in Chapter 17.
■ Stillbirth
■ Low birth weight
■ Preterm birth
■ Intrauterine growth restriction
■ Neonatal withdrawal syndrome (symptoms are drug dependent)
■ Sudden infant death syndrome (SIDS)

Assessment Findings

A variety of screening tools have been proposed, and screening for smoking, alcohol use and illicit drugs is recommended to start at the first prenatal visit. Universal screening of all pregnant women is recommended in a supportive and nonjudgmental manner (Gilbert, 2007). One simple screening tool includes asking the following four questions for a yes or no response, described as Ewing's 4 P's (Taylor, Zaichkin, & Bailey, 2002).

■ Have you ever used alcohol or drugs during this pregnancy?
■ Have you had a problem with drugs or alcohol in the past?

■ Does your partner have a problem with drugs or alcohol?
■ Do you consider one of your parents to have a problem with drugs or alcohol?

A yes answer to any of these questions should trigger further evaluation of habits.

Medical Management (Creasy, Resnik, & Iams, 2004)

■ Refer to multispecialty clinics.
■ Refer to drug treatment programs.
■ Screen for domestic violence.
■ Conduct frequent urine toxicology tests.
■ Use targeted ultrasound to rule out congenital anomalies.
■ Provide patient education.
■ Conduct antepartal testing.

Nursing Actions

Women are more receptive to treatment and lifestyle changes during pregnancy; therefore pregnancy may be a window of opportunity for chemically dependent women to enter treatment. To facilitate this, nurses must be armed with knowledge and information necessary to screen and identify women who abuse substances during pregnancy. Because of the substantial costs and repercussions of drug use during pregnancy for newborns, women, and society it is essential to devise methods of intervention that decrease this risky behavior. It has been proposed that government policies can be viewed as either "facilitative" or "adversarial" (Bornstein, 2003). Facilitative policies improve women's access to prenatal care, food, shelter, and treatment. Adversarial policies propose that women who fail to seek treatment are liable to criminal prosecution and may diminish utilization of prenatal care.

■ Provide health education about the risks to the fetus of substance use during pregnancy and facilitate early diagnosis and appropriate intervention and referral.
■ Laws governing drug screening during pregnancy vary from state to state. Nurses need to be aware of laws and local guidelines for toxicology screening of pregnant women and treatment options and availability of programs, as many treatment programs will not accept pregnant women.
■ Counsel women who test positive for drug or alcohol use and those who smoke during pregnancy to stop and supply referrals to assist with cessation and refer to local treatment centers for pregnant women (Box 7-5).
■ Maintain a nonjudgmental and nonpunitive attitude (Selleck & Redding, 1998), remember addiction is a disease.

BOX 7–5   REFERRALS FOR INFORMATION AND SUPPORT ON QUITTING SUBSTANCE USE DURING PREGNANCY

Alcoholics Anonymous
    www.aa.org
Narcotics Anonymous
    www.na.org
Smoking Cessation
    www.ahrg.gov/consumer/tobacco/quits.htm
    www.helppregnantsmokersquit.com
    www.cancer.org
    www.smokefreefamilies.org
    www.marchofdimes.org

CONCEPT MAP

Preeclampsia

Central Nervous System Irritability

- Headache
- Visual changes
- DTRs + 3
- No clonus

Altered Cardiovascular Function/Vascular Constriction

- Hypertension — B/P 162/102
- Fetal compromise
- +3 pitting edema

Altered Placental Perfusion

- Intrauterine growth restriction
- Decreased fetal heart rate variability
- AFI 4.5

Altered Renal Function

- Proteinuria +2 on urine dipstick
- 24 urine protein 3.4 grams
- Decrease creatinine clearance
- BUN 12 mg/dl
- Uric acid 4.9 mg
- Serum creatinine clearance 2.4 mg/dl

Preeclampsia
Hypertension, proteinuria, edema, elevated liver function tests. Generalized vasospasm and endothelial cell damage decrease perfusion and oxygenation throughout the body causing widespread organ dysfunction.

Altered Hepatic Function

- Nausea
- Epigastric pain
- ATL 35 units/L
- AST 45 units/L

Anxiety
Woman is crying. Woman states she is concerned she and baby are going to die.

Problem No. 1: Central Nervous System Irritability
Goal: Prevent seizures and cerebral edema
Outcome: Patient will remain seizure free and not develop neurological sequelae.

Nursing Actions

1. Monitor CNS changes including headache, dizziness, blurred vision, and scotoma.
2. Maintain seizure precautions.
3. If treated with magnesium sulfate, see critical components box for nursing care of patient on magnesium.
4. Restrict fluids to total of 125 mL/hr or as ordered.
5. Monitor I&O.
6. Assess DTRs.
7. Maintain bedrest in the lateral position.
8. Provide an environment that is conducive to decreased stimulation such as low lights, decreased noise, and uninterrupted rest periods.
9. Teach the patient relaxation techniques.

Problem No. 2: Altered Cardiovascular Function/Vasoconstriction
Goal: Normal blood pressure
Outcome: Blood pressure within acceptable limits, below 140/90 mm Hg

Nursing Actions

1. Monitor BP every hour or more frequently if elevated.
2. Administer antihypertensive medication as ordered related to hypertensive parameters.
3. Assess edema.
4. Assess lungs for pulmonary edema.
5. Maintain bedrest in the left lateral position.

Problem 3: Anxiety Related to Harm for Self and Fetus
Goal: Decreased anxiety
Outcome: Patient verbalizes that she feels less anxious

Nursing Actions

1. Be calm and reassuring in interactions with the patient and her family.
2. Explain all procedures.
3. Explain results of test and procedures.
4. Teach patient relaxation and breathing techniques.
5. Encourage the patient and family to verbalize their feelings regarding recent hemorrhage by asking open-ended questions.

Problem 4: Altered Renal Function
Goal: Maintain adequate renal function.
Outcome: The patient will maintain adequate renal function.

Nursing Actions

1. Monitor and maintain strict I&O.
2. Report urine output <30 mL/hr
3. Check urine protein and specific gravity.
4. Evaluate kidney function tests.
5. Report changes in urine output or worsening kidney function laboratory values to the care provider.
6. Assess edema.

Problem 5: Altered Hepatic Function
Goal: Maintain adequate hepatic function.
Outcome: The patient will maintain adequate hepatic function.

Nursing Actions

1. Assess epigastric pain, right upper quadrant pain, nausea and vomiting
2. Interpret laboratory tests related to liver function (AST, LDH)
3. Report changes in liver function tests to the care provider.

Problem No. 6: Altered Placental Perfusion
Goal: Maintain fetal oxygenation.
Outcome: Assessments of fetal status remain within normal limits.

Nursing Actions

1. Assess FHR baseline, variability, and for abnormal FHR patterns.
2. Provide interventions for intrauterine resuscitation of fetus (IV fluid, O_2, lateral position).
3. Report any abnormal FHR patterns to the care provider.
4. Facilitate antenatal testing.
5. Instruct the woman in daily kick counts.

TYING IT ALL TOGETHER

As the nurse, you evaluate Mallory Polk in triage in the labor and delivery unit. She presented in the triage unit at 8 P.M. at 32 weeks' gestation with complaints of a persistent low dull backache, increased vaginal discharge, and pelvic pressure in her vagina for 2 days with some vaginal spotting this evening when she went to the bathroom. She attributed the discomforts of backache and pulling to working long hours for the past week in arbitration on a "big case" where she is a partner in a large law firm. Mallory is a 42-year-old single African American woman. She is accompanied by her sister Alison, who is visiting for the week from out of state. When placed on the monitor, Mallory is contracting every 5 to 7 minutes that she reports as "menstrual cramping." The FHR is in the 150s baseline with accelerations to 170s with moderate variability. A review of her prenatal record reveals she is a G2 P0 and the pregnancy is a result of in vitro fertilization. She has received regular prenatal visits. She does not smoke or drink alcohol. Her prenatal laboratory results are as follows:

Blood type A+
RPR NR
GBS negative
Hgb 12.4
Hct 32.1
Hepatitis negative

Prenatal Care Summary

Began prenatal care at 10 weeks' gestation and receive regular prenatal care. She conceives after three attempts at in vitro fertilization. She has no prior medical complications and has experienced a normal pregnancy. Her first pregnancy was terminated at 6 weeks of gestation. She is allergic to shellfish and is allergic to sulfa drugs. An ultrasound at 12 weeks confirms a gestational age of 32 weeks.

Detail the aspects of your initial assessment and what you would report to her physician.

Within 40 minutes of arrival, you phone her physician, who is completing a delivery, and report your assessment findings. The physician comes in 10 minutes to evaluate Mallory. Based on her assessment she orders and IV lactated Ringer's 300-mL bolus, a CBC, urinalysis clean catch, does a fetal fibronectin, and does a sterile vaginal exam that reveals her cervix is 2 cm dilated/75% effaced/0 station. Her physician orders a 4-gram magnesium sulfate bolus over 30 minutes, then 2 grams per hour. Betamethasone is to be given 12 mg now and to be repeated in 24 hours. An ultrasound is ordered for fetal size and position. Ampicillin 1 gram is ordered IV every 6 hours. Her physician discussed the plan of care for treatment of preterm labor with Mallory and answers her questions and Mallory agrees to the plan to attempt to stop the contractions and delay delivery.

What are your immediate priorities in nursing care for Mallory?
Discuss the rationale for the priorities.
State nursing diagnosis, expected outcome, and interventions related to this problem.
List Mallory's risk factors for preterm labor.
What teaching would you include?

Within 10 minutes of starting the magnesium sulfate bolus she reports feeling hot and flushed and feels burning at the IV site. After the magnesium sulfate bolus is complete, you start the magnesium sulfate infusion at 2 grams per hour. At midnight, her contractions slow down to every 15 minutes or 4 to 5 contractions/hour. The FHR baseline is 140s with minimal variability and periodic accelerations. An ultrasound reveals the fetus is vertex, estimated fetal weight (EFW) is 1,560 grams, and fetal fibronectin is positive.

What are the assessments for a woman treated for preterm labor on magnesium sulfate?
Discuss the rationale for the assessments.
What teaching would you include in the nursing action plan?

At 7 A.M. when you sign off Mallory is sleeping intermittently. Her contractions are 2 to 3 per hour and the FHR is reassuring. Mallory is very concerned about giving birth to a premature baby. She is concerned that a baby will not survive at this gestation and states, "I have always wanted to be a mother and was so happy when I was finally ready to have a baby and conceived with IVF." She is worried about not being able to return to work over the next few days and weeks, as she has many active cases pending over the next few weeks. She states that she is not ready for the baby to come and has not set up the crib or finished the nursery. She feels guilty she did not come to the hospital sooner and considered the backache as just part of pregnancy discomforts. Before you leave you have requested Mallory be seen that day by the neonatal clinical specialist to review status and care for neonates born prematurely and to have Mallory's sister tour the NICU.

Detail the aspects of your psychosocial assessment for a woman with a high-risk pregnancy.
Discuss the rationale for the assessment.
Discuss nursing diagnosis, nursing actions, and expected outcomes related to this psychosocial assessment.

The next night you come onto you shift at 7 P.M. and care for Mallory again. She remains on the magnesium sulfate and appears to be tolerating the medication. Her magnesium level is 5.6 mEq/L. She still feels warm and somewhat lethargic with sore muscles due to being in bed all day. She is due for her second dose of betamethasone. Her I&O for the past 24 hours are: I: 2,500 mL; O: 2,300 mL. The plan is to wean her off the magnesium sulfate in the next 2 days and transfer her to the antenatal unit in the morning.

Detail the aspects of your ongoing assessment for a woman treated with magnesium sulfate and diagnosed with preterm labor.
Discuss the rationale for the assessment.

At 0320 she reports feeling a gush of fluid from her vagina after a strong contraction. Between her legs is a large amount of clear fluid. The FHR is baseline 140s with minimal variability and accelerations. Mallory appears frightened and anxious. She is crying and her sister is at her side holding her hand and reassuring her.

What are your immediate priorities in nursing care for Mallory?
Discuss the rationale for the priorities.

Within 45 minutes, her physician comes in to see Mallory and does an SVE. She is 5 cm, 90% effaced, and +1 station, and an ultrasound reveals the fetus is vertex. The physician recommends they turn off the magnesium sulfate and anticipate a vaginal birth because of the advanced preterm labor. Mallory agrees with the plan.

■ ■ ■   **Review Questions**   ■ ■ ■

1. The nurse would suspect preeclampsia if which of the following was found during assessment:
   A. Hypertension and diminished reflexes
   B. Ankle edema and ketonuria
   C. Proteinuria and hypertension
   D. Glucosuria and proteinuria

2. Which of the following is an indication to turn off magnesium sulfate in a women managed with preeclampsia?
   A. Blood pressure 190/110 mm Hg
   B. Nausea and vomiting
   C. Epigastric pain
   D. Respiratory rate of 13 breaths/min

3. Type 1 diabetes is associated with
   A. Decreased pancreatic function
   B. Insulin resistance
   C. Inappropriate response to insulin
   D. Absolute insulin deficiency

4. Over the past 25 years, the incidence of preterm birth has:
   A. Declined
   B. Remained the same
   C. Increased

5. An appropriate gestational age to do glucose screening is:
   A. 22 weeks of gestation
   B. 26 weeks of gestation
   C. 30 weeks of gestation
   D. 34 weeks of gestation

6. Smoking during pregnancy increases the risk of:
   A. Low birth weight and prematurity
   B. Neonatal lung disease
   C. Preeclampsia

7. The goal of magnesium sulfate therapy in treating preeclampsia is to:
   A. Reduce blood pressure
   B. Delay delivery
   C. Prevent seizures
   D. Increase placental perfusion

8. Hypoglycemia is defined as a blood glucose below:
   A. 60 mg/dL
   B. 70 mg/dL
   C. 80 mg/dL
   D. 90 mg/dL

9. Management of women with pregestational diabetes should begin:
   A. Before conception
   B. At the end of the first trimester
   C. At the end of 20 weeks
   D. Before the onset of labor

10. An oxygen saturation below _____ is an abnormal finding for a pregnant woman.
    A. 90%
    B. 92%
    C. 95%
    D. 97%

11. The likelihood of dizygotic twinning is affected by:
    A. Advancing maternal age
    B. Use of assisted reproductive technology
    C. Maternal nutritional status

12. Women are more receptive to treatment and lifestyle changes during pregnancy, so pregnancy may be a window of opportunity for chemically dependent women to enter treatment.
    A. True
    B. False

References

American Diabetes Association (ADA). (2004). Gestational diabetes mellitus. *Diabetes Care, 27*; S88–90.

Berkman, N., Thorp, J., Lohr, K., Cary, T., Hartman, K., Gavin, N., Hasselblad, V., & Inicula, A. (2003). Tocolytic treatment for the management of preterm labor: A review of the evidence. *American Journal of Obstetrics and Gynecology, 188*(6), 1648–1659.

Bornstein, B. (2003). Pregnancy, drug testing, and the Fourth Amendment: Legal and behavioral implications: Pregnancy and reproduction issues. *The Journal of Family Psychology, 17*, 220–228.

Centers for Disease Control and Prevention (CDC). (2004a). Pelvic Inflammatory Disease-CDC Fact Sheet, May, 2004. Retrieved from www.cdc.gov/std/PID/STDFact-PID.htm (Accessed June 18, 2009).

Centers for Disease Control and Prevention (CDC). (2004b). STDs & Pregnancy- CDC Fact Sheet, May, 2004. Retrieved from www.cdc.gov/std/STDFact-STDs & Pregnancy.htm (Accessed May, 1, 2007).

Centers for Disease Control and Prevention (CDC). (2005). Sexually Transmitted Disease Surveillance, 2004. Atlanta: U.S. Department of Health and Human Service, September 2005.

Centers for Disease Control and Prevention (CDC). (2006). Sexually Transmitted Diseases Treatment Guidelines 2006. *MMRW* 2006:55 (no. RR-11).

Creasy, R., Resnik, R. & Iams, J. (Eds.). (2004). *Maternal-fetal medicine* (5th ed.). Philadelphia: W. B. Saunders.

Cunningham, F., Leveno, K., Bloom, S., Haut, J., Gilstrap, L., & Wenstrom, K. (2005). *Williams obstetrics* (22nd ed.). New York: McGraw-Hill.

Deglin, J., & Vallerand, A. (2009). *Davis's drug guide for nurses* (11th ed.). Philadelphia: F. A. Davis.

Durham, R. (1998). Strategies women engage in when managing preterm labor at home. *Journal of Perinatology, 18*, 61–64.

Foley, E. (2002). Drug screening and criminal prosecution of pregnant women. *Journal of Obstetric and Gynecologic and Neonatal Nursing, 31*(2), 133–137.

Freda, M., Patterson, E., & Wieczorek, R. (2004). Preterm labor: Prevention and nursing management. In *Continuing education for registered nurses and certified nurse midwives* (3rd ed.). White Plains, NY: March of Dimes.

Gibson, P., Carson, M., & Letterie, G. (2007). Hypertension and pregnancy. emedicine specialties from WEBMD December 13, 2007.

Gilbert, E. (2007). Manual of high risk pregnancy and delivery. St. Louis, MO: C. V. Mosby.

Gregg, A. (2004). Hypertension in pregnancy. *Obstetrics and Gynecology Clinics of North America, 31*, 223–241.

Grey, B. (2006). A ticking uterus. *Lifelines, 10*, 380–389.

Griffith, J., & Conway, D. (2004). Care diabetes in pregnancy. *Obstetrics and Gynecology Clinics of North America, 31*, 243–256.

Hodnett, E. D., & Fredericks, S. (2003). Support during pregnancy for women at increased risk of low birth weight babies. *Cochrane Database of Systematic Reviews* 2003, Issue 3. Art. No.: CD000198. DOI: 10.1002/14651858.CD000198.

Kendrick, J. (2004). *Diabetes in pregnancy* (3rd ed.). White Plains, NY: March of Dimes Nursing Module.

Kröner, C., Turnbull D., & Wilkinson, C. (2001). Antenatal day care units versus hospital admission for women with complicated pregnancy.

Cochrane Database of Systematic Reviews 2001, Issue 4. Art. No.: CD001803. DOI:10.1002/14651858.CD001803.

Magpie Trial Collaborative Group. (2002). Do women with preeclampsia, and their babies, benefit from magnesium sulphate? The Magpie Trial: A randomized placebo-controlled trial. *The Lancet, 359*, 1877–1890.

Maloni, J. A. (1993). Bedrest during pregnancy: Implications for nursing. *Journal of Obstetric, Gynecologic, and Neonatal Nursing, 23*, 422–426.

Maloni, J. A. (1998). Antepartum bedrest: Case studies, research I nursing care. Washington, DC: Association of Women's Health, Obstetric and Neonatal Nurses.

March of Dimes. (2006a). Compendium on preterm birth: Epidemiology and biology of preterm birth. Produced in cooperation with American Academy of Pediatrics, The American College of Obstetricians, and Gynecologists & Association of Women's Health, Obstetric and Neonatal Nurses.

March of Dimes. (2006b). Compendium on preterm birth: Employing systems-based practice for patient care. Produced in cooperation with American Academy of Pediatrics, The American College of Obstetricians and Gynecologists & Association of Women's Health, Obstetric and Neonatal Nurses.

March of Dimes. (2006c). Illicit drug use during pregnancy. Retrieved from www.marchofdimes.com/printableArticles/14332_1169.asp (Accessed June 18, 2009).

March of Dimes. (2008a). Smoking during pregnancy. Retrieved from www.marchofdimes.com/printableArticles/14332_1171.asp (Accessed June 18, 2009).

March of Dimes. (2008b). Drinking alcohol during pregnancy. Retrieved from www.marchofdimes.com/printableArticle/14332_1170.asp (Accessed June 18, 2009).

Martin, J., Hamilton, B., Sutton, P., Ventura, S., Menacker, F., & Kimeyer, S. (2006). Births: Final data for 2004. *National Vital Statistics Reports, 55*(1). Hyattsville, MD: National Center for Health Statistics.

Mattson, S., & Smith, J. E. (Eds.). (2004). *Core curriculum for maternal-newborn nursing* (3rd ed.). St. Louis, MO: Elsevier Saunders.

Mignini, L. E., Villar, J., & Khalid, K. S. (2006). Mapping the theories of preeclampsia: The need for systematic reviews of mechanisms of the disease. *American Journal of Obstetrics and Gynecology, 194*, 317–321.

Nanda, K., Cook, L. A. A., Gallo, M. F., & Grimes, D. A. (2002). Terbutaline pump maintenance therapy after threatened preterm labor for preventing preterm birth. Cochrane Database of Systematic Reviews 2002, Issue 4. Art. No.: CD003933. DOI: 10.1002/14651858. CD003933.

National High Blood Pressure Education Program Working Group (NHBPEP). (2000). Working group report on high blood pressure in pregnancy (NHBPEP Publication No. 00-3029). Washington, DC: National Heart Lung and Blood Institute.

Perkins, J. M., Dunn, J. P., & Jagasia, S. M. (2007). Perspectives in gestational diabetes mellitus: A review of screening, diagnosis, and treatment. *Clinical Diabetes, 25*, 57–62.

Peristats. (2008). National Center for Health Statistics, final natality data. Retrieved from www.marchofdimes.com/peristats (Accessed May 26, 2008).

Peters, R., & Flack, J. (2004). Hypertensive disorders of pregnancy. *Journal of Obstetric, Gynecologic, and Neonatal Nursing, 33*, 209–219.

Queenan, J., Hobbins, J., & Spong, C. (2005). *Protocols in high risk pregnancies*. Malden, MA: Blackwell.

Roberts, D., & Dalziel, S. (2007). Antenatal corticosteroid maturation for women at risk for preterm birth (Cochrane Review). Cochrane Database of Systematic Reviews 2006, Issue 3. Art. No.: CD004454. DOI: 10.1002/14651858.CD004454.pub2.

Selleck, C. S., & Redding, B. A. (1998). Knowledge and attitude of registered nurses toward perinatal substance abuse [Clinical Studies]. *Journal of Obstetric and Gynecologic and Neonatal Nursing, 27*, 70–77.

Simpson, K., Creehan, P., & Association of Women's Health, Obstetrics and Neonatal Nurses. (2008). *Perinatal nursing* (3rd ed.). Philadelphia: Lippincott Williams & Wilkins.

Sibai, B. (2003). Diagnosis and management of gestational hypertension and preeclampsia [An expert's view]. *Obstetrics & Gynecology, 102*, 181–192.

Sibai, B. (2004). Diagnosis, controversies, and management of the syndrome of Hemolysis, Elevated Liver Enzymes, and Low Platelet Count [High Risk Pregnancy Series: An expert's view]. *Obstetrics & Gynecology, 103*, 981–991.

Sosa, C., Althabe, F., Belizán, J., & Bergel, E. (2007). Bed rest in singleton pregnancies for preventing preterm birth (Cochrane Review). In: The Cochrane Library Issue 2, 2007. Cochrane Database of Systematic Reviews 2004, Issue 1. Art. No.: CD003581. DOI: 10.1002/14651858.CD003581.pub2.

Taylor, P., Zaichkin, J., & Bailey, D. (2002). Substance abuse during pregnancy: guidelines for screening. Olympia, WA, 2002, Maternal and Child Health. Retrieved from http://www.doh.wa.gov (Accessed June 18, 2007).

U.S. Department of Health and Human Services. Substance Abuse and Mental Health Administration. Results from the 2007 National Survey on Drug Use and Health: National Findings, Office of Applied Studies, DHHS, publication no. SMA 08-4343, Rockville, MD, 2008 (Accessed September 2, 2009).

The Intrapartal Period

Intrapartum Assessment and Interventions

OBJECTIVES

On completion of this chapter the student will be able to:

☐ Define key terms.
☐ Describe the four stages of labor and the related nursing and medical care.
☐ Demonstrate understanding of supportive care of the laboring woman.
☐ Identify the four P's of labor.
☐ Describe the mechanism of spontaneous vaginal delivery and related nursing care.

Nursing Diagnoses

☐ Pain related to the labor and delivery process
☐ Fear related to unknowns of labor; threat of potential harm to self or fetus
☐ Deficient knowledge of labor process
☐ Risk of ineffective maternal/fetal perfusion related to perfusion in labor
☐ Risk of infection related to vaginal exams after rupture of membranes

Nursing Outcomes

☐ The woman will have decreased pain.
☐ The woman will understand the process and interventions related to labor.
☐ The woman will have decreased fear during labor.
☐ The woman and her partner will express positive feelings regarding their birthing experience.
☐ The woman's vital signs and fetal heart rate remain stable.
☐ The woman will be free of infection.

INTRODUCTION

The **intrapartum period** begins with the onset of regular uterine contractions (UCs) and lasts until the expulsion of the placenta. The process by which this normally occurs is called **labor**. **Childbirth** is the period from the conclusion of the pregnancy to the start of extrauterine life of the infant. This chapter discusses the intrapartum/childbirth process including the factors affecting labor and delivery, progression of labor and delivery, and the nursing care involved.

LABOR TRIGGERS

The question of when and how labor begins has been studied for years. The exact cause of the onset of labor is not completely understood, although there are several theories. Generally it is proposed

that labor is triggered by both maternal and fetal factors (Mattson & Smith, 2004; Simpson & Creehan, 2008).

Maternal Factors

■ Uterine muscles are stretched to the threshold point, leading to release of prostaglandins that stimulate contractions.
■ Increased pressure on the cervix stimulates the nerve plexus, causing release of oxytocin by the maternal pituitary gland, which then stimulates contractions.
■ Estrogen increases, stimulating the uterine response.
■ Progesterone, which has a quieting effect on the uterus, is withdrawn, allowing estrogen to stimulate contractions.
■ Oxytocin stimulates myometrial contractions. Oxytocin and prostaglandin work together to inhibit calcium binding in muscle cells, raising intracellular calcium levels and activating contractions.
■ The oxytocin level surges from stretching of the cervix.

Want to reinforce your reading? Need to review for a test? Listen to this chapter on your accompanying CD.

Fetal Factors

- As the placenta ages it begins to deteriorate, triggering initiation of contractions.
- Prostaglandin synthesis by the fetal membranes and the decidua stimulates contractions.
- Fetal cortisol, produced by fetal adrenal glands, rises and acts on the placenta to reduce progesterone that quiets the uterus, and increases prostaglandin that stimulates the uterus to contract.

FACTORS AFFECTING LABOR

Labor is UCs that bring about effacement and dilation of the cervix. Factors that have been traditionally identified as the essential components in the outcome of labor and delivery include the "**4 P's**":

- Powers (the contractions)
- Passage (the pelvis and birth canal)
- Passenger (the fetus)
- Psyche (the response of the woman)

Powers

Powers refer to the involuntary UCs of labor and the voluntary pushing or bearing down powers that combine to propel and deliver the fetus and placenta from the uterus (see Chapter 9 for assessment of UCs).

Uterine Contractions

- The uterine muscle, known as the myometrium, contracts and shortens during the first stage of labor.
- The uterus is divided into two segments known as the upper segment and the lower segment.
  - *The upper segment composes two-thirds of the uterus and contracts to push the fetus down.*
  - *The lower segment composes the lower third of the uterus and the cervix and is less active, allowing the cervix to become thinner and pulled upward.*
- Uterine contractions are responsible for the dilation (opening) and effacement (thinning) of the cervix in the first stage of labor.
- Uterine contractions are rhythmic and intermittent.

- Each contraction has a **resting phase** or uterine relaxation period that allows the woman and uterine muscle a pause for rest. This pause allows blood flow to the uterus and placenta that was temporarily reduced during the contraction phase. It is during this pause that much of the fetal exchange of oxygen, nutrients, and waste products occurs in the placenta. With every contraction, 500 mL of blood leaves the utero–placental unit and moves back into maternal circulation.
- Uterine contractions are described in the following ways (Fig. 8-1):
  - *Frequency: Time from beginning of one contraction to the beginning of another. It is recorded in minutes (e.g., occurring every 3–4 minutes).*
  - *Duration: Time from the beginning of a contraction to the end of the contraction. It is recorded in seconds (e.g., each contraction lasts 45–50 seconds).*
  - *Intensity: Strength of the contraction. It is evaluated with palpation using the fingertips on maternal abdomen and is described as:*
    - Mild: The uterine wall is easily indented during contraction.
    - Moderate: The uterine wall is resistant to indentation during a contraction.
    - Strong: The uterine wall cannot be indented during a contraction.
- There are three phases of a contraction (see Fig. 8-1):
  - *Increment phase: Ascending or buildup of the contraction that begins in the fundus and spreads throughout the uterus*
  - *Acme phase: Peak of intensity*
  - *Decrement phase; Descending or relaxation of the uterine muscle*
- Contractions facilitate cervical changes (Fig. 8-2).
  - *Dilation and effacement occurs during the first stage of labor when UCs push the presenting part of the fetus toward the cervix, causing it to open and thin out as the musculofibrous tissue of the cervix is drawn upwards (see Fig. 8-2B).*
  - *Dilation is the enlargement or opening of the cervical os.*
    - The cervix dilates from closed (or <1 cm diameter) to 10 cm diameter (see Fig. 8-2C).
    - When the cervix reaches 10 cm dilation it is considered fully or completely dilated and can no longer be palpated on vaginal examination.
  - *Effacement is the shortening and thinning of the cervix.*

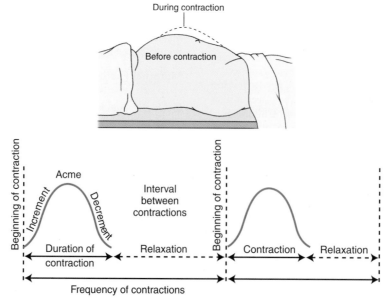

Figure 8-1   Phases, frequency, and duration of a contraction.

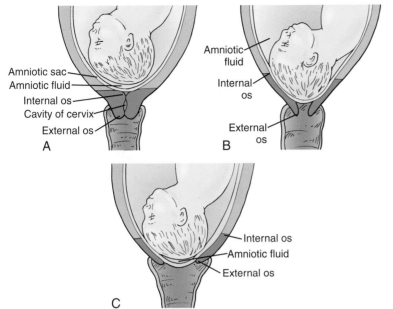

Figure 8-2 Cervical effacement and dilation. *A.* Cervix prior to labor is closed and not effaced. *B.* Cervix in early labor is effaced and starting to dilate. *C.* Cervix is effaced and dilating.

■ The cervix is 2 to 3 cm long and approximately 1 cm thick.
■ The degree of effacement is measured in percentage and goes from 0% to 100%.
■ *Effacement often precedes dilation in a first-time pregnancy. Effacement and dilation progression of the cervix occurs together in subsequent pregnancies.*

Bearing-Down Powers

Once the cervix is fully dilated (10 cm) and the woman feels the urge to push, she will involuntarily bear-down. The urge to push is triggered by the Ferguson reflex, activated when the presenting part stretches the pelvic floor muscles. Stretch receptors are activated, releasing oxytocin, stimulating contractions (Simpson & Creehan, 2008). The bearing-down powers are enhanced when the woman contracts her abdominal muscles and pushes.

Passage

The **passage** includes the bony pelvis and the soft tissues of the cervix, pelvic floor, vagina, and introitus (external opening to the vagina). Although all of these anatomical areas play a role in the birth of the fetus, it is the maternal pelvis that is the greatest determinate in the vaginal delivery of the fetus. The assessment of the size and shape of the pelvis is important. Assessment of the pelvis is performed manually through palpation with a vaginal exam by the care provider during pregnancy.

Pelvis

■ Types of bony pelvis (Fig. 8-3):
■ *Gynecoid (most common type and found in about 50% of women)*
■ *Android*
■ *Anthropoid*
■ *Platypeloid (least common type and found in about 3% of women)*

	Shape	Inlet	Midpelvis	Outlet
Gynecoid				
Android				
Anthropoid				
Platypelloid				

Figure 8-3 Pelvic types: gynecoid, android, anthropoid, and platypelloid.

- The anatomical structure of the pelvis includes the ileum, the ischium, pubis, sacrum, and coccyx (Fig. 8-4A).
- The bony pelvis is divided into:
  - *False pelvis, which is the shallow upper section of the pelvis.*
  - *True pelvis, which is the lower part of the pelvis and consists of three planes: the inlet, the midpelvis, and the outlet (see Fig. 8-4B). The measurement of these three planes defines the obstetric capacity of the pelvis.*
- The pelvic joints include the symphysis pubis, the right and the left sacroiliac joints, and the sacrococcygeal joints.
- The actions of the hormones estrogen and relaxin during pregnancy soften cartilage and increase elasticity of the ligaments, thus allowing room for the fetal head.
- **Station** refers to the relationship of the ischial spines to the presenting part of the fetus and assists in assessing for fetal descent during labor (Fig. 8-5). Station 0 is the narrowest diameter the fetus must pass through during a vaginal birth.

Soft Tissue

- The soft tissue of the cervix effaces and dilates, allowing the descending fetus into the vagina.
- The soft tissue of the pelvic floor muscles helps the fetus in an anterior rotation as it passes through the birth canal.
- The soft tissue of the vagina expands to allow passage of the fetus.

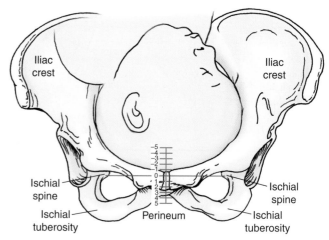

Figure 8-5   Station of presenting part: Fetal head in relation to ischial spines.

Passenger

The **passenger** is the fetus. It is the fetus and its relationship to the passageway that is the major factor in the birthing process. The relationship between the fetus and the passageway includes fetal skull,

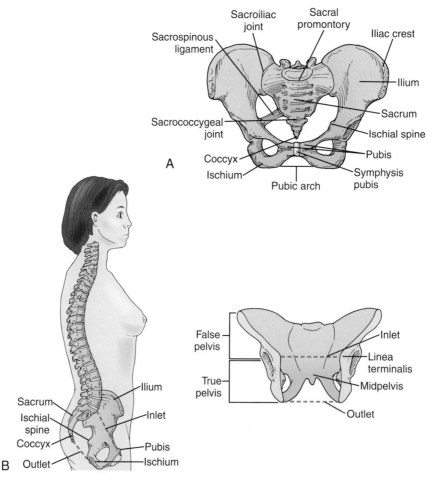

Figure 8-4   Pelvic structures. *A.* Anatomical structures of pelvis. *B.* Pelvic planes.

fetal attitude, fetal lie, fetal presentation, fetal position and fetal size. At the onset of labor, the position of the fetus with respect to the birth canal is critical (Cunningham et al., 2005). In general, in the United States when a fetus is in a position other than cephalic (head first), a cesarean delivery is considered. Size of the fetus alone is less significant in the birthing process than the relationship among fetal size, position, and pelvic dimensions (Mattson & Smith, 2004).

Fetal Skull

■ The fetal head usually accounts for the largest portion of the fetus to come through the birth canal.

■ Bones and membranous spaces help the skull to mold during labor and birth.

■ **Molding** is the ability of the fetal head to change shape to accommodate/fit through the maternal pelvis.

■ The fetal skull is composed of two parietal bones, two temporal bones, the frontal bone, and the occipital bone (Fig. 8-6A and B).

  ■ *The **biparietal diameter (BPD)**, 9.25 cm, is the largest transverse measurement and an important indicator of head size (see Fig. 8-6C).*

  ■ *The membranous space between the bones (sutures) and the fontanels (intersections of these sutures) allows the skull bones to overlap and mold to fit through the birth canal (see Fig. 8-6A and B).*

  ■ *Sutures are used to identify the positioning of the fetal head during a vaginal exam. By identifying the anterior fontanel in relationship to the woman's pelvis, the examiner can determine the position of the head and the degree of rotation that has occurred.*

Fetal Attitude or Posture

Fetal attitude or posture is the relationship of fetal parts to one another. This is noted by the flexion or extension of the fetal joints (Fig. 8-7).

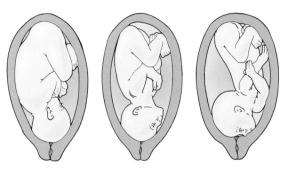

Figure 8-7   Fetal attitude or posture (flexed).

■ At term, the fetus' back becomes convex and the head flexed such that the chin is against the chest. This results in a rounded appearance with the chin flexed forward on the chest, arms crossed over the thorax, the thighs flexed on the abdomen, and the legs flexed at the knees.

■ With proper fetal attitude, the head is in complete flexion in a vertex presentation and passes through the true pelvis easily.

Fetal Lie

Fetal lie refers to the long axis (spine) of the fetus in relationship to the long axis (spine) of the woman.

■ The two primary lies are longitudinal and transverse (Fig. 8-8).
  ■ *In the longitudinal lie, the long axes of the fetus and the mother are parallel (most common).*
  ■ *In the transverse lie, the long axis of the fetus is perpendicular to the long axis of the mother.*
■ A fetus cannot be delivered vaginally in the transverse lie.

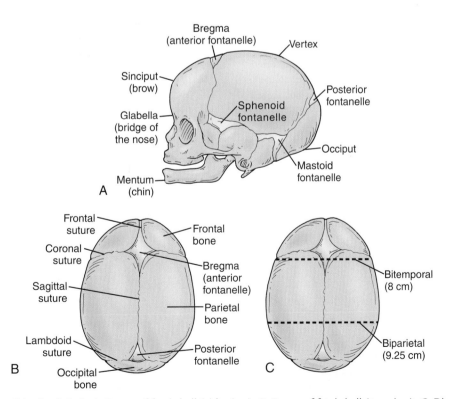

Figure 8-6   Bones of the fetal skull. *A.* Bones of fetal skull (side view). *B.* Bones of fetal skull (top view). *C.* Diameter of fetal skull.

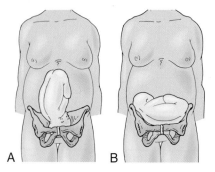

Figure 8-8   Fetal lie. *A.* Longitudinal lie. *B.* Transverse lie.

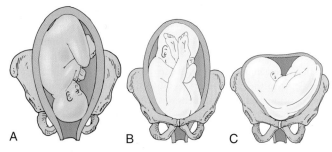

Figure 8-9   Fetal presentation. *A.* Cephalic. *B.* Breech. *C.* Shoulder.

Presentation

Fetal presentation is determined by the part or pole of the fetus that first enters the pelvic inlet. There are three main presentations (Fig. 8-9):

■ Cephalic (head first) (Fig. 8-9A)
■ Breech (pelvis first) (Fig. 8-9B)
■ Shoulder (shoulder first) (Fig. 8-9C)

Presenting Part

The **presenting part** is the specific fetal structure lying nearest to the cervix. It is determined by the attitude or posture of the fetus. Each presenting part has an identified denominator or reference point that is used to describe the fetal position in the pelvis.

■ Cephalic presentations: The presenting part is the head (Fig. 8-10).
  ■ *This accounts for 95% of all births (Mattson & Smith, 2004).*
  ■ *The degree of flexion or extension of the head and neck further classifies cephalic presentations.*
    ■ Vertex presentation indicates that the head is sharply flexed and the chin is touching the thorax. The denominator is the occiput.
    ■ Frontum or brow presentation indicates partial extension of the neck with the brow as the presenting part. The denominator is the frontum.
    ■ Face presentation indicates that the neck is sharply extended and the back of the head (occiput) is arching to the fetal back. The denominator is the mentum-chin.
■ Breech presentations: The presenting part is the buttock and/or feet (Fig. 8-11).

■ *Breech presentations are further classified into:*
  ■ Complete breech: Complete flexion of thighs and legs (see Fig. 8-11A)
  ■ Frank breech: Complete flexion of the thighs and the legs extending over the anterior surfaces of the body (see Fig. 8-11B)
  ■ Footling breech: Extension of one or both thighs and legs so that one or both feet are presenting (see Fig. 8-11C)
■ Transverse presentation: The presenting part is usually the shoulder (see Fig. 8-9C).
  ■ *This usually is associated with a transverse lie.*
■ Compound presentation: The fetus assumes a unique posture usually with the arm or hand presenting alongside the presenting part.

Fetal Position

The **fetal position** is the relation of the denominator or reference point to the maternal pelvis (Fig. 8-13).

■ There are six positions for each presentation: right anterior, right transverse, right posterior, left anterior, left transverse, and left posterior.
■ The occiput is the specific fetal structure for a cephalic presentation (see Fig. 8-9A).
■ The sacrum is the specific fetal structure for a breech presentation (see Fig. 8-9B).
■ The acromion is the specific fetal structure for a shoulder presentation (see Fig. 8-9C).

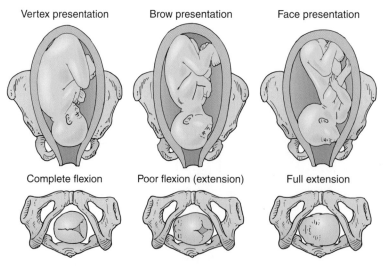

Vertex presentation   Brow presentation   Face presentation

Complete flexion   Poor flexion (extension)   Full extension

Figure 8-10   Cephalic presentation.

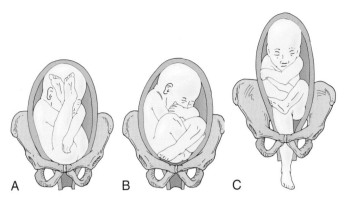

Figure 8-11 Breech presentation. *A.* Frank. *B.* Complete. *C.* Footling.

■ The mentum is the specific fetal structure for the face presentation (see Fig. 8-10 Face presentation).
■ Position is designated by a three-letter abbreviation (Fig. 8-12 & 8-13):
  ■ *First letter: Designates location of presenting part to the left (L) or right (R) of the woman's pelvis (Fig. 8-12 & 8-13).*
  ■ *Second letter: Designates the specific fetal part presenting: occiput (O), sacrum (S), mentum (M), and shoulder (A) (Fig. 8-12 & 8-13).*
  ■ *Third letter: Designates the relationship of the presenting fetal part to the woman's pelvis such as anterior (A), posterior (P), or transverse (T) (Fig. 8-12 & 8-13).*

Psyche

Nursing care of the woman during the intrapartum period addresses not only the physical aspect of care, but also the psychosocial aspect to result in woman's wellness and satisfaction. Preparation of childbirth, both physically and mentally, helps the woman manage labor. This preparation promotes in the woman a sense of security and safety. A woman's experience and satisfaction during the labor and birthing process can be enhanced when there is a coordination of collaborative goals between the woman and health care personnel in the plan of care (Perla, 2002). This is a critical part that influences her self-esteem, self-confidence, her relationship to others, and a general view she holds of life.

Factors that influence the woman's coping mechanism include her culture, expectations, a strong support system, and type of support during labor.

■ Culture
  ■ *Culture influences the woman's reaction to labor expectations and how she interacts with others. Cultural influences are most apparent in the newly immigrated woman. The nurse needs to be culturally aware and sensitive to the needs and practices of the individual.*
  ■ *Nurses need to integrate the woman's cultural and religious values, beliefs, and practices to provide a mutually acceptable plan of care. When the woman feels that the plan of care is one she is actively involved in and integrates her cultural and/or religious values, beliefs, and practices with the decision making, her feeling of safety and control are further facilitated (Cultural Awareness: Culture and Birth Traditions).*

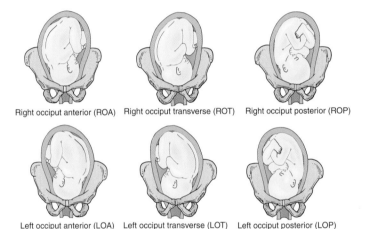

Right occiput anterior (ROA)   Right occiput transverse (ROT)   Right occiput posterior (ROP)

Left occiput anterior (LOA)   Left occiput transverse (LOT)   Left occiput posterior (LOP)

Figure 8-12 Fetal positions left or right of woman's pelvis.

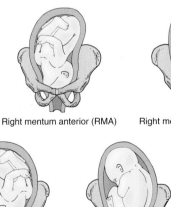
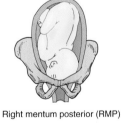

Right mentum anterior (RMA)   Right mentum posterior (RMP)

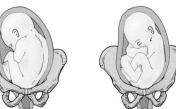

Left mentum anterior (LMA)   Left sacrum anterior (LSA)   Left sacrum posterior (LSP)

Figure 8-13 Fetal part presenting.

CULTURAL AWARENESS: Culture and Birth Traditions

Birth practices vary greatly from culture to culture and within sub-cultures. Each make assumptions about what is safe, healthy, and acceptable in childbirth. Nurses must respond to women and families who make decisions that may differ from our own, related to the use of pain medication in labor, who is with her in labor and their role, and how they respond to labor. The nurse needs to help women formulate their concerns, priorities, and decisions. Behaviors in birth are complex and personal. It is important for nurses to have a general understanding of birth practices of the groups with which they work (Bar-Yam, 1994). Some strategies for providing culturally sensitive care are presented in Chapter 5. Although there is tremendous variation in practices related to childbirth, some generalities may help to guide nurses.

African American/Black

- Often accompanied in labor by a female relative
- Strong extended family support
- Matriarchal support
- Present time orientation
- May vocally express pain

American Indian and Native Alaskan

- Decision-making by families/tribal leaders
- Often stoic; do not make eye contact, limit touch
- Strong spiritual foundation
- May use a medicine man or shaman
- Present time orientation

Asian American and Pacific Islander

- Culturally and linguistically heterogeneous
- Health care decision-making by families
- "Hot/cold" theory of illness (pregnancy considered a "hot" condition, except among Chinese women, who consider it a "cold" condition)
- Vaginal exams and open hospital gowns may be humiliating and upsetting to Southeast Asian women
- Strong extended family support
- Asian fathers may choose not to attend the birth
- Asian Americans have future orientation; Pacific Islanders have a present orientation
- Asians have high respect for others

Hispanic/Latino

- Health care decision-making done by families
- Strong extended family support
- Fathers may choose not to attend the birth
- Present time orientation
- May believe in the "evil eye"
- May moan in a rhythmic way in labor
- May prefer to walk during labor to make the birth faster

White/Caucasian

- Often considered a noncultural group
- Value autonomy and personal decision-making
- Future time orientation
- Focus on achievement

- Expectations
  - *Expectations for the birth experience are related to how childbirth is viewed by the woman (e.g., as a natural process or as a stressful or threatening experience). The nurse should review the woman's expectations to help alleviate fear and to help set realistic goals.*
    - Unrealistic expectations can cause an increase in maternal anxiety.
  - *Past experience and complications of pregnancy, labor, and birth strongly influence women's expectations of labor and response to labor.*
    - Women who have experienced a negative previous birthing experience are at risk for increased anxiety; women who experienced a positive previous birthing experience have lower anxiety levels.
  - *Current pregnancy experience with difficulty conceiving, an unplanned pregnancy, or a high-risk pregnancy may increase a woman's anxiety and fears.*
- Support system
  - *The woman's perception of being able to maintain control during labor and delivery is an important contributing factor to a positive and favorable evaluation of childbirth. This includes control of pain perception, control over emotions and actions, and being able to influence decisions while being an active participant (Mackey, 1995).*
  - *Studies have shown that with a support person, be it a family member, friend, doula or professional such as a nurse, the patient experiences a decrease in anxiety and has a feeling of being in more control. This results in a decrease in interventions, a significantly lower level of pain, and an enhanced overall maternal satisfaction (Hodnett, Gates, Hofmeyr, & Sakala, 2007).*
  - *Nursing care of women in labor should incorporate the following types of support and interventions:*
    - Emotional support, including continuous presence, reassurance, and praise
    - Information about labor progress and advice regarding coping techniques
    - Comfort measures (e.g., comforting touch, massage, warm baths/showers, promoting adequate fluid intake and output)
    - Advocacy, including assisting the woman in articulating her wishes to others
- Labor support
  - *Since the middle of the 20th century, a majority of women have given birth in a hospital rather than at home, even in poorer, less developed countries. Access to continuous care and support during labor has become the exception rather than the routine in the hospital setting. Concerns about the consequent dehumanization of women's birth experiences have resulted in demands for a return to continuous, one-to-one support by women for women during labor (Fig. 8-14) (Evidence-Based Practice: Continuous Labor Support for Women During Childbirht).*
  - *Two complementary theoretical explanations have been offered for the effects of labor support on childbirth outcomes (Hodnett, Gates, Hofmeyr, & Sakala, 2007). Both explanations hypothesize that labor support enhances labor physiology and woman's feelings of control and competence.*
    - The first theoretical explanation considers possible mechanisms when support during labor is used in stressful, threatening, and disempowering clinical birth environments. During labor women may be uniquely vulnerable to unfamiliar environmental influences; current obstetric care frequently subjects women to institutional routines, high rates of intervention, unfamiliar personnel, and lack of

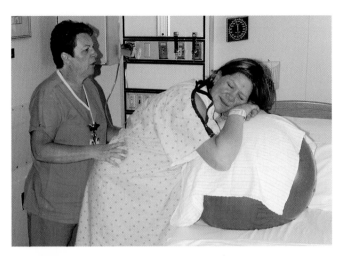

Figure 8-14   Woman receiving labor support from her nurse.

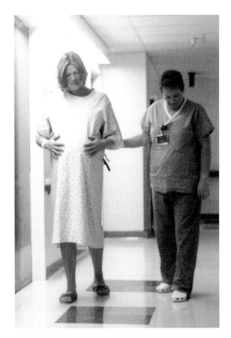

Figure 8-15   Woman walking in labor with her nurse.

privacy. These conditions may have an adverse effect on the progress of labor and on the development of feelings of competence and confidence; this may in turn impair adjustment to parenthood and establishment of breast-feeding, and increase the risk of depression. This response may, to some extent, be buffered by the provision of support and companionship during labor.

■ The second theoretical explanation does not focus on a particular type of birth environment. It describes two pathways, enhanced passage of the fetus through the pelvis and soft tissues, and decreased stress response, by which labor support may reduce the likelihood of operative birth and subsequent complications, and enhance women's feelings of control and satisfaction with their childbirth experiences (Hodnett, 2002). Enhanced fetopelvic relationships may be accomplished by encouraging mobility and effective use of gravity, supporting women to assume their preferred positions and recommending specific positions for specific situations. Studies of the relationships among fear and anxiety, the stress response and pregnancy complications have shown that anxiety during labor is associated with high levels of the stress hormone epinephrine in the blood, which may lead to abnormal fetal heart rate (FHR) patterns in labor, decreased uterine contractility, a longer active labor phase with regular well-established contractions and low Apgar scores (Lederman, 1986). Emotional support, information and advice, comfort measures, and advocacy may reduce anxiety and fear and associated adverse effects during labor.

■ Anxiety (a sense of uneasiness in response to a vague unspecific threat) can interfere with labor and increase nausea and crying, as well as interfering with the ability to focus.

■ Fear (a painful uneasy feeling in response to an identifiable threat) can be fear related to the unknown, fear of injury to self and fetus, or fear of pain. Fear can decrease UCs and enhance the perception of pain. Procedures and an unfamiliar environment can result in a sense of loss of control and feeling of helplessness. Women in labor can feel abandoned (Mattson & Smith, 2004).

■ *Nurses can help and support women to be actively involved in their own care by allowing time for discussion, listening to worries and concerns, and offering information to help women gain increased self-determination in the context of care (Nordgren & Fridlund, 2001).*

Position

Discussion of the influence on labor often includes a fifth **"P,"** referred to as maternal position during labor and birth. The woman's position has an effect on both the anatomical and physiological adaptations to labor.

■ During the first stage of labor an upright position (walking, sitting, kneeling, or squatting) and/or a lateral position is encouraged (Fig. 8-15).

■ *These positions are used to decrease the compression of the maternal descending aorta and ascending vena cava that could result in a compromised cardiac output. Compression of these vessels can lead to supine hypotension, resulting in decreased placental perfusion (Fig. 8-16).*

■ *The upright position has shown benefits of aiding in the descent of the infant and more effective contractions that result in shorter labor (Gupta, Hofmeyr, & Smyth, 2004).*

■ *Frequent position changes are associated with a reduction of fatigue, an increase of comfort, and improved circulation to both mother and fetus.*

■ During the second stage of labor, the upright position has been shown to increase the pelvic outlet and better aligns the fetus with the pelvic inlet (Simkin & Ancheta, 2000).

■ *The position most used in births in the United States is the lithotomy position.*

THE PROCESS OF LABOR

Signs of Impending Labor

A few weeks before labor, changes occur that indicate the woman's body is preparing for the onset of labor. These changes are also referred to as premonitory signs of labor. These signs are:

■ **Lightening:** This refers to the descent of the fetus into the true pelvis that occurs approximately 2 weeks before term in

Evidence-Based Practice: Continuous Support for Women During Childbirth

Hodnett, E., Gates, S., Hofmeyr, G., & Sakala, C. (2007). Continuous support for women during childbirth. Cochrane Database of Systematic Reviews 2007, Issue 3, Art. No. CD003766. DOI: 10.1002/1465185.CD003766.pbb2.

In recent decades in hospitals worldwide, continuous support during labor has become the exception rather than the routine. Concerns about the consequent dehumanization of women's birth experiences have led to calls for a return to continuous support by women for women during labor.

Objective of Systematic Review

Primary: To assess the effects, on women and their babies, of continuous, one-to-one intrapartum support compared with the usual care. Secondary: To determine whether the effects of continuous support are influenced by (1) routine practices and policies in the birth environment that may affect a woman's autonomy, freedom of movement, and ability to cope with labor; (2) whether the caregiver is a member of the staff of the institution; and (3) whether the continuous support begins early or later in labor.

Selection Criteria

All published and unpublished randomized controlled trials comparing continuous support during labor with usual care.

Main Results

Sixteen trials involving 13,391 women met inclusion criteria and provided usable outcome data. Primary comparison: women who had continuous intrapartum support were likely to have a slightly shorter labor, and were more likely to have a spontaneous vaginal birth and less likely to have intrapartum analgesia or to report dissatisfaction with their childbirth experiences. Subgroup analyses: In general, continuous intrapartum support was associated with greater benefits when the provider was not a member of the hospital staff, or when it began early in labor and in settings in which epidural analgesia was not routinely available.

Summary

Continuous support in labor increased the chance of a spontaneous vaginal birth, had no identified adverse effects, and women were more satisfied.

Supportive care during labor may involve emotional support, comfort measures, information, and advocacy. These may enhance normal labor processes as well as women's feelings of control and competence, and thus reduce the need for obstetric intervention. The review of studies included 16 trials, from 11 countries, involving more than 13,000 women in a wide range of settings and circumstances. Women who received continuous labor support were more likely to give birth "spontaneously," i.e., give birth with neither cesarean birth nor vacuum nor forceps. In addition, women were less likely to use pain medications, were more likely to be satisfied, and had slightly shorter labors.

Common elements of this care include emotional support (continuous presence, reassurance, and praise); information about labor progress; and advice regarding coping techniques, comfort measures (comforting touch, massage, warm baths/showers, promoting adequate fluid intake and output); and advocacy (helping the woman articulate her wishes to others).

A systematic review examining factors associated with women's satisfaction with the childbirth experience suggests that continuous support can make a substantial contribution to this satisfaction. When women evaluate their experience, four factors predominate: the amount of support from caregivers, the quality of relationships with caregivers, being involved with decision-making, and having high expectations or having experiences that exceed expectations (Hodnett, 2002).

Authors' Conclusions and Implications for Practice

Continuous support during labor should be the norm, rather than the exception. All women should be allowed and encouraged to have support people with them continuously during labor. In general, continuous support from a caregiver during labor appears to confer the greatest benefits when the provider is not an employee of the institution, when epidural analgesia is not routinely used, and when support begins in early labor.

Every effort should be made to ensure that women's birth environments are empowering, nonstressful, afford privacy, communicate respect, and are not characterized by routine interventions that add risk without clear benefit.

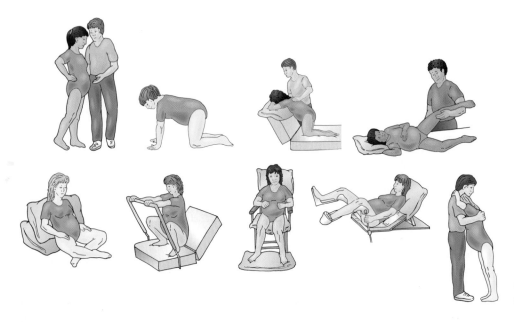

Figure 8-16   Positions for labor and pushing.

first-time pregnancies. The woman may feel she can breathe more easily but may experience urinary frequency from increased bladder pressure. In subsequent pregnancies, this may not occur until labor begins.

■ **Braxton-Hicks** contractions: These are irregular UCs that do not result in cervical change and are associated with false labor.
■ Cervical changes: The cervix becomes soft (ripens) and may become partially effaced and begin to dilate.
■ Surge in energy: Some women may experience a burst of energy or feel the need to put everything in order.
■ Gastrointestinal changes: Less commonly, some women may experience a 1- to 3-pound weight loss and some experience diarrhea, nausea, or indigestion preceding labor.
■ Backache: The woman may experience low backache and sacroiliac discomfort due in part to the relaxation of the pelvic joints.
■ **Bloody show:** The woman may experience a brownish or blood-tinged cervical mucus discharge referred to as bloody show.

Assessment of Rupture of the Membranes

■ **Spontaneous rupture of the membranes (SROM)** may occur before the onset of labor but typically occurs during labor. Once the membranes have ruptured, the protective barrier to infection is lost and ideally the woman should deliver within 24 hours to reduce the risk of infection to her and her fetus.
■ Assessing the status of membranes
  ■ *Nitrazine paper: Nitrazine paper is placed in a visible pool of fluid around the cervix. The paper turns blue when in contact with amniotic fluid.*
  ■ *Ferning: A sterile speculum exam may be performed to confirm rupture of membranes (ROM).*
    ■ A sample of fluid in the upper vaginal area is obtained.
    ■ The fluid is placed on a slide and assessed for "ferning pattern" under a microscope.
    ■ A ferning pattern confirms ROM.

Nursing Actions

■ Assess the amniotic fluid for color, amount, and odor.
  ■ *Normal amniotic fluid is clear or cloudy with a normal odor that is similar to that of ocean water.*
  ■ *Fluid can be meconium stained and this needs to be reported to the care provider, as this may be an indication of fetal compromise in utero.*
■ Assess the FHR.
  ■ *There is an increase risk of umbilical cord prolapse with ROM.*
  ■ *There is a higher risk of umbilical cord prolapse when the presenting part is not engaged.*

■ Document the date and time of SROM, characteristic of fluid, and FHR.

ONSET OF LABOR

As the woman comes closer to term pregnancy, the uterus becomes more sensitive to oxytocin and the contractions increase in frequency and intensity. This can be an anxious time for the woman and family in trying to determine if she needs to proceed to the birthing center. An understanding of true versus false labor can help to alleviate some of these fears (Table 8-1).

True Labor Versus False Labor

■ True labor contractions occur at regular intervals and increase in frequency, duration, and intensity.
■ True labor contractions bring about changes in cervical effacement and dilation.
■ False labor is irregular contractions with little or no cervical changes.

Guidelines for Going to the Birthing Facility

■ When to go to the birthing facility depends greatly on the past history of pregnancies, location of birth center, and risk status of the pregnancy.
■ By law, all pregnant women have access to medical care regardless of their ability to pay (Box 8-1).
■ A general rule of thumb for first-time pregnancy with no risk factor is to wait until contractions are 5 minutes apart, lasting 60 seconds, and are regular.
■ The woman should go to the birthing center when:
  ■ *The membrane ruptures, or "bag of waters" break.*
  ■ *The woman is experiencing intense pain.*
  ■ *There is an increase of bloody show.*

MECHANISM OF LABOR

The mechanism of labor known as **cardinal movements of labor** is the positional changes that the fetus goes through to best navigate the birth process (Fig. 8-17).

■ Engagement: When the greatest diameter of the fetal head passes through the pelvic inlet; can occur late in pregnancy or early in labor (see Fig. 8-17A)

TABLE 8–1 TRUE VERSUS FALSE LABOR

CHARACTERISTICS	TRUE LABOR	FALSE LABOR
CONTRACTIONS	Regular contractions that increase in frequency, intensity, and duration	Irregular or regular mild contractions with no increase in frequency, intensity, and duration
DISCOMFORT	Begins in the back and radiates to the lower abdomen and the front.	Felt in the middle of the abdomen or groin area. Can be mentally and physically tiring.
CERVICAL CHANGES	Progressive cervical dilation and effacement	Little or no cervical change
BLOODY SHOW	Usually present and increases with cervical changes	None present
ACTIVITY	Activity such as walking may increase intensity of contraction.	Activity or position change often lessens contractions.

BOX 8–1   EMERGENCY MEDICAL TREATMENT AND ACTIVE LABOR ACT

The Emergency Medical Treatment and Active Labor Act (EMTALA) is a federal regulation that was enacted to ensure treatment for a woman seeking care in an emergency or if she thinks she is in labor regardless of her ability to pay. Nurses who work in the labor and delivery unit(s) of the hospital need to be familiar with EMTALA regulations (Angelini & Mahlmeister, 2005). In general, the criteria for admission to the hospital for labor are cervical dilation to 3–4 cm and/or ruptured membranes (Cunningham et al., 2005).

■ Descent: Movement of the fetus through the birth canal during the first and second stage of labor (see Fig. 8-17A)

■ Flexion: When the chin of the fetus moves toward the fetal chest; occurs when the descending head meets resistance from maternal tissues; results in the smallest fetal diameter to the maternal pelvic dimensions; normally occurs early in labor (see Fig. 8-17A)

■ Internal rotation: When the rotation of the fetal head aligns the long axis of the fetal head with the long axis of the maternal pelvis; occurs mainly during second stage of labor (see Fig. 8-17B)

■ Extension: Facilitated by resistance of the pelvic floor that causes the presenting part to pivot beneath the pubic symphysis and the head to be delivered; occurs during the second stage of labor (see Fig. 8-17C)

■ External rotation: During this movement, the sagittal suture moves to a transverse diameter and the shoulders align in the anteroposterior diameter. The sagittal suture maintains alignment with the fetal trunk as the trunk navigates through the pelvis (see Fig. 8-17D).

■ Expulsion: The shoulders and remainder of the body are delivered (see Fig. 8-17E)

STAGES OF LABOR AND CHILDBIRTH

Labor or parturition is the process in which the fetus, placenta, and membranes are expelled through the uterus. The care of women and families during labor and delivery requires astute and ongoing assessments of the bio–psycho–social adaptation of the woman and fetus. Because childbirth is a natural process, care should move forward on a continuum from noninvasive to least invasive intervention and from nonpharmacological to pharmacological interventions according to the desires of the woman and assessment of health care providers based on individual clinical situations (Simpson & Creehan, 2008).

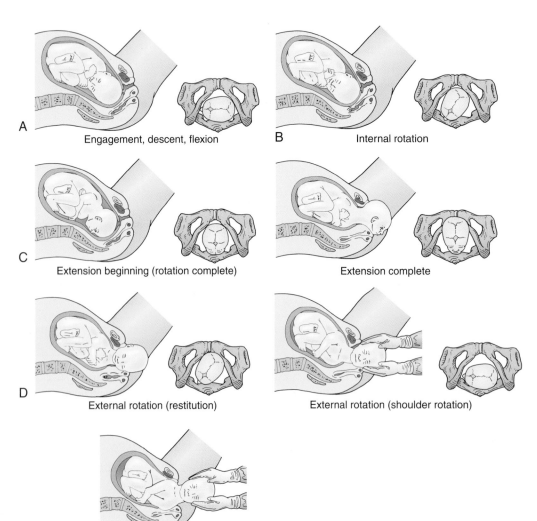

A   Engagement, descent, flexion

B   Internal rotation

C   Extension beginning (rotation complete)

Extension complete

D   External rotation (restitution)

External rotation (shoulder rotation)

E   Expulsion

Figure 8-17   Cardinal movements of labor. *A.* Engagement and flexion. *B.* Internal rotation. *C.* Extension. *D.* External rotation. *E.* Expulsion.

In the United States in 2003, 99% of all births were delivered in hospitals, 91.4% were delivered by physicians, and 8% of the births were delivered by midwives (Martin et al., 2005). Because most babies are delivered in the hospital by physicians, nurses in the intrapartal setting have a key role in providing comprehensive and individualized care for women and their families.

Labor and birth is divided into four stages (Table 8-2):

- **Stage 1** begins with onset of labor and ends with complete cervical dilation.
- **Stage 2** begins with complete dilation of cervix and ends with delivery of baby.
- **Stage 3** begins after delivery of baby and ends with delivery of placenta.
- **Stage 4** begins after delivery of the placenta and is completed 4 hours later; it is the immediate postpartum period.

Stage 1

The first stage of labor is defined as the progression of cervical changes. This stage is divided into three phases: latent phase, active phase, and transition. Characteristics of the first stage of labor are:

- It begins with onset of true labor and ends with complete cervical dilation (10 cm) and complete effacement (100%).
- Stage 1 is longest stage, typically lasting 12 hours for primigravidas and 8 hours for multigravidas.
- There are normally tremendous variations in lengths of labor (Cunningham et al., 2005).
- The bag of waters or fetal membranes usually ruptures during this stage
- The woman's cardiac output increases.
- The woman's pulse may increase.
- Gastrointestinal motility decreases, which leads to increase in gastric emptying time (Mattson & Smith, 2004).
- The woman experiences pain associated with UCs that result in the dilation and effacement of the cervix.
- The first stage has three phases: the latent, active and transition phases (see Table 8-2).

Assessment

Assessment during all phases of the first stage of labor includes:

- Maternal vital signs
- FHR and UCs
- Cervical changes
- Fetal position and descent in the pelvis
- The woman's response to labor and pain

Nursing Actions

Nursing actions during all phases of the first stage of labor are related to:

- Diet and hydration
- Activity and rest
- Elimination
- Comfort
- Support and family involvement
- Education
- Safety
- Documentation of labor admission and progression (Figs. 8-18 and 8-19)

First Phase

The **first phase of labor**, or **latent phase**, is the early and slower part of labor with an average length of 8.6 hours for primiparous

---

CRITICAL COMPONENT

Supportive Activities and Comfort Measures in Labor

Labor support is a repertoire of techniques used to help women with the process of childbirth (Wood & Carr, 2003). Providing support and comfort is one of the primary activities of nurses and includes:

Emotional Support

- Sustaining physical presence, eye contact
- Verbal encouragement, reassurance, and praise
- Listen to woman and family

Physical Support

- Comfort measures such as ice chips, fluids, food, and pain medications
- Hygiene including mouth care, pericare, and changing soiled linens
- Assistance with position changes and ambulation
- Reassuring touch, massage
- Application of heat and cold
- Hydrotherapy in shower and tub, if no ROM
- Calm environment (dim lighting, quiet, music, minimize interruptions)

Informational Support

- Provide information on the progress of labor.
- Explain all procedures.
- Communicate in lay language so the woman and her family understands.
- Use interpreters as needed.

Advocacy

- Support decisions made by the woman and her family.
- Ensure respect for the woman's decisions.
- Manage the environment, which includes visitors.

Support of the Partner and Family

- Offer support and praise.
- Role model therapeutic behaviors.
- Assist the partner with food and rest.
- Provide breaks if desired or needed.

(Wood & Carr, 2003)

---

and 5.3 hours for multiparous woman. Women in this phase are usually both excited and apprehensive about the start of labor. They are talkative and able to relax with the contractions. Many women choose to stay home during this phase, although some women are admitted to the birth center during this time. Characteristics of this phase are:

- Cervical dilation from 0 to 3 cm with effacement from 0 to 40%.
- Contractions occur every 5 to 10 minutes, lasting 30 to 45 seconds, and mild intensity. Women often describe them as feeling like strong menstrual cramps.

Medical Interventions

- Order laboratory tests, which may include complete blood count (CBC), blood type and Rh, urinalysis, syphilis screening, HBsAg, HIV, and possible drug screening.
- Order IV or saline lock.
- Order intermittent fetal monitoring or continuous fetal and uterine monitoring.

TABLE 8-2 STAGES OF LABOR

	FIRST STAGE OF LABOR			SECOND STAGE OF LABOR	THIRD STAGE OF LABOR	FOURTH STAGE OF LABOR
PHASE	LATENT PHASE	ACTIVE PHASE	TRANSITION PHASE			
DILATION	0–3 cm	4–7 cm	8–10 cm	10 cm to delivery	From birth of baby until expulsion of the placenta	Immediate postpartum period
EFFACEMENT	0%–40%	40%–80%	80%–100%	100%		
LENGTH OF PHASE	6–24 hours	3–6 hours	20–60 minutes	10 minutes to several hours	5–7 minutes, up to 20 minutes	Immediate postpartum period; 4 hours
CONTRACTION FREQUENCY	Every 5–30 minutes	Every 2–5 minutes	Every 2–3 minutes	Every 1–3 minutes	Irregular	
CONTRACTION STRENGTH	Mild to moderate 25–40 mm Hg by IUPC	Moderate to strong 50–70 mm Hg by IUPC	Strong 70–90 mm Hg by IUPC	Strong, increase to expulsive 80–100 mm Hg by IUPC	Mild	
CONTRACTION DURATION	30–45 seconds	45–70 seconds	45–90 seconds	60–90 seconds	30–60 seconds	
CONTRACTION PATTERN	Irregular	Regular	Regular	Minimal rest between UCs	Irregular	
SHOW AMOUNT AND COLOR	Scant Mucoid, blood-tinged	Scant to moderate Mucoid, bloody	Moderate to heavy Bloody	Increase bloody show	Gush of blood with placental separation	
DESCENT OF THE FETUS, NULLIPARA	0 station	−2 to 0/+1/+2	0 to +2/+3	0 to +3 to birth of baby		
DESCENT OF THE FETUS, MULTIPARA	−3 to 0 station	−2 to +1/+2	−1 to +2/+3	0 to +3 to birth of baby		
SUMMARY OF MATERNAL BEHAVIORS	Excited, talkative; pain is well-controlled; open to suggestions and follows directions easily	More serious and inner-directed; doubtful of her ability to control pain; desiring companionship and encouragement; has difficulty following directions	Describes pain as severe; fears loss of control; is irritable; has difficulty communicating; may have nausea and vomiting; perspires; may shake or tremble and feel the need to push	May be fatigued or sleepy initially, the urge to bear down, grunting, may be swearing or screaming, loses ability to focus or concentrate, irritable, may feel burning with crowning of fetal head	Relief with completion of birth, laughing, crying, talking, interest in fetus	Excited, talkative, hungry and thirsty, holds and inspects newborn

Source: Wood & Carr (2003).

Labor and Delivery Admission Record

PT. NAME: __________ AGE: __________ CARE PROVIDER: __________

ADMIT DATE/TIME: __________

EDC	LMP	Weeks of Gestation	Gravida	Para	Term	Preterm	Spontaneous Abortion	Elective Abortion	Living	Stillborn	C-Section	VBAC

T	P	R	BP	Height	Weight	Pre-Pregnant weight	Weight Gain	How Admitted	Accompanied By

Date/Time Care Provider Notified	Date/Time Seen By Care Provider	Reason for Admission

Onset of Labor   Contraction Frequency (Min)

Dilatation (cm)   Effacement (%)   Station

Contraction Duration (Sec)   Contraction Quality
None Mild Moderate Strong

Pelvic Exam By:

Pain Level Assessment: *Pain scale 0–10*

Admission Membranes: Intact Ruptured Bulging Unknown

Fern: N/A Negative Positive Equivocal

AROM/SROM (Date/Time):

Amniotic Fluid:
Amount: None N/A Copious Large Moderate Small Scant
Color: N/A Clear Bloody Meconium Heavy Light Particulate
Odor: None N/A Normal Foul
Amniotic Fluid Comments:

Vaginal Bleeding: None Normal Frank bleeding
Describe Vaginal Bleeding:

Mental Status: Alert Anxious Confused

Feeding Preference: Breast Bottle Breast/bottle Undecided

Support Person: None Husband Partner Other
Support Person(s) Name:

Anesthesia Plans: None Local Epidural Spinal General Pudendal Paracervical
Anesthesia Plans Other:
Anesthesia Class: Yes No Yes, Previous Pregnancy

Attended Prenatal Class: Yes No Yes, Previous Pregnancy

Labor Teaching Initiated: Yes No N/A
Fetal Well-being Yes No N/A
Labor Progress Yes No N/A
Pain Relief Measures Yes No N/A
Other

Nutritional screen:
[ ] N/A
[ ] History of Diabetes/Gestational Diabetes
[ ] History of Eating Disorder
[ ] Multiple Pregnancy
[ ] Special Diet/Vegetarian Diet
[ ] Pt. is 18 Years Old or Younger
[ ] Failure to Gain at Least 1/2 lb. per Wks. of Gestation
[ ] Food Allergies
[ ] Other __________

Describe Last Solid Intake (Include Date/Time):

Describe Last Fluid Intake (Include Date/Time):

In-Pt. Dietary Referral Entered in Computer: Yes No N/A   **In-Pt. Dietary Referral Entered in Computer:** Yes No N/A

Medication Allergy: Yes No
Medication Allergy Detail:

Food Allergies: Yes No
Food Allergy detail:

Latex Allergy: Yes No
Describe Latex Reaction:

Allergy Sticker on Chart: Yes N/A   **Allergy Band on Patient:** Yes N/A

Prenatal Vitamins This Pregnancy: Yes No   **Anticoagulants This Pregnancy:** Yes No   Describe:

For current prescription/over the counter medications taken during pregnancy see Home Medication Order Sheet.

Prescription/over the counter medications previously taken during pregnancy:

Addressograph

Figure 8-18 Labor and delivery admission sheet.

(continued on next page)

Labor and Delivery Admission Record (continued)

PT. NAME: _____

GBS Yes	**Drug Use:** Denies Yes *If Yes, Describe:*
Results: Negative Results	**Drug Use Comments:**
Positive Date:	
Tested: No Unknown	**Contact Lenses:** Yes No Soft Hard Lenses Lenses
	Lenses Lenses In Out
Blood **Rhogam** **This**	
Type/Rh: Pregnancy: N/A Yes No No Record	**Glasses:** Yes No **Dentures:** Yes No
Immune Negative Non-Reactive	**Body Piercing:** Yes No **Body piercing**
Rubella: Non-immune **HBsAg:** Positive **RPR:** Reactive	**Location/Removed:**
Unknown Unknown Unknown	
	Support System After Birth: Family Friends Community None
Hemoglobin = _____ g/dl Initials: _____ **HIV:** Non-Reactive	**If None, Social Service Referral Entered In**
Reference Range: 11–14 g/dl (pregnancy) Reactive	**Computer:** Yes No N/A
Heart Disease: Yes No **Hypertension:** Yes No	**History of** Denies Emotional Physical Sexual *If Other,*
	Abuse: Other _____ *Describe*
MVP: Yes No **Diabetes:** Yes No	**Social Service Referral**
	Entered in Computer: Yes No N/A
Asthma: Yes No **DVT:** Yes No	
	Special Needs: None Spiritual Cultural Emotional *If Other,*
Blood Transfusion: Yes No	Other _____ Hearing/vision impaired: Yes No *Describe*
Blood Transfusion Reason/Yr:	
	Social Service **Pastoral Service**
Sexually Denies Chlamydia Syphilis Gonorrhea	**Referral Entered** **Referral Entered**
Transmitted HIV HPV/Genital Warts Herpes	**in Computer:** Yes No N/A **in Computer:** Yes No N/A
Diseases: Other _____	
	Interpreter needed? Yes No Primary language: _____
Exposure to Infectious Denies Measles Mumps HIV/AIDS	
Disease This Pregnancy: Chicken Pox TB Hepatitis	**Psychosocial Comments:**
Other	
	Room Orientation: EFM Bed Phone Call Light Visitors Computer
Cervical Denies D & C LEEP Cervical biopsy	
Procedures: Laser Cryo/Cautery	**Does the Patient Have an Advance Directive?**
Other	

History of Major Illness or Surgery:		**If No Copy on Chart, Remind Pt.**
	If Yes, is Yes	**to Have Family Member Bring** Referral Yes
Patient History Detail:	Yes Copy in	**Copy AND Send Advance** Entered in
	Chart? No	**Directive Referral to Pastoral** Computer: No
Past Pregnancy None PIH Cystitis Pyelitis Preterm Labor		**Services**
Complications: Preterm Birth Anemia Rh Sensitization		
Positive GBS Other _____	If No, Does Pt. Yes	If Yes, Was Yes Referral Yes
Comments:	No Want Additional	Referral Sent Entered in
	Information or No	to Pastoral No Computer: No
Complications None PIH Cystitis Preterm Labor	Assistance?	Care?

Complications None PIH Cystitis Preterm Labor	**Disposition** Sent Home Kept with Pt. Valuables in Security Office
Current Anemia Rh sensitization	**of Valuables:** Pt. Encouraged to Take Valuables Home
Pregnancy: Placental abnormalities	Other _____
Comments: Other _____	**Valuables Comments:**
Fetal Assessments None Non-Stress Test OCT	**Pt. Wants Other Physician or Family Notified:** Yes No
Done This Pregnancy: CVS BPP US Amnio	
Previous Labor Durations:	**Other Physician/Family Notified:**
Sibling History:	
Family N/A Adopted Heart Disease HTN Diabetes Cancer	
History: Bleeding Disorder Other _____	
Family History	
Comments:	

Smoke Denies <5 per day 5–10 per day	**Alcohol** Denies Occasional 3–5 Drinks/Week 6 or More Drinks/Week	
Use/Frequency: >10 per day >20 per day	**Use:**	

Morse Fall Scale Score:	**Initiate Care Plan if:**	**Immunization History**
[ ] < 45, low fall risk; initiate appropriate interventions	[ ] Anticipated physiological fall risk	Vaccines: Influenza Yes No Date ____
[ ] > 50, high fall risk; initiate appropriate interventions	[ ] Unanticipated physiological fall risk	Pneumonia Yes No Date ____
[ ] 4 medications associated with increased fall risk;	[ ] Accidental fall risk	Tetanus Yes No Date ____
high fall risk; initiate appropriate interventions		PPD Yes No Date ____

Nursing _____	Requests cord blood banking: Y N
Assessment _____	Cord blood banking type: ☐ NA
Summary: _____	☐ St. Louis Cord Blood Bank
	☐ Private cord blood bank

Addressograph

Patient Name:		Physician/CNM:		

		DATE:				KEY
		TIME:				**Variability**
Cervix	Dilation					Ab = Absent (undetectable)
	Effacement					Min = Minimal (>0 out 5 bpm)
	Station					Mod = Moderate (6–25 bpm)
Fetal Heart	Baseline Rate					Mar = Marked (>25 bpm)
	Variability					**Accelerations**
	Accelerations					+ = Present and appropriate
	Decelerations					for gestational age
	STIM/pH					= Absent
	Monitor Mode					**Decelerations**
Uterine Activity	Frequency					E = Early
	Duration					L = Late
	Intensity					V = Variable
	Resting Tone					P = Prolonged
	Monitor Mode					**Stim/pH**
	Oxytocin milliunits/min					+ = Acceleration in response
	Pain					to stimulation
	Coping					= No response to stimulation
	Maternal Position					Record number for scalp pH
	O2/LPM/Mask					**Monitor mode**
	IV					A = Auscultation/Palpation
	Nurse Initials					E = External u/s or toco

Key (continued):

Monitor mode
A = Auscultation/Palpation
E = External u/s or toco
FSE - Fetal spiral electrode
IUPC = Intrauterine pressure
catheter
Frequency of uterine activity
 = None
Irreg = Irregular
Intensity of uterine activity
M = Mild
Mod = Moderate
Str = Strong
By IUPC = mm Hg
Resting tone
R = Relaxed
By IUCP = mm Hg
Coping
W = Well
S = Support provided
For pain use 0–10 scale
Maternal position
A = Ambulatory
U = Upright
SF = Semi-Fowler's
RL = Right lateral
LL = Left lateral
MS = Modified Sims'

Narrative notes:

Figure 8-19   Labor documentation.

Nursing Actions (see Clinical Pathway)

■ Admit to the labor unit and orient the woman, her partner, and family to the labor room. Review prenatal record for estimated date of delivery (EDD) and prior obstetrical history (pregnancy, births, abortions and living children) review allergies; medications; trends in vital signs and weight gain, chronic conditions or pregnancy-related complications; and biochemical and infectious disease laboratory test results, for example, Group B streptococcus (GBS) status (see Fig. 8-18).

■ Review childbirth plan and discuss the woman's expectations.

■ Teach and reinforce relaxation and breathing techniques.

■ Obtain laboratory tests as per orders.

■ Start IV or insert saline lock, if ordered.

■ Review the woman's report of onset of labor.

■ Assess and record the following (see Fig. 8-18 and Clinical Pathway):
   ■ *Maternal vital signs*
   ■ *FHR*
   ■ *Uterine contractions*
   ■ *Cervical dilation and effacement; and fetal presentation, position, and station by performing a sterile vaginal examination (Box 8-2).*
   ■ *Status of membranes*
   ■ *Amniotic fluid for color, amount, consistency, and odor*
   ■ *Vaginal bleeding or bloody show for amount and characteristics of vaginal discharge*

BOX 8–2   STERILE VAGINAL EXAM

Intrapartal Sterile Vaginal Exam

To perform a vaginal exam, the labia are separated with a sterile gloved hand. Fingers are lubricated with a water-soluble lubricant. The first and second fingers are inserted into the introitus; the cervix is located and the following parameters are assessed (Fig. 8-20):

■ Cervical dilation: This measurement estimates the dilation of the cervical opening by sweeping the examining finger from the margin of the cervical opening on one side to that on the other.

■ Cervical effacement: This measurement estimates the shortening of the cervix from 2 cm to paper thin measured by palpation of cervical length with the fingertips. The degree of cervical effacement is expressed in terms of the length of the cervical canal compared to that of an unaffected cervix. When it is reduced by one-half (1 cm) it is 50% effaced. When the cervix is thinned out completely, it is 100% effaced.

■ Position of cervix: Relationship of the cervical os to the fetal head and is characterized as posterior, midposition, or anterior.

■ Station: Level of the presenting part in the birth canal in relationship to the ischial spines. Station is 0 when the presenting part is at the ischial spines or engaged in the pelvis.

■ Presentation: Cephalic (head first), breech (pelvis first), shoulder (shoulder first)

■ Fetal position: Locate presenting part and specific fetal structure to determine fetal position in relation to the maternal pelvis.

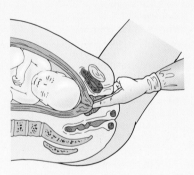

Figure 8-20   Sterile vaginal exam.

BOX 8–3   LEOPOLD'S MANEUVERS

The purpose of Leopold's maneuvers is to inspect and palpate the maternal abdomen to determine fetal position, station, and size (Fig. 8-21).

■ The first maneuver is to determine what part of the fetus is located in the fundus of the uterus.

■ The second maneuver is to determine location of the fetal back.

■ The third maneuver is to determine the presenting part.

■ The fourth maneuver is to determine the location of the cephalic prominence.

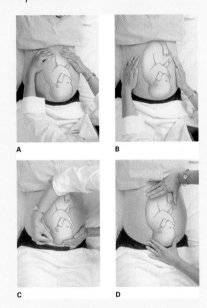

Figure 8-21   Leopold's maneuver.

Source: Mattson & Smith (2004).

■ *Fetal position with Leopold maneuver (Box 8-3)*
■ *Deep tendon reflexes*
■ *Signs of edema*
■ *Heart and lung sounds*
■ *Emotional status*
■ *Pain and discomfort*
■ Review laboratory results, note blood Rh status hematocrit and hemoglobin and dipstick urine for glucose and protein.
■ Document allergies, history of illness, and last food intake.
■ Encourage fluid intake; food may or may not be restricted.

■ Provide comfort measures (see Critical Component: Supportive Activities and Comfort Measures in Labor and section on non-pharmacological management of discomfort).
■ Encourage the woman to walk as much as possible by:
    ■ *Explaining the importance of walking in facilitating labor progression and fetal descent and rotation and in making UCs more efficient*
    ■ *Walking with the woman, which can provide a comforting and reassuring presence and distraction*
■ Assess cultural needs and incorporate beliefs in the nursing care and delivery plan.
■ Establish a therapeutic relationship through active listening and providing labor support (Box 8-4).
■ Incorporate understanding of the couple's maturity level, educational level, and previous experience into nursing care.
■ Review the labor plan with the woman and her partner.
■ Inquire about concerns and questions the woman and/or her partner have concerning the labor and birth process.
■ Provide clear explanations and updates on progress.

Second Phase

The **second phase** (dilation to 7 cm), also referred to as the **active phase** of labor, averages 3 to 6 hours in length. It is typically shorter for multigravidas. Women in this phase may have decreased energy and experience fatigue. They become more serious and turn attention to internal sensations. As labor progresses most women turn inward. Characteristics of this phase are:

- The cervix dilates, on average, 1.2 cm/hr for primiparous women and 1.5 cm/hr for multiparous women.
- Cervical dilation progresses from 4 cm to 7 cm with effacement of 40% to 80%.
- Fetal descent continues.
- Contractions become more intense, occurring every 2 to 5 minutes with a duration of 45 to 60 seconds.
- Discomfort increases, and this is typically the time the woman comes to the birth center or hospital if she has not done so already.

Medical Interventions

- Rupture membranes if not previously ruptured.
- Perform internal monitoring with application of internal fetal electrode and/or uterine transducer, if necessary.
- Order pain medication or epidural anesthesia.
- Evaluate progression in labor.
- Evaluate fetal status.

Nursing Actions (see Clinical Pathway)

- Monitor FHR and contractions every 15 to 30 minutes.
- Monitor maternal vital signs every 2 hours; every 1 hour if ROM.
- Perform intrapartal vaginal exam as needed to assess cervical changes and fetal descent.
- Assess pain (location and degree).
- Administer analgesia as per orders and desire of woman.
- Evaluate effectiveness of epidural or other pain medication.
- Monitor intake and output (I&O), hydration status, and for nausea and vomiting.
- Encourage intake of fluids and ice chips.
- Offer clear explanations and updates of progress.
- Promote comfort measures (see Critical Component: Supportive Activities and Comfort Measures in Labor).
- Assist with elimination needs as bladder distension can hinder fetal descent.
- Encourage breathing and relaxation methods (see Box 8-4).
  - *Review and reinforce relaxation techniques.*
  - *Maintain eye contact and physical proximity to the woman.*
  - *Develop a rhythm and breathing style to deal with each contraction.*
  - *Use a direct and gentle voice and have a calm and confident manner.*
  - *Use touch of massage if acceptable to the woman.*
- Communicate the woman's progress and status with the care provider.
- Incorporate the support person in care of patient by:
  - *Role modeling supportive behaviors*
  - *Offering support and praise*
  - *Assisting partner with food and rest*
  - *Providing breaks if desired or needed*

- Explain procedures being done.
- Assess the environment for adjustments to be made; typically decrease stimulation with dim lighting and decrease noise and interruptions.
- Provide reassurance, updates on progress, and positive reinforcement.

Third Phase

The third phase (dilation to 10 cm), or **transition phase,** is usually the most difficult but shortest of the first stage of labor. In transition, women are easily discouraged, irritable, and may be overwhelmed and panicky. They often feel and act out of control. Characteristics of this phase are:

- Cervical dilation from 8 to 10 cm with complete (100%) effacement
- Contractions every 1 to 2 minutes lasting 60 to 90 seconds and intense
- Exhaustion and increased difficulty concentrating
- Increase of bloody show
- Nausea and vomiting
- Backache
- Trembling
- Diaphoresis
- Strong urge to bear down or push

Medical Interventions

- Perform amniotomy (AROM) if not previously done.
- Order pain medications, if desired.

Nursing Actions (see Clinical Pathway)

- Assess FHR and UCs every 15 minutes.
- Encourage woman to breathe during contractions and rest between contractions by staying with patient and breathing with her (see Box 8-4).
- Assess I&O and for bladder distention.
- Assist the woman with voiding.
- Promote comfort measures (see Critical Component: Supportive Activities and Comfort Measures in Labor).
- Attend to the hygiene needs of the woman such as mopping her brow and face, providing pericare, and changing chux.
- Assist with breathing and relaxation methods by demonstrating breathing through demonstration and reinforcement.
- Communicate the woman's progress and status with the care provider.
- Prepare the room and couple for delivery.
  - *Familiarize the woman and support people with usual routine and keep informed of what to expect.*
  - *Open the delivery tray.*
  - *Turn on the infant radiant warmer.*
- Use brief explanations, as the woman's focus is narrowed.
- Remain in the room with the woman and family.
- Provide encouragement and reassurance to the woman and her support person(s).
  - *Keep them apprised of labor progress, such as changes in cervical dilation.*
  - *Compliment them on their effective breathing and relaxation techniques.*

BOX 8–4 STANDARD OF PRACTICE. AWHONN PRACTICE STATEMENT: PROFESSIONAL NURSING SUPPORT OF LABORING WOMEN

Association for Women's Health, Obstetric and Neonatal Nurses (AWHONN) maintains that continuously available labor support by a professional registered nurse is a critical component to achieve improved birth outcomes. AWHONN views labor care and labor support as powerful nursing functions, and believes it is incumbent on health care facilities to provide an environment that encourages the unique patient–nurse relationship during childbirth. Only the registered nurse combines adequate formal nursing education and clinical patient management skills with experience in providing physical, psychological, and sociocultural care to laboring women. The registered nurse facilitates the childbirth process in collaboration with the laboring woman. The nurse's expertise and therapeutic presence influence patient and family satisfaction with the labor and delivery experience. Evidence supports women who are provided with continuously available support during labor experience improved labor and delivery outcomes compared with those who labor without a skilled support person. The support provided by the professional registered nurse should include:

- Assessment and management of the physiological and psychological processes of labor
- Provision of emotional support and physical comfort measures
- Evaluation of fetal well-being during labor
- Instruction regarding the labor process
- Patient advocacy and collaboration among members of the health care team
- Role modeling to facilitate family participation during labor and birth
- Direct collaboration with other members of the health care team to coordinate patient care

Source: AWHONN (2000a).

Stage 2

The woman enters the **second stage** of labor when cervical dilation is complete (10 cm) (see Table 8-2). This stage ends with the birth of the baby (Fig. 8-22). Women in the second stage may have a burst of energy, be more focused, and may feel like they are able to actively participate in facilitating birth with active pushing efforts. Characteristics of this stage are:

- Typically last 50 minutes for primigravidas and 20 minutes for multigravidas, although a second stage of several hours is normal.
- Woman may feel an intense urge to push or bear-down when the baby reaches the pelvic floor.
  - *Studies have shown that bearing-down in the second stage is less tiring and more effective when begun after the woman has the urge to do so instead of beginning to push without an urge to (Roberts, 2002, 2003).*
- Contractions are intense, occurring every 2 minutes and lasting 60 to 90 seconds in duration.
- Bloody show increases.
- The perineum flattens and the rectum and vagina bulge.

Labor Position and Bearing-Down

Variation in practice exists in positioning of women during the second stage of labor. Many women maintain a semirecumbent

position but there are benefits to a more upright position. Along with the timing of the bearing-down efforts, which include the spontaneous versus the directed pushing, the way a woman pushes has also been studied. Two types have been studied for the effects on the fetus: the closed-glottis (Valsalva maneuver) and the open-glottis pushing (see Evidence-Based Practice: Guideline of Nursing Management of Second Stage of Labor). The results are that fetal hypoxia and acidosis have been associated with the prolonged breath holding (closed glottis) and forceful pushing efforts. No significant differences have been found in the duration of the second stage of labor with the timing and how a woman pushes (Mayberry et al., 2000).

Medical Interventions

- Prepare for delivery.
- Perform episiotomy if necessary (Fig. 8-23 and Box 8-5).
- Assist the woman in the birthing of her child.

Nursing Actions (see Clinical Pathway)

- Instruct the woman to bear down with the urge to push (see Evidence-Based Practice).
- Monitor for fetal response to pushing; check FHR 5-15 minutes or after each contraction.
- Provide comfort measures (see Critical Component: Supportive Activities and Comfort Measures in Labor).
- Support and encourage woman's spontaneous pushing efforts.
- Attend to perineal hygiene as needed, as the woman may pass stool with pushing.
- Give praise and encouragement of progress made.
- Encourage rest between contractions by breathing with the patient and therapeutic touch.
- Review and reinforce pushing technique by:
  - *Maintaining eye contact*
  - *Developing a rhythm and pushing style to deal with each contraction that maximizes the woman urge to push*
  - *Use direct, simple, and focused communication, avoiding unnecessary conversation.*
- Advocate on the woman's behalf for her desires of the delivery plan.
- Assist the support person and partner.
  - *Role model supportive behaviors.*
  - *Offer support, praise, and encouragement.*
  - *Assist with food and rest and provide breaks.*

Third Stage

The **third stage** of labor begins immediately after the delivery of the fetus and involves separation and expulsion of the placenta and membranes (see Table 8-2). As the infant is born, the uterus spontaneously contracts around its diminishing contents. This sudden decrease in uterine size is accompanied by a decrease in the area of placental implantation. This results in the decidual layer separating from the uterine wall. Placental separation typically occurs within a few minutes after delivery. Once the placenta separates from the wall of the uterus, the uterus continues to contract until the placenta is expelled (Fig. 8-25). This process typically takes 5 to 20 minutes post delivery of the baby and occurs spontaneously. Signs that signify the impending delivery of the placenta include:

- Upward rising of the uterus into a ball shape
- Lengthening of the umbilical cord at the introitus
- Sudden gush of blood from the vagina

Normal blood loss for a vaginal birth is approximately 500 mL. The placenta, membranes, and cord are examined by the care provider for completeness and anomalies.

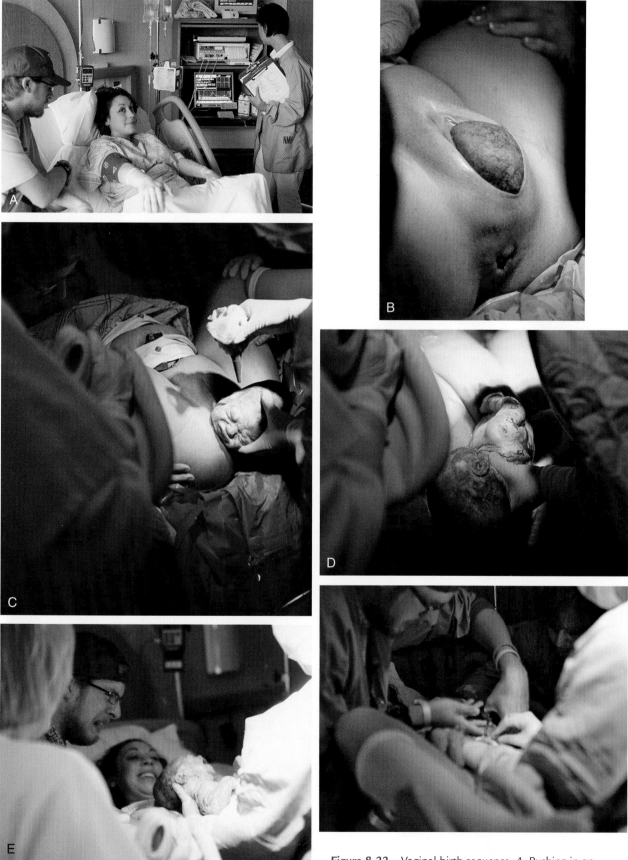

Figure 8-22 Vaginal birth sequence. *A.* Pushing in an upright position allows the use of gravity to promote fetal descent. *B.* Crowning. *C.* Birth of the head. *D.* Birth of the shoulders. *E.* The infant is shown to the new parents. *F.* The baby's father cuts the umbilical cord.

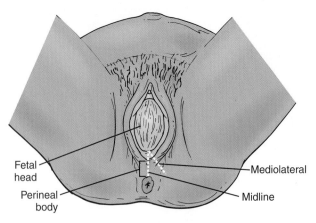

Figure 8-23   Episiotomy locations.

BOX 8–5   EPISIOTOMY AND LACERATIONS

An **episiotomy** is an incision in the perineum to provide more space for the presenting part at delivery (see Fig. 8-23). Routine use of episiotomy at delivery is no longer typical.

A median or midline episiotomy is at the midline and tends to heal more quickly with less discomfort.

A medilateral episiotomy is cut at a 45-degree angle to the left or right and may be used for a large infant. It tends to heal more slowly, causes greater blood loss, and is more painful.

Lacerations are tears in the perineum that may occur at delivery (see Fig. 8-24):

A first-degree laceration involves the perineal skin and vaginal mucous membrane

A second-degree laceration involves skin, mucous membrane, and fascia of the perineal body.

A third-degree laceration involves skin, mucous membrane, and muscle of the perineal body and extends to the rectal sphincter.

A fourth-degree laceration extends into the rectal mucosa and exposes the lumen of the rectum.

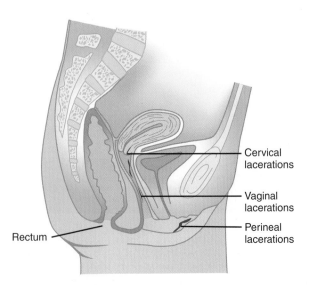

Figure 8-24   Potential locations of lacerations.

Evidence-Based Practice: AWHONN Evidence-Based Clinical Practice Guideline: Nursing Management of Second Stage of Labor

AWHONN. (2000b). Evidence-Based Clinical Practice Guideline, Nursing Management of the Second Stage of Labor. Clinical Practice Recommendation. Washington, DC: Author.

Association of Women's Health, Obstetric and Neonatal Nurses (AWHONN) clinical practice recommendations for management of pushing include:

■ Assess the woman's knowledge of pushing techniques, expectations for pushing, presence of Ferguson's reflex (urge to bear down), and readiness to push as well as the fetal presentation, position, and station.

■ Encourage open glottis pushing for 4 to 6 seconds followed by a slight exhale, repeating this pattern for five or six pushes per contraction. Open glottis refers to spontaneous, involuntary bearing down accompanying the forces of the uterine contraction and is usually characterized by expiratory grunting or vocalizations. This spontaneous method usually involves five or six pushes of 4 to 6 seconds' duration with each contraction.

■ Whenever possible, discourage the traditional practice of breath holding for 10 seconds with each contraction. Closed glottis pushing, also referred to as the Valsalva technique, involves a voluntary or directed strenuous bearing-down effort against a closed glottis for at least 10 seconds. This method usually involves two to three pushes of 10 seconds each during a contraction.

■ Provide birthing aids such as birthing balls, squat bars, birthing stools, and cushions to support the woman and the pelvis.

■ Evaluate the effectiveness of pushing efforts and descent of the presenting part.

■ Support and facilitate the woman's spontaneous pushing efforts.

■ Evaluate the effectiveness of upright or other positions on fetal descent, rotation, and maternal–fetal condition.

■ Upright positioning for the second stage of labor refers to the patient's position sitting with the head of the bed at a 45-degree angle or greater, squatting, kneeling, or standing during the second stage of labor. Benefits of upright positioning include: pelvic diameter may be increased by 30%, shortened duration of second stage, pain may be decreased, and perineal trauma may be decreased.

■ Ferguson's reflex is a physiological response of the woman, activated when the presenting part of the fetus is at least at +1 station; it is usually accompanied by spontaneous bearing-down efforts. Pushing efforts may be delayed until the Ferguson reflex is present.

■ Delayed pushing is waiting for fetal descent and or initiation of Ferguson's reflex before pushing begins in the second stage of labor. Delayed pushing is also referred to as "laboring down," "passive pushing," and "rest and descend."

■ Delayed pushing may also be appropriate for women with epidural anesthesia/analgesia who do not feel the urge to push.

Medical Interventions

■ At delivery, the neonate is often placed skin to skin on mother's abdomen.

■ Await delivery of the placenta.

■ Inspect the placenta after delivery.

■ Order pain medications if necessary.

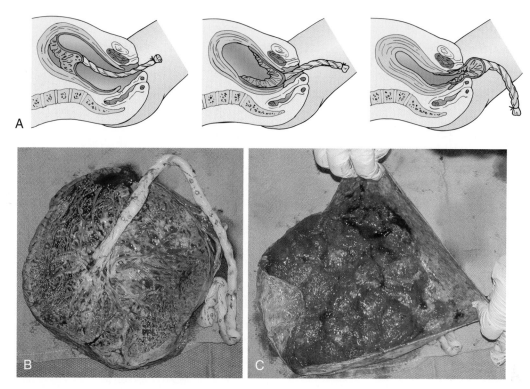

Figure 8-25 *A.* Delivery of the placenta. *B.* Delivered placenta (fetal side). *C.* Inside of placenta (maternal side).

Nursing Actions (see Clinical Pathway)

■ Assess maternal vital signs every 15 minutes.
■ Encourage the woman to breathe with contractions and relax between contractions.
■ Encourage mother–baby interactions by providing immediate newborn contact, if the newborn is stable (Critical Component: Newborn Family Attachment).
■ Administer pain medications as per order.
■ Complete documentation of the delivery (Fig. 8-26).
■ Documentation of delivery includes labor summary, delivery summary for mother and baby, infant information, infant resuscitation and documentation of personnel in attendance.
■ Explain all forthcoming procedures.
■ Stay with the woman and her family.

CRITICAL COMPONENT

Newborn–Family Attachment

An important goal during the fourth stage is the newborn–family attachment. This is promoted by allowing early contact with the newborn, encouragement of eye contact and touch, and also by allowing time to hold the newborn. Positive maternal bonding behaviors include making eye contact, touching and talking to the baby, and other positive behaviors such as smiling and cuddling the newborn. This is often the best time to institute breastfeeding. The newborn may remain in the labor and delivery room with the family for all of the immediate recovery period (Fig. 8-27).

Fourth Stage

The **fourth stage** begins with the delivery of the placenta and typically ends within 4 hours or with the stabilization of the mother.

After the placenta delivers, the primary mechanism by which hemostasis is achieved at the placental site is vasoconstriction produced by a well contracted myometrium. During this stage, the nurse is caring for both the woman and her newborn child. This stage also begins the postpartum period (see Chapter 12 for a discussion of postpartum period).

Medical Interventions

■ Repair the episiotomy or laceration (see Box 8-5 and Fig. 8-24).
■ Inspect the placenta.
■ Assess the fundus for firmness.
■ Order oxytocin, Methergine, or prostaglandin as needed.
■ Order pain medications, if necessary.

Nursing Actions (see Clinical Pathway)

■ Assess the uterus for position, tone, and location, intervening with fundal massage as necessary.
■ Assess lochia for color, amount, and clots.
■ Administer oxytocin as per orders.
■ Explain all procedures.
■ Assist the care provider with repair of lacerations and/or episiotomy.
■ Assess maternal vital signs every 15 minutes.
■ Monitor perineum for unusual swelling or hematoma formation.
■ Apply ice packs to the perineum.
■ Monitor for bladder distention.
    ■ *Assist the woman to the bathroom.*
■ Assess for return of full motor–sensory function if epidural or spinal anesthesia is used.
■ Assess pain and medicate as per orders.
■ Stay with the mother and family.
■ Offer congratulations and reassurance on a job well done to the woman and family.

Delivery/Newborn Record

LABOR SUMMARY	Time	Date

Regular contractions began: _____
Time of Oxytocin start: _____
BOW ruptured: _____
(best estimate) 4cm: _____
10cm: _____

Labor description:
☐ spontaneous   ☐ AROM for induction
☐ augmented, oxytocin   ☐ no labor
☐ induced, oxytocin

☐ Cervical ripening agent _____
☐ **IUPC**
☐ **Amino infusion**
   Previous C/S: ☐ No   **VBAC** ☐ No
              ☐ Yes   **attempted:** ☐ Yes

Analgesics: before delivery
drug   dose   time
_____ _____ _____
_____ _____ _____
_____ _____ _____

Steroids for lung maturity: Date ____ Time ____ Date ____ Time ____
Antibiotic started: (prior to birth): ☐ <4 hrs ☐ 4 hrs ☐ >24 hrs
   Why: ☐ GBS Pending / Preterm   # Doses before birth _____
        ☐ Cardiac prophylaxis
        ☐ Fever / Chorioamnionitis
        ☐ Other: _____
Peak maternal temp ☐ <99.5   ☐ 99.5–101.9   ☐ 102

Amniotic fluid rupture:
☐ Spontaneous
☐ Artificial
Color:
☐ Clear
☐ Light mec. (stain)
☐ Medium mec.
☐ Thick mec.
☐ Cloudy
☐ Bloody

Fetal monitoring in labor:
☐ Auscultation only
☐ External monitor
☐ Internal monitor
☐ Both
☐ IFM site

Labor analgesia:
☐ none   ☐ epidural
☐ narcotic   ☐ both
☐ ____ cervical dil@epid

DELIVERY SUMMARY		

Baby [____] **of a** [____] **gestation**
      Birth Order   Plurality

	Time	Date
DELIVERY:		
PLACENTA:		
C/S start time:		
Uterine incis. time:		
C/S finish time:		

INFANT	(circle)	Boy	Girl

Weight _____ lb _____ gm
Length _____ in _____ cm
Head circ _____ in _____ cm

Delivery Outcomes: **Feeding:**
☐ live birth admitted for regular care   ☐ Breast
☐ live birth admitted to trans. nursery   ☐ Bottle
☐ live birth admitted to NICU
☐ neonatal death in delivery room   Gest. Age @
☐ fetal death before admission   Delivery
☐ fetal death after admission

I.D. BAND #: [_____]
Bands Checked by:
_____ RN _____ RN

Cord Blood to Lab: ☐ Yes   ☐ No
Cord Gases Sent: ☐ Yes   ☐ No
Specimen to Lab: ☐ Type _____
Culture to Lab: ☐ Type _____

GROUP B STREP SCREEN	APGAR SCORE		Cord around neck X

Universal Risk Factors
☐ Previous GBS infected infant
☐ urine cx for GBS in current pregnancy

Culture Based
☐ negative
☐ positive
☐ not available

Risk Based (Intrapartum)
☐ No risk factors
☐ < 37 weeks
☐ ROM 18 hours
☐ Maternal temp 100.4

	1 min	5 min
Heart Rate		
Respiratory Effort		
Muscle Tone		
Reflex Irritability		
Color		
TOTAL		

Umbilical Vessel Number: [____]

☐ Voided in DR
☐ Stool in DR

RESUSCITATION		

Respirations: ☐ Spontaneous
              ☐ Delayed _____ min
              ☐ Narcan Given
Check ALL that apply: Time: _____
☐ suction   Dose: _____
☐ oxygen   Route: _____
☐ mask vent   By whom: _____
☐ intubation for resuscitation **For Meconium Babies:**
☐ chest compression   ☐ Not intubated
☐ medications   ☐ Intubated – Below Cords
☐ volume   ☐ Intubated – Meconium noted

Note: _____
_____
_____
_____
_____

DELIVERY–MOTHER		

Method of Delivery: **Episiotomy/Laceration:**
☐ Vertex, Vaginal   ☐ None
☐ Breech, Vaginal   ☐ Median
☐ Cesarean Section   ☐ Mediolateral
☐ Vacuum   ☐ Laceration
☐ Forceps   ☐ Repaired

PLACENTA:
☐ Spontaneous
☐ Assist
☐ Manual
Abnormalities:

Medications at Delivery:
drug   dose   time
Pitocin IV IM _____ units _____
_____ _____ _____
_____ _____ _____

PEDIATRICIAN:

Newborn attended by _____ RN/MD
☐ Newborn admitted time: _____ am/pm
MR # _____   Pat # _____
Pediatrician notified of delivery: K # _____
   Name _____ MD
   Date _____ Time _____ am/pm
   Via _____ by _____

DELIVERING PHYSICIAN/CNM:	APN/NICU STAFF AT DELIVERY:	ANESTHESIOLOGIST:
ASSIST MD/CNM:	OB/RN AT DELIVERY:	RN SIGNATURE DATE/TIME:

Patient's Data/Addressograph

Figure 8-26   Documentation of delivery.

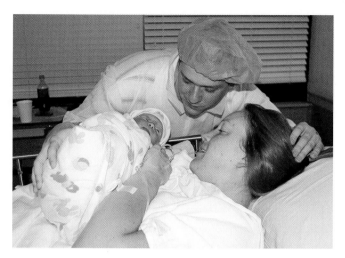

Figure 8-27 Newly delivered baby in the delivery room with family.

■ Encourage mother–baby interaction by:
  ■ *Providing immediate newborn contact*
  ■ *Assisting with early breastfeeding, if desired*
  ■ *Pointing out the newborn's quiet, alert state*
■ Monitor newborn status, including temperature, heart and respiratory rates, skin color, adequacy of peripheral circulation, type of respiration, level of consciousness, and tone and activity every 30 minutes.
■ Provide an opportunity for the support person to interact with newborn.

THE NEWBORN

Newborn transition and initial care typically occur in the labor and delivery room. Initial assessments can be safely done with the infant skin-to-skin on the mother's abdomen after delivery, if the infant is stable. Apgar scores should be obtained at 1 minute and 5 minutes after birth. If the 5-minute Apgar score is less than 7, additional scores should be assigned every 5 minutes up to 20 minutes. Temperature, heart and respiratory rates, skin color, adequacy of peripheral circulation, type of respiration, level of consciousness, tone, and activity should be monitored and recorded at least every 30 minutes until the newborn's condition has remained stable for at least 2 hours.

The **Apgar score** is a rapid assessment of five physiological signs that indicate the physiological status of the newborn and includes (Table 8-3):

■ Heart rate based on auscultation
■ Respiratory rate based on observed movement of chest
■ Muscle tone based on degree of flexion and movement of extremities
■ Reflex irritability based on response to tactile stimulation
■ Color based on observation

Each component is given a score of 0, 1, or 2. An Apgar score of 0 to 3 indicates severe distress, a score of 4 to 6 indicates moderate difficulty with transition to extrauterine life, and a score of 7 to 10 indicates stable status. The Apgar score is not used to determine the need for resuscitation, nor is it predictive of long-term neurological outcome of the neonate (American Academy of Pediatrics [AAP] & American College of Obstetrics and Gynecology [ACOG], 2006). Rather it is a rapid, objective, convenient shorthand for reporting the status of the newborn and the response to resuscitation immediately after birth.

At every delivery, there should be one person who is solely responsible for assessment of the neonate response to the birth and who has the capacity to initiate resuscitation of the neonate if needed. Only 1% of neonates need extensive resuscitation at birth (American Heart Association [AHA] & AAP, 2006). A comprehensive discussion of the newborn's transition to extrauterine life, physical assessment, and routine procedures are presented in Chapter 15.

One of the first procedures after birth is newborn identification. Perinatal nurses must be meticulous when recording the identification band number, birth and newborn information, and applying identification bands to mothers and newborns. Institutional policies for newborn identification and newborn safety may vary. Routinely two medications are administered to newborns:

■ Erythromycin ointment is administered to the eyes as prophylaxis to prevent gonococcal and *Chlamydia* infections.
■ Vitamin K is administered via intramuscular injection to prevent hemorrhagic disease caused by vitamin K deficiency.

Newborn care is discussed in Chapter 15.

MANAGEMENT OF DISCOMFORT DURING LABOR AND DELIVERY

Pain in childbirth is a universal experience and considered a normal occurrence. Pain associated with labor has been described as one of the most intensely painful experiences possible. Labor pain differs from other conditions in which pain is experienced in several ways (Table 8-4).

Understanding the cause and characteristics of pain in the labor and delivery setting helps the nurse develop a plan of care for the

TABLE 8–3 NEONATAL APGAR SCORE			
	SCORE		
SIGN	**0**	**1**	**2**
RESPIRATORY EFFORT	Absent	Slow, irregular	Good cry
HEART RATE	Absent	Slow, below 100 bpm	Above 100 bpm
MUSCLE TONE	Flaccid	Some flexion of extremities	Active motion
REFLEX ACTIVITY	None	Grimace	Vigorous cry
COLOR	Pale, blue	Body pink, blue extremities	Completely pink

TABLE 8–4	LABOR PAIN VERSUS OTHER KINDS OF PAIN	
LABOR PAIN	**OTHER PAIN**	
Part of normal process	Often indicates disease or injury	
Source of pain is known and purposeful.	Source of pain may be unknown and be the result of tissue damage.	
There is time for preparation with understanding and skills to assist in managing pain.	Pain may be sudden onset or chronic.	

woman in each stage of the labor process. Factors influencing pain response include both the physical and psychosocial:

- Rate of cervical dilation and strength of contractions
- Size and position of fetus impacts length of labor.
- Sleep deprivation and exhaustion from long labor increases pain perception.
- Culture of the woman influences her response to labor and pain. Pain behaviors are culturally bound (see Cultural Awareness: Culture and Birth Traditions).
- The woman's labor support system can affect her anxiety level and perception of pain.
- Previous birth experiences may increase or decrease anxiety.
- Childbirth preparation may decrease anxiety and decrease pain.
- The womans' expectations influence her satisfaction with her birth experience (Evidence-Based Practice: Maternal Satisfaction).

Pain in childbirth is transmitted from the periphery of the body along nerve pathways to the brain. This pain is attributable to:

- Uterine contractions resulting in uterine pain from a decrease in blood supply to the uterus

- Increased pressure and stretching of the pelvic structures resulting in the pulling and expansion of ligaments, muscle, and peritoneum
- Cervical dilation and stretching resulting in the stimulation of the nerve ganglia

Evidence-Based Practice: Maternal Satisfaction

Florence, D., & Palmer, D. (2003). Therapeutic choices for the discomforts of labor *Journal of Perinatal & Neonatal Nursing, 17* (4), 238.

Hodnett, E. (2002). Pain and women's satisfaction with the experience of childbirth: A systematic review. *American Journal of Obstetrics and Gynecology, 186*(5), S160–S172.

Research has shown that maternal satisfaction post-birth is influenced by the degree of pain endured, but is far more influenced by whether the actual birth event met the woman's personal expectations (Hodnett, 2002). Satisfaction with the labor experience is based on variables that include cultural influence, previous experiences, communication from family and providers, and prenatal education (Florence & Palmer, 2003).

Gate Control Theory of Pain

The use of the gate control theory of pain can be applied to the process of labor and birth (Fig. 8-28). This theory states that sensation of pain is transmitted from the periphery of the body along ascending nerve pathways to the brain. Because of the limited number of sensations that can travel along these pathways at any given time, an alternate activity can replace travel of the pain sensation, thus closing the gate control at the spinal cord and reducing pain impulses traveling to the brain. Based on this premise, the application of pressure to certain areas of the body, the cutaneous stimulation such as effleurage (gentle stroking of the abdomen), or the use of heat or cold can have a direct effect on closing the gate, which then limits the transmission of pain. A similar gating mechanism can be found in the descending nerve fibers from the hypothalamus and cerebral cortex. Strategies such as breathing, focusing, and visual and auditory stimulation may affect whether pain impulses reach the level of conscious awareness.

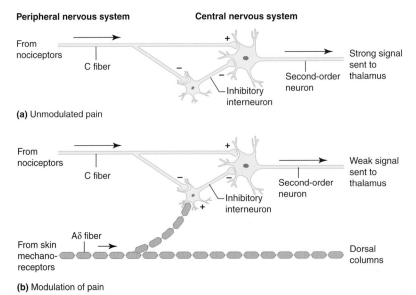

Figure 8-28   Gate control theory of pain modulation. *A.* Normally C-fibers carrying slow pain signals block inhibitory interneurons and transmit their signals across the synapse unimpeded. *B.* A-delta fibers carrying pleasurable signals from touch excite inhibitory interneurons, which then block the transmission of slow pain signals (+ equals transmission, – equals no transmission).

Nonpharmacological Management of Labor Discomfort

Nonpharmacological management of labor discomfort includes preparation by the woman for childbirth, cutaneous stimulation, thermal stimulation, mental stimulation, and the presence of a support person. It is essential that nurses have a repertoire of strategies to manage discomfort and pain during labor. A willingness to try a variety of strategies, adapt those that are effective, and modify and abandon those that are not effective are important aspects of care. Usually no one strategy works for very long in labor, making flexibility and adaptability key qualities for labor nurses.

■ Childbirth preparation methods: Education and explanation of birth process is offered through classes to the woman and her support person before the delivery time. In these classes, the woman and her partner learn about pregnancy, the labor process, the painful aspects of labor, and methods to help relieve the discomforts of pregnancy and childbirth. Some of the major methods of childbirth preparation include:
  ■ *Dick-Read method: Advocates birth without fear by education and environmental control and relaxation.*
  ■ *Lamaze: Promotes psychoprophylaxis with conditioning and breathing.*
  ■ *Bradley: This is husband-coached childbirth and support by working with and managing the pain rather than being distracted away from it.*
  ■ *Relaxation and breathing techniques: Varied breathing patterns that promote relaxation and avoidance of pushing before complete cervical dilation. Most childbirth preparation methods teach some form of relaxation and breathing techniques (Fig. 8-29). Most women are taught to take a deep breath at the beginning of the contraction to signal the onset of the contraction and then to breathe slowly during the contraction. As labor pain increases, the woman may need to breathe in a more rapid and shallow manner. On occasion, a woman will experience hyperventilation from this type of breathing. Symptoms are related to respiratory alkalosis and include tingling of the fingers or circumoral numbness, light-headedness, or dizziness. This undesirable side effect can be eliminated by having the woman breathe into a bag or cupped hands. This causes her to rebreathe carbon dioxide and reverses the respiratory alkalosis.*

■ Cutaneous stimulation: Massage by self such as effleurage. **Effleurage** is done by lightly stroking the abdomen in rhythm with breathing during contractions. Another form of cutaneous stimulation is back massage and/or counterpressure to the sacral area by another. Counterpressure is exerted to the sacral area with the heel of the hand or fist to relieve the sensation of intense pain in the back caused by internal pressure of the fetal head. This increased internal pressure by the fetal head is often associated with the posterior position of the fetus during labor. As labor advances, women may not want to be touched.

■ Thermal stimulation: Application of warmth or cold such as use of warm showers or ice packs. The use of hydrotherapy via whirlpools, warm baths, or showers is very effective and promotes relaxation and comfort. This may reduce the woman's anxiety and promote well-being, causing a reduction in catecholamine production, which interferes with uterine contractility. Application of cold may release musculoskeletal pain and the numbing effect of cold may decrease the sensation of pain.

■ Mental stimulation: Focal points, imagery, and music help the woman to concentrate on something outside her body. This helps her to focus away from the pain. With imagery, the woman is encouraged to bring into her mind a picture of a relaxing scene.

■ Support person: A significant other and/or a doula provides emotional support and physical comfort and aids in a beneficial form of care. Research has shown that support early in labor significantly relieves pain, improves outcomes, decreases interventions and complication rates, and thus enhances overall maternal satisfaction (Simkin & O'Hara, 2002).

Pharmacological Management of Labor Discomfort

Pharmacological management of discomfort and pain in labor requires the nurse to assess the woman's preferences for pain management throughout labor. The decision to use pain medication in labor should be made by the woman in collaboration with her physician or midwife. The unique circumstances of every labor influence the experience and perception of pain (Simpson & Creehan, 2008).

■ Assessment of pain is an essential part of nursing care.
  ■ *The standard 0 to 10 pain scale is insufficient for assessment of labor pain.*
  ■ *Assessment of labor pain should include intensity, location, pattern, and degree of distress for the woman.*
■ The use of medication in the relief of pain during labor falls into two major categories:
  ■ *Analgesia (Table 8-5)*
  ■ *Anesthesia (Table 8-6).*
■ Basic principles when using analgesia include:
  ■ *Labor should be established.*
  ■ *Medication should provide relief to the woman with minimal risk to the baby.*
    ■ Neonatal depression may occur if medication is given within an hour before delivery.
    ■ Women with a history of drug abuse may have a lessened effect from pain medication and require higher doses.

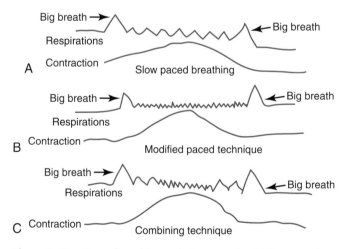

Figure 8-29 Space breathing technique graph. *A.* Slow-paced breathing is with big breath at beginning and end of contraction; the typical rate is fewer than 10 breaths per minute *B.* Modified paced breathing is with a big breath at the beginning and end of the contraction and rapid shallow breaths that are comfortable for the woman at a rate of about twice normal respirations. *C.* Combining technique. Big breath at the beginning and end of the contraction with more rapid and shallow breathing at the peak of the contraction.

TABLE 8–5 ANALGESIC MEDICATIONS IN LABOR

MEDICATION	CLASS	SIDE EFFECTS	NURSE INTERVENTION
Morphine 5 mg–10 mg IM 2 mg–5 mg IV	Opioid	CNS depression Neonatal respiratory depression	Avoid use when close to delivery time (about 1 hour).
Meperidine (Demerol) 50 mg–100 mg IM 25 mg–50 mg IV	Opioid	CNS depression Neonatal respiratory depression	Avoid use close to delivery time (about 1 hour).
Butorphanol (Stadol) 2 mg–4 mg IM 0.5 mg–2 mg IV Nalbuphine (Nubain) 10 mg IM or IV	Opioid agonist-antagonist	No respiratory depression in woman or neonate	Check maternal history for drug abuse. Do not give to drug dependent woman due to possible precipitation of sudden withdrawal response in woman and baby. Monitor effective response.
Sublimaze (Fentanyl) May be used in conjunction with regional anesthesia	Short acting opioid antagonist Crosses the placenta rapidly	FHR changes Hypotension Maternal/fetal/neonatal CNS depression Respiratory depression	Monitor for side effects such as sedation, nausea, vomiting, itching. Monitor respiratory rate and effort.
Promethazine (Phenergan) 25 mg–75 mg IM 25 mg–50 mg IV Hydroxyzine (Vistaril) 25–100 mg IM or Z tract	Ataractics	Drowsiness Agonist effect of narcotics	Monitor effective response. Potentiates narcotic effect.
Naloxone (Narcan)	Antagonist-used to reverse narcotic effect May be used to relieve maternal itching and respiratory depression		Review appropriate dosing for adult vs. newborn.

Sources: Faucher & Brucker (2000); Florence & Palmer (2003); Spratto & Woods (2006).

- Basic principles for anesthesia include:
  - *Local anesthesia is used at the time of delivery for episiotomy and repair.*
  - *Regional anesthesia is used during labor and at delivery.*
    - Regional anesthesia includes the pudendal block, epidural block, and spinal block.
  - *Regional or general anesthesia is used for cesarean deliveries (Chapter 12 addresses care of cesarean birth women.)*

Epidural Anesthesia

Epidural anesthesia is one of the most common forms of pain relief during labor used in the United States. **Epidural anesthesia** involves the placement of a very small catheter and injection of local anesthesia and or analgesia between the fourth and fifth vertebrae into the epidural space. A **combined spinal epidural analgesia (CSE)** involves the injection of local anesthetic and/or analgesic into the subarachnoid space. Some patients may be able to ambulate with this type of anesthesia, hence it is referred to as a "walking epidural." Because of the widespread use of epidural anesthesia in labor, AWHONN has generated evidence-based practice guidelines for care of pregnant women receiving regional anesthesia/analgesia (AWHONN, 2001b).

- More than half of the women undergoing labor in the United States use this method each year (Buckley, 2005). Some research shows that epidural analgesia is associated with a lower rate of spontaneous vaginal delivery, a higher rate of instrumental (e.g., vacuum suction and/or forceps) vaginal delivery, longer labors, and increased incidence of intrapartum fevers and/or suspected sepsis (Buckley, 2005). A review of the evidence has concluded that research about the effects of regional anesthesia/analgesia on the progress of labor is inconclusive (AWHONN, 2001b).
- Elevations in maternal temperature associated with regional anesthesia have been reported, but the causes are unclear whether it is a response to infection versus a response to sympathetic blockade. It may be associated with decreased maternal hyperventilation, reduced perspiration, and altered thermoregulatory transmission.
- A wide variety of medications and dosing regimens are used for regional analgesia/anesthesia. Nurses are responsible for knowing general information about classification of these medications, their actions, potential side effects, and complications (AWHONN, 2001a).

TABLE 8–6 ANESTHESIA IN LABOR AND DELIVERY

TYPE OF ANESTHESIA	TIME GIVEN AND EFFECTS	ADVERSE EFFECTS	NURSING IMPLICATIONS
LOCAL: Anesthetic injected into perineum at episiotomy site	Second stage of labor, immediately before delivery Anesthetizes local tissue for episiotomy and repair	Risk of a hematoma Risk of infection	Monitor for: Return of sensation to area Increased swelling at site of injection
REGIONAL: **Pudendal Block:** Anesthetic injected in the pudendal nerve (close to the ischial spines) via needle guide known as "trumpet".	Second stage of labor, prior to time of delivery Anesthetizes vulva, lower vagina and part of perineum for episiotomy and use of low forceps	Risk of local anesthetic toxicity Risk of a hematoma Risk of infection	Monitor for: Return of sensation to area Increased swelling Signs and symptoms of infection Urinary retention
Epidural Block: Anesthetic injected in the epidural space: Located outside the dura mater between the dura and spinal canal via an epidural catheter	First stage and/or second stage of labor Can be used for both vaginal and cesarean births Has the potential of 100% blockage of pain Can be used with opioids such as Sublimaze to allow walking during first stage of labor and effective pushing in second stage of labor	Most common complication is hypotension Other side effects include nausea, vomiting, pruritis, respiratory depression, alterations in FHR	**Pre-anesthesia care** Obtain consent. Check lab values—especially for bleeding or clotting abnormalities, platelet count. IV fluid bolus with normal saline or lactated Ringer's. Ensure emergency equipment is available. **Post-procedure care.** Monitor maternal vital signs and FHR every 5 min initially and after every re-bolus then every 15 minutes and manage hypotension or alterations in FHR. Urinary retention is common and catheterization may be needed. Assess pain and level of sensation and motor loss. Position woman as needed (on side to prevent inferior vena cava syndrome) Assess for itching, nausea and vomiting, and headache and administer meds PRN. When catheter discontinued, note intact tip when removed.
Spinal Block: Anesthetic injected in the subarachnoid space	Second stage of labor or in use for cesarean section. Rapid acting with 100% blockage of sensation and motor functioning. Can last up to 3 hours.	Adverse effects are similar to the epidural with the addition of a spinal headache. A blood patch often provides relief.	Interventions are same as for epidural. Monitor site for leakage of spinal fluid or formation of hematoma. Observe for headache.

Continued

TABLE 8–6   ANESTHESIA IN LABOR AND DELIVERY—CONT'D

TYPE OF ANESTHESIA	TIME GIVEN AND EFFECTS	ADVERSE EFFECTS	NURSING IMPLICATIONS
GENERAL ANESTHESIA: Use of IV injection and/or inhalation of anesthetic agents that render the woman unconscious.	Used mainly in emergency cesarean birth	Risk for fetal depression Risk for uterine relaxation Risk for maternal vomiting and aspiration	Obtain consent. Ensure woman is NPO. IV with large-bore needle. Place indwelling urinary catheter. Administer medications to decrease gastric acidity as ordered such as antacids: Bicitra or Proton pump inhibitor: Protonix. Place wedge to hip to prevent vena cava syndrome. Assist with supportive care of newborn.

Sources: AWHONN (2001a and b); Pitter & Preston (2001); Spratto & Woods (2006).

CRITICAL COMPONENT

Epidural Anesthesia

■ Nurses monitor, but not manage, the care of woman receiving epidural anesthesia.
■ Catheter dosing of intermittent and continuous infusion of regional analgesia/anesthesia is outside the scope of registered nursing.
■ Only qualified, licensed anesthesia providers should perform insertion, injection, increasing, or decreasing rates of a continuous infusion.

(AWHONN, 2001a)

■ Responsibilities of nurses caring for women receiving regional anesthesia/analgesia are assessment, monitoring, and interventions to minimize complications.
■ After the stabilization of the patient after regional anesthesia, the nurse monitors the woman's vital signs, mobility, level of consciousness, and perception of pain, as well as fetal status.

Nursing Actions Before the Epidural

Nursing actions are based on AWHONN guidelines (2001a):

■ Determine the woman's and her family's knowledge and concerns about epidural anesthesia.
■ Consult with obstetrical and anesthesia care providers when the woman requests epidural anesthesia.
■ Assess and document baseline blood pressure, pulse, respiratory rate, and temperature.
■ Assess FHR to confirm a normal FHR pattern; if indeterminate or abnormal report to the physician or midwife.
■ Encourage the patient to void before initiation of epidural anesthesia.
■ Administer an IV bolus as ordered to decrease incidence of hypotension.

Nursing Actions During Administration of Epidural Anesthesia

■ Assist the anesthesia provider, anesthesiologist, or nurse anesthetist (CRNA) with placement of the epidural, including placement of patient in the lateral position with head flexed toward chest, or sitting position with head flexed on chest, elbows on knees and feet supported on stool (AWHONN, 2001a) (Fig. 8-30A and B).

Nursing Actions After Epidural Administration (AWHONN, 2001a)

■ Check blood pressure and FHR every 5 minutes for 15 minutes after initiation or rebolus of epidural, as up to 40% of women may experience hypotension, then every 15 minutes or according to agency protocols.
  ■ *Hypotension is defined as systolic blood pressure less than 100 mm Hg or 20% decrease on blood pressure from preanesthesia levels.*
  ■ *Notify the anesthesia provider if the patient becomes hypotensive.*
■ Assess pulse and respiratory rate with the blood pressure.
■ If patient-controlled analgesia (PCA) is used, reinforce information on infusion device as needed; report any onset of dense motor blockade.
■ Facilitate lateral or upright positioning with uterine displacement to help avoid supine hypotension.
■ Assess for effectiveness of the epidural and the woman's pain levels and description of pain (Critical Component: Epidural Anesthesia).
  ■ *Notify the anesthesia provider of inadequate pain relief.*
■ Assess for sedation if opioid medication is administered with local anesthesia, as drowsiness can occur in up to 50% of women who receive combination local/opioid analgesia.
■ Assess the level of motor blockade according to agency criteria.
  ■ *If the patient receives an epidural that allows ambulation. Before ambulation, the nurse assesses somatosensory status, motor strength, and ability to ambulate.*
■ Monitor for pruritis, as up to 90% of women who receive opioids in epidural have itching.
  ■ *For severe itching medicate prn per orders.*

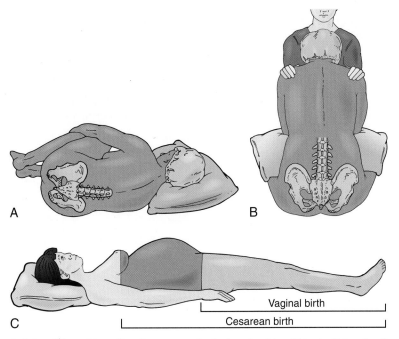

Figure 8-30   Lateral *(A)* and sitting *(B)* positions for placement of spinal and epidural block. *C.* Levels of anesthesia necessary for vaginal and cesarean births.

■ Monitor for nausea and vomiting (up to 50% of women experience this and may be treated with antiemetics prn).

■ Assess for post-procedural headache, as it occurs in up to 3% of women related to leakage of spinal fluid with inadvertent puncture. If this occurs, it should be reported to the anesthesia provider.

■ Assess the woman for urinary retention, as this occurs in most women who receive epidural anesthesia because of decreased motor function.
  ■ *Catheterization is typically necessary.*

■ Assess the partner's or support person's response to epidural pain relief and answer questions (see Evidence-Based Practice: Expectant Fathers and Labor Epidurals).

■ Monitor uterine contractions as uterine activity may slow for up to 60 minutes after epidural placement.

■ Monitor for signs and symptoms of intravascular injection including:
  ■ *Maternal tachycardia or bradycardia*
  ■ *Hypertension*
  ■ *Dizziness*
  ■ *Tinnitus (ringing in the ears)*
  ■ *Metallic taste in the mouth*
  ■ *Loss of consciousness*

If intravascular injection occurs the anesthesia care provider should be immediately notified and care includes administering oxygen, fluids, and medication as ordered. Initiating CPR may be necessary

■ A higher level of anesthesia is necessary for a cesarean birth than for labor (see Fig. 8-30C).

Evidence-Based Practice: Expectant Fathers and Labor Epidurals

Chapman, L. (2000). Expectant fathers and labor epidurals. *Maternal Child Nursing*, 25, 133–138.

A qualitative research study using grounded theory methodology was conducted with the aim to describe and explain the expectant father's experience during labor and birth when epidural anesthesia/analgesia is used for labor pain management. Based on the research data a theory, "cruising through labor," was developed. The epidural labor process different from nonepidural labor and is comprised of six phases:

■ Holding out
■ Surrendering
■ Waiting
■ Getting
■ Cruising
■ Pushing

Expectant fathers explained that before the epidural they felt like they were "losing" their partner as the increasing pain caused the woman to focus inward and away from interaction with those in the labor room. The expectant fathers explained that they felt a loss of connection with their partner and a loss of control. They felt that the pain of labor overtook their partner and was all encompassing. The men further explained that they felt helpless, frustrated, anxious, and a sense of losing her to the pain of labor.

The men explained that the labor nurse played a significant role in supporting them during this time. The major supportive behaviors by the nurse were:

■ Remaining in the labor room
■ Explaining what was happening to their partner
■ Including the men in the care of their partner

Expectant fathers reported that once the epidural was administered and the woman experienced relief from labor pain, they saw a dramatic change in their partner's behavior. They often stated "She's back," that she was comfortable and able to interact with those around her. One man stated, "She wasn't in pain. Her color was back. Her pain was gone. She wasn't throwing up. She was back. She was comfortable."

Men further explained that the effects of the epidural in decreasing the degree of labor pain allowed the men to shift their focus from labor pain management to enjoying the labor and birthing experience (Fig. 8-31).

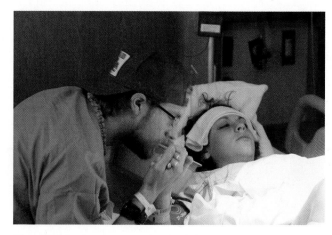

Figure 8-31   Partners experiencing labor together.

Clinical Pathway for Intrapartal Maternal and Fetal Assessment

	Active Labor	Second Stage Labor (Active Pushing)	Third Stage of Labor (Delivery of Placenta)	Fourth Stage of Labor (Immediate Postpartum)
Maternal Vital Signs	P, R, BP every hour; temp every 2 hours unless ROM then every hour	P, R, BP every hour; temp every 2 hours unless ROM then every hour	P, R, BP every 15 minutes	P, R, BP every 15 minutes
FHR	Every 15–30 minutes*	Assessment every 5–15 minutes*	NA	Initiate neonatal transition care
Uterine Activity	Every 15–30 minutes**	Assessment every 5–15 minutes**	NA	NA Fundal and lochia checks every 15 minutes
Pain Status	Every 30 minutes	Assessment every 15 minutes	Assessment every 15 minutes	Assessment every 15 minutes
Response to Labor	Every 30 minutes	Assessment every 15 minutes	Assessment every 15 minutes	
Comfort Measures	Every 30 minutes	Assessment every 15 minutes	Assessment every 15 minutes	Assessment every 15 minutes
Position	Every 30 minutes	Assessment every 15 minutes		
Vaginal Exam/ Fetal Station/ Progress in Descent	As needed	As needed, at least every 30 minutes	NA	NA
Intake and Output	Every 8 hours	Assess bladder distension		Assess bladder distension

P, pulse; R, respirations, BP, blood pressure; FHR, fetal heart rate.
*FHR characteristics include baseline rate, variability, and presence or absence of accelerations and periodic or episodic decelerations.
**Uterine activity included contraction frequency, duration, intensity, and uterine resting tone.
Source: AWHONN (2008).

TYING IT ALL TOGETHER

As the nurse, you admit Margarite Sanchez to the labor and delivery unit. She arrived in the triage unit at midnight in early labor. She presented with uterine contractions that were 5 minutes apart for 3 hours. Patient is a 28-year-old G3 P1 Hispanic woman. She is 39 weeks' gestation. José, her husband, has accompanied her to the unit. Two years ago, she had a normal spontaneous vaginal delivery NSVD after an 18-hour labor for a baby girl, Sonya that was 7 lbs., 3 oz.

Her cervix is now 4 cm/80%/0 station and fetal position is left occiput anterior (LOA).

Prenatal Labs
Blood type O+
RPR NR
GBS negative
Hgb
Hct
Hepatitis negative
Vital signs: Blood pressure 110/60; pulse 84 bpm; respiratory rate 18; temperature 98.6°F (37°C).

Prenatal Care Summary

Began prenatal care at 10 weeks of gestation and received regular prenatal care. She gained 22 pounds during pregnancy, and her current weight is 164 lbs. She is 5 feet, 4 inches. She has no prior medical complications and has experienced a normal pregnancy. Her first pregnancy ended in miscarriage at 8 weeks' gestation. She has no allergies to food or medication. She does not have a birth plan and states, "I just hope for a normal delivery and a health baby."

Detail the aspects of your initial assessment.

EFM reveals a FHR pattern that is normal with a FHR baseline of 140s moderate variability with accelerations to 160s × 20 seconds. She is uncomfortable with contractions and rates her pain at 5. She requests ambulation, as she feels more comfortable with walking.

At 0120 she has SROM for a large amount of clear amniotic fluid. FHR is baseline 130s with moderate variability, and accelerations and contractions are every 3 minutes and feel moderate to palpation. Her SVE reveals her cervix is 5 cm/90/0 station. She is very uncomfortable with contractions but does not want pain medication at this time. José appears anxious and at a loss for how to help his wife.

What are your immediate priorities in nursing care for Margarite and José Sanchez?
Discuss the rationale for the priorities.
What teaching would include?
State nursing diagnosis, expected outcome, and interventions related to managing her labor pain.
What are appropriate interventions to manage her labor pain nonpharmacologically?

At 2 A.M. Margarite is increasingly uncomfortable with contractions and cries out that she can no longer take the pain. Her cervical exam is 6/100/0. She requests pain medication and is given a dose of Nubain at 0215 for pain relief in active labor. José asks how much longer the labor will be and when the baby will be born.

Detail the aspects of your ongoing assessment.
What are your current priorities in nursing care for Margarite Sanchez? Discuss the rationale for the priorities.
Further teaching would include the following:
State nursing diagnosis, expected outcome, and interventions related to this problem.

At 0410 Margarite is very uncomfortable with contractions and cries out that she feels more pressure. She vomits a small amount of bile-colored fluid, and is perspiring and breathing hard with contractions. Her cervical exam is 8/90/0. She requests pain medication and is given a dose of Nubian at 0440 for pain relief in transition.

What are appropriate interventions?

At 0630 Margarite reports an urge to bear down and push with contractions and is very uncomfortable with contractions and cries out that she feels more pressure. Her sterile vaginal exam (SVE) reveals she is 10 cm/100% and +1 station. She has a strong urge to push with contractions that are every 2 minutes and strong to palpation. The fetal heart rate is 130s with moderate variability and the FHR drops to 90 bpm × 40 seconds with pushing efforts.

What are your immediate priorities in nursing care for Margarite Sanchez?
Discuss the rationale for the priorities.
What does the FHR indicate?
Teaching would include the following:
State nursing diagnosis, expected outcome, and interventions related to managing her labor pain.

Margarite continues to bear down, using open glottis pushing with contractions and the fetal head is descending with contractions. The fetal heart rate is 130s with moderate variability and the FHR drops to 90 bpm × 40 seconds with pushing efforts. At 7:30 A.M. Margarite is increasingly unfocused with contractions and states, "I can't push.... call my doctor to get the baby out!" José is at her side holding her hand and encouraging her pushing efforts.

What are your immediate priorities in nursing care for Margarite Sanchez?
Discuss the rationale for the priorities.

At 0815 Margarite continues to bear down with contractions and the fetal head is descending with contractions. The FHR is 130s with moderate variability and the FHR drops to 90 bpm × 40 seconds with pushing efforts. Margarite is focused with contractions. The fetal head is starting to crown with pushing efforts

What are your immediate priorities in nursing care for Margarite Sanchez?
Discuss the rationale for the priorities.

Her doctor comes into the labor and delivery room and she delivers a baby boy at 0839, with a second-degree perineal laceration. Her son weighs 3800 grams and 1- and 5-minute Apgar scores are 8 and 9.

Both Margarite and José begin to cry when their son is born and José holds his son and hugs his wife. The placenta is delivered apparently intact at 0845. Both Margarite and her son are stable and you initiate immediate postpartum and transition care for the mother and baby.

■ ■ ■ Review Questions ■ ■ ■

1. The primary reason for administering Nubain to a woman in active labor is to:
   A. Slow uterine contractions
   B. Relieve nausea and vomiting
   C. Relieve pain
   D. Promote dilation

2. Labor pain in active labor is primarily caused by:
   A. Cervical dilation
   B. Uterine contractions
   C. Fetal descent
   D. Perineal tearing

3. Passenger, as one of the 4 P's of labor, refers to:
   A. The position of the mother
   B. The passage of the vagina
   C. The fetal descent in the pelvis
   D. The fetus

4. Nurses manage the care of patients receiving regional anesthesia:
   A. True
   B. False

5. Supportive activities in labor are:
   A. Interventions ordered by care provider
   B. Techniques used to help women in labor
   C. Derived from adhering to birth plan
   D. Pharmacological interventions

6. An involuntary urge to push is most likely a sign of:
   A. Malposition of the fetus
   B. Transition to active labor
   C. Low fetal station
   D. Imminent delivery

7. False labor is characterized by:
   A. Irregular uterine contractions and cervical change
   B. Back pain that radiates to the lower abdomen
   C. The presence of bloody show
   D. Irregular contractions with no cervical change

8. Women who have a support person with them in labor are more likely to:
   A. Have epidural anesthesia
   B. Have a precipitous labor
   C. Experience fewer birth complications
   D. Experience more interventions

9. A sterile vaginal exam reveals that the woman is 5 cm/80% effaced/0 station. Based on this exam the woman is:
   A. In the transition phase
   B. In the latent phase
   C. In the active phase

10. A common side effect of epidural anesthesia in labor includes:
    A. Maternal hypotension
    B. Maternal hypertension
    C. Variable decelerations in the FHR
    D. Hypertonic labor pattern

References

American Academy of Pediatrics (AAP) and American College of Obstetrics and Gynecology (ACOG). (2006). The Apgar score. *Pediatrics* 117(4), 1444–1447.

American Heart Association (AHA) & American Academy of Pediatrics (AAP). (2006). *Textbook of neonatal resuscitation* (5th ed.) Elk Grove, IL: American Academy of Pediatrics

Angelini, D., & Mahlmeister, L. (2005). Liability in triage: Management of EMTALA regulations and common obstetric risks. *Journal of Midwifery & Women's Health, 50*(6), 472–478.

Association of Women's Health, Obstetric and Neonatal Nurses (AWHONN). (2000a). *Professional nursing support of laboring women.* AWHONN Practice Statement. Washington, DC: Author.

Association of Women's Health, Obstetric and Neonatal Nurses (AWHONN). (2000b). *Nursing management of the second stage of labor.* Evidence-Based Clinical Practice Guideline. Washington, DC: Author.

Association of Women's Health, Obstetric and Neonatal Nurses (AWHONN). (2001a). *Role of the registered nurse in the care of the pregnant woman receiving analgesia/anesthesia by catheter techniques (epidural, intrathecal, spinal, PCEA catheters).* AWHONN Clinical Position Statement. Washington, DC: Author.

Association of Women's Health, Obstetric and Neonatal Nurses (AWHONN). (2001b). *Nursing care of the woman receiving analgesia/anesthesia in labor.* Evidence-Based Clinical Practice Guideline. Washington, DC: Author.

Association of Women's Health, Obstetric, and Neonatal Nurses (AWHONN). (2008). *Fetal heart rate monitoring: Principles and practice* (4th ed.). Washington, DC: Author.

Bar-Yam, N. B. (1994). Learning about culture: A guide for birth practitioners. *International Journal of Childbirth, 9*(2), 8–10.

Buckley, L. (2005). Evidence-based care sheet: *Epidural analgesia in labor & childbirth.* Glendale, CA: Cinahl Information Systems, January 11, 2005.

Chapman, L. (2000). Expectant fathers and labor epidurals. *Maternal Child Nursing, 25,* 133–138.

Cunningham, F., Leveno, K., Bloom, S., Hauth, J., Gilstrap, L., & Wenstrom, K. (2005). *Williams obstetrics* (22nd ed.). New York: McGraw-Hill.

Faucher, M., & Brucker, M. (2000). Intrapartum pain: Pharmacologic management [Clinical Issues: Pharmacology Update in Obstetric and Gynecologic Nursing]. *Journal of Obstetric, Gynecologic, and Neonatal Nursing, 29*(2), 169–180.

Florence, D., & Palmer, D. (2003). Therapeutic choices for the discomforts of labor. *Journal of Perinatal & Neonatal Nursing, 17*(4), 238.

Gupta, J., Holmeyr, G., & Smyth, R. (2006). Position in the second stage of labour for women without epidural anaesthesia. *Cochrane Database of Systematic Reviews* 2004, Issue 1. Art. No.: CD002006. DOI: 10.1002/14651858.CD002006.pub2.

Hodnett, E. (2002). Pain and women's satisfaction with the experience of childbirth: A systemic review. *American Journal of Obstetrics and Gynecology, 186*(5), S160–S172.

Hodnett, E., Gates, S., Hofmeyr, G., & Sakala, C. (2007). Continuous support for women during childbirth. *Cochrane Database of Systematic Reviews* 2007, Issue 3. Art. No.: D003766. DOI: 10.1002/14651858.CD003766.pub2.

Lederman, R. (1986). Maternal anxiety in pregnancy: Relationship to health status. *Annual Review of Nursing Research, 2,* 27–61.

Mackey, C. (1995). Women's evaluation of their childbirth performance. *Maternal-Child Nursing Journal, 23*(2), 57–72.

Martin, J., Hamilton, B., Sutton, P., Ventura, S., Menacker, F., & Munson, M. (2005). Births: Final Data for 2003. *National Vital Statistics Reports, 54*(2). Hyattsville, MD: National Center for Health Statistics.

Mattson, S., & Smith, J. E. (2004). *Core curriculum for maternal-newborn nursing.* (3rd ed.). St. Louis, MO: Elsevier Saunders.

Mayberry, L., Wood, S., Strange, L., Lee, L., Heisler, D., & Neilsen-Smith, K. (2000). *Second-stage labor management: Promotion of evidence-based practice and a collaborative approach to patient care.* Washington, DC: Association of Women's Health, Obstetric and Neonatal Nurses.

Nordgren, S., & Fridlund, B. (2001). Patients' perceptions of self-determination as expressed in the context of care. *Journal of Advanced Nursing, 35*(1), 117–125.

Perla, L. (2002). Patient compliance and satisfaction with nursing care during delivery and recovery. *Journal Nursing Care Quality, 16*(2), 60–66.

Pitter, C., & Preston, R. (2001). Modern pharmacologic methods in labor analgesia. *International Journal of Childbirth Education*, 16(2), 15–19.

Roberts, J. (2002). The 'push' for evidence: Management of the second stage. *Journal of Midwifery & Women's Health, 47*(1), 2–15.

Roberts, J. (2003). A new understanding of the second stage of labor: Implications for nursing care. *Journal of Obstetric, Gynecologic, and Neonatal Nursing, 32*(6), 794–801.

Simkin, P., & Ancheta, R. (2000). *The labor progress handbook: Early intervention to prevent and treat dystocia*. Oxford: Blackwell Science.

Simkin, P., & O'Hara, M. (2002). Nonpharmacologic relief of pain during labor: Systemic reviews of five methods. *American Journal of Obstetrics & Gynecology, 186*(5), S131–S159.

Simpson, K., Creehan, P., & Association of Women's Health, Obstetrics and Neonatal Nurses (AWHONN). (2008). *Perinatal nursing* (3rd ed). Philadelphia: Lippincott Williams & Wilkins.

Spratto, G., & Woods, A. (2006). *2006 PDR nurse's drug handbook*. Clifton Park, NY: Delmar.

Wood, S., & Carr, K. (2003). *The art and science of labor support*. White Plains, NY: March of Dimes.

Fetal Heart Rate Assessment

OBJECTIVES

On completion of this chapter, the students will be able to:

- ☐ Define terms used in electronic fetal monitoring (EFM).
- ☐ Identify the modes of fetal monitoring, auscultation, and EFM.
- ☐ Describe the components of fetal heart rate (FHR) patterns essential to interpretation of monitor strips.
- ☐ Articulate the physiology of FHR accelerations and decelerations.
- ☐ Identify normal and abnormal FHR patterns and correct nursing actions based on monitor strip interpretations.

Nursing Diagnoses

- ☐ Knowledge deficit related to fetal monitoring
- ☐ Impaired fetal gas exchange related to:
  - ☐ Umbilical cord compression
  - ☐ Placental insufficiency
- ☐ Risk of fetal injury related to:
  - ☐ Unrecognized hypoxemia
  - ☐ Hypoxia
  - ☐ Acidemia

Nursing Outcomes

- ☐ The pregnant woman and family will verbalize basic understanding of fetal monitoring.
- ☐ Nursing actions to decrease risk of fetal injury will be initiated if abnormal FHR patterns are present.

INTRODUCTION

This chapter is an introduction to basic electronic fetal monitoring (EFM) concepts. Fetal heart rate (FHR) monitoring was introduced more than three decades ago. It continues to be the primary method for intrapartum fetal surveillance despite concerns about its efficacy and ability to improve neonatal outcomes (Freeman, 2002). EFM is a technique for fetal assessment based on the fact that the FHR reflects fetal oxygenation (Simpson & Creehan, 2008). The goal of fetal monitoring is the ongoing assessment of fetal oxygenation (Feinstein, Torgersen, & Atterbury, 2003). Current practice indicates that EFM is used for virtually all women during labor in the United States. Interpretation of EFM is essential in the assessment of maternal and fetal well-being in antepartal and intrapartal settings. Assessment of FHR in intrapartal period is the focus of this chapter.

Nurses are expected to independently assess, interpret, and intervene related to interpretations of EFM patterns. Assessments and interactions with women and their families are individualized and are geared to providing information and explanation, reduce anxiety, and assisting the woman with breathing and relaxation. Clear and accurate communication with care providers and the perinatal team is essential for optimizing perinatal outcomes.

TERMINOLOGY RELATED TO FETAL ASSESSMENT

Definitions used in this chapter are from the National Institute of Child Health and Human Development (NICHD) Research Planning Workshop (1997) and the 2008 National Institute of Child Health and Human Development Workshop Report on Electronic Fetal Monitoring: Update on Definitions, Interpretation, and Research Guidelines. There is currently a movement to standardize language for FHR interpretation because of variations in language used at present. It is critical for Labor Units to select one set of definitions for FHR patterns for all types of professional communication (Simpson 2004a; AWHONN 2009) (Table 9-1 and Box 9-1).

TABLE 9–1   TERMINOLOGY RELATED TO FETAL HEART RATE ASSESSMENT

TERMINOLOGY	DEFINITION
BASELINE FHR	Mean fetal heart rate (FHR) rounded to increments of 5 beats per minute (bpm) during a 10-minute window, excluding accelerations and decelerations.
BASELINE VARIABILITY	Fluctuations in the baseline FHR that are irregular in amplitude and frequency. The fluctuations are visually quantified as the amplitude of the peak to trough in beats per minute. It is determined in a 10-minute window, excluding accelerations and decelerations. It reflects the interaction between the fetal sympathetic and parasympathetic nervous system. ■ Absent: Amplitude range is undetectable ■ Minimal: Amplitude range is visually undetectable ≤ 5 bpm ■ Moderate: Amplitude from peak to trough 6 bpm to 25 bpm ■ Marked: Amplitude range >25 bpm
ACCELERATIONS	Visually apparent, abrupt increase in FHR above the baseline. The peak of the acceleration is ≥15 bpm over the baseline FHR for ≥15 seconds and <2 minutes. ■ Before 32 weeks' gestation an acceleration is ≥10 beats over the baseline FHR for ≥10 seconds. **Prolonged accelerations** are ≥2 minutes, but ≤10 minutes.
DECELERATION	Transitory decrease in the FHR from the baseline. ■ **Early deceleration** is a visually apparent gradual decrease in FHR below the baseline. The nadir (lowest point) of the deceleration occurs at the same time as the peak of the UC. In most cases the onset, nadir, and recovery of the deceleration are coincident or mirror the contraction ■ **Variable deceleration** is a visually apparent abrupt decrease in the FHR below baseline the decrease in the FHR is FHR is ≥15 bpm lasting ≥15 seconds and <2 minutes in duration ■ **Late deceleration** is a visually apparent gradual decrease of FHR below the baseline. Nadir (lowest point) of the deceleration occurs after the peak of the contraction. In most cases the onset, nadir, and recovery of the deceleration occurs after the respective onset, peak and end of the UC. ■ **Prolonged deceleration** is a visually apparent abrupt decrease in FHR below baseline that is ≥15 bpm lasting ≥2 minutes but ≤10 minutes. ■ **Sinusoidal pattern** is defined as having a visually apparent smooth sine-like wave like undulating pattern in FHR baseline with a cycle frequency of 3–5/min that persists for ≥ 20 minutes
TACHYCARDIA	Baseline FHR of >160 bpm lasting 10 minutes or longer.
BRADYCARDIA	Baseline FHR of <110 bpm lasting for 10 minutes or longer.
NORMAL FHR	FHR pattern that reflects a favorable physiological response to the maternal fetal environment.
ABNORMAL FHR	FHR pattern that reflects an unfavorable physiological response to the maternal fetal environment.

Sources: NICHD (2008); AWHONN (2009), ACOG (2010) Macones et al (2008).

MODES OR TYPES OF FETAL AND UTERINE MONITORING

Auscultation

Auscultation is use of the Doppler or fetoscope (a listening device) to assess the FHR by listening (Fig. 9-1).

■ This method can detect the baseline, rhythm, increase, and decrease in the FHR.

■ This method can only interpret Category I and Category II FHR characteristics as all Category III patterns include assessment of FHR variability not possible with intermittent auscultation (IA).
■ This method is not to be confused with EFM.
   ■ *EFM provides a continuous printout of information on FHR.*
   ■ *Doppler ultrasound and fetoscopes do not provide a continuous printout.*

Research evidence supports the use of intermittent auscultation (IA) as a method of fetal surveillance during labor for low-risk pregnant

BOX 9–1 COMMON ABBREVIATIONS FOR ELECTRONIC FETAL MONITORING

bpm	beats per minute
ED	Early deceleration
EFM	Electronic fetal monitoring
FHR	Fetal heart rate
FSE	Fetal scalp electrode
IA	Intermittent auscultation
IUPC	Intrauterine pressure catheter
LD	Late deceleration
LTV	Long-term variability
MVU	Montevideo units
PD	Prolonged deceleration
STV	Short-term variability
TOCO	Tocodynamometer
VAS	Vibroacoustic stimulation
UC	Uterine contractions
US	Ultrasound
VD	Variable deceleration
VE	Vaginal examination

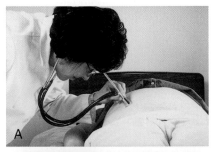

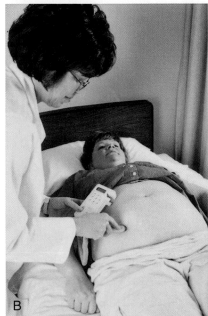

Figure 9-1   Auscultation of fetal heart rate. *A.* Fetoscope. *B.* Doppler ultrasound stethoscope.

women (Lyndon & Ali, 2008; Feinstein, Sprague, & Trepanier, 2008). See Figure 9-6 for Decision-Making in FHR Assessment. Box 9-2 provides the Clinical Position Statement of the Association of Women's Health, Obstetric and Neonatal Nurses (AWHONN) with regard to fetal heart monitoring.

Palpation of Contractions

■ The frequency, duration, tone, and intensity of contractions can be assessed by palpation.
  ■ *Palpation of uterine contractions is done by the nurse placing her fingertips on the fundus of the uterus and assessing the degree of tension as the contractions occur.*
  ■ *The intensity of contractions is measured at the peak of the contraction and are rates as:*
    ▩ Mild or 1+ (easily dented)
    ▩ Moderate or 2+ (can slightly indent)
    ▩ Strong or 3+ (cannot indent uterus)

External Electronic Fetal and Uterine Monitoring

External electronic fetal and uterine monitoring uses an ultrasound device to detect FHR and a pressure device to assess uterine activity (Fig. 9-2 and Box 9-3).

■ The FHR is measured via an ultrasound transducer.
  ■ *External EFM detects FHR baseline, variability, accelerations, and decelerations, but it cannot detect short-term variability (STV).*
■ Contractions are measured via a **tocodynamometer**, an external uterine monitor.
  ■ *The relative frequency, duration of uterine contractions (UCs), and relative resting tone can be measured by this method.*
  ■ *External uterine monitors cannot measure pressure/intensity.*
  ■ *Pressure/intensity of the contraction must be estimated by palpation of contractions.*

Internal Electronic Fetal and Uterine Monitoring

Internal electronic fetal monitoring uses an electrode that is applied to the presenting part of the fetus to directly detect the FHR. A pressure sensor is placed in the uterine cavity and directly measures uterine contractions (Fig. 9-3 and Box 9-4).

BOX 9–2 AWHONN FETAL HEART MONITORING CLINICAL POSITION STATEMENT

The professional organization for perinatal nursing states "AWHONN supports the assessment of the laboring woman and her fetus through the use of auscultation, palpation and/or electronic monitoring techniques .... to assess and promote maternal and fetal well being". AWHONN "does not support the use of EFM as a substitute for appropriate professional nursing care and support of women in labor" (AWHONN, 2008, p. 1).

The policy statement recommends ongoing education in the interpretation of fetal assessment. The policy recommends that guidelines are developed in facilities specifying modes and frequency of fetal assessment as well as policies that address communication and collaboration essential to providing quality care and optimizing patient outcomes.

Source: AWHONN (2008).

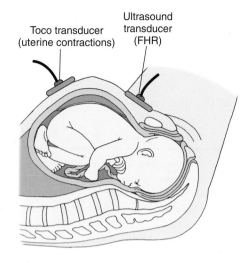

Figure 9-2   External monitoring showing placement of the ultrasound and tocodynamometer.

BOX 9–3   GUIDELINES FOR PLACEMENT OF AN EXTERNAL ELECTRONIC FETAL MONITOR

Explain the procedure to the woman and her family. For example: *"The monitor records your baby's heart rate, uterine contractions, and tells us the baby's response to uterine contractions. We place 2 monitors on your abdomen and secure them with belts. You can move around in bed and we will adjust the monitors."*

FHR	UCs
Use Leopold's maneuver to locate fetal back. Apply ultrasound gel to FHR ultrasound transducer and place it on the woman's abdomen at the location of the fetus's back and move the transducer until clear signal and FHR is heard. Secure with monitor belt.	Place the uterine activity sensor (tocodynamometer) in the fundal area where the contraction feels strongest to palpation. Secure the monitor with a belt.

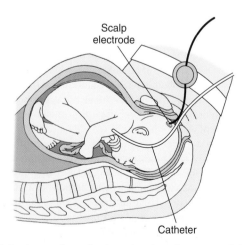

Figure 9-3   Internal monitoring, showing placement of the fetal scalp electrode and intrauterine pressure catheter.

BOX 9–4   GUIDELINES FOR PLACEMENT OF AN INTERNAL ELECTRONIC FETAL MONITOR

Explain the procedure to the woman and her family. For example: *"The internal fetal scalp electrode allows us to directly monitor you baby's heart rate. It is clipped on the babies' scalp with a vaginal exam and the monitor is attached to your leg. You can still move around and go to the bathroom."*
"The intrauterine pressure catheter tells us exactly how strong your contractions are. It is a direct measurement of the pressure of your contractions. It is placed in your uterus with a vaginal exam."

FHR	UCs
Placement of the FSE requires skills and techniques of vaginal examination and EFM as well as risks, limitations and contraindications (primarily preexisting infections such as herpes or HIV). For placement of FSE, a vaginal exam is performed and the guide tube with the electrode is advanced and attached to the presenting part of the fetus.	Placement of an IUPC is an invasive procedure where the nurse should have knowledge and understanding of indications and contraindications and risks of internal monitoring. For placement of the IUPC, the manufacturer directions are reviewed as there are several types of IUPC with different set up guidelines. The IUPC in the guide tube are inserted in the vagina with a vaginal exam and the catheter is advanced through the cervix into the uterus.

- FHR is measured via an internal fetal scalp electrode (FSE).
  - *Internal EFM detects FHR baseline, variability, short-term variability, and long-term variability accelerations, decelerations, and FHR dysrhythmias.*
  - *It is attached to the presenting part of the fetus by the nurse or care provider.*
- Contractions are measured via an **intrauterine pressure catheter (IUPC).**
  - *IUPC provides an objective measure of the pressure of contractions expressed as mm Hg*
  - *IUPC monitoring can detect actual frequency, duration, and strength of UCs and resting tone in mm Hg.*
  - ***Peak pressure*** *is the maximum uterine pressure during a contraction measured with an IUPC.*
  - *The IUPC is inserted by the care provider. Some institutions may have protocols for nurses to insert IUPCs.*
- Monitor paper is used for EFM (Fig. 9-4).
  - *Each dark vertical line represents 1 minute.*
  - *Each lighter vertical line represents 10 seconds.*
  - *FHR is recorded on the top grid of the paper.*
  - *Uterine contractions are recorded on the lower grid.*

AWHONN STANDARDS FOR FREQUENCY OF ASSESSMENT OF FHR

Frequency of FHR assessment is based on assessment of risk status, stage of labor, ongoing clinical assessment (AWHONN, 2008a; Lyndon & Ali, 2009) (Box 9-5).

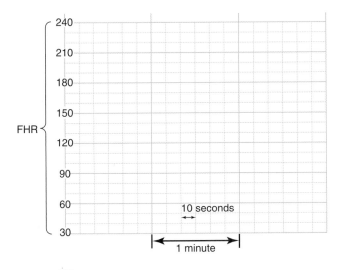

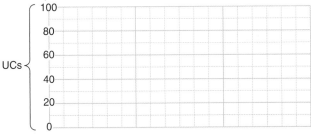

Figure 9-4 Monitor paper indicating timing on grid.

BOX 9–5 AWHONN STANDARDS FOR FREQUENCY FOR FHR ASSESSMENT

Intermittent Auscultation (IA)
■ Absence of risk factors:
  ■ Latent phase every 1 hour
  ■ Active phase every 5-15 minutes
  ■ Second stage every 5-15 minutes
■ Risk factors present:
  ■ Continuous EFM is recommended

This method can only interpret Category I and Category II FHR characteristics as all Category III patterns include assessment of FHR variability not possible with intermittent auscultation (IA).

Electronic Fetal Monitoring (EFM)
■ Absence of risk factors:
  ■ Latent phase every 1 hour
  ■ Active phase every 30 minutes
  ■ Second stage every 15 minutes
■ Risk factors present:
  ■ Latent phase every 30 minutes
  ■ Active phase every 15 minutes
  ■ Second stage every 5 minutes

A full description of the EFM tracing require a qualitative and quantitative description of baseline FHR, variability, accelerations, decelerations, changes in FHR patterns, and uterine contractions.

Sources: AWHONN (2008); Feinstein, Sprague, & Trepanier (2008); Lyndon & Ali (2008).

■ The frequency of assessment increases when:
  ■ *Indeterminate or abnormal FHR characteristics are heard*
  ■ *Before and after rupture of membranes or administration of medication.*
■ When indeterminate or abnormal characteristics are heard, electronic FHR monitoring is used to:
  ■ *Clarify pattern interpretation*
  ■ *Assess variability*
  ■ *Further assess fetal status*
■ In the presence of risk factors continuous EFM is recommended and the FHR should be evaluated:
  ■ *Every 15 minutes in the active phase*
  ■ *Every 5 minutes while pushing*
■ It is common practice for all women to at least have a baseline EFM tracing of at least 20 minutes at the time they are first evaluated in labor.
■ Routine continuous FHR monitoring remains controversial. Refer to Evidence-Based Practice: Continuous Electronic Heart Rate Monitoring for Fetal Assessment During Labor.

Evidence-Based Practice: Continuous Electronic Heart Rate Monitoring for Fetal Assessment During Labor

Thacker, S., Stroup, D., & Chang, M. Continuous Electronic Heart Rate Monitoring for Fetal Assessment during Labor. (Cochrane Review In: The Cochrane Library Issue 1, 2006 Oxford: Update Software)

A review was conducted to compare the efficacy and safety of routine continuous EFM of labor with intermittent auscultation using the results of published randomized controlled trials (RCTs). Nine RCTs were included in the review, including more than 18,000 subjects. None of the nine RCTs demonstrated a statistically significant decrease in the number of births with a 1-minute Apgar score below 4 and perinatal mortality with EFM. A statistically significant decrease was associated with EFM for neonatal seizures. No significant differences were observed in a 1-minute Apgar score below 4-7, rate of admission to neonatal intensive care units, and perinatal deaths. An increase in the rate of cesarean deliveries and operative vaginal deliveries was noted with EFM. The risk of cesarean deliveries was highest in low-risk pregnancies. The reviewers concluded that "the use of routine EFM has no measurable impact on morbidity and mortality." In view of the increase in cesarean sections and operative vaginal deliveries, the benefit of the reduction in neonatal seizures must be evaluated and the decision reached jointly by the woman and care provider as to the use of EFM or IA during labor.

INFLUENCES ON FETAL HEART RATE

An understanding of FHR physiology aids in the interpretation of FHR patterns. The FHR responds to multiple physiological factors. The following sections review the influences on the FHR (Fig. 9-5).

Utero-Placental Unit

At term, about 10% to 15% of maternal cardiac output (600–750 mL) perfuses the uterus per minute. Oxygenated blood from the mother is delivered to the intervillous space in the placenta via the uterine arteries. Maternal–fetal exchange of oxygen, carbon dioxide, nutrients, waste products, and water occurs in the intervillous space across the membranes that separate fetal and maternal circulations. Oxygen and carbon dioxide diffuse across the membranes rapidly and efficiently.

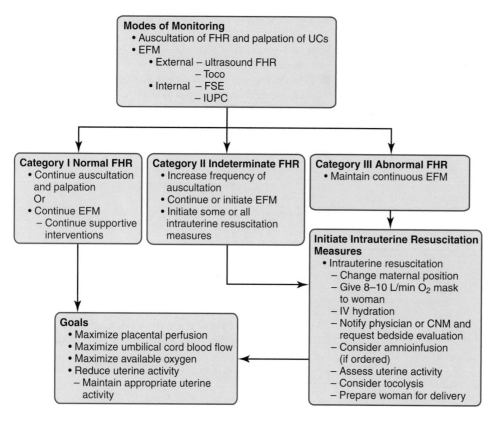

Figure 9-5   Decision-making in FHR assessment.

■ Effective transfer of oxygen and carbon dioxide between fetal and maternal blood streams is dependent on:
  ■ *Adequate uterine blood flow*
  ■ *Sufficient placental area*
  ■ *Unconstricted umbilical cord*
■ Appropriate oxygenation to the fetus depends on:
  ■ *Adequate oxygenation of the mother*
  ■ *Adequate blood flow to the placenta*
  ■ *Adequate uteroplacental circulation*
  ■ *Adequate umbilical circulation*
  ■ *The fetus's own innate ability to initiate compensatory mechanisms to regulate the FHR (Lyndon & Ali, 2008)*
■ Additional factors in the fetal environment that influence fetal oxygenation include:
  ■ *Uteroplacental function*
  ■ *Uterine activity*
  ■ *Umbilical cord issues*
  ■ *Maternal physiological function*
■ Having a basic understanding of the extrinsic influence on FHR, such as normal physiological changes in pregnancy, uterine and placental blood flow, and umbilical blood flow improves the nurse's ability to assess FHR patterns (Feinstein, Torgersen, & Atterbury, 2003).
■ The influences related to labor are discussed in Chapter 10.

Autonomic Nervous System

Parasympathetic Nervous System

■ Parasympathetic stimulation decreases the heart rate.
■ The parasympathetic nervous system is primarily mediated by vagus nerve innervating sinoatrial (SA) and atrioventricular (AV) nodes in the heart.

■ Vagus nerve stimulation slows FHR and helps maintain variability.
  ■ *Variability develops at 28 to 30 weeks of gestation.*

Sympathetic Nervous System

■ Sympathetic nervous system (SNS) stimulation increases the FHR.
■ Nerves are distributed widely in the fetal heart and stimulation produces an increase in strength of fetal heart contraction.
■ SNS is responsible for long-term baseline variability.
■ Action occurs through release of norepinephrine.
■ SNS may be stimulated during hypoxemia.

Baroreceptors

■ Baroreceptors are stretch receptors in the aortic arch and the carotid arch which detect pressure changes
■ They provide a protective homeostatic mechanism for regulating heart rate by stimulating a vagal response and decreasing FHR, fetal blood pressure, and cardiac output

Central Nervous System (CNS)

■ CNS is the integrative center responsible for variations in FHR and baseline variability related to fetal activity
■ CNS regulates and coordinates autonomic activities
■ Mediates cardiac and vasomotor reflexes
■ Responds to fetal movement

Chemoreceptors

■ Chemoreceptors are located in the aortic arch and the central nervous system (CNS).

■ They respond to changes in fetal O_2 and CO_2 and pH levels. Decreased O_2 and increased CO_2 cause peripheral chemoreceptors to stimulate the vagal nerve and slow the heart rate and central chemoreceptors respond to an increased heart rate and an increased blood pressure.

Hormonal Regulation

■ The fetus responds to a decrease in O_2 or uteroplacental blood flow by releasing hormones that maximize blood flow to vital organs such as the heart, brain, and adrenals.

■ Epinephrine, norepinephrine, catecholamines, and vasopressin facilitate hemodynamic changes in response to changes in fetal oxygenation. Fetal hypoxia causes a release of epinephrine and norepinephrine that increases FHR and blood pressure. Vasopressin increases blood pressure in response to hypoxia.

■ Renin–angiotensin secreted by the kidneys produce vasoconstriction in response to hypovolemia.

FETAL RESERVES

Placental reserve describes the reserve oxygen available to the fetus to withstand the transient changes in blood flow and oxygen during labor (Feinstein, Torgesen, & Atterbury, 2003).

■ In a healthy maternal-fetal unit, the placenta provides oxygen and nutrients beyond the baseline needs of the fetus.

■ When oxygen is decreased, blood flow is deferred to vital fetal organs to compensate.

■ When placental reserves of oxygen are decreased or depleted, the fetus may not be able to adapt to or tolerate decreased oxygen that occurs during a labor contraction.

■ Fetal adaptation to the stresses of labor occurs through homeostatic mechanisms.

■ *Prolonged or repeated hypoxemia may deplete reserves resulting in decompensation.*

■ *Interpretation of FHR data requires the ability to differentiate three types of fetal responses:*
  ■ Nonhypoxic reflex responses such as FHR accelerations
  ■ Compensatory responses to hypoxemia, such as variable decelerations
  ■ Impending decompensation responses such as late decelerations (Feinstein, Torgersen, & Atterbury, 2003)

NICHD Criteria for Interpretation of FHR Patterns

A variety of systems and terminology have been used in the interpretation of FHR patterns. The FHR should be interpreted within the context of the overall clinical circumstances. Clinical conditions that impact FHR patterns include gestational age, prior results of fetal assessment, medications, maternal medical conditions, and fetal conditions. FHR patterns are dynamic and transient and require frequent assessment (Fig. 9-6). A careful review of current evidence has resulted in a new recommendation for FHR interpretation in the intrapartum period from NICHD based on a three-tier category system (Critical Component: Three-Tier FHR Interpretation System).

■ Category I FHR tracings are normal. They are strongly predictive of a well oxygenated, nonacidotic fetus with a normal fetal acid–base balance. They may be followed in a routine manner and no action is required

■ Category II FHR tracings are indeterminate. They are not predictive of abnormal fetal acid–base status, yet there is not adequate evidence to classify them as category I or III. They require evaluation and continued surveillance and reevaluation in the context of the clinical circumstances.

■ Category III FHR tracings are abnormal. They are predictive of abnormal fetal acid–base status and require prompt evaluation. Depending on the clinical situation, intrauterine resuscitation should be initiated.

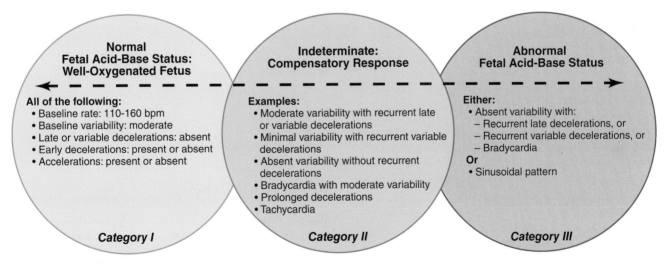

Dynamic Physiologic Response Model

Figure 9-6 Alterations in FHR patterns by dynamic physiologic response.

CRITICAL COMPONENT

Three-Tier FHR Interpretation System

Category I Normal

FHR tracings include **all** of the following:

- Baseline rate 110–160 bpm
- Baseline variability moderate
- Late or variable deceleration absent
- Early decelerations absent or present
- Accelerations absent or present

Category II Indeterminate

FHR tracings include all FHR tracings not categorized as category I or III.
    They include **any** of the following:

- Bradycardia not accompanied by absent variability
- Tachycardia
- Minimal baseline variability
- Absent baseline variability not accompanied by recurrent decelerations
- Marked baseline variability
- Absence of induced accelerations after fetal stimulation
- Recurrent variable decelerations with minimal or moderate variability
- Prolonged decelerations ≥2 minutes but ≤10 minutes
- Recurrent late decelerations with moderate variability
- Variable decelerations with other characteristics such as slow return to baseline "overshoots" or "shoulders"

Category III Abnormal

FHR tracings that are **either**:

- Absent variability with any of the following:
    - Recurrent late decelerations
    - Recurrent variable decelerations
    - Bradycardia
- Sinusoidal pattern

(Macones et al., 2008)

CRITICAL COMPONENT

Older Terminology and Criteria for FHR Assessment: Reassuring and Nonreassuring FHR

Older terminology and criteria for FHR assessment is presented in this box as some clinical agencies may not have changed over to newer terminology.

- **Reassuring FHR** is a normal FHR pattern that reflects a favorable physiologic response to maternal-fetal environment. A reassuring pattern includes:
    - Baseline between 110 and 160 bpm with average variability
    - Presence of accelerations
    - Absence of late or variable or prolonged deceleration
- **Nonreassuring FHR** is an abnormal FHR pattern that reflects an unfavorable physiological response to the maternal–fetal environment. Nonreassuring patterns are associated with adverse neonatal outcomes. Any one of the following signs lasting more than 15 minutes are nonreassuring FHR:
    - Persistent decreased variability
    - Tachycardia when accompanied by decreased variability
    - Persistent decreased variability
    - Persistent late decelerations (>50% of contractions)
    - Recurrent prolonged decelerations
    - Variable decelerations
        - Associated with decreasing variability
        - Variables with slow return of FHR to baseline
        - Variables >70 bpm variables with tachycardia
- **Ominous patterns** are associated with increased risk of fetal academia. These patterns include:
    - Absent variability with:
        - Tachycardia
        - Bradycardia <80 bpm
        - Recurrent late decelerations
        - Recurrent variable decelerations of increasing depth and duration
    - Minimal variability with:
        - Tachycardia with variable or late decelerations
        - Bradycardia with variable or late decelerations
        - Recurrent late decelerations
        - Recurrent variable decelerations of increasing depth and duration.

- Older terminology focusing on reassuring, nonreassuring and ominous FHR patterns may still be used in clinical settings. Refer to Critical Component: Older Terminology and Criteria for FHR Assessment: Reassuring and Nonreassuring FHR.

*F*HR PATTERN INTERPRETATION

Three major areas are assessed when interpreting FHR pattern: FHR baseline, periodic and episodic changes, and uterine activity.

- Interpretation of FHR baseline includes:
    - *Baseline rate*
    - *Baseline variability*
    - *Accelerations*
    - *Tachycardia*
    - *Bradycardia*
    - *Short-term and long-term variability (these are no longer differentiated)*
- Interpretation of periodic and episodic changes includes:
    - *Decelerations (early, variable, late, and prolonged)*

- Interpretation of uterine activity includes:
    - *Frequency*
    - *Duration*
    - *Intensity*
    - *Resting tone*
    - *Relaxation time between UCs*

Baseline Fetal Heart Rate

Baseline FHR is the mean fetal heart rate (FHR) rounded to increments of 5 beats per minute (bpm) during a 10-minute window excluding accelerations, decelerations, or marked variability (Fig. 9-7).

Characteristics

- The normal range is 110 to 160 bpm.

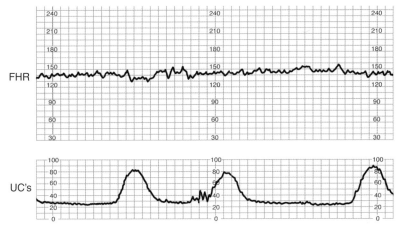

Figure 9-7 Normal fetal heart rate with average variability. *Top.* Fetal heart rate. *Bottom.* Contractions.

CRITICAL COMPONENT

Intrauterine Resuscitation Interventions

When an indeterminate or abnormal FHR pattern is identified, initial assessment may include:

- Perform cervical exam to assess for:
  - Umbilical cord prolapse
  - Rapid cervical dilation
  - Rapid descent of fetal head
- Assess uterine activity for uterine tachysystole.
- Assess maternal vital signs especially:
  - Maternal temperature for maternal fever
  - Maternal blood pressure for hypotension

Interventions for indeterminate or abnormal FHR patterns are referred to as **intrauterine resuscitation**. These interventions maximize intravascular volume, uterine perfusion, placental exchange, and oxygen delivery to the fetus (Lyndon & Ali, 2009; Simpson, 2004b; Simpson & Creehan, 2008; Simpson & James, 2005). Interventions include:

- Maternal position change (left or right lateral) to minimize or correct cord compression and decrease frequency of UCs and improve uterine blood flow
- Administration of IV bolus of fluid of at least 500 mL of lactated Ringer's to maximize maternal intravascular volume and improve uteroplacental perfusion
- Correct maternal hypotension with positioning, hydration, and ephedrine prn

- Administration of O$_2$ at 10 L/min via non rebreather face mask to improve fetal oxygen status
- Reduction of uterine activity if UCs are too frequent, as there may be insufficient time for blood to perfuse placenta.
  - Decrease or discontinue oxytocin.
  - Remove cervical ripening agent, if possible
  - Terbutaline may be used to relax the uterus.
- Amnioinfusion has been used to resolve variable FHR deceleration by correcting umbilical cord compression as a result of oligohydramnios.
  - Amnioinfusion is a procedure in which a saline solution at room temperature is introduced transcervically via an IUPC to correct the FHR decelerations associated with cord compression and/or decreased amniotic fluid (Simpson & Creehan, 2008).
- Alteration in pushing efforts, or stopping pushing, or pushing with every other or every third UC to provide time for fetus to recover when FHR is indeterminate or abnormal during the second stage.
- Support the woman and her family to decrease anxiety or pain, and improve uterine blood flow and maximize oxygenation to fetus.

Abnormal FHR patterns are associated with fetal acidemia.

- The presence of one of the abnormal patterns warrants immediate bedside evaluation by a physician who can initiate a cesarean birth (Simpson, 2008).

Medical Management

- Assess the baseline over a 10-minute period.

Nursing Actions

- Assess baseline over 10-minute period.

Baseline Variability

Baseline variability is the fluctuations in the baseline FHR that are irregular in amplitude and frequency. It is the most important predictor of adequate fetal oxygenation during labor. The fluctuations

are visually quantified as the amplitude of the peak and trough in bpm. Current guidelines from NICHD describe variability as a summation of long-term variability (LTV) and short-term variability (STV) and make no distinction between STV and LTV.

- Cycles portray the peak to trough (rise and fall) of the heart rate within its baseline range over a minute.
- Variability reflects the interaction between the fetal sympathetic and parasympathetic nervous system.
- The presence of variability reflects well functioning and well oxygenated autonomic nervous system and confirms that the fetus is not in metabolic acidosis.

■ **Short term variability** (STV) is the change in the FHR from one beat to the next.
  ■ *STV is measured from the R to R of the intervals of cardiac cycles.*
  ■ *The presence of STV reflects fetal reserves and its presence is a positive sign of fetal well-being.*
  ■ *STV is measured with the use of an internal fetal scalp electrode (FSE).*
  ■ *Current guidelines do not distinguish between LTV and STV*
■ **Long term variability** (LTV) is the changes in FHR range or fluctuations in the FHR baseline.

Characteristics

Variability is described as follows:

■ **Absent:** Amplitude range is undetectable (Fig. 9-8)
■ **Minimal:** Amplitude range undetectable ≤5 bpm (bpm) range (Fig. 9-9)
■ **Moderate:** Amplitude from peak to trough 6 bpm to 25 bpm (Fig. 9-10)
■ **Marked:** Amplitude range greater than 25 bpm (Fig. 9-11)

Causes

■ The FHR is influenced by the autonomic nervous system.
  ■ *The sympathetic system increases the FHR.*
  ■ *The parasympathetic system decreases the FHR.*
  ■ *This push and pull effect produces the moment-to-moment fluctuations in the FHR called variability (Feinstein, Torgersen & Atterbury, 2003).*

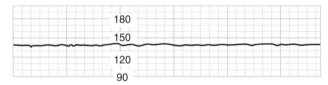

Figure 9-8   Absent variability.

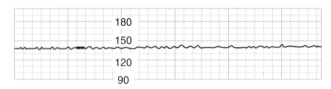

Figure 9-9   Minimal variability.

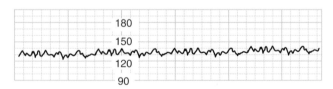

Figure 9-10   Moderate variability.

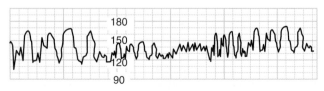

Figure 9-11   Marked variability.

Medical Management

■ Evaluate FHR for abnormal pattern and consider delivery.

Nursing Actions

■ Assess, classify, and document FHR variability.
■ Report decreased variability to care provider.

Fetal Tachycardia

■ Tachycardia may be a sign of early fetal hypoxemia, especially with decreased variability and decelerations.
■ If tachycardia persists above 200 to 220 bpm fetal demise may occur
■ A number of causes of fetal tachycardia, such as maternal fever, do not reflect a risk of acidemia.

Characteristics

■ **Tachycardia** is a FHR above 160 bpm that lasts for at least 10 minutes (Fig. 9-12).
■ It is often accompanied by a decreased or absent baseline variability due to the relationship to the increased parasympathetic and sympathetic tone.

Causes

■ Maternal related causes:
  ■ *Fever*
  ■ *Infection*
  ■ *Chorioamnionitis*
  ■ *Dehydration*
  ■ *Anxiety*
  ■ *Anemia*
  ■ *Medications such as betasympathomimetic, sympathomimetic, ketamine, atropine, phenothiazines, and epinephrine*
  ■ *Illicit drugs*
■ Fetal related causes:
  ■ *Infection or sepsis*
  ■ *Activity/stimulation*
  ■ *Compensatory effort following acute hypoxemia*
  ■ *Chronic hypoxemia*
  ■ *Fetal tachyarrhythmia*
  ■ *Cardiac abnormalities*
  ■ *Anemia*

Medical Management

■ Treat the underlying cause of tachycardia such as antibodies for infection or fluids for dehydration.
■ Consider delivery.

Nursing Actions

■ Assess maternal vital signs (particularly temperature and pulse), as maternal fever and tachycardia increase FHR.
■ Initiate interventions to decrease maternal temperature, if elevated.
  ■ *Give medications as ordered (i.e., antibiotics, antipyretics)*
  ■ *Use ice packs to decrease maternal fever.*

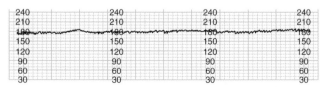

Figure 9-12   Fetal tachycardia.

■ Assess hydration by checking skin turgor, mucous membranes, urine specific gravity, and intake and output.
  ■ *Hydrate the woman by oral intake and/or IV fluids.*
■ Reduce anxiety by explaining, reassuring, and encouraging.
■ Assess FHR variability and consider need for position change or oxygen to promote fetal oxygenation.
■ Decrease or discontinue oxytocin.
■ Notify the physician or midwife.

Fetal Bradycardia

■ **Fetal bradycardia** is a baseline FHR of less than 110 bpm.
■ Unresolved bradycardia may result in fetal hypoxia and needs immediate intervention.
■ A decreased FHR can lead to decreased cardiac output, which causes a decrease in umbilical blood flow that leads to decreased oxygen to the fetus, causing fetal hypoxia.
■ Bradycardia may be tolerated by the fetus if the FHR remains above 80 bpm with variability.
■ Bradycardia with normal variability may be benign.
■ Bradycardia with loss of variability or late decelerations is associated with current or impending fetal hypoxia (NICHD, 1997).
■ Sudden, profound bradycardia is an obstetrical emergency

Characteristics

■ FHR less than 110 bpm for more than 10 minutes (Fig. 9-13).

Causes

■ Maternal related:
  ■ *Supine position*
  ■ *Dehydration*
  ■ *Hypotension*
  ■ *Acute maternal cardiopulmonary compromise*
  ■ *Rupture of uterus or vasa previa*
  ■ *Placental abruption*
  ■ *Medications such as anesthetics and adrenergic receptors*
■ Fetal related:
  ■ *Fetal response to hypoxia*
  ■ *Umbilical cord occlusion*
  ■ *Acute hypoxemia*
  ■ *Late or profound hypoxemia*
  ■ *Hypothermia*
  ■ *Chronic fetal head compression*
  ■ *Fetal bradyarrhythmias*

Medical Management

■ Intervene related to the cause of bradycardia.
■ Consider delivery.

Nursing Actions

■ Confirm if EFM is monitoring FHR versus maternal HR.
■ Assess fetal movement.
■ Assess the fetal response to fetal scalp stimulation. This is done when FHR is between contractions.
■ Perform a vaginal exam and assess for a prolapsed cord.

■ Assess maternal vital signs (especially blood pressure).
■ Assess hydration and hydrate prn to reduce UCs and promote fetal oxygenation
■ Depending on FHR variability and other FHR characteristics consider:
  ■ *Maternal position change (left or right lateral) to promote fetal oxygenation*
  ■ *Discontinuing oxytocin to reduce UCs*
  ■ *Giving oxygen 8 to 10 L/min by mask to promote fetal oxygenation*
  ■ *Modifying pushing to every other contraction or stop pushing until the FHR recovers to promote fetal oxygenation*
  ■ *Supporting the woman and her family*
  ■ *Notifying the physician or midwife*

Minimal or Absent Variability

■ Decreased variability can occur when the fetus is in a sleep cycle.
■ Decreased variability can be significant for the presence of fetal hypoxia or acidosis.
■ Decreased variability in the presence of FHR decelerations is associated with low Apgar scores and acidosis.

Characteristics

■ Minimal or absent variability, less than 0 to 5 bpm (see Figs. 9-8 and 9-9)

Causes

■ Maternal related:
  ■ *Supine hypotension*
  ■ *Cord compression*
  ■ *Uterine tachysystole*
  ■ *Drugs (prescription, illicit drugs, alcohol)*
■ Fetal related:
  ■ *Fetal sleep*
  ■ *Prematurity*

Medical Management

■ Consider artificial rupture of membranes (AROM) for more invasive monitoring (FSE).
■ Manage cause of decreased variability.
■ Consider delivery.

Nursing Actions

■ Change the maternal position to promote fetal oxygenation.
■ Assess fetal response to fetal scalp stimulation or vibroacoustic stimulation (VAS).
■ Assess hydration. Give IV bolus to reduce uterine activity and promote uterine perfusion.
■ Discontinue oxytocin to reduce uterine activity.
■ Deliver oxygen to the woman (8–10 L/min by mask) to promote fetal oxygenation.
■ Consider more invasive monitoring such as internal FSE.
■ Support the woman and her family.
■ Notify the physician or midwife.

Periodic and Episodic Changes

■ **Periodic changes** are accelerations or decelerations in the FHR that are in relation to uterine contractions and persist over time.
■ Periodic changes include accelerations and four types of decelerations: early, variable, late, and prolonged.

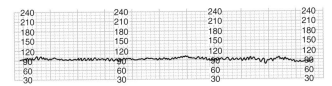

Figure 9-13 Fetal bradycardia.

■ **Episodic changes** are acceleration and deceleration patterns not associated with contractions.

■ Accelerations are the most common episodic change.

Fetal Heart Rate Accelerations

■ The presence of FHR accelerations is predictive of adequate central fetal oxygenation and reflects the absence of fetal acidemia. They identify a well oxygenated fetus and require no intervention. The absence of FHR accelerations, however, does not reliably predict fetal acidemia.

Characteristics

■ **FHR accelerations** are the visually abrupt, transient increases (onset to peak <30 seconds) in the FHR above the baseline (Fig. 9-14).

■ They are 15 beats above the baseline and last from 15 seconds to less than 2 minutes.

■ The peak of the acceleration is ≥15 bpm over the baseline FHR for ≥15 seconds and <2 minutes.

■ Before 32 weeks' gestation, accelerations are defined as acceleration ≥10 bpm or greater over the baseline FHR for ≥10 seconds.

■ Prolonged accelerations are ≥2 minutes, but ≤ 10 minutes.

Causes

■ Sympathetic response to fetal movement

■ Transient umbilical vein compression

Medical Management

■ None

Nursing Actions

■ Record accelerations in the woman's labor chart.

Fetal Heart Rate Decelerations

Fetal heart rate decelerations are transitory decreases in the FHR baseline. They are classified as early, variable, late, and prolonged decelerations.

■ They are classified according to their shape, timing, and duration in relationship to the contraction.

■ Decelerations are defined as **recurrent** when they occur with at least 50% of UCs over a 20-minute period

■ Decelerations are defined as **intermittent** when they occur with fewer than 50% of UCs over a 20-minute period.

Early Decelerations

■ **Early decelerations** are visually apparent, usually symmetrical, with a gradual decrease and return of FHR associated with a UC (Fig. 9-15).

■ They do not occur early or before the contraction starts; thus, this term is something of a misnomer.

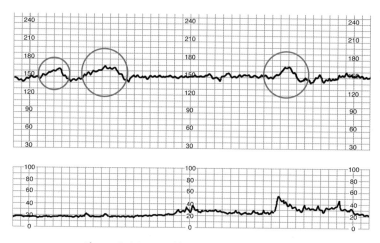

Figure 9-14 Fetal heart rate accelerations.

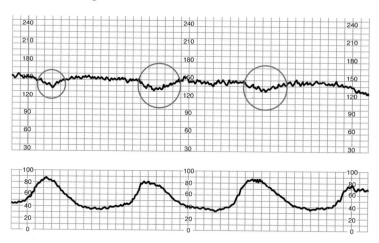

Figure 9-15 Early decelerations.

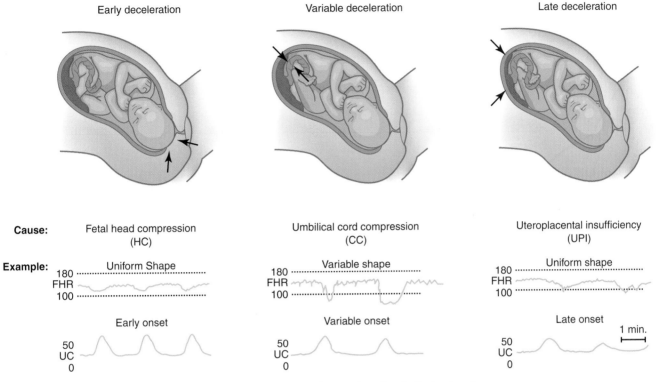

Figure 9-16   Causes and examples of periodic decelerations.

Characteristics

- The **nadir** (the lowest point of the deceleration) occurs at the peak of the contraction.
- Generally the onset, nadir, and the recovery mirror the contraction.

Causes

- When a UC occurs, the fetal head is subjected to pressure that stimulates the vagal nerve
- Fetal head compression resulting in increased intracranial pressure, decreased transient cerebral blood flow, and corresponding decrease in PO_2 with stimulation of cerebral chemoreceptor (Fig. 9-16)

Medical Management

- None

Nursing Actions

- Early decelerations are benign and no intervention is needed.

Variable Decelerations

- A **variable deceleration** is a visually apparent abrupt decrease in the FHR.
- They are the most common decelerations seen in labor
- When variable decelerations persist over time, fetal tolerance is confirmed by the presence of variability or accelerations in the FHR (Feinstein, Torgersen, & Atterbury, 2003).
- An acceleration that precedes or follows the deceleration is a shoulder. It is a compensatory response to hypoxemia and is an increase in the FHR of 20 bpm for <20 seconds.

Characteristics

- They can be periodic or episodic and may vary in duration, depth or nadir, and timing in relation to UCs (Fig. 9-17).
- The decrease in FHR is ≥15 bpm lasting ≥15 seconds and <2 minutes in duration
- The shape can be a U, W, or V.
- The depth of the deceleration is not related to fetal hypoxemia or acidosis.
- They can mimic early or late decelerations.
- An overshoot or rebound overshoot is a gradual smooth acceleration in FHR of 10 to 20 bpm for >60 to 90 seconds.
- Characteristics of normal variable decelerations include:
    - *Duration of <60 seconds*
    - *Rapid return to baseline*
    - *Accompanied by normal baseline and variability*
- Characteristics of indeterminate or abnormal variable decelerations include:
    - *Prolonged return to baseline*
    - *Persistence to less than 60 bpm and >60 seconds*
    - *Presence of overshoots tachycardia*
    - *Repetitive overshoots and absent variability.*

Causes

- Umbilical cord occlusion
- Umbilical cord compression triggers a vagal response that slows the FHR, usually related to decreased cord perfusion.
- This results in initial compression of the umbilical vein (decreased PO_2 and chemoreceptor stimulation) then compression of the more muscular umbilical arteries (fetal hypertension with resultant baroreceptors stimulation; remember that hypertension is often accompanied with a corresponding drop in heart rate) (see Fig. 9-16).

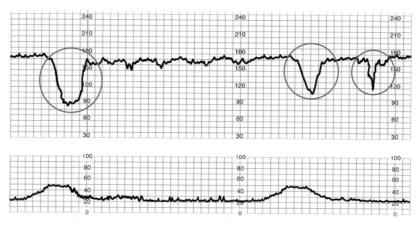

Figure 9-17 Variable decelerations.

■ Prolonged cord compression produces a decrease in PO_2 with direct myocardial depression, adrenal activation, and rebound tachycardia (note: rebound tachycardia does not always occur).

■ Variable decelerations can also occur with sudden descent of the vertex late in active phase of labor (i.e., head compression).

■ These appear different from early decelerations in that they are usually not repetitive nor smooth or regular in shape.

Medical Management

■ Consider amnioinfusion.

■ Consider tocolytics.

■ Consider delivery.

Nursing Actions (See Critical Component: Intrauterine Resuscitation Interventions)

■ Change the maternal position to promote fetal oxygenation.

■ Perform SVE to evaluate cord and labor progress and perform fetal scalp stimulation.

■ Perform amnioinfusion if ordered to alleviate umbilical cord compression by increasing volume of fluid in uterus and thereby correcting umbilical cord compression (Critical Component: Amnioinfusion).

■ Administer O_2 (10 L/min by mask) to promote fetal oxygenation.

CRITICAL COMPONENT

Amnioinfusion

Amnioinfusion is a therapeutic option when there are recurrent variable decelerations as a result of decreased amniotic fluid. During amnioinfusion, room temperature normal saline is infused into the uterus transcervically via an intrauterine pressure catheter to increase intraamniotic fluid to cushion the umbilical cord and reduce cord compression.

   Indications: Variable deceleration

   Contraindications: Vaginal bleeding, uterine anomalies, and active infection

   Careful monitoring of maternal and fetal response is needed; documentation of fluid infused is also important to avoid iatrogenic polyhydramnios.

(Lyndon & Ali, 2008)

■ Decrease or discontinue oxytocin consider need for tocolytic to reduce UCs.

■ Consider more invasive monitoring.

■ Modify pushing.

■ Support the woman and her family to decrease anxiety or pain.

■ Notify the physician or midwife.

■ Plan for delivery and care of the neonate.

Late Decelerations

■ **Late deceleration** is a visually apparent symmetrical gradual decrease of FHR associated with UCs.

■ Late decelerations can be a sign of fetal intolerance to labor.

■ Fetal tolerance of late decelerations is assessed by evaluating the baseline, presence of variability, and the presence of accelerations.

Characteristics

■ Onset is gradual with onset to nadir ≥30 seconds (Fig. 9-18).

■ Nadir (lowest point) of the deceleration occurs after the peak of the contraction.

■ In most cases the onset, nadir, and recovery of the deceleration occurs after the respective onset, peak, and end of the UC.

■ Nadir decreases 10 to 20 bpm and rarely 30 to 40 bpm (Freeman, Garite, & Nageottee, 2003).

Causes

■ Reflect fetal response to transient or chronic uteroplacental insufficiency

■ Related to decreased availability of O_2 because of uteroplacental insufficiency (see Fig. 9-16)

■ Suppression of the fetal myocardium

■ Late decelerations are not completely understood

   ■ *Usually related to placental insufficiency (in which case they are often accompanied by decreased or absent FHR variability)*

   ■ *Late decelerations with moderate variability reflect a compensatory response and are not associated with significant fetal acidemia.*

   ■ *Late decelerations with minimal or absent variability reflect hypoxia and represent a risk of significant fetal acidemia.*

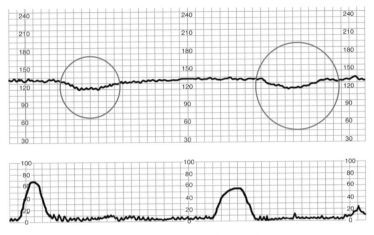

Figure 9-18 Late decelerations.

- *Can be related to aorto-caval compression or obstetrical anesthesia, in which case they are usually accompanied by moderate FHR variability and can be corrected by position change or improving maternal blood pressure. This latter type of late deceleration is sometimes referred to as a "**reflex late deceleration.**"*
- *Fetal hypoxia stimulates chemoreceptors when it is acute (i.e., recently occurring) and if prolonged, results from direct myocardial depression.*
- *Maternal related factors associated with decreased uteroplacental circulation include:*
  - Hypotension from regional anesthesia, supine positioning, or maternal hemorrhage
  - Maternal hypertension, gestational or chronic
  - Placental changes affecting gas exchange such as postmaturity or placental abnormalities
  - Decreased maternal hemoglobin or oxygen saturation from severe anemia or cardiopulmonary disease
  - Uterine tachysystole

Medical Management

- Interventions are directed at causes of late decelerations.
- Consider tocolytics.
- Consider delivery.

Nursing Actions (See Critical Component: Intrauterine Resuscitation Interventions)

- The degree to which the deceleration is abnormal depends on the status and response of the fetus after the deceleration (see Fig. 9-18).
- Change the maternal position to promote fetal oxygenation.
- Discontinue oxytocin (consider terbutaline) to reduce uterine activity.
- Assess hydration. Give an IV bolus to promote fetal oxygenation.
- Consider fetal scalp stimulation or VAS to assess fetal status.
- Administer O_2 (10 L/min by mask) to promote fetal oxygenation.
- Consider more invasive monitoring.
- Support the woman and her family.
- Notify the physician or midwife.
- Plan for delivery and care of the neonate.

Prolonged Decelerations

- **Prolonged deceleration** is a visually apparent abrupt decrease in FHR below baseline that is ≥15 bpm, lasting ≥2 minutes but <10 minutes (see Fig. 9-19).
- Prolonged decelerations that are not recurrent and are preceded and followed by normal baseline and moderate variability are not associated with fetal hypoxemia

Characteristics

- Episodic decelerations that last >2 minutes and <10 minutes
- May be abrupt or gradual

Causes

- May be any mechanism that causes a profound change in the fetal O_2
- Interruption of uteroplacental perfusion
  - *Tachysystole*
  - *Maternal hypotension*
  - *Abruptio placenta*
- Interruption of umbilical blood flow
  - *Cord compression*
  - *Cord prolapse*
- Vagal stimulation
  - *Profound head compression*
  - *Rapid fetal descent*

Medical Management

- Treat the cause of prolonged deceleration.
- Consider amnioinfusion.
- Consider tocolytics.
- Consider delivery.

Nursing Actions (See Critical Component: Intrauterine Resuscitation Interventions)

- Assess baseline variability preceding and following deceleration.
- Change the maternal position to improve fetal oxygenation.
- Discontinue oxytocin (consider terbutaline) to decrease the UCs.

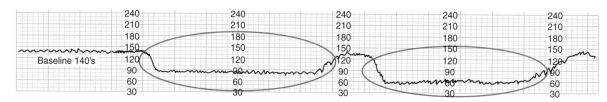

Figure 9-19   Prolonged deceleration.

- Administer O$_2$ to the woman (10 L/min by mask) to promote fetal oxygenation.
- Assess hydration. Give an IV bolus to promote fetal oxygenation.
- Perform SVE to assess labor and cord, and perform scalp stimulation.
- Perform amnioinfusion, if ordered, to alleviate umbilical cord compression.
- Consider more invasive monitoring.
- Support the woman and her family.
- Notify the physician or midwife.
- Plan for delivery and care of the neonate.

Combined Decelerations

- **Combined deceleration** patterns are decelerations that are difficult to classify, such as a variable deceleration that has a late deceleration (Fig. 9-20).
- Interventions performed for one pattern should help to alleviate other patterns.

Characteristics

- Interpretation and assessment of the pattern should be based on the most abnormal pattern.

Causes

- Combined decelerations occur because multiple mechanisms can impact the FHR.
- Combined patterns most frequently occur at the end of the first stage of labor and are associated with tachysystole of the uterus (Feinstein, Torgersen, & Atterbury, 2003).

Medical Management

- Manage the cause of deceleration.

Nursing Actions (See Critical Component: Intrauterine Resuscitation Interventions)

- Interventions are related to the presumed primary cause of the decelerations.
- In combined patterns, the more abnormal pattern defines the interventions used.
- When complex decelerations occur, assessment of FHR baseline, variability, and accelerations is used to evaluate fetal tolerance of labor (Feinstein, Torgerson, & Atturbury, 2003).

Uterine Activity and Contraction Patterns

Uterine activity is an integral part of fetal monitoring interpretation. Interpretation of the FHR pattern is done in concurrence with uterine activity. Interpretation of uterine activity includes assessment of contractions frequency, duration, intensity, and uterine resting tone (Fig. 9-21). Uterine activity can be monitored by palpation or via an IUPC.

- **Frequency of contractions** is determined by counting number of contractions in a 10-minute period, counting from the start of one contraction to the start of the next contraction in minutes. It is recorded in minutes (i.e., frequency of contractions is every 3 minutes).
- **Duration of contractions** is measured by counting from the beginning to the end of one contraction and measured in seconds. Because contractions often vary in their duration, this is often calculated for several contractions and expressed as a range.

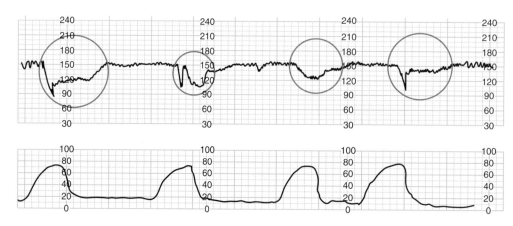

Figure 9-20   Combined deceleration.

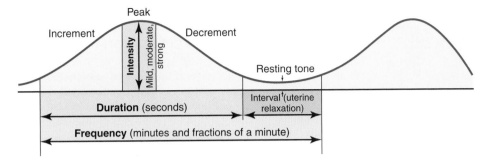

Figure 9-21 Example of contraction frequency, duration, intensity, and resting tone.

- **Intensity** is strength of the contraction and measure by palpation, or internally by an IUPC in mm Hg
- **Resting tone** is the pressure in the uterus between contractions. It is measured by an IUPC when internal fetal monitoring is used or by palpation when an external monitor is used. It is described as the number of mm Hg when the uterus is not contracting when an IUPC is being used and as "soft" if the uterus feels relaxed by palpation.
- **Normal:** 5 or fewer contractions in 10 minutes averaged over a 30-minute window
- **Tachysystole:** More than 5 contractions in 10 minutes over a 30-minute window

Tachysystole

- **Tachysystole** also may be referred to as **hyperstimulation** is excessive uterine activity (Fig. 9-22).
  - *Contraction patterns that may contribute to fetal hypoxia.*
  - *Tachysystole should be treated regardless of fetal response.*
  - *Tachysystole can result in decreased uteroplacental blood flow and result in indeterminate or abnormal fetal heart rate patterns.*

Characteristics of Tachysystole

- More than 5 contractions in 10 minutes
- Contractions lasting 2 minutes or longer

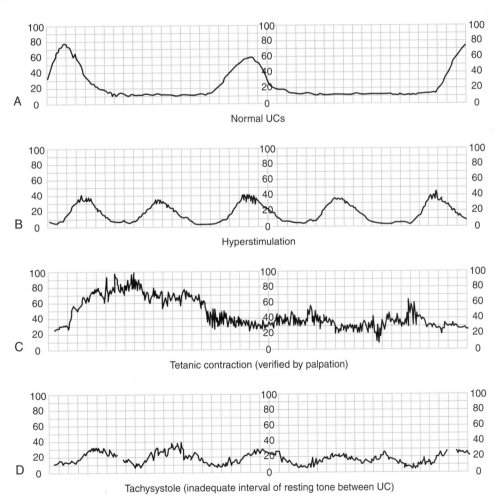

Figure 9-22 Examples of UC patterns. *A.* Normal UCs. *B.* Tachysystole (<5 UCs 10 minutes). *C.* Tachysystole (tetanic contraction verified by palpation). *D.* Tachysystole (inadequate interval of resting tone between UC).

■ Contractions occurring within 1 minute of each other
■ Increasing resting tone greater than 20 to 25 mm Hg, peak pressure greater than 80 mm Hg or Montevideo units greater than 400

Causes

■ Tachysystole can be spontaneous or stimulated labor.
■ Most commonly tachysystole can be caused by medications used for cervical ripening, induction, and augmentation of labor.

Medical Management

■ Manage cause of tachysystole (e.g., discontinuing oxytocin, removing cervical ripening medication). See Chapter 10.

Nursing Actions

■ Reducing uterine activity can be accomplished with a variety of interventions such as the following (these practices are known as intrauterine resuscitation):
  ■ *Changing maternal position*
  ■ *Providing hydration*
  ■ *Using IV fluid bolus*
  ■ *Reducing maternal anxiety or pain*
  ■ *Administering a tocolytic (terbutaline)*
  ■ *Support woman and family*

Assessment of fetal acid–base status is beyond the scope of this chapter on basic FHR interpretation. Monitoring of the preterm fetus and multiple gestations, fetal arrhythmias, and dysrhythmias and sinusoidal pattern is also beyond the scope of this chapter. Resources are cited for more in-depth exploration and advanced concepts in fetal monitoring. Antenatal fetal surveillance and testing is discussed in Chapter 6.

DOCUMENTATION OF ELECTRONIC MONITORING INTERPRETATION-UTERINE ASSESSMENT

Documentation of fetal monitoring consists of the elements described in Critical Component: Assessment and Documentation of Electronic Fetal Monitoring and Uterine Activity (Fig. 9-23).

CRITICAL COMPONENT

Assessment and Documentation of Electronic Fetal Monitoring

FHR	UC
External/ultrasound	External/tocodynamometry
■ FHR baseline ■ Baseline variability ■ Presence of accelerations ■ Periodic or episodic decelerations	■ Frequency ■ Duration ■ Palpate strength of UCs and resting tone
Internal/fetal scalp electrode	Internal/intrauterine pressure catheter
■ FHR baseline ■ Variability (STV/LTV) ■ Presence of accelerations ■ Periodic or episodic decelerations ■ FHR dysrhythmias	■ Frequency ■ Duration ■ Strength of uterine contractions and resting tone (in mm Hg)

FETAL HEART RATE		CONTRACTIONS	
BASELINE VARIABILITY	PERIODIC PATTERN	FREQUENCY In Minutes	INTENSITY
Ab = Absent	L = Late	I = Irregular	M = Mild
Min = ≤5 bpm	V = Variable	∅ = Absent	Mod = Moderate
Mod = 6–25 bpm	E = Early		S = Strong
Mark = >25 bpm	A = Accelerations		
		MONITOR MODE	
		E = External	
	* Refer to DAILY NURSES'	I = Internal	
		D = Doppler	
* Indicates further documentation in DAILY NURSES' NOTES			

Date/Time								
FHR	Monitor Mode							
	Baseline FHR							
	Baseline Variability							
	Periodic Pattern							
Contractions	Frequency							
	Duration							
	Intensity							

Figure 9-23   Example of FHR documentation.

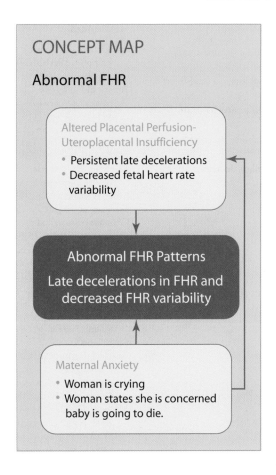

Problem No. 1: Abnormal FHR
Goal: Improve placental perfusion
Outcome: Fetus will remain well perfused and oxygenated.

Nursing Actions

1. Perform cervical exam to assess cord prolapse, rapid cervical dilation, or rapid descent of the fetal head.
2. Assess uterine activity for uterine tachysystole.
3. Assess maternal vital signs, especially temperature, for maternal fever, and blood pressure for hypotension.
4. Change maternal position (left or right lateral).
5. Administer IV bolus of fluid
6. Administer of O$_2$ at 10 L/min via face mask
7. Consider decrease or discontinue oxytocin.
8. Consider use of terbutaline
9. Alteration in pushing efforts, or stopping pushing, or pushing with every other or every third UC to provide time for fetus to recover when FHR is abnormal during second stage.
10. Request an immediate bedside evaluation by a physician or midwife.

Problem No. 2: Anxiety related to harm for fetus
Goal: Decreased anxiety
Outcome: Patient verbalizes that she feels less anxious

Nursing Actions

1. Be calm and normal in interactions with the patient and her family.
2. Explain all procedures and interventions.
3. Explain current fetal status.
4. Assist patient with breathing and relaxation techniques.
5. Encourage the patient and her family to verbalize their feelings regarding concern for fetus
6. Remain with the patient and her family.

■ ■ ■ **Review Questions** ■ ■ ■

1. Which of the following descriptions indicates a normal fetal heart rate:
   A. Baseline rate of 170 bpm, decreased variability, no fetal heart rate decelerations.
   B. Baseline rate of 150 bpm, average variability, accelerations to 170 bpm for 20 seconds.
   C. Baseline rate of 150 bpm, decreased variability, no fetal heart rate decelerations.
   D. Baseline rate of 130 bpm, average variability, decreases after uterine contractions.

2. Potential causes of late decelerations include:
   A. Maternal fever
   B. Umbilical cord compression
   C. Uteroplacental insufficiency
   D. Fetal activity

3. The goal of maternal position changes for an abnormal fetal heart rate is:
   A. Maximizing uterine blood flow
   B. Increasing uterine contractions
   C. Maximizing maternal oxygenation
   D. Increasing maternal movement

4. Assessment of uterine contractions with an intrauterine pressure catheter includes:
   A. Frequency, duration, intensity, and resting tone
   B. Frequency, duration, and intensity
   C. Intensity only
   D. Labor progress

5. Fetal heart rate should be assessed in a low risk woman in active labor:
   A. Every 5 minutes
   B. Every 10 minutes
   C. Every 15 minutes
   D. Every 30 minutes

References

Association of Women's Health Obstetric and Neonatal Nurses Fourth Edition (AWHONN) (2009), *Fetal Heart Monitoring Principles and Practices,* Washington, DC

American College of Obstetrics and Gynecologists (2010), *Management of Intrapartum Fetal Heart Rate Tracing, Practice Bulletin #116,* Obstetrics and Gynecology (116, 5) pg 1232-1240

Feinstein, N., Sprague, A., & Trepanier, M. (2008). *Fetal heart rate auscultation* (2nd ed.) Washington, DC: Association of Women's Health, Obstetric and Neonatal Nurses.

Feinstein, N., Torgersen, K., & Atterbury, J. (2003). *AWHONN's fetal heart monitoring principles and practices* (3rd ed.). Washington, DC: Association of Women's Health, Obstetric and Neonatal Nurses.

Freeman, R. (2002). Problems with intrapartum fetal heart rate monitoring interpretation and patient management. *American College of Obstetricians and Gynecologists, 100*(4), 813–826.

Freeman, R., Garite, T., & Nageottee, M. (2003). *Fetal heart rate monitoring* (3rd ed.). Philadelphia: Lippincott Williams & Wilkins.

Lyndon, A. & Ali, L. U. (Eds.) (2009). *Fetal heart rate monitoring: Principles and practice* (4th ed.). Dubuque, IA: Kendal/Hunt.

National Institute of Child Health and Human Development. (1997). Electronic fetal heart rate monitoring: Research guidelines for interpretation. *Journal of Obstetric Gynecology and Neonatal Nursing, 26*(6), 635–640.

National Institute of Child Health and Human Development Research Planning Workshop. (1997). Electronic fetal heart rate monitoring: Research guidelines for interpretation. *American Journal of Obstetrics and Gynecology, 177*(6), 1385–1390.

Macones, G., Hankins, G., Spong, C., Hauth, J., & Moore, T. (2008). The 2008 National Institute of Child Health and Human Development Workshop Report on Electronic Fetal Monitoring: Update on Definitions, Interpretation, and Research Guidelines. *Journal of Obstetric, Gynecologic and Neonatal Nurses, 37,* 510–515.

Simpson, K. (2004a). Standardized language for electronic fetal heart rate monitoring. *American Journal of Maternal/Child Nursing, 29*(5), 336.

Simpson, K. (2004b). Fetal assessment in the adult intensive care unit. *Critical Care Nursing Clinics of North America, 16,* 233–242.

Simpson, K. (2009). *Cervical ripening and induction and augmentation of labor* (3rd ed., updated). Washington, DC: Association of Women's Health, Obstetric and Neonatal Nurses.

Simpson, K., Creehan, P., & Association of Women's Health, Obstetric and Neonatal Nurses (2008). *Perinatal nursing* (3rd ed.). Philadelphia: Lippincott Williams & Wilkins.

Simpson, K., & James, D. (2005). Efficacy of intrauterine resuscitation techniques in improving fetal oxygen status during labor. *American College of Obstetricians and Gynecologists, 105*(6), 1362–1368.

Thacker, S., Stroup, D., & Chang, M. (2006). *Continuous electronic heart rate monitoring for fetal assessment during labor.* Cochrane Review. The Cochrane Library Issue 1, 2006 Oxford: Update Software

High-Risk Labor and Birth

Nursing Diagnoses

- ■ Risk of maternal injury related to interventions implemented for dystocia
- ■ Risk of maternal injury related to obstetrical emergencies
- ■ Risk of fetal injury related to complications of labor and birth
- ■ Anxiety related to labor and birth complications.

Nursing Outcomes

- ■ The woman will understand the causes of dystocia and interventions to achieve a normal labor pattern.
- ■ The woman will give birth without maternal or fetal injury.
- ■ The woman will give birth to healthy infant without complications.
- ■ The woman verbalizes understanding of the situation and plan of care and uses effective coping methods.

INTRODUCTION

The majority of pregnant women go into labor spontaneously and have a normal labor and spontaneous vaginal birth. However, interventions to initiate or accelerate labor and birth are increasingly common. This chapter presents problems encountered during labor and birth and interventions related to those complications. Nurses have a key role in identification of complications and implementing nursing actions in response to them to improve maternal and neonatal outcomes.

DYSTOCIA

Dystocia is defined as a long, difficult, or abnormal labor. It is diagnosed when there is an alteration in the progress of labor related to cervical dilation and/or descent of the fetus. Dystocia is the most common reason for primary cesarean sections (Queenan, Hobbins, & Spong, 2005). It is associated with the same factors that influence normal labor the 4 P's discussed in Chapter 8:

- ■ **Powers** of labor (uterine contractions [UCs])
- ■ **Passenger** (fetal aspects/position)
- ■ **Passage** (pelvis)
- ■ **Psychological** response of the woman.

Dysfunctional labor is abnormal UCs that prevent the normal progress of cervical dilation or descent of the fetus. Abnormal uterine activity typically has a hypertonic or hypotonic pattern. The American College of Obstetricians and Gynecologists (ACOG, 1995) currently suggests two practical classifications of abnormal labor in the active phase:

- ■ Protraction disorders: Slower than normal labor
- ■ Arrest disorders: Complete cessation of UCs

The primary issues impacting nursing care with regard to dystocia are related to uterine factors, which are described in this chapter. Other factors are presented in Chapter 8. Risk factors for dystocia include:

- ■ Congenital uterine abnormalities such as bicorniate uterus
- ■ Malpresentation of the fetus such as occiput posterior, or face presentation
- ■ Cephalopelvic disproportion
- ■ Tachysystole of the uterus with oxytocin
- ■ Maternal fatigue and dehydration

Want to reinforce your reading? Need to review for a test? Listen to this chapter on your accompanying CD.

- Administration of analgesia or anesthesia early in labor
- Extreme maternal fear or exhaustion, which can result in catecholamine release interfering with uterine contractility.

Hypertonic Uterine Dysfunction

Hypertonic uterine dysfunction is uncoordinated uterine activity. Contractions are frequent and painful but ineffective in promoting dilation and effacement. When this occurs in early labor it may be referred to as **prodromal labor**. Women who experience hypertonic uterine dysfunction are at risk for exhaustion related to the prolonged labor and the fetus is at risk for fetal intolerance of labor and asphyxia related to decreased placental profusion.

Risk Factors

- Nulliparous woman are more subject to abnormal early labor.

Assessment Findings

- Painful, frequent, UCs with inadequate uterine relaxation between UCs with little cervical changes (Fig. 10-1B).
- May be indeterminant or abnormal fetal heart rate (FHR) related to prolonged labor and inadequate uterine relaxation

Medical Management

- Evaluate labor progress.
- Evaluate cause of labor dysfunction.
- Hydrate to improve uterine perfusion and coordination of UCs.
- Provide pain management to allow the woman to sleep and prevent exhaustion.

Nursing Actions

- Promote rest to try to break the pattern of frequent but ineffective UCs. The pattern typically becomes effective when the woman sleeps for a period of several hours and awakens in a normal labor pattern of active labor. Methods used to promote uterine rest are:
  - *Administration of pain medication such as Demerol or morphine as per order to decrease labor contractions and allow the uterus to rest*
  - *Promotion of relaxation*
    - Warm shower or tub bath
    - Quiet environment
    - Minimal interruptions to allow for long period of sleep
- Hydrate the woman with IV or PO fluids if tolerated. Dehydration can result in dysfunctional labor.
- Assess FHR and UCs.
- Evaluate labor progress with a sterile vaginal exam (SVE).
- Inform the woman and family of the progress of labor and explain interventions.
- Inform the care provider of the woman's response and progress in labor.

Hypotonic Uterine Dysfunction

Hypotonic uterine dysfunction occurs when the pressure of the UC is insufficient (IUPC pressure <25 mm Hg) to promote cervical dilation and effacement (Gilbert & Harmon, 2003). Typically, the woman makes normal progress during the latent phase of labor, but during active labor the UCs become weaker and less effective for cervical changes and labor progress (see Fig. 10-1A). The woman is at risk for exhaustion and infection related to the prolonged labor and the fetus is at risk for fetal intolerance of labor and asphyxia.

Risk Factors

- Multiparous women often have more problems in the active phase.
- Extreme fear may result in catecholamine release, interfering with uterine contractility.

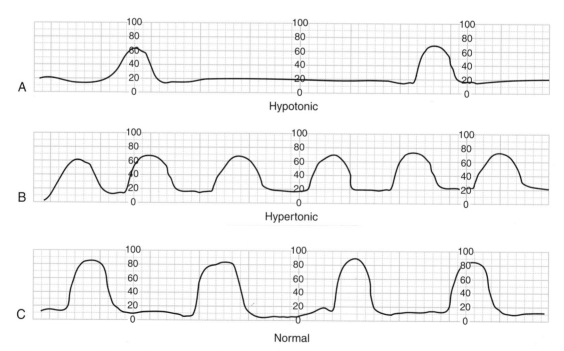

Figure 10-1 Hypertonic versus hypotonic versus normal uterine contractions. *A.* Hypotonic uterine contraction pattern. *B.* Hypertonic uterine contraction pattern. *C.* Normal uterine contraction pattern.

Assessment Findings

- Decreased frequency, strength, and duration of UCs
- Little or no cervical change
  - *Less than 0.5 cm/hr progress in cervical dilation for a primiparous woman in active labor*
  - *Less than 1.0 cm/hr progress in cervical dilation for a multiparous woman in active labor*
- Increased fear and anxiety levels

Medical Management

- Evaluate labor progression.
- Determine the cause of the dysfunction.
- Determine obstetrical interventions:
  - *Augment labor with oxytocin.*
  - *Perform amniotomy.*
  - *Perform cesarean birth when other interventions have failed or when there are signs of fetal intolerance of labor.*

Nursing Actions

- Assess uterine activity.
- Assess maternal and fetal status.
- Stimulate uterine activity to achieve a normal labor pattern using the following methods:
  - *Ambulate and change the position of the woman to promote comfort and labor progress.*
  - *Hydrate with IV or PO as per orders as dehydration can result in dysfunctional labor.*
  - *Administer IV fluids to maximize maternal fluid volume, to correct maternal hypotension and improve placental perfusion.*
  - *Augment labor with oxytocin as per order.*
- Evaluate labor progress with SVE.
- Inform the woman and the family of the progress of labor and explain interventions.
- Provide emotional support. Anxiety levels can increase due to prolonged labor; increased anxiety and fear can interfere with effective UCs.
- Maintain good aseptic technique to minimize the risk of infection if ROM.
  - *Minimize the vaginal exam.*
  - *Maintain perineal cleanliness.*
- Inform the care provider of the woman's response and progress in labor.

Precipitous Labor

Precipitous labor is a labor that lasts fewer than 3 hours from onset of labor to birth. Women who experience a precipitous labor often have higher anxiety and pain levels related to the rapid and intense labor experience. Precipitous labor and/or birth places the woman at risk for postpartum hemorrhage related to uterine atony or lacerations. It places the fetus/neonate at risk for hypoxia and at risk for central nervous system (CNS) depression related to hypoxia from the rapid birth.

Risk Factors

- Grand multiparity
- History of precipitous labor

Assessment Findings

- Hypertonic UCs (tetanic UCs) that are occurring every 2 minutes or more frequently, lasting greater than 60 seconds and strong (Fig. 10-2).
- FHR pattern may be indeterminate or abnormal and nursing actions are based on FHR pattern (see Chapter 9).
- Rapid cervical dilation such that labor is less than 3 hours.

Medical Management

- Prepare for and stand by for precipitous birth.

Nursing Actions

- Remain in the room with the woman since birth is often very rapid with precipitous labor.
- Monitor FHR and UCs every 15 minutes.
- Monitor labor progress and cervical change closely with sterile vaginal exams (SVEs).
  - *Assess the cervix if the woman states she feels pressure or feels like "the baby is coming." It may be a sign of impending birth.*
- Support the woman and the family. This type of labor can be frightening, overwhelming, and painful.
- Anticipate potential maternal postpartum complications such as hemorrhage and lacerations.
- Anticipate potential neonatal complications such as hypoxia and CNS depression related to rapid birth.
- Prepare for delivery

Inadequate Expulsive Forces

Inadequate expulsive forces occur in the second stage of labor when the woman is not able to push or bear-down. It was previously thought that limiting the second stage to 2 hours was essential to decrease fetal morbidity and mortality. It is now known that waiting beyond 2 hours is safe for the fetus and the 2-hour time frame is no longer clinically valid (Simpson & Creehan, 2008).

- The fetus is at higher risk for asphyxia related to prolonged second stage of labor.
- The woman with a prolonged second stage, beyond 4 hours, is at risk for operative vaginal birth and perineal trauma (Simpson & Creehan, 2008).

Risk Factors

- Maternal exhaustion
- Epidural anesthesia because woman may not feel the urge to push

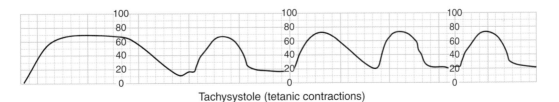

Tachysystole (tetanic contractions)

Figure 10-2 Tetanic uterine contractions.

Assessment Findings

- Inadequate or ineffective pushing with little or no descent of the fetal head with expulsive pushing efforts
- Potential for indeterminate or abnormal FHR

Medical Management

- Evaluate the woman's progress, maternal–fetal status, and likelihood of vaginal birth.
- Augment with oxytocin.
- Assist birth with vacuum or forceps.
- Perform cesarean birth when other interventions are ineffective or signs of fetal intolerance to labor.

Nursing Actions

- Assess fetal descent.
- Evaluate fetal response to expulsive pushing.
- Facilitate the second stage of labor by doing the following:
  - *Coaching the woman in bearing-down efforts*
  - *Minimizing the Valsalva maneuver (by using open glottis push strategies)*
  - *Maintaining adequate pain relief for the woman with labor epidurals*
  - *Changing the maternal position to a more upright position to facilitate fetal descent*
  - *Supporting the woman's involuntary pushing efforts*

Fetal Dystocia

Fetal dystocia may be caused by excessive fetal size, malpresentation, multifetal pregnancy, or fetal anomalies. The fetus can move through the birth canal most effectively when the head is flexed and is presenting anterior to the woman's pelvis (occiput anterior position). This allows the smallest diameter of the fetal head to enter the maternal pelvis and the most flexible part of the fetal body, the back of the neck, to adapt to the curve of the birth canal. When the fetal position is other than flexed and vertex or the fetus is large in comparison to the maternal pelvis, labor may be difficult and vaginal birth a challenge. Complications of fetal dystocia are:

- Neonatal asphyxia related to prolonged labor
- Fetal injuries, such as bruising
- Maternal lacerations
- Cephalopelvic disproportion (CPD) (Critical Component: Cephalopelvic Disproportion)

CRITICAL COMPONENT

Cephalopelvic Disproportion (CPD)

Cephalopelvic disproportion is a condition in which the size, shape, or position of the fetal head prevents it from passing through the lateral aspect of the maternal pelvis or when the maternal pelvis is of a size or shape that prevents the descent of the fetus through the pelvis. A diagnosis of CPD often necessitates a cesarean birth. CPD can rarely be diagnosed until labor has progressed for some time.

The success of any labor depends on the complex interrelationship of several factors:

- Fetal size, presentation, and position
- Size and shape of the maternal pelvis
- Quality of the UCs

Risk Factors

- Abnormal fetal presentation or position such as face, brow, or breech (Table 10-1)
- Fetal anomalies, such as hydrocephalus, and/or any other fetal anomaly that interferes with fetal descent through the birth canal
- Fetal macrosomia; birth weight greater than 4500 g

Assessment Findings

- FHR may be heard above the umbilicus versus in the lower uterine segment; this is a sign that the fetus may be in position other than vertex.
- The SVE reveals a buttocks or face when malpresentation is the cause of dystocia.
- The presenting part is not engaged in the maternal pelvis.
- There is no fetal descent through the pelvis.

Medical Management

- Confirm the fetal position with vaginal exams and ultrasound.
- Determine the type of obstetrical interventions such as use of vacuum extractor, forceps, or need for cesarean birth.

Nursing Actions

- Perform Leopold's maneuver as described in Chapter 8 to determine the fetal position.
- Assess the location of the FHR.
- Assess the fetal position with SVE.
- Alert the primary care provider if there is any question regarding fetal presentation, position, or absence of fetal descent.

Pelvic Dystocia

Pelvic dystocia is related to the contraction of one or more of the three planes of the pelvis. During the prenatal period, the care provider determines the general pelvic size and configuration by vaginal examination. Pelvic measurements are not typically done; instead, descent and engagement of fetal head in labor indicate adequate pelvic inlet. A key point in the outcome of labor is dependent on the interrelationship of the size and shape of the pelvis, fetal size, presentation and position, and quality of the UCs (see Critical Component: Cephalopelvic Disproportion).

The three contractions of the pelvic planes are:

- Inlet contraction occurs when the widest part of the pelvis is small.
- Midpelvis contraction related to prominent ischial spines, convergent pelvic side walls, and a narrow sacrosciatic notch may result in arrest of descent of the vertex.
- Outlet contraction can be estimated by measuring the transverse diameter of the pelvis. Normally, the anteroposterior diameter is 14 cm.

Risk Factors

- Small pelvis
- Abnormal pelvic shape

Assessment Findings

- Delayed descent of fetal head

TABLE 10–1 MALPRESENTATION OF THE FETUS

MALPRESENTATION	DESCRIPTION	IMPLICATIONS
OCCIPUT POSTERIOR	The occiput of the fetus is in the posterior portion of the pelvis rather than the anterior. As the fetus moves through the birth canal, the occiput bone presses on the woman's sacrum. Rotation of fetal head may occur during fetal descent	Prolonged labor and prolonged second stage Severe back pain
FACE PRESENTATION	Fetal head is in extension rather than flexion as it enters the pelvis	Labor and pushing may be prolonged. Cesarean delivery may be indicated. The neonate's face may have extensive bruising.
BROW PRESENTATION	Fetal head presents in a position midway between full flexion and extreme extension. This causes the largest diameter of the head to engage in the pelvis	Prolonged second stage of labor.
SHOULDER PRESENTATION/ COMPOUND PRESENTATION	Shoulder presentation: The fetal spine is vertical to the maternal pelvis. Compound presentation: One or more fetal extremities accompany the presenting part.	Higher risk of prolapsed cord. Cesarean delivery is typically indicated.

Continued

TABLE 10–1 MALPRESENTATION OF THE FETUS—CONT'D

MALPRESENTATION	DESCRIPTION	IMPLICATIONS
BREECH PRESENTATIONS		
Frank breech	Frank breech: Thighs flexed alongside body, feet are close to the head	Dysfunctional labor Fetal injury Increased risk of prolapsed cord Typically cesarean birth is indicated
Complete breech	Complete breech: One or both knees are flexed.	
Footling breech (single)	Footling breech: Either one (single footling) or both (double footling) feet present before the buttocks.	
Footling breech (double)		

Medical Management

■ Evaluate the pelvis for contraction of one or more of the planes of the pelvis.
■ Evaluate the descent and engagement of the fetal head.

Nursing Actions

■ Perform SVE to evaluate the progress of labor and fetal descent.

LABOR INTERVENTIONS

The majority of pregnant women go into labor spontaneously at term (37–42 weeks gestation) and progress through the labor and birth experience without complications. Increasingly, the approach to labor has shifted from a natural process to one that should be "managed" by the woman, nurse, and care provider. Management of labor has resulted in an increase in labor interventions including induction of labor (which may also include cervical ripening) and augmentation to speed up labor. This section reviews interventions to induce (initiate) and augment (strengthen) labor.

Labor interventions are medically indicated when either the condition or safety of the woman or fetus would be improved with birth. Because spontaneous labor is associated with fewer complications than induced labor, induction of labor without a medical indication is discouraged.

Despite risks to the woman and fetus (such as increased rates of cesarean birth), labor interventions such as elective induction are at an all-time high. Because of the potential risks associated with induction of labor, elective induction should be undertaken only after fully informing the woman of risks and benefits and establishing a gestational age of 39 weeks or greater. The nurse providing care for the woman during cervical ripening, induction, or augmentation of labor should be aware of the indications, actions, expected results, and potential risks of each agent. Before any agent is used, maternal status and fetal well-being should be established and cervical status should be assessed and documented (Simpson, 2009).

Labor Induction

Induction of labor is the deliberate stimulation of UCs before the onset of spontaneous labor. According to the National Center for Health Statistics, the rate of induction of labor has increased significantly during the past 15 years from an induction rate of 9.5% in 1990 to 22.3% in 2005, more than a 100% increase (Martin et al., 2007). The nurse may face a dilemma when women are admitted for induction or cervical ripening without documented indications for the induction. It is the nurse's responsibility to ensure that the woman is fully informed by her provider before beginning a procedure (Simpson, 2009; Simpson & Creehan, 2008).

Induction of labor is a complex intervention that leads to a "cascade of interventions" that typically include:

■ Intravenous (IV) fluids
■ Bed rest
■ Continuous electronic fetal monitoring
■ Increased pain medication use and epidural anesthesia
■ Amniotomy
■ Prolonged stay in the labor unit (Simpson, 2009; Simpson & Atterbury, 2003; Simpson & Creehan, 2008)

A number of methods of induction of labor have been proposed as effective in initiating labor. When the decision has been made to induce labor, the next important question raised is how to induce labor. When deciding on the method of induction of labor, certain clinical factors are considered, including:

■ Parity
■ Status of membranes: Ruptured or intact
■ Status of the cervix: Favorable or unfavorable
■ History of previous cesarean births

All these factors or clinical situations are thought to be important to a provider in making the decision about which method of labor induction should be used. Labor induction is thought to be less successful when the cervix is unfavorable (not ripe). It is more successful in parous women than in nulliparous women. Little attention has been given to the combination of these factors, which may be important to women and clinicians when attempting to make informed decisions about induction of labor (Kelly, Alfirevic, Hofmeyr, Kavanagh, Neilson, & Thomas, 2009).

Oxytocin Induction

A pharmacological method for induction of labor is administration of oxytocin. Oxytocin is the most common induction agent used worldwide to initiate labor. It has been used alone, in combination with amniotomy, or after cervical ripening with other pharmacological or nonpharmacological methods. Before the introduction of prostaglandin agents, oxytocin was used as a cervical ripening agent as well.

■ Endogenous oxytocin is a peptide synthesized by the hypothalamus that is transported to the posterior lobe of the pituitary gland, where it is released in the maternal circulation in response to vaginal and cervical stretching. The release of oxytocin stimulates UCs.
■ Synthetic oxytocin is identical to endogenous oxytocin.
■ Considerable controversy exists related to dose and rate increase intervals when oxytocin is used for induction of labor.

There was a trend to use higher doses of oxytocin termed "active management of labor" (Box 10-1). This dosing regimen is based on research

---

BOX 10–1 PRINCIPLES OF ACTIVE MANAGEMENT OF LABOR

The original research on active management of labor included only nulliparous women in spontaneous, active labor (O'Driscoll, Jackson, & Gallagher, 1970). The following is the summary of their findings:
■ True labor was defined as UCs with either bloody show, spontaneous rupture of membranes, or 100% cervical effacement.
■ Women received 1:1 labor care from the midwife or nurse.
■ Amniotomy was preformed if membranes did not rupture spontaneously once labor was diagnosed.
■ If cervical dilation did not proceed at 1 cm/hour, oxytocin was administered at beginning at 6 mU/min and increasing by 6 mU/min every 15 minutes until adequate labor was established (maximum dose 40 mU/min).

The principles of active management have not been shown to decrease the cesarean birth rate in the United States.

conducted in the 1970s in Dublin, Ireland. However, current evidence supports lower dose infusions (Simpson, 2002), with research reporting more successful vaginal births, fewer operative vaginal deliveries, and less tachysystole and lower cesarean birth rates. Continued increases in oxytocin rates over a long period during induction can result in oxytocin receptor desensitization or down-regulation, making oxytocin less effective in producing normal UCs (Simpson & Creehan, 2008).

Indications

- Post-term pregnancy
- Pregnancy-induced hypertension
- Preclampsia/eclampsia
- Maternal medical conditions (e.g., diabetes mellitus, renal disease, chronic pulmonary disease, chronic hypertension)
- Premature rupture of membranes
- Chorioamnionitis
- Fetal compromise (such as fetal growth restriction)
- Fetal demise
- History of rapid labors/distance from the hospital
- Psychosocial considerations

Contraindications

- Any contraindications for vaginal birth (Critical Component: Contraindications for Augmentation or Induction of Labor)

CRITICAL COMPONENT

Contraindications for Augmentation or Induction of Labor

- Complete placenta previa or vasoprevia
- Abnormal fetal position
- Umbilical cord prolapse
- Previous vertical (classical) uterine scar or prior transfundal uterine scar
- Active genital herpes
- Pelvic abnormalities

Risks Associated with Inductions

- Tachysystole leading to indeterminate or abnormal FHR pattern is the primary complication of oxytocin in labor (Critical Component: Tachysystole).
- Side effects of oxytocin use are primarily dose related; tachysystole and subsequent FHR decelerations are common side effects (ACOG, 1999) (Critical Component: Administering Oxytocin in Labor).
- Water intoxication can occur with high concentrations of oxytocin with large quantities of hypotonic solutions but usually only with prolonged administration with at least 40 mU/min.

Assessment Findings

- The woman understands the indication for induction.
- Assessment findings and prenatal records reflect an indication for induction.

Medical Management

- Advise of indication for induction of labor and order induction of labor as per institutional protocol.
- Be available to respond to complications.

CRITICAL COMPONENT

Tachysystole

Tachysystole, sometimes referred to as hyperstimulation, is excessive uterine activity and is the most concerning side effect of oxytocin because it can result in a progressive adverse effect on fetal status (Simpson & Creehan, 2008) (Fig. 10-3). UCs cause an intermittent decrease in blood flow in the intervillous space where oxygen exchange occurs. The decreased intervillous blood flow associated with tachysystole leads to decreased oxygen to the fetus (Simpson & Creehan, 2008). Tachysystole can result in progressive deterioration in fetal status and hypoxemia that result in an abnormal fetal heart rate. Tachysystole may result in abruptio placenta or uterine rupture, which are rare complications (ACOG, 1999).

Tachysystole is defined as:

- Five or more UCs in 10 minutes over a 30-minute window
- A series of single UCs lasting 2 minutes or longer
- UCs occurring within 1 minute of each other

Nursing actions for tachysystole with normal FHR pattern:

- Maternal repositioning
- IV fluid bolus of at least 500 mL of lactated Ringer's solution
- Decrease rate of oxytocin infusion by at least half if no response to above measures.
- Discontinue oxytocin if the pattern persists.

Nursing actions for tachysystole with an indeterminate or abnormal FHR pattern would also include (Lyndon & Ali, 2008):

- Maternal repositioning
- IV fluid bolus of at least 500 mL of lactated Ringer's solution
- Decrease rate of oxytocin infusion by at least half
- Discontinue oxytocin if pattern persists
- Maternal position change
- O$_2$ at 10 L/min by mask
- Notify the provider.
- Consider terbutaline if no response to above measures.

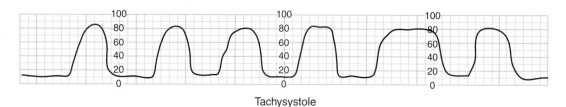

Tachysystole

Figure 10-3 Uterine tachysystole (hyperstimulation).

CRITICAL COMPONENT

Administering Oxytocin in Labor

- Oxytocin is administered intravenously and is piggybacked to a mainline IV solution at the port most proximal to the venous site (Fig. 10-4).
- Oxytocin is *always* infused via a pump.
- There is variation in the concentrations of oxytocin, and it should be prepared by the pharmacy, as it is a high-alert medication.
- Typical concentrations are:
  - 10 units of oxytocin in 1000 mL of lactated Ringer's result in an infusion rate of 1 mU/min = 6 mL/hr.
  - 20 units of oxytocin in 1000 mL of lactated Ringer's result in an infusion rate of 1 mU/min = 3 mL/hr.
- Current dose recommendations are for low-dose oxytocin starting at 0.5 mU/min and increasing the dose by 1–2 mU/min every 30–60 minutes until adequate labor progress is achieved (i.e., cervical effacement or cervical dilation of 0.5–1 cm/hr) and regular UCs every 2–3 minutes lasting 45–60 seconds.
- Nursing responsibilities during oxytocin infusion involve careful titration of the drug to the maternal and fetal response.
  - The titration process includes decreasing dosage rates or discontinuing infusion when UCs are too frequent.
  - Discontinuing oxytocin when FHR is abnormal (Simpson, 2009; Simpson & Creehan, 2008).
  - Increasing doses when UCs are inadequate; however, the lowest possible dose should be used to achieve labor progress (Simpson & Atterbury, 2003).
- Once active labor is established oxytocin should be discontinued to avoid downregulation
- Maternal–fetal response to oxytocin is the primary consideration (Simpson & Creehan, 2008).
  - Avoid tachysystole because it frequently results in indeterminate or abnormal fetal heart rate pattern.
  - Continuous EFM is typically used with oxytocin administration.
  - In the absence of risk factors intermittent auscultation is permitted with evaluation of FHR and UCs at least every 30 minutes in active labor and every 15 minutes in the second stage.
  - For indeterminate or abnormal FHR pattern interventions include the following actions:
    - Change maternal position.
    - Initiate IV hydration.
    - Administer O₂ by mask at 10 L/min.
    - Decrease or discontinue oxytocin.
    - If decreasing dose, dose should be lowered by half.
    - Notify the provider and request bedside evaluations for abnormal FHR.

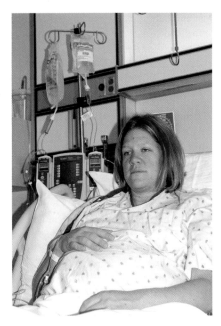

Figure 10-4 Intravenous oxytocin administration.

Nursing Actions

- Review prenatal record with woman indication for induction of labor
- Administer low-dose oxytocin starting at 0.5 mU/min (current dose recommendations) and increase the dose by 1 to 2 mU/min every 30 to 60 minutes (see Critical Component: Administering Oxytocin in Labor).
- In the absence of risk factors evaluate and document FHR at least every 30 minutes in active labor and every 15 minutes in the second stage via intermittent auscultation or electronic fetal monitoring (EFM).
- In the presence of risk factors continuous EFM is recommended and FHR should be evaluated and documented every 15 minutes in active labor and every 5 minutes in the second stage
- Monitor strength, frequency, and duration as an indicator of oxytocin efficacy.
- Evaluate uterine resting tone by palpation or IUPC pressure below 20 mm Hg to ensure uterine relaxation between contractions.
- Decrease or discontinue oxytocin in the event of uterine tachysystole or indeterminate or abnormal fetal status. The current recommendation when decreasing oxytocin is to lower the dose by half.
- Assess FHR in response to UCs (see Chapter 9).
- For indeterminate or abnormal FHR pattern interventions include the following actions:
  - *Change maternal position.*
  - *IV bolus of at least 500 mL of lactated Ringer's*
  - *Administer O₂ by mask at 10 L/min.*
  - *Decrease or discontinue oxytocin.*
  - *Notify the provider and request a bedside evaluation if the FHR is abnormal.*
- Monitor labor progress with SVE.
- Assess the character and amount of amniotic fluid
- Assess the character and amount of bloody show
- Assess the maternal response including level of discomfort and effectiveness of pain management and labor support.

■ Assess input and output (I&O) for fluid overload; output should mirror intake.

Cervical Ripening

The cervix, composed of connective tissue, is typically closed until labor begins. At the onset of labor it undergoes rapid changes including ripening, effacement, and dilation (Fig. 10-5). Cervical ripening is the process of physical softening and opening of the cervix in preparation for labor and birth. Because cervical status is the most important predictor of successful induction of labor, cervical status is assessed before induction of labor. Typically, cervical status is assessed via the Bishop score (Table 10-2). A score of 6 or more is considered favorable for successful induction of labor.

If the cervix is not ripe (a Bishop score of less than 6) and it is medically indicated that the labor needs to be induced, a mechanical or pharmacological cervical ripening agent may be used. These agents can also sometimes stimulate labor.

Mechanical Cervical Ripening

Mechanical cervical ripening methods are devices that are inserted through the vagina and into the cervix to dilate the cervix. These methods have a lower risk of tachysystole compared to pharmacological methods. Examples of mechanical cervical ripening methods are:
■ Laminaria, lamicil, or dilapan
  ■ *These materials expand by absorbing fluid from the cervical tissues and cause the cervix to dilate and release local prostaglandin.*
■ Balloon catheters
  ■ *The balloon is inflated after insertion into the cervix and causes pressure on the cervix and lower uterine segment and the release of prostaglandin.*

Indications

■ When the woman has little or no cervical effacement (Simpson, 2002)

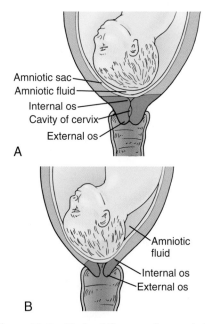

Amniotic sac
Amniotic fluid
Internal os
Cavity of cervix
External os
A

Amniotic fluid
Internal os
External os
B

Figure 10-5   Unripe (*A*) versus ripe cervix (*B*).

■ When pharmacological methods are contraindicated, such as women with prior uterine incision

Risks Associated with Mechanical Cervical Ripening

■ The infection rate is higher.

Assessment Findings

■ The cervix is unripe based on SVE and Bishop score.
■ Prenatal record reflects indications for induction.

Medical Management

■ The physician or midwife places the mechanical dilators, which usually stay in place for 6 to 12 hours before being removed by the care provider.

Nursing Actions

■ Assess onset of UCs.
■ Assess FHR.
■ Assess maternal temperature, as the woman is at higher risk for infection.
■ Assess for rupture of membranes and vaginal bleeding.
■ Record the type of dilator and number of dilators or the size of the balloon placed.
■ Assess maternal and fetal status as per institutional policy.

Pharmacological Methods of Cervical Ripening

Pharmacological methods of cervical ripening in preparation for induction of labor may use one of a variety of hormonal preparations (Table 10-3). These preparations, which are placed in or near the cervix, produce cervical ripening by causing softening and thinning of the cervix. Occasionally these agents can stimulate labor contractions. A review of research on the use of prostaglandins concluded there is an improvement in labor stimulation in vaginal birth rates in 24 hours, no increase in operative birth rates, and significant improvements in cervical favorability within 24 to 48 hours when using prostaglandins (Kelly, Kavanagh, & Thomas, 2003).

Indications

■ See indications for induction.

Risks Associated with Pharmacological Methods of Cervical Ripening

■ Tachysystole of the uterus (see Critical Component: Uterine Tachysystole)

Assessment Findings

■ Unripe cervix based on SVE and Bishop score of less than 6
■ Prenatal record reflecting indication for induction

Medical Management

■ Determine the need for cervical ripening.
■ Insert the pharmacological agent.
  ■ *Administration of the agent should be done at or near the labor and birthing unit.*

Nursing Actions

■ Evaluate the prenatal record for indications and contraindications for induction (see Critical Component: Contraindications to Augmentation and Induction of Labor)

TABLE 10–2   BISHOP SCORE TO ASSESS CERVICAL RIPENESS

SCORE	DILATION (CM)	EFFACEMENT (%)	STATION	CONSISTENCY	POSITION OF CERVIX
0	Closed	0–30	–3	Firm	Posterior
1	1-2	40–50	–2	Medium	Midposition
2	3-4	60–70	–1, 0	Soft	Anterior
3	≥5	≥80	+1, +2	–	–

Source: Bishop (1964).

TABLE 10–3   PHARMACOLOGICAL CERVICAL RIPENING AGENTS

MEDICATION	Prepidil PGE$_2$ (Dinoprostone Gel)	Cervidil (Dinoprostone Insert)	Misoprostol PGE$_1$ (Cytotec)
DOSE	0.5 mg gel is placed below cervical os with speculum exam, can be repeated every 6 hours × 3 doses	10 mg controlled released vaginal insert with string for removal after 12 hours	25 mcg inserted in the posterior vaginal fornix. A recent review reports the possibility of rare but serious adverse events, particularly uterine rupture, with misoprostil use. *Oral administration is not recommended. Further research is needed to establish the ideal route of administration and dosage, and safety. (Hofmeyr & Gülmezoglu, 2003)
NURSING ACTIONS	Woman should remain recumbent for 30 minutes after dose. Continuous FHR and UC monitoring for 30 minutes–2 hours after dose Oxytocin should be delayed for 6–12 hours after dose	Woman should remain supine or lateral position for 2 hours after insert. Continuous FHR and UC monitoring while medication is in place and for 15 minutes after removal Oxytocin should be delayed for 30–60 minutes after removal	Continuous FHR and UC monitoring. Oxytocin should be delayed until at least 4 hours after last dose
CONTRAINDICATIONS	Previous cesarean section or uterine scar	Previous cesarean section or uterine scar	Previous cesarean section or uterine scar
ACTIONS	Uterine activity within 1 hour and peak dose 4 hours; tachysystole can occur within 1 hour in up to 5% of patients.	UCs after 5–7 hours, tachysystole can occur within 1 hour in up to 5% of patients. Remove if tachysystole or indeterminate or abnormal FHR.	Wide variations in onset of UCs. Peak action 1–2 hours. Tachysystole more common with misoprostol than with prostaglandins or oxytocin

Source: Simpson (2009).

■ Document baseline cervical exam with SVE.
■ Monitor FHR and uterine activity as indicated based on medication and institutional policies.

Stripping the Membranes

Stripping the membranes is digital separation of the chorionic membrane from the wall of the cervix and lower uterine segment during a vaginal exam done by a primary care provider to stimulate labor. The exact mechanism of action is unclear but it is commonly believed it releases prostaglandins and also may cause maternal oxytocin release. It is most effective in first-time pregnancies with an unripe cervix. However, there is little scientific evidence of the efficacy of stripping the membranes.

■ The procedure is usually done in the care providers' office.
■ The care provider is responsible for explaining the procedure and its risks.
■ The FHR should be assessed before and after the procedure.
■ The woman might experience some spotting after the procedure.
■ The woman might experience mild cramping immediately after the procedure.

Indications

■ See indications for oxytocin induction.

Risks Associated with Stripping of the Membranes

■ Infection
■ Bleeding from undiagnosed placental problem
■ Unplanned rupture of membranes (ROM)

Assessment Findings

■ Intact membranes
■ Presenting part engaged

Medical Management

■ Stripping the membranes is done by the primary care provider during a SVE by inserting a finger into the cervix and sweeping the finger around the cervix to separate the membrane from the cervix.

Amniotomy

Amniotomy is the artificial rupture of membranes (AROM). The membranes are ruptured with an amnihook during a SVE (Fig. 10-6).

■ Amniotomy is most typically used to augment or shorten labor but may also be used to induce labor. There is insufficient evidence to support the value of this as a sole intervention for induction (Bricker & Luckas, 2000).
■ This procedure is done by the primary care provider.
■ It is most effective in multiparous women who are dilated to 2 cm or more
■ Amniotomy in early labor increases the risk of cesarean birth for abnormal FHR.

Indications

■ To stimulate labor

Contraindications

■ Fetal head not engaged in the maternal pelvis

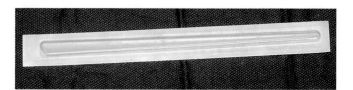

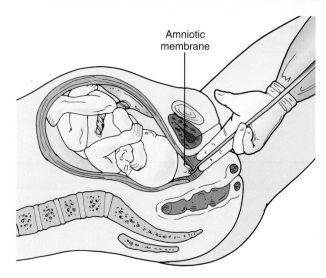

Figure 10-6   Amnihook and AROM procedure.

Risks Associated with Amniotomy

■ Intra-amniotic infection
■ Umbilical cord prolapse when presenting part is not engaged
■ Bleeding from undiagnosed placental abnormality
■ Severe variable decelerations

Assessment Findings

■ The woman leaks amniotic fluid vaginally.

Medical Management

■ The procedure is done by the primary care provider with a SVE when head is engaged in the pelvis.

Nursing Actions

■ Assess the FHR before and after the amniotomy because of the risk of umbilical cord prolapse.
■ Offer comfort and support to the woman, as the procedure may be uncomfortable.
■ Assess the color, amount, and odor of amniotic fluid.
■ Document the time of the AROM.
■ Assess maternal temperature every 4 hours.
■ Administer pericare, as the woman continues to leak fluid after AROM.
■ Typically nurses do not perform an amniotomy. There may be individual institutional policies allowing nurses to perform AROM under specific criteria.

Labor Augmentation

Wide variations in labor progress and duration occur among women in labor and there is no consensus among experts as to the appropriate length of labor. Many providers believe there is benefit to decreasing the length of labor through augmentation with oxytocin (Simpson, 2002). The rate of augmentation of labor has increased 50% over the last decade, to a current rate of at least 18% (Martin et al., 2006). Generally, maternal–fetal status and individual clinical situations are the basis for labor management decisions.

Labor augmentation is the stimulation of ineffective UCs after the onset of spontaneous labor to manage labor dystocia. All of the principles of oxytocin induction apply to the use of oxytocin for augmentation of labor.

Lower doses of oxytocin are required for augmentation of labor because cervical resistance is lower in women in labor who have some cervical effacement and dilation. This may not be indicated in induction protocols, as some protocols have been influenced by research on active management of labor (see Box 10-1).

Indications

■ To strengthen and regulate UCs
■ To shorten the length of labor

Contraindications

■ See Critical Component: Contraindications for Induction or Augmentation of Labor.

Risks Associated with Augmentation

■ Tachysystole leading to an indeterminate or abnormal FHR pattern is primary complication of oxytocin in labor (see Critical Components: Tachysystole).

Assessment Findings

■ Prolonged labor
■ Inadequate UCs and inadequate labor progress

Medical Management

■ Determine the need for labor augmentation.
■ Be available to respond to complications of use of oxytocin in labor for augmentation.

Nursing Actions

■ Administer low-dose oxytocin starting at 0.5 mU/min and increasing the dose by 1–2 mU/min every 30–60 minutes as recommended.
■ Monitor FHR and UCs. FHR and UCs are typically continuously monitored but intermittent monitoring is within the standard of care (see Chapter 9).
■ Follow the same principles of nursing care for induction of labor (see Critical Component: Tachysystole and Critical Component: Administering Oxytocin in Labor).
■ Decrease or discontinue oxytocin in the event of uterine tachysystole or indeterminate or abnormal fetal heart rate.

OPERATIVE VAGINAL DELIVERY

Operative vaginal delivery is a vaginal birth that is assisted by a vacuum extraction or forceps. Since 1996, the rate of cesarean birth has increased and the percentage of operative vaginal deliveries with either forceps or vacuum extraction has decreased 45% over 10 years, from 9.4% to 5.2% (Martin et al., 2006). Indications for operative

vaginal delivery are to improve maternal or fetal status by shortening the second stage of labor. Facilitating birth and shortening the second stage of labor can be performed only by care providers with hospital privileges for these procedures. Although sometimes indicated, operative vaginal birth is not without risk of complications to the woman and the fetus. Specific guidelines for the use of forceps and vacuum extraction are provided and use of only one method, either forceps or vacuum, for an individual patient is recommended. If attempts are unsuccessful, the physician proceeds with a cesarean birth

Vacuum-Assisted Delivery

Vacuum-assisted delivery or vacuum extraction is a birth involving the use of a vacuum cup on the fetal head to assist with delivery of the fetal head (Fig. 10-7). The cup is placed on the fetal head and suction is increased gradually until a seal is formed. Gentle traction is then applied to deliver the fetal head (Fig. 10-8).

The rate of vacuum-assisted delivery, which had increased by 77% between 1989 (3.5%) and 1997 (6.2%), has since decreased by one third, to 4.1% for 2004 (Martin et al., 2006). Some advantages to the use of vacuum over forceps include:

■ Easier application
■ Less anesthesia required
■ Less maternal soft tissue damage
■ Fewer fetal injuries

Current guidelines for vacuum application are:

■ The fetal head needs to be engaged and the cervix completely dilated.
■ There should be a maximum of three attempts for a period of 15 minutes: The "three-pull rule."
■ Cup detachment from the fetal head (pops off of the vacuum) is a warning sign that too much pressure or ineffective force is being exerted on the fetal head.
■ The physician should proceed with a cesarean birth when vacuum attempts are not successful.

Indications

■ Suspicion of immediate or potential fetal compromise
■ Need to shorten the second stage for maternal benefit

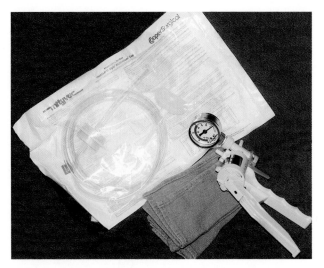

Figure 10-7 Vacuum device.

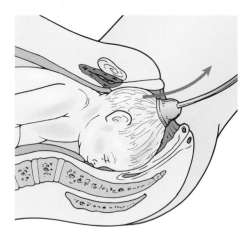

Figure 10-8   Vacuum delivery.

■ Prolonged second stage
  ■ *Nulliparous woman with lack of continuing progress for 3 hours with regional anesthesia, or for 2 hours without anesthesia*
  ■ *Multiparous woman with lack of continuous progress for 2 hours with regional anesthesia, or for 1 hour without regional anesthesia (ACOG, 2000)*

Risks for the Woman

■ Vaginal and cervical lacerations
■ Extension of episiotomy
■ Hemorrhage related to uterine atony, uterine rupture
■ Bladder trauma
■ Perineal wound infection

Risks for the Newborn

■ Cephalohematoma (15%) and increased risk of jaundice (Fig. 10-9)
■ Intracranial hemorrhage and retinal hemorrhage
■ Scalp lacerations or bruising (10%)

Assessment Findings

■ Fetus at 36 weeks' gestation and the fetal head is engaged, at least at 0 station in the maternal pelvis (Cunningham et al., 2005).

Medical Management

■ Explain the procedure and obtain the woman's consent.
■ Place the vacuum appropriately.
■ After three unsuccessful attempts, proceed with a cesarean birth.

Nursing Actions

■ Assess the woman's comfort level.
■ Educate and reassure the woman and her family.
■ Anticipate potential complications for the woman and the newborn.
■ Pump up the vacuum pump manually to the pressure indicated on the pump, not to exceed 500 to 600 mm Hg.
■ Pressure should be released between contractions.
■ The vacuum procedure should be timed from insertion of the cup into the vagina until the birth and the cup should not be on the fetal head for longer than 15 to 20 minutes (Simpson & Creehan, 2008).
  ■ *Adherence to the guidelines for the vacuum device related to pressure and maximum time will minimize the nurse's liability in vacuum-assisted vaginal births.*

Forceps-Assisted Delivery

Forceps-assisted birth is one in which an instrument is used to assist with delivery of the fetal head, typically done to improve the health of the woman or the fetus. The rate of forceps delivery has decreased over the last 20 years from 5.55% to only 1.1% (Martin et al., 2006). Outlet forceps are used when the head is visible on the perineum and the skull has reached the pelvic floor, and rotation is less than 45 degrees (Fig. 10-10). Low forceps is used when the skull is at +2 station or lower in the maternal pelvis and not on the pelvic floor and rotation is greater than 45 degrees (ACOG, 2000) (Fig. 10-11). Only outlet and low forceps are currently recommended for use in assisting delivery.

Indications

■ The fetal head engaged and the cervix is completely dilated.
■ There is suspicion of immediate or potential fetal compromise.
■ To shorten the second stage for maternal benefit (e.g., maternal exhaustion and/or fetal compromise)
■ Prolonged second stage
  ■ *Nulliparous woman with lack of continuing progress for 3 hours with regional anesthesia, or for 2 hours without anesthesia*
  ■ *Multiparous woman with lack of continuous progress for 2 hours with regional anesthesia, or for 1 hour without regional anesthesia.*
■ High level of regional anesthesia that inhibits pushing
■ Maternal cardiac or pulmonary disease that contraindicates pushing efforts

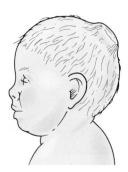

Figure 10-9   Cephalohematoma.

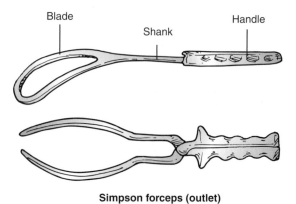

Simpson forceps (outlet)

Figure 10-10   Outlet forceps.

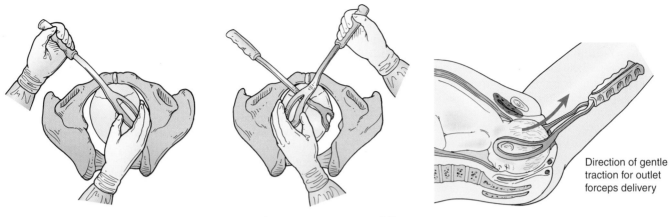

Direction of gentle traction for outlet forceps delivery

Figure 10-11 Forceps delivery.

Risks for the Woman

- Vaginal and cervical lacerations
- Extension of episiotomy
- Hemorrhage related to uterine atony, uterine rupture
- Perineal hematoma
- Bladder trauma
- Perineal wound infection

Risks for the Newborn

- Cephalohematoma
- Nerve injuries including craniofacial and brachial plexus injuries
- Skin lacerations or bruising
- Skull fractures
- Intracranial hemorrhage

Assessment Findings

- The cervix is completely dilated and the membranes are ruptured.
- The fetal head is engaged.
- The woman has adequate anesthesia.

Medical Management

- Use only on a fetus that is at least 36 weeks' gestation.
- Explain the procedure and obtain the woman's consent.
- Place forceps appropriately.

Nursing Actions

- Assess the woman's anesthesia level and comfort level.
- Insert a straight catheter to empty the bladder to decrease the risk of bladder trauma and increase room for the fetal head and forceps.
- Provide emotional support for the woman and her partner, since use of forceps can increase the anxiety level.
- Document the type of forceps, number of applications, and time of application.
- Anticipate potential complications for the woman and the neonate.

OPERATIVE BIRTH

Cesarean birth is a common operation performed on women, with reported rates varying across the world (Fig. 10-12). In developed countries, cesarean birth accounts for 21.3% of births in the

United Kingdom; 23% in Northern Ireland; 23.3% in Australia; 30.2% in the United States; and more than 50% in some private hospitals in Chile, Argentina, Brazil, and Paraguay (Viswanathan et al., 2006). The benefits and harms of elective cesarean birth, repeat cesarean birth, and vaginal birth after cesarean (VBAC) are under vigorous debate. Because cesarean birth accounts for 30.2% of births in the United States, Chapter 12 is devoted to care of cesarean woman and their families.

Vaginal Birth After a Cesarean

Vaginal birth after a cesarean (VBAC) is used to describe labor and vaginal birth in a woman who has had a prior cesarean birth. This is sometimes referred to a trial of labor after cesarean or TOLAC. Evidence suggests that benefits of VBAC outweigh risks in women with lower uterine transverse cesarean birth who have no contraindications for a vaginal birth. Benefits of VBAC include shorter recovery time and overall lower morbidity and mortality, including less blood loss, fewer infections, and fewer thromboembolic problems (ACOG, 2004). According to ACOG, most women with one previous cesarean birth with a low transverse incision are candidates for

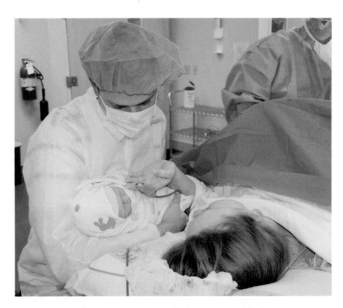

Figure 10-12 Family in cesarean birth.

vaginal birth after cesarean birth and should be counseled about VBAC and offered a trial of labor (ACOG, 2004). However, VBAC rates have fallen 67% since 1996 (Martin et al., 2006). This is reported to be related to more conservative ACOG practice guidelines, legal pressure, and the continuing debate over the harms and benefits of vaginal birth compared with cesarean birth and an increase in repeat cesarean births. Regardless of the reason for the previous cesarean birth, once a woman has had a cesarean birth there is a more than 90% chance that subsequent deliveries will be by cesarean (Martin et al., 2006). VBAC is associated with a small but important risk of uterine rupture, and that risk increases with the number of previous cesarean births.

Indications

- One or two prior low transverse cesarean births with no other uterine scars
- Clinically adequate pelvis
- Physician and OR team immediately available to perform emergent cesarean birth.

Contraindications

- Prior vertical (classical) or T-shaped uterine incision or other uterine surgery (Fig. 10-13)
- Previous uterine rupture
- Pelvic abnormalities
- Medical or obstetric complications that preclude a vaginal birth
- Inability to perform an emergent cesarean birth if necessary because of insufficient personnel such as surgeons, anesthesia, or facility
- Two prior uterine scars and no vaginal births

Risks Associated with VBAC

- Uterine rupture and complications associated with uterine rupture (1%)
  - *Waiting for spontaneous labor and avoiding use of prostaglandins and oxytocin reduces the risk of uterine rupture*

Assessment Findings

- Records confirm prior transverse uterine scar.

Medical Management

- Explain the risks and benefits of VBAC.
- The physician and surgical team must be available to perform a cesarean birth if necessary.

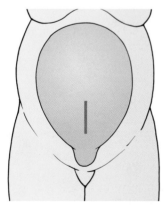

Figure 10-13   Vertical uterine incision.

Nursing Actions

- Review the prenatal record for documentation of prior uterine scar because VBAC is contraindicated in vertical uterine incisions.
- Monitor closely and continuously uterine activity and FHR (Simpson & Creehan, 2008).
- Assess the progress of labor.
- Provide information, reassurance, and support to the woman.
- Report any complaints of severe pain and be alert to signs of uterine rupture such as vaginal bleeding and ascending station of fetal presenting part.

POST-TERM PREGNANCY

A **post-term pregnancy** is one that has a gestational period of 42 completed weeks or more from the first day of the last menses (if the menstrual cycle is 28 days). The actual cause of post-term pregnancy is unclear; the etiology and pathophysiology are not completely understood (Gilbert, 2007). For 5% to 10% of pregnant women, their pregnancies continue beyond 294 days (42 completed weeks) and are described as being "post-term" or "postdate" (Cunningham et al., 2005). Both the woman and infant are at increased risk of adverse events when the pregnancy continues beyond term. After 41 weeks, neonatal and postneonatal death risk increase significantly (Gülmezoglu, Crowther, & Middleton, 2006).

Obstetric problems associated with post-term pregnancy include:

- Induction of labor with an unfavorable cervix
- Cesarean birth
- Prolonged labor
- Postpartum hemorrhage
- Traumatic birth

It is likely that some of these unwanted outcomes result from intervening when the uterus and cervix are not ready for labor.

First-trimester pregnancy ultrasound is associated with a reduced incidence of post-term pregnancy, possibly by avoiding incorrect dating and misclassification of postdates. Induction of labor is widely practiced to try to prevent the problems mentioned above and to improve the health outcome for women and their infants.

- Labor induction may itself cause problems, especially when the cervix is not ripe.
- The ideal timing for induction of labor is not clear. In the past, there was a tendency to await spontaneous labor until 42 completed weeks.
- Current practice is to induce labor between 41 and 42 weeks.

The gestational age and the cervix being unfavorable (unripe) may affect the success of the induction of labor and result in an increase in cesarean birth rates.

- When the cervix is favorable (usually a Bishop score of 6 or more), induction is often carried out via oxytocin and AROM.
- If the cervix is not favorable, usually a prostaglandin gel or tablet is placed in the vagina or cervix to ripen the cervix and to initiate the UCs and labor. Many protocols are used with varying repeat intervals and transition to oxytocin and amniotomy depending on the onset of UCs and progress of cervical dilatation.

Risks Associated with Post-term Pregnancy

- Prolonged pregnancy causes a decrease in amniotic fluid volume and may impact fetal status because amniotic fluid cushions the fetus and cord from pressure and injury and amniotic fluid volume is an indicator of placental function.

■ As the placenta begins to age, there are increased areas of infarction and deposition of calcium and fibrin within its tissue. This creates decreased placental reserve (Fig. 10-14).

■ Meconium-stained fluid occurs in 25% to 30% of post-term pregnancies. This creates an increased risk for meconium aspiration of the neonate at birth (Cunningham et al., 2005).

■ There is an increased risk of fetal macrosomia as the fetus increases in size approximately 1 ounce per day after term.

Assessment Findings

■ Indeterminate or abnormal FHR related to decreased amniotic fluid and uteroplacental insufficiency with aging placenta
■ Meconium-stained fluid
■ Women report increased anxiety and frustration with prolonged pregnancy
■ Fetal macrosomia

Medical Management

■ Antenatal surveillance
■ Induction of labor

Nursing Actions

■ Review the plan of care with the woman.
■ Confirm post dates on the prenatal record.
■ Anticipate management with induction of labor and possible cervical ripening agents.
■ Monitor FHR because of increased incidence of uteroplacental insufficiency.
■ Assess amniotic fluid for amount and meconium staining with ROM (Concept Map for post-term pregnancy and labor induction).

OBSTETRICAL EMERGENCIES

Obstetrical emergencies are urgent clinical situations that place either the maternal or fetal status at risk for increased morbidity and mortality. Intrapartum emergencies may be related to one or more maternal,

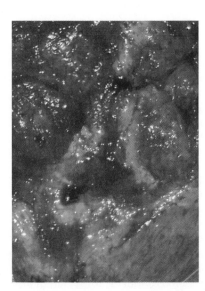

Figure 10-14 Calcified placenta are white areas in placenta.

fetal, uterine, cord, and/or placental factors. The physiological effects of intrapartum emergencies on the woman and fetus may create rapid deterioration in oxygenation and perfusion. Intrapartum emergencies may place the woman and fetus at risk of exceeding their oxygen and perfusion reserves (Curran, 2003). Interventions are directed to stabilization of maternal status, which in turn stabilizes fetal status.

Shoulder Dystocia

Shoulder dystocia refers to difficulty encountered during delivery of the shoulders after the birth of the head. The anterior shoulder or more rarely both shoulders become impacted above the pelvic rim. The first sign is a retraction of the fetal head against the maternal perineum after delivery of the head, sometimes referred to a **turtle sign**. This impaction of the fetal shoulders may lead to a prolonged delivery time of more than 60 seconds. Shoulder dystocia is an obstetric emergency that can result in serious fetal morbidity and even mortality if not recognized and successfully managed. Neonatal morbidity includes:

■ Brachial plexus injuries
■ Clavicle fracture
■ Neurological injury
■ Asphyxia
■ Death

Reduction in the interval of time from delivery of the head to the body is crucial to fetal outcome. Most experts note that more than a 5-minute delay in head to body interval may result in fetal acidosis (Simpson & Creehan, 2008). The incidence of shoulder dystocia ranges from reports of 0.6% to 1.4% (ACOG, 2002). Most cases of shoulder dystocia cannot be accurately predicted or prevented (Cunningham et al., 2005; Simpson & Creehan, 2008).

Risk Factors Associated with Shoulder Dystocia

■ Fetal macrosomia
■ Maternal diabetes
■ History of shoulder dystocia
■ Prolonged second stage
■ Excessive weight gain
■ Postdates pregnancy

Risks Associated with Shoulder Dystocia

■ Delay in delivery of the shoulders results in compression of the fetal neck by the maternal pelvis which impairs fetal circulation and results in possible increased intracranial pressure, anoxia, asphyxia, and brain damage.
■ Brachial plexus injury and clavicle fracture in the neonate can also occur.
■ Maternal complications include lacerations, infection, bladder injury, or postpartum hemorrhage.

Assessment Findings

■ The first sign is a retraction of the fetal head against the maternal perineum after delivery of the head, sometimes referred to as turtle sign.
■ Delay in delivery of shoulders after delivery of head.

Medical Management

■ Downward traction may be applied to the fetal head with suprapubic pressure.
■ Extend the midline episiotomy to obtain room for maneuvers.

- The McRoberts maneuver is a reasonable initial approach.
- The Woods corkscrew maneuver progressively rotates the posterior shoulder 180 degrees to disimpact the anterior shoulder.
- Deliver the posterior shoulder by sweeping the posterior arm across the fetus' chest followed by delivery of the arm.
- Most shoulder dystocias are resolved by using the above maneuvers.
- The Zavanelli maneuver is cephalic replacement into the pelvis and then cesarean delivery, for catastrophic cases only (ACOG, 2002).
- Planned cesarean birth to prevent shoulder dystocia may be considered for suspected fetal macrosomia with an estimated fetal weight exceeding 5000 grams in women without diabetes and 4500 grams in women with diabetes (ACOG, 2002).

Nursing Actions

- Explain the situation to the woman and the family and explain the interventions to resolve dystocia and importance of woman's assistance with maneuvers.
- Request assistance, as additional nurses may be needed to implement maneuvers to resolve dystocia.
- Insert a straight catheter to woman to empty the bladder if it is distended to make more room for the fetus.
- A variety of techniques may be used to free the impacted shoulder from beneath the symphysis pubis; suprapubic pressure can be applied (Fig. 10-15). Apply pressure directly behind pubic bone or laterally to the pubic bone to dislodge anterior shoulder and push it beneath the symphysis.
- The McRoberts maneuver consists of sharply flexing the thigh toward the maternal abdomen to straighten the sacrum (Fig. 10-16).
- Use of fundal pressure is controversial and not indicated in shoulder dystocia.
- Notify the neonatal team.
- Prepare for neonatal resuscitation.
- Document the series of interventions and clinical events with time intervals (Simpson & Creehan, 2008).

Prolapse of the Umbilical Cord

Prolapse of the umbilical cord is when the cord lies below the presenting part of the fetus (Fig. 10-17). The cord may prolapse in front of the presenting part, into the vagina, or through the introitus. **Occult prolapse** is when the cord is palpated through the membranes but does not drop into the vagina. When cord prolapse occurs it is typically with AROM or SROM when the presenting part is not

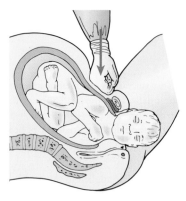

Figure 10-15   Suprapubic pressure.

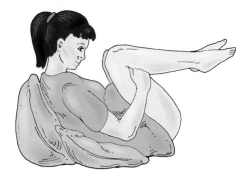

Figure 10-16   McRoberts maneuver.

engaged in the pelvis. The cord becomes entrapped against the presenting part and circulation is occluded, resulting in FHR bradycardia. A loop of cord may be palpated or visualized in the vagina. An emergency cesarean birth is typically done to improve neonatal outcomes with a prolapsed cord.

Risk Factors for Prolapse of the Umbilical Cord

- Malpresentation of the fetus (such as breech)
- Unengaged presenting part
- Polyhydramnios
- Small or preterm fetus
- Multiple gestation
- High parity

Risks Associated with Prolapse of the Umbilical Cord

- Total or partial occlusion of the cord, resulting in rapid deterioration in fetal perfusion and oxygenation (Curran, 2003)

Assessment Findings

- Sudden fetal bradycardia (i.e., prolonged decelerations).
- Prolapsed umbilical cord that may be felt with a SVE or visualized in or protruding from the vagina.

Medical Management

- Vaginal birth or operative vaginal delivery may be attempted if birth is imminent.
- Perform emergency cesarean section.

Nursing Actions

- Occlusion of the cord may be partially relieved by lifting the presenting part off the cord with a vaginal exam. The examiner's hand remains in the vagina, lifting the presenting part off the cord until delivery by cesarean (Fig. 10-18).
- Request assistance and notify the medical provider.
- Explain the situation to the woman and family and that interventions are necessary to expedite delivery.
- Explain to the woman the importance of her assistance.
- Recommend position changes such a knee–chest position or Trendelenburg to try to relieve pressure on the occluded cord (Fig. 10-19).
- Administer O_2 at 10 L/min by mask.
- Give IV fluid hydration bolus.
- Discontinue oxytocin.
- Administer a tocolytic agent to decrease uterine activity.
- Prepare for emergency delivery. If birth is imminent, the provider may proceed with vaginal delivery. If birth is not imminent, anticipate and prepare for emergency cesarean section.

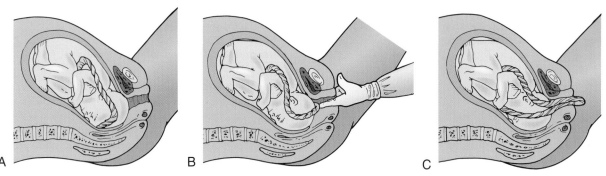

Figure 10-17   Prolapsed cord. *A.* Occult. The cord cannot been seen or felt during a vaginal examination. *B.* Complete. During a vaginal examination, the cord is felt as a pulsating mass. *C.* Frank. The cord precedes the fetal head or feet and can be seen protruding from the vagina.

Rupture of the Uterus

Rupture of the uterus is a partial or complete tear in the uterine muscle.

- In complete uterine rupture, all of the layers of the uterine wall are separated.
- In incomplete uterine rupture (uterine dehiscence), the uterine muscle is separated but the visceral peritoneum is intact.

Signs and symptoms of uterine rupture are related to internal hemorrhage and reflected in both the maternal and fetal status, in relationship to the extent of the rupture.

- The condition usually becomes evident because of signs of fetal compromise and maternal hypovolemia related to hemorrhage.
- If the fetal presenting part is in the pelvis, loss of station may occur which is detected with a vaginal exam.

Maternal and fetal survival depends on prompt identification and surgical intervention.

- Fetal mortality with uterine rupture is reported at 50% to 70%.
- Maternal mortality is 5%.

Risks Associated with Rupture of the Uterus

- The greatest risk factor is previous cesarean section (Cunningham et al., 2005); others are previous vertical uterine scar, multifetal gestation, and uterine tachysystole.

- Potential effects on woman and fetus include hypovolemic shock, infection, hypoxemia, acidosis, neurological damage, and possible death.
- Maternal complications are primarily due to hypovelemia as a result of hemorrhage.
- Complications to the fetus may be due to uteroplacental insufficiency, placental abruption, cord compression, asphyxia, and/or hypovolemia.

Assessment Findings

- Maternal assessment findings may include signs and symptoms of hypovolemic shock such as:
  - *Hypotension*
  - *Tachypnea*
  - *Tachycardia*
  - *Pallor*
- Severe tearing sensation, burning "stabbing" pain and contractions
- Vaginal bleeding
- Fetal response is related to hemorrhage and placental separation and may include late decelerations, loss of FHR variability, fetal bradycardia, or even loss of FHR.
- Ascending station of the fetal presenting part

Medical Management

- Perform emergency cesarean birth.
  - *Control maternal hemorrhage.*
  - *Hysterectomy may be necessary.*
- Transfusions may be needed.

Nursing Actions

- Request assistance and notify the medical provider.
- Stabilize the woman with O$_2$ and IV fluids.

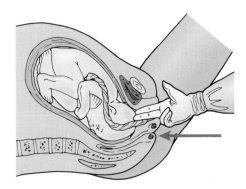

Figure 10-18   Vaginal examination with prolapsed cord, lifting presenting part off the cord.

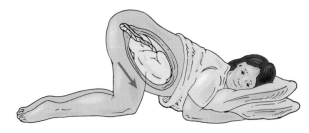

Figure 10-19   Knee–chest position with prolapsed cord.

■ Prepare for emergency cesarean birth.
■ Explain the situation to the woman and her family, that interventions that will expedite delivery, and the importance of their assistance.

Amniotic Fluid Embolism

Amniotic fluid embolism (AFE) is a rare but often fatal complication that occurs during pregnancy, labor and birth, or the first 24 hours post-birth. An embolism forms when the amniotic fluid that contains fetal cells, lanugo, and vernix enters the maternal vascular system and results in cardiorespiratory collapse. This is discussed more completely in Chapter 14.

Disseminated Intravascular Coagulation

Disseminated intravascular coagulation (DIC) is a syndrome that occurs when the body is breaking down blood clots faster than it can form a clot. This quickly depletes the body of clotting factors, leads to hemorrhage, and can rapidly lead to maternal death. Women who experience DIC are transferred to critical care unit and a perinatologist manages the care. This is discussed more completely in Chapter 14.

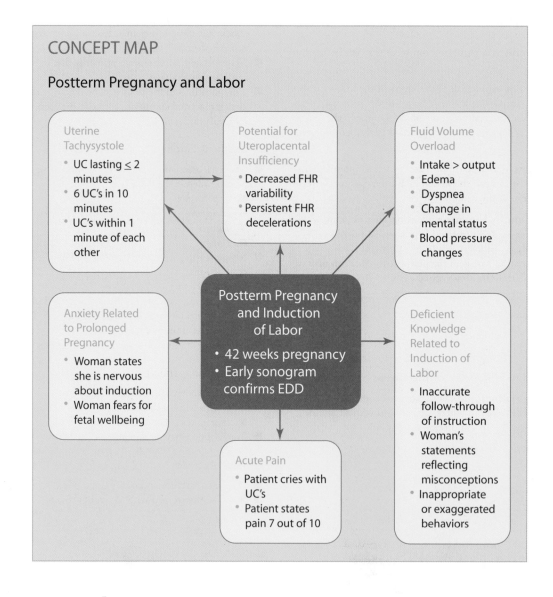

CONCEPT MAP

Postterm Pregnancy and Labor

Uterine Tachysystole
- UC lasting ≤ 2 minutes
- 6 UC's in 10 minutes
- UC's within 1 minute of each other

Potential for Uteroplacental Insufficiency
- Decreased FHR variability
- Persistent FHR decelerations

Fluid Volume Overload
- Intake > output
- Edema
- Dyspnea
- Change in mental status
- Blood pressure changes

Postterm Pregnancy and Induction of Labor
- 42 weeks pregnancy
- Early sonogram confirms EDD

Anxiety Related to Prolonged Pregnancy
- Woman states she is nervous about induction
- Woman fears for fetal wellbeing

Deficient Knowledge Related to Induction of Labor
- Inaccurate follow-through of instruction
- Woman's statements reflecting misconceptions
- Inappropriate or exaggerated behaviors

Acute Pain
- Patient cries with UC's
- Patient states pain 7 out of 10

Problem No. 1: Uterine tachysystole
Goal: Decreased uterine activity
Outcome: Patient will have decreased contractions.

Nursing Actions

1. Evaluation of uterine contraction strength, frequency, and duration by palpation or IUPC
2. Evaluation of uterine resting tone by palpation or IUPC pressure below 20 mm Hg
3. Assessment of fetal heart rate in response to uterine contractions
4. Turn oxytocin down or off in the event of uterine tachysystole or indeterminate or abnormal fetal heart rate.
   ■ Maternal position change
   ■ IV bolus of at least 500 mL of lactated Ringer's
   ■ O_2 administration by mask at 10 L/min
   ■ If no response consider terbutaline.

Problem No. 2: Knowledge deficit related to induction of labor
Goal: Patient understands indication and process of labor induction
Outcome: Patient states she understands indication and process of induction of labor

Nursing Actions

1. Explain all procedures
2. Encourage verbalization of questions.
3. Practice active listening.
4. Provide emotional support.
5. Make needed referrals to social services and mental health specialists if needed

Problem 3: Anxiety related to prolonged pregnancy
Goal: Decreased anxiety
Outcome: Patient verbalizes that she feels less anxious

Nursing Actions

1. Be calm and reassuring in interactions with the patient and her family.
2. Explain all information repeatedly related to procedures.
2. Provide autonomy and choices.
4. Encourage patient and family to verbalize their feelings regarding prolonged pregnancy by asking open-ended questions.
5. Explore past coping strategies.

Problem 4: Fluid volume overload related to prolonged oxytocin
Goal: Fluid balance
Outcome: Patient maintains fluid balance.

Nursing Actions

1. Assess I&O.
2. Maintain IV fluids as ordered.
3. Calculate intake of all fluids.
4. Measure output including emesis and urine.
5. Assess edema.
6. Auscultate the lung sounds.

Problem No. 5: Acute pain related to UCs
Goal: Decreased pain
Outcome: Patient will state that pain is improved.

Nursing Actions

1. Assess level, location, and type of pain.
2. Sustaining physical presence, eye contact
3. Verbal encouragement, reassurance, and praise
4. Comfort measures such as ice chips, fluids, food, and pain medications
5. Hygiene including mouth care, pericare, and changing chux
6. Assistance with position changes
7. Reassuring touch, massage
8. Application of heat and cold
9. Hydrotherapy shower and tub if no ROM
10. Provide an environment that is conducive to relaxation such as low lights, decreased noise.
11. Teaching patient relaxation and breathing techniques.

Problem No. 6: Potential for uteroplacental insufficiency indeterminate or abnormal FHR
Goal: Maintain normal FHR
Outcome: FHR baseline is normal with variability and accelerations pattern are within normal limits.

Nursing Actions

1. Assess FHR baseline variability and for decelerations.
2. Turn oxytocin down or off.
3. Change the mother's position.
4. IV bolus of at least 500 mL of lactated Ringer's
5. O_2 at 10 L/min by mask
6. Notify the provider.
7. Request bedside evaluation if the FHR is abnormal.

TYING IT ALL TOGETHER

As a labor and delivery nurse, this is your second shift caring for Mallory Polk. She is a 42-year-old, single, African American attorney whom you admitted yesterday at 32 weeks' gestation with the diagnosis of preterm labor. She was treated with magnesium sulfate and betamethasone. Tonight when you came on your shift at 7 P.M. she remained on magnesium sulfate but was contracting regularly and at 3:20 A.M. had SROM for clear fluid. At 4:00 A.M. her cervix was 5 cm/90%/+1. At that time the magnesium sulfate was discontinued and normal spontaneous vaginal birth is anticipated because of advanced preterm labor. Over the next hour Mallory is contracting every 2 to 3 minutes and is coping well with uterine contractions. Her sister, Allison, is at the bedside providing labor support. The FHR baseline is 140s, with average variability, occasional accelerations and no FHR decelerations. At 5:15 A.M. Mallory feels the urge to have a bowel movement and you do an SVE. Her vaginal exam reveals that she is 10 cm/100%/+1.

Who needs to be notified of your significant assessment findings?
What would you report?

Within 15 minutes of your report her physician arrives and confirms your assessment that Mallory is completely dilated and her doctor wants her to start to push. You coach Mallory to begin pushing with her next contraction.

What are your priorities in nursing care for Mallory?
Discuss the rationale for the priorities.
State nursing diagnosis, expected outcome, and interventions related to this problem.
What would you anticipate as Mallory's teaching needs?

Over the next hour Mallory's contractions slow to every 7 minutes and she is pushing with open glottis pushing and feels the urge to bear down with the peak of contractions. A sterile vaginal exam reveals that she is completely dilated and descent of the fetal head is +2 station. You request the physician to come to the bedside to evaluate fetal descent. After her physician evaluates Mallory, she requests oxytocin augmentation to increase the frequency of her contractions. You initiate oxytocin augmentation at 1 mU/min per physician orders.

Discuss the risk associated with oxytocin augmentation.
Outline nursing actions when caring for a patient with oxytocin augmentation.
What teaching would include related to oxytocin augmentation?

Within 30 minutes of starting the oxytocin Mallory is having UCs every 1 to 2 minutes lasting 45 to 55 seconds moderate to palpation with a relaxed uterus between contractions. The FHR baseline is in the 140s with variable decelerations to 90s for 40 seconds with UCs, and FHR variability is moderate.

What are your priorities in nursing care?
Discuss the rationale for the priorities and nursing actions.
What are your nursing actions based on your assessment?
State nursing diagnosis, expected outcomes.

Over the next hour, Mallory's contractions are every 3 to 4 minutes and she is pushing with contractions and has a strong urge to bear down with contractions. The FHR is 140s with moderate variability and variable decelerations to 100 bpm for 30 seconds with contractions and open glottis pushing. Her SVE reveals fetal descent to +3 station.

What are your immediate priorities in nursing care for Mallory?
Discuss the rationale for the priorities.

■ ■ ■   Review Questions   ■ ■ ■

1. Which nursing action can improve uterine blood flow, increase umbilical cord circulation, improve maternal oxygenation, and decrease uterine activity?
   A. Administering oxygen to the mother
   B. Changing the woman's position
   C. Discontinuing oxytocin
   D. Infusing intravenous fluids

2. A laboring woman reports spontaneous rupture of membranes and you assess severe decelerations in the FHR. Examination reveals a cord in the vagina. The first nursing action is to:
   A. Manually elevate the presenting part
   B. Administer a tocolytic agent
   C. Administer an IV fluid bolus
   D. Empty the patient's bladder

3. An increased risk for shoulder dystocia is associated with:
   A. Preterm labor
   B. Maternal diabetes
   C. VBAC
   D. Previous precipitous birth

4. Vacuum extractor cup placement on the fetal head should not exceed:
   A. 5 minutes
   B. 10 minutes
   C. 20 minutes
   D. 30 minutes

5. A high probability of successful induction is associated with a Bishop score of:
   A. Greater than 4
   B. Greater than 6
   C. Less than 4
   D. Less than 6

References

American College of Obstetricians and Gynecologists (ACOG). (1995). *Dystocia and the augmentation of labor.* Technical Bulletin No. 218, December, 1995. Washington, DC: Author.

American College of Obstetricians and Gynecologists (ACOG). (1999). *Induction of labor.* Practice Bulletin No. 10, 2002. Washington, DC: Author.

American College of Obstetricians and Gynecologists (ACOG). (2000). *Operative vaginal delivery.* Practice Bulletin No. 17, June 2000. Washington, DC: Author.

American College of Obstetricians and Gynecologists (ACOG). (2002). *Shoulder dystocia.* Practice Bulletin No. 40, November, 2002. Washington, DC: Author.

American College of Obstetricians and Gynecologists (ACOG). (2004). *Vaginal birth after previous cesarean delivery.* Practice Bulletin No. 54, July, 2004. Washington, DC: Author.

Bishop, E. H. (1964). Pelvic scoring for elective induction. *Obstetrics and Gynecology, 24,* 266–268.

Bricker, L, & Luckas, M. (2000). Amniotomy alone for induction of labour. Cochrane Database of Systematic Reviews 2000, Issue 4. Art. No.: CD002862. DOI: 10.1002/14651858.CD002862.

Cunningham, F., Leveno, K., Bloom, S., Hauth, J., Gilstrap, L., & Wenstrom, K. (2005). *Williams obstetrics* (22nd ed.). McGraw-Hill: New York.

Curran, C. (2003). Intrapartum emergencies. *Journal of Obstetric, Gynecologic & Neonatal Nursing, 32,* 802–813.

Gilbert, E., & Harmon, J. (2003). *Manual of high risk pregnancy and delivery*. St. Louis, MO: C. V. Mosby.

Gülmezoglu, A. M., Crowther, C. A., & Middleton, P. (2006). Induction of labour for improving birth outcomes for women at or beyond term. Cochrane Database of Systematic Reviews 2006, Issue 4. Art. No.: CD004945. DOI: 10.1002/14651858.CD004945.pub2.

Hofmeyr, G. J., & Gülmezoglu, A. M. (2003). Vaginal misoprostol for cervical ripening and induction of labour. Cochrane Database of Systematic Reviews 2003, Issue 1. Art. No.: CD000941. DOI: 10.1002/14651858. CD000941.

Kelly, A. J., Alfirevic, Z., Hofmeyr, G. J., Kavanagh, J., Neilson, J. P., & Thomas, J. (2009). Induction of labour in specific clinical situations: Generic protocol. (Protocol) Cochrane Database of Systematic Reviews 2009, Issue 2. Art. No.: CD003398. DOI: 10.1002/14651858.CD003398. pub2.

Kelly, A. J., Kavanagh, J., & Thomas, J. (2003). Vaginal prostaglandin (PGE2 and PGF2a) for induction of labour at term. Cochrane Database of Systematic Reviews 2003, Issue 4. Art. No.: CD003101. DOI: 10.1002/14651858.CD003101.

Lyndon, A., & Ali, L. U. (Eds.) (2008). *Fetal heart rate monitoring: Principles and practice* (4th ed.). Dubuque, IA; Kendal/Hunt.

Martin, J., Hamilton, B., Sutton, P., Ventura, S., Menacker, F., Kimeyer, S., & Munson, M. (2007). Births: Final data for 2005. *National Vital Statistics Reports*; 56, Hyattsville, MD: National Center for Health Statistics 1–104.

Nurses Association of American College of Obstetrics and Gynecologists (NAACOG). (1991). *Inpatient obstetrics certification review manual*. Washington, DC: Author.

O'Driscoll, K., Jackson, R. J., & Gallagher, J. (1970). Active management of labour and cephalopelvic disproportion. *Journal of Obstetrics and Gynecology of the British Commonwealth*, 77, 385–389.

Queenan, J., Hobbins, J., & Spong, C. (2005). *Protocols in high risk pregnancies*. Malden, MA: Blackwell.

Simpson, K. (2009). *Cervical ripening and induction and augmentation of labor* (3rd ed., updated). Washington, DC: Association of Women's Health, Obstetric and Neonatal Nurses.

Simpson, K., & Atterbury, J. (2003). Trends and issues in labor induction in the United States: Implications for clinical practice. *Journal of Obstetric, Gynecologic & Neonatal Nursing*, 32, 767–779.

Simpson, K., Creehan, P., & Association of Women's Health, Obstetric and Neonatal Nurses (AWHONN). (2008). *Perinatal nursing* (3rd ed.). Philadelphia: Lippincott Williams & Wilkins

Viswanathan, M., Visco, A., Hatmann, K., Wechter, M., Gartlehner, G., Wu, J., et al. (2006). Cesarean delivery on maternal request. Evidence Repost/Technology Assessment No. 133 (Prepared by the RTI International-University of North Carolina Evidence-Based Practice Center under Contract No. 290-02-0016.) ARHQ Publication No. 06-E009. Rockville, MD: Agency for Healthcare Research and Quality. March 2006.

Intrapartum and Postpartum Care of Cesarean Birth Families

11

OBJECTIVES

On completion of this chapter, student will be able to:

☐ Define key terms.
☐ Identify factors that place a woman at risk for cesarean birth.
☐ Discuss the preoperative nursing care and medical and anesthesia management for cesarean births.
☐ Describe the intraoperative nursing care and medical and anesthesia management for cesarean births.
☐ Discuss the postoperative nursing care of cesarean birth families.
☐ Identify potential intraoperative and postoperative complications related to cesarean birth and nursing actions to reduce risk.

Nursing Diagnosis

■ At risk for low self-esteem related to perceived failure of life event
■ At risk for injury related to surgical procedure and effects of anesthesia
■ At risk for fluid volume deficit related to blood loss and oral fluid restriction
■ At risk for acute pain related to surgical trauma
■ At risk for infection related to tissue trauma or prolonged rupture of membranes
■ At risk for altered parent–infant attachment related to surgical intervention

Nursing Outcomes

■ Parents will verbalize factors that contributed to the need for cesarean birth.
■ The woman will experience an uncomplicated intraoperative period and postoperative recovery.
■ The woman will have adequate urinary output and lochia within normal limits.
■ The woman will verbalize a pain level below 3 on a pain scale of 0 to 10.
■ The woman will be afebrile and the abdominal incisional site will be free of signs of infection.
■ The parents will hold the infant close to the body and care for infant needs.

INTRODUCTION

Cesarean birth, also referred to as cesarean section or C-section (C/S), is an operative procedure in which the fetus is delivered through an incision in the abdominal wall and the uterus. Approximately one-third of pregnant couples experience a cesarean birth. The percentage of cesarean births has increased from 20.7% in 1996 to 30.2% in 2005 and reflects a 46% increase over a 10-year period (Hamilton, Martin, & Ventura, 2006; Martin et al., 2006). This increase is partially attributed to:

■ A decrease in vaginal birth after cesarean section (VBAC) rates from 30.1 per 100 live births of women with previous cesarean section in 1996 to 10.6 in 2003 (Menacker, 2005).
■ An increase in the number of **cesarean delivery on maternal request (CDMR)**. **CDMR** is a cesarean section that is performed at the request of the woman before the start of labor

and in the absence of maternal or fetal medical conditions that present a risk for labor (Grossman et al., 2006).

The needs and experiences of cesarean birth couples are distinctly different from those of couples who experience a vaginal birth. The experiences are also different for couples who experience a planned cesarean birth related to being a repeat cesarean birth versus an unplanned cesarean birth related to fetal intolerance of labor. These differences include:

■ Increased length of hospitalization
■ Longer period of physical recovery
■ Increased pain
■ Increased negative emotional responses to the childbirth experience

Women who experience an unplanned cesarean birth may experience feelings of guilt and failure for not being able to have a vaginal birth. These feelings have decreased as the rates of cesarean births have increased and cesarean births have become more common.

Want to reinforce your reading? Need to review for a test? Listen to this chapter on your accompanying CD.

Evidence-Based Practice: Cesarean Delivery on Maternal Request

National Institutes of Health (2006). NIH State-of-the-Science Conference: Cesarean Delivery on Maternal Request.

Responding to the increased rates of cesarean delivery on maternal request (CDMR), NIH conducted a systematic literature review and a three-day conference focusing on the risks and benefits of CDMR. The panel reached the following conclusions:

■ "There is insufficient evidence to evaluate fully the benefits and risks of CDMR as compared to planned vaginal delivery, and more research is needed.

■ Until quality evidence becomes available, any decision to perform a CDMR should be carefully individualized and consistent with ethical principles.

■ Given the risk of placenta previa and accreta rise with each cesarean delivery, CDMR is not recommended for women desiring several children.

■ CDMR should not be performed prior to 39 weeks of gestation or without verification of lung maturity, because of the significant danger of neonatal respiratory complications."

INDICATIONS FOR CESAREAN BIRTH

The major medical indications for a cesarean birth are:

■ Dystocia, difficult childbirth or dysfunctional labor, that is caused by:
  ■ *Ineffective uterine contractions that lead to prolonged first stage of labor*
  ■ *Cephalopelvic disproportion (CPD) which occurs when the maternal bony pelvis is not large enough or appropriately shaped to allow for fetal descent*
■ Previous cesarean birth
■ Malpresentaion or malposition of fetus such as:
  ■ *Breech presentation*
  ■ *Transverse lie*
  ■ *Persistent occipitoposterior position*
■ Fetal intolerance of labor/nonreassuring fetal heart rate
■ Placental abnormalities such as:
  ■ *Complete placenta previa*
  ■ *Marginal or partial placenta previa with hemorrhage*
  ■ *Complete abruptio placenta*
  ■ *Partial abruptio placenta with significant blood loss*
■ Previous uterine surgery
  ■ *Surgeries that involved an incision through the myometrium of the uterus*
■ Maternal health factors such as:
  ■ *Cardiac diseases*
  ■ *Severe hypertension*
  ■ *Severe diabetes mellitus*

CLASSIFICATION OF CESAREAN BIRTHS

Cesarean births are classified into two major groupings of scheduled (planned) and unscheduled (unplanned).

■ Scheduled cesarean births occur before the onset of labor. Common reasons for a scheduled cesarean birth are:

■ *Previous cesarean birth*
■ *Maternal or fetal health conditions that place the woman or fetus at risk during labor and/or vaginal birth*
■ *Malpresentation, such as breech presentation, diagnosed before labor*
■ *Cesarean delivery on maternal request (CDMR)*
■ Unscheduled cesarean births are divided into emergent, urgent, and non-urgent.
  ■ *Emergent cesarean birth indicates an immediate need to deliver the fetus (e.g., prolapse of umbilical cord or rupture of uterus).*
  ■ *Urgent cesarean birth indicates a need for rapid delivery of the fetus such as with malpresentation diagnosed after labor has begun or placenta previa with mild bleeding and fetal heart rate within normal limits.*
  ■ *Non-urgent cesarean birth indicates a need for cesarean birth related to such complications as failure to progress (cervix does not fully dilate) and failure to descend (fetus does not descend through the pelvis) with stable FHR.*

RISKS RELATED TO CESAREAN BIRTH

Maternal deaths in the United States related to cesarean birth have decreased due to improved surgical techniques, anesthetic care, and the availability of blood transfusions and antibiotic therapy, but still pose a risk to both the woman and her fetus. Women who experience a cesarean birth are at higher risk for postpartum infection, hemorrhage, and thromboembolic disease (Hacker, Moore, & Gambone, 2004). Neonates are at higher risk for respiratory morbidity (Chestnut, 2006).

PREOPERATIVE CARE

It is common in the United States for cesarean births to be performed in the obstetrics department and for labor and delivery nurses to care for the family throughout the perioperative experience.

Preoperative care may vary based on the urgency of the cesarean birth

Scheduled Cesarean Birth

Couples are encouraged to complete the preadmission hospital paperwork, which includes consent form for cesarean birth and conditions of admission, before the day of the scheduled cesarean birth. Diagnostic laboratory work, such as complete blood count (CBC), platelet count, urinalysis, blood type, and cross match, are completed a few days before admission. Couples are admitted to the labor and birthing unit the day of surgery (Fig. 11-1).

Medical Management

■ Explain the reason for the cesarean birth and what it involves before hospital admission and obtain surgical consent.
■ Schedule the surgery.
■ Order presurgery diagnostic laboratory tests, such as CBC, blood type, and Rh.
■ Send the prenatal record and orders to the birthing unit to be placed in the woman's hospital chart.

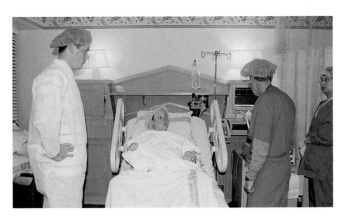

Figure 11-1 Couple awaiting scheduled cesarean section.

Anesthesia Management

■ The anesthesiologist or certified registered nurse anesthetist (CRNA) meets with the couple during the admission process and before the woman is transferred to the operating room.

■ The anesthesiologist or CRNA reviews the prenatal record.

■ The anesthesiologist or CRNA completes an anesthesia history and physical and discusses anesthesia options with the couple and answers their questions regarding anesthesia and the procedure.

■ The anesthesiologist or CRNA determines, based on the woman's history, physical, and clinical signs, if a platelet count is required before administration of epidural or spinal (American Society of Anesthesiologists Task Force, 2007).

Nursing Actions

■ Complete the appropriate admission assessments and required preoperative forms.
  ■ *Expected findings*
    ■ Couples may have an increased level of anxiety related to the surgery and method of anesthesia.
      ■ *Anxiety may be related to this being the woman's first surgical experience and fears of the unknown for self and fetus.*
      ■ *The expectant father may have concerns about injury to his partner and/or child.*
    ■ Couples are excited about the upcoming birth of their child.
    ■ Couples have questions and concerns regarding the cesarean birth and method of anesthesia.
    ■ Vital signs are within normal limits, with a mild increase in blood pressure related to increased anxiety.

■ Obtain a baseline fetal heart rate monitor strip.
  ■ *Expectant findings*
    ■ Reassuring fetal heart rate

■ Review the prenatal chart for factors that place the woman at risk during or after cesarean birth and ensure that physician and anesthesiologist or CRNA are aware of risk factors such as low platelet count.

■ Ensure that all required documents, such as prenatal record, current laboratory reports, and consent forms, are in the woman's chart.

■ Verify that the woman has been NPO for 6 to 8 hours before surgery (American Society of Anesthesiologists Task Force, 2007).

■ Complete the surgery checklist, which includes removal of jewelry, eyeglasses/contact lenses, and dentures. Eyeglasses can be given to the expectant father to bring into the operating room so the woman can use them to see her newborn baby.

■ Explain to the couple what they can expect before, during, and after the cesarean birth.

■ Draw blood for laboratory testing as per orders.

■ Start an IV line and administer an IV fluid preload as per orders.

■ Insert a Foley catheter as per order. Insertion may be done in the operating room after placement of the spinal or epidural.

■ Shave the abdominal and pubic regions with electric clippers.

■ Administer preoperative medications per orders.
  ■ *This might include sodium citrate to neutralize stomach acids.*

■ Prepare the expectant father or the support person who plans to be present for the birth for the experience by providing appropriate surgical garb to wear in the operating room.

■ Instruct the expectant father or the support person as to where he or she will sit and what he or she can anticipate regarding sights, sounds, and smells typical of an operating room.

■ Provide emotional support for the couple as they wait to be transferred to the operating room.

CRITICAL COMPONENT

IV Fluid Preload before Anesthesia

An I.V. fluid preload of 500–1,000 mL is given before administration of spinal or epidural anesthesia to increase fluid volume and decrease risk of hypotension related to effects of anesthetic agent.

(American Society of Anesthesiologists Task Force, 2007 and AWHONN, 2001)

Unscheduled Cesarean Birth

Unscheduled cesarean births are usually due to an urgent or emergent cause such as fetal intolerance of labor or placental problems. The woman and her family are usually highly anxious and have fears that either the woman and/or infant are in danger of a negative birthing outcome.

■ Emergent cesarean births require immediate preparation of the woman for surgery with minimal time to spend explaining what is happening to the woman and her fetus. The woman and her partner or support person need an opportunity to debrief during the immediate postpartum period.

■ Urgent and non-urgent cesarean births allows the time necessary to explain fully what and why a cesarean birth is required, but the couple still needs time in the postpartum unit to review the events leading up to the cesarean birth.

Medical Management

■ Determine the need for a cesarean birth.

■ Explain the reason for the cesarean birth.

■ Explain the surgical procedure and obtain consent.

Anesthesia Management

■ The anesthesiologist or CRNA completes an anesthesia history and physical and discusses anesthesia options with the woman. This may not occur until the woman is transferred to the operating room based on the amount of time from the decision for need of cesarean birth and transfer to the operating room.

- The anesthesiologist or CRNA explains the procedure for type of anesthesia and addresses the woman's and her partner's or support person's questions and concerns.
- The anesthesiologist or CRNA determines the need for a platelet count.

Evidence-Based Practice: Predictive Relationship of Preoperative Anxiety with Postoperative Satisfaction

Hobson, J., Slade, P., Wrench, I., & Power, L. (2006). Preoperative anxiety and postoperative satisfaction in women undergoing elective cesarean section. *International Journal of Obstetric Anesthesia, 15,* 18–23.

The aim of this study was to determine the predictive relationship of preoperative anxiety with postoperative maternal satisfaction. The sample included 85 women scheduled for elective cesarean birth. Degree of anxiety, social support, and aspects of preoperative preparation were measured within 24 hours of the scheduled cesarean birth. Postoperative measures included the maternal satisfaction scale for cesarean section, recovery from cesarean section scale, and postoperative discharge summary form.

Results from this study indicate that the lower the preoperative anxiety the higher the postoperative maternal satisfaction. They also indicate that postoperative satisfaction was highest when the woman was highly satisfied with the preoperative information provided by the anesthesiologist and when the woman's perceived support by her partner was high.

Implications of this study for evidence-based practice in enhancing the woman's satisfaction with her birthing experience are the importance of providing preoperative information to the woman and facilitating support to the woman from her partner.

Nursing Actions

- Notify the anesthesia department and perioperative department of the impending cesarean birth.
- Initiate continuous electronic fetal heart rate monitoring.
  - *Expected findings*
    - Nonreassuring fetal heart rate when the cesarean section is related to fetal intolerance of labor
- Administer oxygen when indicated (i.e., signs of fetal distress).
- Alert neonatal personnel of the impending cesarean birth.
- Assess the woman's vital signs.
  - *Expected findings*
    - The woman's blood pressure is elevated related to anxiety level.
    - There is a potential increase in temperature and pulse rate due to infection and/or dehydration related to prolonged labor and rupture of membranes
- Start an IV and administer IV fluid preload as per orders.
- Complete and witness surgical and anesthesia consent forms.
- Insert a Foley catheter as per order. Insertion may be done in the operating room after placement of the spinal or epidural.
- Assess the couple's emotional response to the need for a cesarean birth.
  - *Expected findings*
    - Couples may experience high levels of anxiety based on fear of injury to the woman and/or unborn child.
    - Couples are not emotionally or mentally prepared for cesarean birth.

- Couples have a knowledge deficit regarding cesarean birth and anesthesia options.
- Couples ask questions regarding cesarean birth and anesthesia options.
- Shave the abdominal and pubic regions with electric clippers.
- Ensure that all required documents are in the patient's chart.
- Complete the surgical checklist.
- Ensure that the laboratory tests are completed as per orders.
- Reinforce reason for cesarean section and address questions.
- Provide emotional support to the couple and family members.
- Review with the couple what to expect during and after the cesarean birth.
- Explain that the woman may feel pressure or pulling as her baby is being born.
- Prepare the expectant father or support person who plans to attend the birth as to what to anticipate in the operating room and provide him or her with proper surgical garb to wear in operating room.

*I*NTRAOPERATIVE CARE

The cesarean birth often is the first surgical experience for most women and can increase the anxiety level for both the woman and her partner. Couples are anxious irrespective of whether this is a scheduled or unscheduled cesarean birth. To help decrease the anxiety level, ideally, the nurse who admitted the woman for a scheduled cesarean section or the nurse who cared for the couple during labor continues to care for them during the surgery as the circulating nurse.

Complications

Intraoperative complications are rare owing to the advances in obstetrical anesthesia and surgical techniques. Women who are healthy during pregnancy are at low risk for complications. Intraoperative complications include:

- Hemorrhage
- Bladder, ureters, and bowel trauma
- Maternal respiratory depression related to anesthesia
- Maternal hypotension related to anesthesia which increases the risk for fetal distress
- Inadvertent injection of the anesthetic agent into the maternal blood stream
  - *The woman experiences ringing in her ears, metallic taste in her mouth, and hypotension that can lead to unconsciousness and cardiac arrest (Schwartz, 2006).*

Anesthesia Management

- Determine the method of anesthesia.
  - *The determination of type of anesthesia is based on which one:*
    - Is the safest and most comfortable for the woman
    - Has the least effect on the fetus/neonate
    - Provides the optimal conditions for the surgery (Hughes, Levinson, & Rosen, 2002).
  - *Method of anesthesia (Fig. 11-2)*
    - Spinal anesthesia is the preferred method for scheduled cesarean sections or for laboring women who do not have an epidural in place. Spinal anesthesia, which is faster to place, provides a full sensory and motor block.

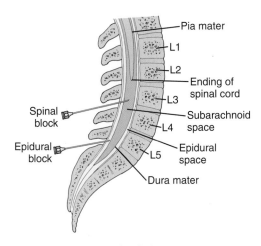

Figure 11-2 Spinal and epidural placements.

- Epidural anesthesia is used for laboring women who have an epidural in place for labor pain management and then require a cesarean birth. Women with epidurals may feel tugging and pulling during the procedure because epidurals are not as dense and do not provide full sensory and motor block.
- General anesthesia, which is rarely used and carries increased risks, is indicated in the following situations:
  - *Rapid delivery is imperative*
  - *Severe hemorrhage*
  - *Seizures*
  - *Failed spinal*
  - Gastric aspiration leading to pneumonitis is a potential complication of general anesthesia.
- Contraindications for epidural or spinal anesthesia
  - *The woman's refusal or inability to cooperate with the procedure*
  - *Increased intracranial pressure*
  - *Infection at the site of needle insertion*
  - *Low platelet count*
  - *Uncorrected maternal hypovolemia (Chestnut, 2006)*
- Administration of anesthesia by the anesthesiologist or CRNA
  - *Bupivacaine is the preferred anesthetic agent for spinal and epidural blocks.*
  - *Preservative-free morphine is administered intrathecally to provide postoperative analgesia (Kuczkowski, Reisner, & Lin, 2006).*

Medication

Preservative-Free Morphine

- Indication: Severe pain
- Action: Alters perception of and response to painful stimuli and produces generalized CNS depression.
- Common side effects: Respiratory depression, itching, hypotension, nausea and vomiting, and urinary retention
- Route and dose: Administered intrathecally by Anesthesiologist or CRNA; 5–10 mg

(Data from Deglin & Vallerand, 2009)

- Maintain a left uterine displacement before, during, and after administration of anesthesia to decrease the risk of aortocaval compression related to compression on the aorta and inferior vena cava due to weight of the gravid uterus (Chestnut, 2006).
- Monitor vital signs and oxygen saturation.

- *Expected findings*
  - Vital signs and oxygen saturation within normal limits with potential mild increase in blood pressure due to anxiety
  - Hypotension following administration of the anesthetic agent
- Monitor level of anesthesia and effectiveness of anesthesia.
- Administer oxytocin after the delivery of the placenta.
- Administer antibiotics when indicated.

CRITICAL COMPONENT

Maternal Respiratory Depression Related to Intrathecal Morphine

Severe respiratory depression (3% occurrence) is a life-threatening adverse reaction to intrathecal morphine.

- Naloxone and resuscitative equipment need to be available whenever intrathecal morphine is administered and during the 24 hours postoperative after injection.
- Respiratory rate and level of sedation are monitored for the first 24 hours postoperative after administration.
- An initial dose of 0.4–2 mg of naloxone is administered intravenously for severe respiratory depression. Dose can be repeated every 2–3 minutes for a total of 10 mg.
- Respiratory resuscitation is initiated immediately and continued until normal respiratory function returns.

Medical Management

- Operative techniques:
  - *There are two primary operative techniques used for cesarean births.*
  - *The preferred technique is the **Pfannestiel incision** or "bikini cut." This is a transverse skin incision at the level of the mons pubis with a transverse incision in the lower uterine segment (Fig. 11-3).*
  - *The **classical cesarean delivery** technique is rare and is used in emergent cesarean births when immediate delivery is critical. A vertical midline incision is made into the abdominal wall with a vertical incision in the upper segment of the uterus (see Fig. 11-3).*
  - *The neonate is delivered through the uterine and abdominal incisions (Fig. 11-4).*

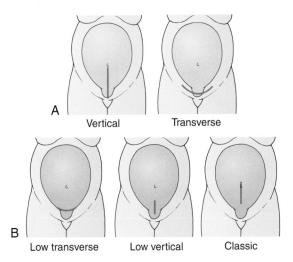

Figure 11-3 Abdominal wall and uterine incisions for cesarean births. *A.* Skin (abdominal wall) incisions. Vertical and transverse (Pfannenstiel) incisions. *B.* Uterine wall incisions. Low transverse, low vertical, classic.

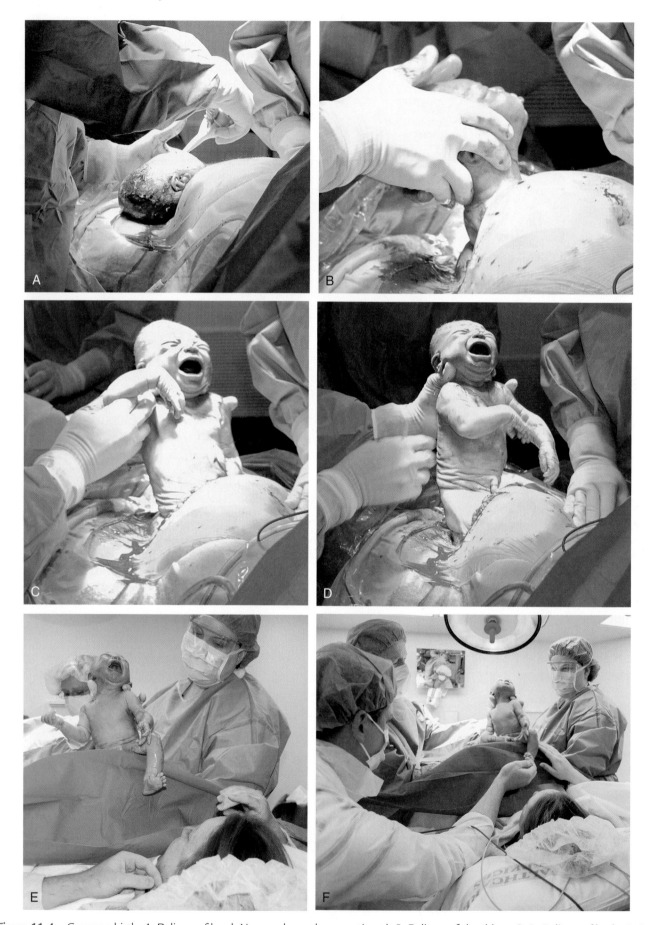

Figure 11-4 Cesarean birth. *A.* Delivery of head. Nose and mouth are suctioned. *B.* Delivery of shoulders. *C, D.* Delivery of body. *E, F.* Mom and dad meeting their daughter.

- *The placenta is manually removed.*
- *The uterus is lifted out of the abdominal cavity and the uterine incision is repaired.*
- *Abdominal tissues and incision are repaired.*

Nursing Actions

- Assist the woman onto the operating table and place a rolled blanket under her right buttock to facilitate maintaining a left uterine displacement.
- Continue external fetal heart rate monitoring until abdominal preparation is initiated.
- Remove the internal scalp electrode after abdominal preparation and before delivery.
  - *Expected findings*
    - Reassuring fetal heart rate unless nonreassuring fetal heart rate was indication for cesarean birth
- Assist the woman into the proper position for epidural or spinal anesthesia.
- Reposition the woman after epidural or spinal anesthesia in a supine position with a left lateral tilt to decrease the pressure from the uterus on the inferior vena cava and to maintain placental perfusion.
- Apply the grounding device.
- Secure the woman to the operating room table with a strap over her upper legs.
- Check equipment used for the newborn to ensure it is in working order and all supplies are readily available for care of the neonate.
- Assess the couple's response to the cesarean birth.
  - *Expected findings*
    - Anxiety levels increase related to operating room environment and impeding surgery.
    - Couples may have concerns related to potential injury to the woman from anesthesia and/or surgery.
    - The woman may feel abdominal pressure as the neonate is being delivered.
- Position the expectant father or support person on a stool next to the woman's head.
- Instruct the expectant father or support person as to what he or she can and cannot touch.
- Instruct the expectant father or support person to remain seated on the stool.
- Provide emotional support to the woman and her partner or support person.
- Perform the duties of the circulating nurse.
- Provide care for the neonate. This is done by the neonatal personnel (neonatal nurse, nurse practitioner, and/or neonatologist) who are present for the birth.
- Perform Apgar scoring. This is completed by the neonatal personnel.
  - *Expected findings*
    - The neonate's 1- and 5-minute Apgar scores are 7 or above unless there is fetal intolerance of labor before the birth.
- Record the time of delivery of the neonate and delivery of the placenta.
- Complete identification bands and place on the neonate and parents before the neonate leaves the operating room.
- Ensure that the new mother has an opportunity to see and touch her newborn and that the new father or support person has an opportunity to hold the newborn before taking the newborn to the nursery. In some birthing units the neonate, if stable, remains in the operating room and is transferred to the maternity recovery room with the woman and her partner.
- Transfer unstable neonates to the nursery and encourage the new father or support person to accompany the newborn to the nursery. Neonatal personnel are responsible for transferring unstable neonates.
- Address parents' questions regarding the health of their newborn.
- Complete intraoperative nursing notes.

CRITICAL COMPONENT

Universal Protocol for Preventing Wrong Patient, Wrong Site, Wrong Person Surgery

Joint Commission Standard PC 13.20 EP 9 states that "the site, procedure, and patient are accurately identified and clearly communicated using active communication techniques, during a final verification process such as time-out before the start of any surgical or invasive procedure" (Joint Commission, 2003).

The operating room circulating nurse assists in actively verifying that this is the correct patient and procedure when "time-out" is called immediately before the epidural or spinal procedure begins and immediately before the surgical incision is made to verify that it is the correct site, procedure, and patient.

POSTOPERATIVE CARE

The recovery time following a cesarean birth is longer compared to vaginal delivery due to the tissue trauma related to surgical intervention. The usual hospital stay is 3 to 5 days, with full recovery taking 6 weeks or longer.

Complications

Women who enter pregnancy in a healthy state and experienced a healthy pregnancy are at low risk for complications. Women who experience a prolonged labor, multiple interventions such as internal monitoring, or who have experienced prolonged rupture of membranes are at high risk for postoperative complications. Postoperative complications include:

- Hemorrhage
- Deep vein thrombosis
- Pulmonary embolism
- Paralytic ileus
- Hematuria related to bladder trauma
- Infections of the bladder, endometrium, and incisional site.

First 24 Hours After Birth

Medical Management

- Assess the woman for involutional changes and signs of potential complications.
- Medical orders are usually standardized. These orders include:
  - *IV therapy*
  - *Medications such as analgesics and stool softeners*
  - *Antibiotic therapy for the woman at risk for infection related to prolonged rupture of membranes, prolonged labor, or elevated temperature during labor*
  - *Progression of diet*
  - *Removal of the Foley catheter*
  - *Activity level*

Anesthesia Management

■ Accompany the woman to the recovery unit and provide a verbal report to nurse.

■ Remove the epidural catheter.

■ Order pain medications.

■ Order PRN medication to counteract side effects of intrathecal morphine.

Nursing Actions

After a cesarean birth, most women recover in the labor and birthing recovery unit versus the post anesthesia unit. Nursing actions are similar to care of women with vaginal birth with addition to and/or emphasis on the following:

■ Review prenatal, labor and intrapartal records for risk factors.

■ Monitor vital signs as per protocol.

   ■ *Monitor respiratory rate and level of sedation every hour for the first 24 hours after administration of intrathecal morphine.*

■ Monitor the level of sensation.

■ Monitor for side effects of intrathecal morphine and provide appropriate interventions. The primary side effects and interventions are:

   ■ *Pruritus (80%): Administer medication as per order such as naloxone or diphenhydramine.*

   ■ *Nausea/vomiting (53%): Administer medication as per order such as naloxone or metoclopramide.*

   ■ *Urinary retention (43%) that occurs after removal of catheter: Administer naloxone or catheterize as per orders*

   ■ *Respiratory depression (3%): Administer oxygen as needed and/or naloxone as per orders (Hughes, Levinson, & Rosen, 2002).*

■ Monitor for side effects/complications of anesthesia. These are:

   ■ *Postpartum hemorrhage related to uterine atony*

   ■ *Seizures*

   ■ *Neurological deficits (e.g., prolonged decreased sensation in legs)*

   ■ *Post dural puncture headaches*

   ■ *Newborn respiratory depression*

■ Assess the fundus and lochia as per protocol.

■ Assess the abdominal dressing for signs of bleeding.

■ Monitor for signs of hemorrhage.

■ Monitor urinary output per Foley catheter.

■ Regulate IV fluids as per order.

   ■ *Oxytocin is usually added to IV fluids to reduce the risk of postpartum hemorrhage related to uterine atony.*

■ Monitor the level of anesthesia.

■ Observe for side effects/adverse reactions related to intrathecal morphine.

■ Assist the woman into a comfortable position for infant feeding. Breastfeeding mothers may be more comfortable in a side lying position or using the football hold, which prevents pressure on her abdomen.

■ Assist woman with infant care.

■ Provide emotional support by actively listening to the couple recalling their birth experience and by addressing their questions and concerns.

Expected Assessment Findings

■ Vital signs are within normal limits.

■ Lochia is scant to moderate.

■ The fundus is firm and midline and generally 1 to 2 cm above the umbilicus.

■ The abdominal dressing is dry.

■ The catheter is draining clear/yellow urine.

■ *Blood in the urine occurs when there has been trauma to the bladder.*

■ The IV site is free of signs of infiltration or inflammation.

■ The pain level is below 3 on a pain scale of 0 to 10.

■ The woman gradually regains full motor and sensory function as the effects of anesthetic agent decrease.

   ■ *The woman sits at the bedside for short periods of time.*

■ The woman may experience itching, nausea, or decreased respirations related to side effects of morphine.

   ■ *Itching and nausea are the most common side effect of morphine.*

     ■ Itching varies from a facial rash to a full body rash. Antihistamines are given to promote comfort.

■ The woman feeds (breast or bottle) her newborn with assistance.

■ The partner assists in care of the newborn.

■ The couple may be tired and need time to rest.

■ Women with unplanned cesarean births may experience guilt feelings or a sense of failure or disappointment.

■ Couples with unplanned cesarean births may ask questions about the cesarean birth and the events leading up to it.

■ The couple will want time alone with their newborn child.

■ The couple will call family and friends informing them of the birth.

24 Hours Postoperative to Discharge

Medical Management

■ Assess the woman for involutional changes and signs of potential postoperative complications.

■ Remove abdominal dressing. The dressing is usually removed on the first postoperative day.

■ Provide discharge instructions.

Nursing Actions

Nursing actions are similar to the care of women with vaginal birth with addition to and/or emphasis on the following:

■ Monitor vital signs as per protocol.

■ Assess breath sounds.

■ Instruct the woman to deep breathe and cough every 2 hours.

■ Instruct the woman on the use of an incentive spirometer if ordered.

■ Assess postoperative pain and medicate as indicated.

■ Assess the fundus and lochia as per protocol. Use gentle pressure when assessing the fundus due to the woman's abdomen being tender.

■ Monitor for signs of hemorrhage and infection.

■ Assess the abdominal dressing or surgical wound for drainage and signs of infection.

■ Administer antibiotics as per order. Women who experience a prolonged labor, prolonged rupture of membranes, or increased temperature may be placed on antibiotic therapy.

■ Remove the Foley catheter as per orders when the woman is able to ambulate to bathroom. This generally occurs 8 to 12 hours post surgery.

■ Assist the woman with ambulation and encourage her to ambulate to reduce risk of abdominal pain related to gas buildup.

■ Encourage fluid intake to assist in hydration.

■ Discontinue IV fluids per order when the woman is able to take fluids by mouth and the fundus and lochia are within normal limits.

■ Assess bowel sounds and advance to a regular diet as per order based on the presence of bowel sounds and absence of nausea and vomiting.

- Provide information on nutrition to promote tissue healing.
- Assist the woman into a comfortable position for infant feeding. Breastfeeding mothers may be more comfortable in a side lying position or football hold, which prevents pressure on her abdomen.
- Assist the woman with infant care.
- Provide opportunities for the couple to ask questions about their cesarean birth experience.
- Facilitate mother–infant attachment by bringing the infant to the woman and ensuring the woman's comfort.
- Instruct the family that they need to assist the woman with infant care and housework as she needs 6 weeks to recover from surgery.
- Provide teaching on infant care, postoperative care, and postpartum care.
- Remove staples before discharge per protocol.

Expected Assessment Findings

- Vital signs are within normal limits.
  - *Temperature elevations may be a sign of infection.*
- Breath sounds are clear.
- The woman deep breathes and coughs every 2 hours while awake.
- The pain level is 3 or below on a pain scale of 0 to 10 with the use of nonpharmacological and pharmacological interventions.
- The fundus is firm and midline at one finger breadth below the umbilicus.
- The lochia is scant to moderate.
- The abdominal incision is clean, intact, and free of signs of infection.
- The woman spontaneously voids at least 200 mL within 4 to 6 hours of removal of the Foley catheter.
- The woman ambulates to the bathroom and in hallways.
- Bowel sounds are present.
- The woman reports passing gas.
- The woman is able to tolerate oral fluids and food.
- Negative Homans' sign.
- The mother is able to feed her newborn with assistance.
- The couple cares for the needs of their newborn.
- The woman may remain in the taking-in phase longer related to her focus being on pain control and integration of the birthing experience.
- Couples talk about their cesarean birth experience with staff, family, and friends.

Clinical Pathway for Scheduled Cesarean Birth

Focus of Care	Preoperative	Intraoperative	Postoperative First 24 Hours	Postoperative 24 Hours to Discharge
Assessments	Review prenatal record for risk factors. Complete admission assessments as per protocol. Assess the couple's emotional responses. Completes the surgical checklist.	Vital signs are monitored by the anesthesiologist or CRNA. Apgar score on neonate by neonatal personnel. Assess the neonate per protocol.	Monitor VS, usually every hour x 4; and then every 4 hours. Monitor respirations and sedation level as per post intrathecal morphine administration protocol — usually every hour for the first 24 hours. Assess the level and location of pain. Assess abdominal dressing for bleeding and/or drainage. Monitor intake and output. Monitor ability to void. Monitor for signs of potential postpartum hemorrhage. Review laboratory test reports such as H&H, CBC. Monitor for signs of potential infections. Complete post-anesthesia assessments. Assess for adverse reaction related to intrathecal morphine such as decreased respirations, itching, and vomiting and intervene as per protocol.	Assess as per protocol, usually every 4 hours. Assess incisional site for drainage and signs of infection. Assess for signs of urinary disturbances.
Activity Level	Ambulatory until Foley inserted	Bed rest	Bed rest until complete return of motor and sensory sensation/function. Following return of motor and sensory sensation, the woman is assisted in short walks and sitting in chair or on bedside. Assistance is required for peri-care and ADLs.	Up ad libitum Encourage the woman to ambulate to reduce risk of gas pains. May require assistance with pericare and ADLs.
Education	Provide information on surgical procedure, anesthesia, and what to expect during cesarean birth and postoperatively.	Provide information to the woman and her support person on woman's and fetus's/neonate's condition.	Begin teaching on care of the neonate and of the woman's needs during the postpartum period.	Continue teaching and preparing the couple for discharge. Provide postoperative discharge teaching.

Clinical Pathway for Scheduled Cesarean Birth —cont'd

Focus of Care	Preoperative	Intraoperative	Postoperative First 24 Hours	Postoperative 24 Hours to Discharge
Elimination	Insert the Foley catheter and connect to continuous drainage.	Insert the Foley catheter if not done previously. Connect the Foley catheter to continuous drainage.	Connect the Foley catheter to continuous drainage for the first 8–12 hours. Remove the Foley catheter as per orders. Assist the woman to the bathroom and measure voidings.	Assist the woman to the bathroom and measure voidings.
Emotional Needs	The couple may be anxious and excited. Provide emotional support and address questions and concerns. Keep the couple informed on surgical time.	The couple may be anxious and excited. Address the couple's concerns and questions. Provide an opportunity for the couple to see and touch the neonate before transferring the neonate to the nursery. Encourage the new father or support person to accompany the neonate to the nursery.	Couples may be excited and tired. Address the couple's concerns regarding cesarean birth and the woman's and neonate's condition. Provide opportunities for the couple to share their experience and emotional responses to the birth.	Provide opportunities for couples to share their thoughts and feelings regarding the birthing experience and care of their neonate.
Medications	Administer preoperative medications as per protocol.	The CRNA or anesthesiologist administers antibiotics as indicated. The CRNA or anesthesiologist administers oxytocin.	Administer medications as per orders (i.e., stool softener, vitamins).	Administer medications as per orders (i.e., stool softeners, vitamins).
Nutrition	NPO Insert IV. Administer IV fluid preload.	NPO IV fluids	NPO and advancing to regular diet. IV fluids until bowel sounds are present and the woman is tolerating fluids by mouth.	Diet as tolerated. Provide information on the role of nutrition in postpartum recovery and breastfeeding.
Pain Management	CRNA or anesthesiologist meets with the couple to discuss anesthesia options.	The CRNA or anesthesiologist inserts the epidural catheter. The CRNA or anesthesiologist administers anesthetic agents via epidural catheter. The CRNA or anesthesiologist remove the epidural catheter.	Intrathecal morphine administered via epidural catheter by CRNA or anesthesiologist after the birth of the neonate Administer interventions including medications for treatment of intrathecal morphine side effects such as pruritus and nausea/vomiting. The anesthesiologist or CRNA responsible for prescribing medication for pain management and treatment of intrathecal morphine side effects.	PO analgesic prescribed by obstetrician. Provide information on relaxation and breathing techniques Offer comfort measures such as positioning or a warm blanket.

TYING IT ALL TOGETHER

You are assigned to care for a couple who is scheduled to have a repeat cesarean birth. Lisa is a gravida 2 para 1, 25-year-old woman. Her husband, Joe, is 27 years old and plans to accompany Lisa in the operating room. Their first cesarean birth was due to CPD. Lisa and Joe have a healthy 3-year-old daughter, Sara, who is excited about having a baby brother.

Describe the nursing action for the preoperative period.

You transfer the couple to the operating room on the labor and birthing unit. You will be the circulating nurse. Spinal anesthesia is used for the cesarean birth.

Describe the major nursing action during the intraoperative period.
Describe the anesthesia management during this period of time.

Lisa experiences an uncomplicated cesarean birth and delivers a 3800-gram baby boy with Apgar scores of 9 and 9. Lisa and her son are transferred to the OB recovery room where you continue to care for the family. Lisa plans to breastfeed her son.

Describe the major nursing actions during the immediate postoperative recovery period.

The following day you are assigned to Lisa and her family in the postpartum unit. The shift report indicates that Lisa's lungs are clear, BS positive, fundus firm at 1 above U. Lisa ambulated to the bathroom and voided 450 mL. She is tolerating fluids. Her H & H are 30 and 10.2. She is having difficulty with breastfeeding. She complained of pain of 6 on a 10-point pain scale.

List the expected assessment findings for this period of time.
Discuss the nursing actions based on the shift report.
Discuss the major nursing action for couples and their newborn in preparation for discharge.

■ ■ ■ Review Questions ■ ■ ■

1. Indication for a cesarean delivery on maternal request is:
   A. Nonreassuring fetal heart rate
   B. Placenta previa
   C. Woman's desire to have a cesarean birth versus vaginal birth
   D. Obstetrician preference for cesarean delivery

2. The experiences of cesarean birth parents differ from those of vaginal birth parents in which of the following?
   A. Emotional responses to the childbirth experience
   B. Ability to breastfeed
   C. Nutritional needs
   D. Maternal hormonal changes

3. In the operating room, the circulating nurse calls a "time-out" before the surgery begins. The purpose of the time out is to:
   A. Confirm that the surgeon is ready to begin.
   B. Verify that it is the correct site, procedure, and patient.
   C. Verify that the anesthesia is adequate.
   D. Confirm that the neonatal team is in attendance

4. The most serious complication of the use of intrathecal morphine in the first 24 hours postoperative is:
   A. Urinary retention
   B. Nausea and itching
   C. Decreased sensation in legs
   D. Respiratory depression

5. You are assigned to take care of a woman, Lisa, who is 24 hours postoperative after an emergent cesarean birth related to fetal intolerance of labor. Lisa tells you that she is upset about having a cesarean birth. Your best initial nursing action is to:
   A. Inform her she has a healthy newborn.
   B. Inform her that most women experience disappointment in having a cesarean birth.
   C. Ask her to tell you more about her feelings.
   D. Explain why she had a cesarean birth.

References

American Society of Anesthesiologists Task Force. (2007). *Anesthesiology, 106*, 843–863.

Association of Women's Health, Obstetric and Neonatal Nursing (AWHONN). (2001). *Evidence-Based Clinical Practice Guideline: Nursing care of the woman receiving regional analgesia/anesthesia in labor.* Washington, DC: Author.

Chestnut, D. (2006). Cesarean delivery on maternal demand: Implications for anesthesia providers. *International Journal of Obstetric Anesthesia, 15*, 269–272.

Deglin, J., & Vallerand, A. (2009). *Davis's drug guide for nurses* (11th ed.). Philadelphia: F. A. Davis.

Grossman, G., Joesch, J., & Tanfer, K. (2006). Trends in maternal request cesarean delivery from 2001 to 2004. *The American College of Obstetricians and Gynecologists, 108*, 1506–1516.

Hacker, N., Moore, J., & Gambone, J. (2004). *Essentials of obstetrics and gynecology* (4th ed). Philadelphia: W.B. Saunders.

Hamilton, B., Martin, J., & Ventura, S. (2006). Births: Preliminary data for 2005. *National Vital Statistics Reports, 55*, 1–20 [online]. Hyattsville, MD: National Center for Health Statistics. Retrieved from www.cdc.gov/nchs/products/pubs/pubd/hestats/prelimbirths05/prelimbirths05.htm (Accessed September 19, 2009).

Hobson, J., Slade, P., Wrench, I., & Power, L. (2006). Preoperative anxiety and postoperative satisfaction in women undergoing elective cesarean section. *International Journal of Obstetric Anesthesia, 15*, 18–23.

Hughes, S., Levinson, G., & Rosen, M. (2002). *Shnider and Levinson's anesthesia for obstetrics* (4th ed.). Philadelphia: Lippincott, Williams & Wilkins.

Joint Commission (2003). Universal protocol for preventing wrong site, wrong procedure, wrong person surgery. Retrieved from www.jointcommission.org/patientsafety/universalprotocol/(Accessed September 19, 2009).

Kuczkowski, M., Reisner (Ed), L., & Lin, D. (2006). Anesthesia for cesarean section. In D. Chestnut (Ed), *Obstetric anesthesia: Principles and practice* (3rd ed.). Philadelphia: C. V. Mosby.

Martin, J., Hamilton, B., Sutton, P., Ventura, S., Menacker, F., & Kirmeyer, S. (2006). Final data for 2004. *National Vital Statistics Reports, 55*, 1–20. Retrieved from www.cdc.gov/nchs/data/nvsr/nvsr55/nvsr545_11.pdf (Accessed September 19, 2009).

Menacker, F. (2005). Trends in cesarean rates for first time and repeat cesarean rates in low risk women: United States. *National Vital Statistics Reports, 54*, 1-12. Retrieved from www.cdc.gov/nchs/nvsr/nvsr54/nvsr54_04.pdf (Accessed September 19, 2009).

National Institutes of Health (2006). NIH State-of-the-Science Conference: Cesarean Delivery on Maternal Request. Retrieved from www.consensus.nih.gov/2006/2006CesareanSOS027main.htm (Accessed September 19, 2009).

Schwartz, A. (2006). Learning the essentials of epidural anesthesia. *Nursing 2006, 36*, 44–49.

Postpartum Physiological Assessments and Nursing Care

OBJECTIVES

On completion of this chapter, the student will be able to:

☐ Define key terms.
☐ Describe the physiological changes that occur during the postpartum period.
☐ Identify the critical elements of assessment and nursing care during the postpartum period.
☐ Describe the critical elements of discharge teaching.

Nursing Diagnosis

☐ At risk for infection related to tissue trauma
☐ At risk for fluid volume deficit related to uterine atony
☐ At risk for impaired urinary elimination related to decreased sensation; tissue trauma
☐ At risk for constipation related to hormonal effects on smooth muscles
☐ At risk for knowledge deficit regarding health promotion post-birth related to lack of information

Nursing Outcomes

☐ The woman will remain free from symptoms of infection.
☐ The woman's fundus will remain firm with scant to moderate lochia.
☐ The woman will spontaneously void within 6 to 8 hours post-birth.
☐ The woman will eat a diet high in fiber and roughage and will drink a minimum of 8 glasses of fluid per day.
☐ The woman will verbalize an understanding of major components of health promotion.

INTRODUCTION

The **postpartum** is the 6-week period after childbirth. It is a time of rapid physiological changes within the woman's body as it returns to a pre-pregnant state. Women who enter pregnancy in a healthy state and experience a low-risk pregnancy and labor and birth are at low risk for complications during the postpartum period.

CRITICAL COMPONENT

Physiological Aspect of Postpartum Nursing Care

The focus of the physiological aspect of postpartum nursing care is:
- Assessing for early signs of potential complications
- Health promotion
- Family education

THE REPRODUCTIVE SYSTEM

The reproductive system, which includes the uterus, cervix, vagina, and perineum, undergoes dramatic changes during the 6 weeks after the birthing experience. Women are at risk for hemorrhage and infection. Nursing assessments and interventions are aimed at reducing these risks.

Uterus

After delivery of the placenta, the uterus begins the process of **involution**, by which the uterus returns to a pre-pregnant size, shape, and location; and the placental site heals. This occurs through uterine contractions and atrophy of the uterine muscle. Primiparous women usually do not experience discomfort related to uterine contractions during the postpartum period. Multiparous women or women who are

Want to reinforce your reading? Need to review for a test? Listen to this chapter on your accompanying CD.

breastfeeding may experience "afterpains" during the first few postpartum days. **Afterpains** are moderate to severe cramp-like pains that are related to the uterus working harder to remain contracted and/or to the increase of oxytocin that is released in response to infant suckling.

The uterus needs to be in a contracted state during the postpartum period to decrease the risk of postpartum hemorrhage. The contracted uterine muscle compresses the open vessels at the placental site and decreases the amount of blood loss.

Nursing Actions

■ Assess the uterus for location, position, and tone of the fundus.
  ■ *After the third stage of labor, assess the uterus:*
    ■ Every 15 minutes for the first hour
    ■ Every 30 minutes for the second hour
    ■ Every 4 hours for the next 22 hours
    ■ Every shift after the first 24 hours (Scoggin, 2004)
    ■ More frequently if the assessment findings are not within normal limits
  ■ *Before assessment:*
    ■ Inform the woman that you will be palpating her uterus.
    ■ Explain the procedure.
    ■ Instruct the woman to void.
    ■ Provide privacy.
    ■ Lower the head and foot of the bed so that the woman is in a supine position and flat.
  ■ *Support the lower uterine segment by placing one hand just above the symphysis pubis (Fig. 12-1).*
  ■ *Locate the fundus with the other hand using gentle downward pressure.*
  ■ *Determine the tone of the fundus: Firm (contracted) or soft (boggy).*
    ■ A boggy uterus indicates that the uterus is not contracting and places the woman at risk for excessive blood loss. If the uterus is boggy the nurse should:
      ■ *Massage the fundus with the palm of the hand.*
      ■ *Give oxytocin as per the physician's or midwife's orders.*
      ■ *Notify the physician or midwife if the uterus does not respond to massage.*

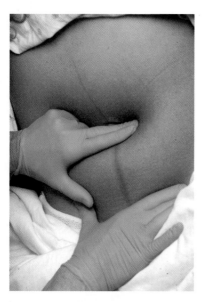

Figure 12-1   Nurse supporting lower uterine segment while assessing the postpartum uterus.

  ■ *Measure the distance between the fundus and umbilicus with your fingers.*
    ■ Each finger breadth equals 1 cm.
  ■ *Determine the position of the uterus.*
    ■ A uterus that is shifted to the side may indicate a distended bladder.
    ■ A distended bladder interferes with uterine contractibility, which places the woman at risk for uterine atony and increases her risk of hemorrhage.
    ■ The immediate action is to explain to the patient the need for her to void and to assist her to the bathroom. Reassess the uterine position after the woman has voided and returned to her bed.
  ■ *Expected assessment findings (Fig. 12-2):*
    ■ Immediately after birth of the placenta, the uterine fundus is located at the umbilicus and is firm and midline.
    ■ 1 to 2 hours after birth of the placenta, the fundus is midway between umbilicus and symphysis pubis and is firm and midline.
    ■ 12 hours after birth of the placenta, the fundus is located 1 cm above the umbilicus and is firm and midline.
    ■ 24 hours after birth of placenta, fundus is located at 1 cm below the umbilicus and is firm and midline.
    ■ The uterus descends 1 cm per day; by day 10 the fundus has descended into the pelvis and is not palpable.
■ Document the location, position, and tone of the fundus and nursing interventions.
  ■ *Sample charting: Fundus firm in midline position at U/2*

CRITICAL COMPONENT

Boggy Uterus

■ A boggy uterus is a sign that the uterus is not in a contracted state.
■ Risk of excessive blood loss and/or hemorrhage is increased.
■ The immediate action is to massage the fundus with the palm of your hand in a circular motion until firm and reevaluate within 30 minutes
■ If the uterus does not respond to massage, follow the standing order for oxytocin and notify the physician or midwife.

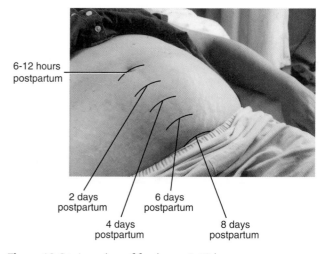

6-12 hours postpartum

2 days postpartum

4 days postpartum

6 days postpartum

8 days postpartum

Figure 12-2   Location of fundus at 6–12 hours postpartum, 2, 4, 6, and 8 days postpartum.

Medication

Oxytocin (Syntocinon)

- Indication: Postpartum control of bleeding
- Action: Stimulates uterine smooth muscle to produce uterine contraction
- Adverse reactions with IV use: Coma, seizures, hypotension, water intoxication
- Route and doses: 10 units in a liter of IV solution or 10 units IM

(Data from Deglin & Vallerand, 2009)

The Endometrium

The **endometrium**, the mucus membrane that lines the uterus, undergoes regeneration after the birth of the placenta through the process of necrosis of the superficial layer of the decidua and regeneration of the decidua basalis into endometrial tissue. **Lochia**, a bloody discharge from the uterus that contains sloughed off necrotic tissue, undergoes changes that reflect the healing stages of the uterine placental site (Table 12-1). Uterine contractions constrict the vessels around the placental site and help decrease the amount of blood loss. Primary complication is **endometritis,** which is an infection of the endometrial tissue (see Chapter 14).

Nursing Actions

- Assess lochia each time the uterus is assessed.
  - *Lower the peripad for inspection and determine the amount of lochia.*
    - The amount of flow is determined by the amount of lochia on a perineal pad after 1 hour (Association of Women's Health, Obstetric and Neonatal Nurses [AWHONN], 2006).
  - *Lochia is assessed as scant, light, moderate, or heavy (Fig. 12-3).*
    - Scant is less than 1 inch on the pad.
    - Light is less than 4 inches on the pad.
    - Moderate is less than 6 inches on the pad.

Scant: Blood only on tissue when wiped or 1- to 2-inch stain

Light: 4-inch or less stain

Moderate: Less than 6-inch stain

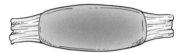

Heavy: Saturated pad

Figure 12- 3   Comparison of heavy, moderate, and scant lochia on pads.

  - Heavy is when the pad is saturated within one hour (AWHONN, 2006).
- Assess for clots.
  - *It is common for lochia to contain clots which occur when the lochia has been pooling in the lower uterine segment.*
  - *Small clots should be noted in the patient chart.*
  - *Large clots can interfere with uterine contractions.*
  - *Large clots should be weighed and findings reported to the physician or midwife.*
    - 10 grams equals 10 milliliters of blood loss.
  - *Expected assessment findings (see Table 12-1)*

TABLE 12–1   STAGES AND CHARACTERISTICS OF LOCHIA

STAGE	TIMEFRAME	EXPECTED FINDINGS	DEVIATIONS FROM NORMAL
LOCHIA RUBRA	Day 1–3	Bloody with small clots Moderate to scant amount Increased flow on standing or breastfeeding Fleshy odor	Large clots Heavy amount; saturates pad within 15 minutes (sign of possible hemorrhage) Foul odor (sign of infection) Placental fragments
LOCHIA SEROSA	Day 4–10	Pink or brown color Scant amount Increased flow during physical activity Fleshy odor	Continuation of rubra stage after day 4 Heavy amount; saturates pad within 15 minutes (sign of possible hemorrhage) Foul odor (sign of infection)
LOCHIA ALBA	Day 10	Yellow to white in color Scant amount Fleshy odor	Bright red bleeding (sign of possible late postpartum hemorrhage) Foul odor (sign of infection)

CRITICAL COMPONENT

Excessive Bleeding

- Heavy lochia is a sign of excessive bleeding and/or postpartum hemorrhage.
- Assess the tone of uterus.
- If the uterus is boggy, massage.
- If the uterus is boggy and displaced to the side, instruct the patient to void and reevaluate.
- If firm, change the pad and reevaluate in 15 minutes.
- In case of continued excessive bleeding, notify the physician or midwife.

- Patient education
  - *Teach the woman how to assess the uterus and explain the normal involutional process.*
  - *Teach the woman how to massage her uterus if boggy and instruct her to notify the nurse while in the hospital and health care provider after discharge.*
  - *Provide information regarding "afterpains."*
    - Uterine cramps are caused by the contraction and relaxation of the uterus as it decreases in size.
    - Afterpains occur within the first few days and last 36 hours.
    - They occur more commonly with multiparous women and increase with each additional pregnancy/birth.
    - The condition may increase when breastfeeding during the first few postpartum days.
    - A distended bladder can increase afterpains.
    - Comfort measures:
      - *Empty bladder*
      - *Warm blanket to abdomen*
      - *Analgesia (ibuprofen is commonly used for postpartum discomfort)*
      - *Relaxation techniques*
  - *Provide information on the stages of lochia.*
  - *Explain that the flow of lochia can increase when getting up in the morning or after sitting for prolonged periods of time due to vaginal pooling of lochia, or from excessive physical activity.*
  - *Instruct the woman to notify the nurse, physician, or midwife if she experiences:*
    - A sudden increase in the amount of lochia
    - Bright red bleeding after the rubra stage
    - Foul odor
  - *Provide information for reducing the risk of infection.*
    - Instruct the patient to change the peripad frequently because lochia is a medium for bacterial growth.
- Document the stage and amount of lochia and nursing interventions.
  - *Sample charting: Scant amount of lochia serosa; teaching provided on stages of lochia*

Medication

Ibuprofen (Motrin)

- Indication: Mild to moderate pain
- Action: Decreased pain and inflammation
- Common side effects: Headaches, constipation, dyspepsia, nausea, vomiting, edema
- Route and dose: PO; 600–800 mg every 6 hours PRN

(Data from Deglin and Vallerand, 2009)

Vagina and Perineum

- The vagina and perineum experience changes related to the birthing process ranging from mild stretching and minor lacerations to major tears and episiotomies.
- The woman may experience mild to severe pain depending on the degree and type of vaginal and/or perineal trauma.
- The primary complication is infection at the lacerations or episiotomy sites.
- The vagina and perineum undergo healing and restoration during the postpartum period.

Nursing Actions

- Assess the perineum every shift using the acronym REEDA (redness, edema, ecchymosis, discharge, approximation of edges of episiotomy or laceration).
  - *Explain the procedure.*
  - *Provide privacy.*
  - *Assist the woman to her side.*
  - *Lower the peripad and separate the buttocks to expose the perineum for assessment.*
- Expected assessment findings:
  - *Mild edema*
  - *Minor ecchymosis*
  - *Approximation of the edges of the episiotomy or laceration*
  - *Mild to moderate pain*
- Assess for discomfort.
- Provide comfort measures:
  - *Apply ice to the perineum for the first 24 hours to decrease edema and provide an anesthetic effect.*
  - *Encourage the woman to lie on her side to decrease pressure on perineum.*
  - *Instruct the woman to tighten her gluteal muscles as she sits down and to relax muscles after she is seated. This helps cushion the perineum and increases comfort when assuming a sitting position.*
  - *Instruct the woman to wear peripads snugly to prevent rubbing.*
  - *Instruct the woman to take Sitz baths starting 24 hours after delivery twice a day for 20 minutes to promote circulation, healing, and comfort.*
  - *Administer analgesia per the physician's or midwife's order.*
  - *Administer a topical anesthetic per the physician's or midwife's order.*
- Reduce the risk for infection.
  - *Instruct the woman to use a peribottle with warm water and rinse the perineum after elimination.*
  - *Instruct the woman to change the peripad frequently due to lochia being a medium for bacterial growth.*
  - *Instruct the woman to properly dispose of soiled pads and to wash her hands.*
- Document findings and interventions.
  - *Sample charting: Perineum intact with no signs of bruising or edema. Patient reports a 2 on the pain scale of 0–10. An ice pack is applied to the perineum.*

BREASTS

During pregnancy, the breasts undergo changes in preparation for lactation. Around the third postpartum day all women, breastfeeding and non-breastfeeding, experience some degree of primary breast engorgement. **Primary engorgement**, which is an increase in the vascular and lymphatic system of the breasts, precedes the initiation of milk production. The woman's breasts become larger, firm, warm, and tender and the woman may feel a throbbing pain in the breasts. Primary engorgement subsides within 24 to 48 hours. Women who breastfeed experience **subsequent breast engorgement** related to distention of milk glands that is relieved by having the baby suckle or by expressing milk. The primary complication is **mastitis**, which is an infection of the breast (see Chapter 14).

Colostrum, a clear, yellowish fluid, precedes milk production. It is higher in protein and lower in carbohydrates than breast milk. It contains immunoglobulins G and A that provides protection for the newborn during the early weeks of life.

Lactation is further addressed in Chapter 16.

CRITICAL COMPONENT

Mastitis

- Mastitis is an inflammation or infection of the breast.
- The infection may be due to bacterial entry through cracks in nipples.
- Symptoms: Fever, malaise, unilateral breast pain, and tenderness in the infected area
- Treatment: Antibiotic therapy, analgesia, rest, and hydration
- The woman should continue to breastfeed or pump her breasts as per the physician's or midwife's recommendation.

Nursing Actions for the Breastfeeding Woman

- Assess the breasts for engorgement.
  - *Inspect the breasts for signs of engorgement: tenderness, firmness, warmth, and/or enlargement.*
  - *Expected assessment findings:*
    - In the first 24 hours postpartum, the breasts are soft and nontender.
    - On postpartum day 2, the breasts are slightly firm and nontender.
    - On postpartum day 3, the breasts are firm, tender, and warm to touch.
- Assess the nipples for signs of irritation and nipple tissue breakdown.
  - *Signs of irritation and tissue breakdown are cracked, blistered, or reddened areas. (See Chapter 16 for interventions to decrease risk of nipple irritation and breakdown.)*
- Assess for mastitis.
  - *Inspect the breasts for localized tenderness to touch, increased warmth, and redness.*
  - *Note signs of increased temperature and feeling of malaise.*
  - *Report signs and symptoms of mastitis to the physician or midwife.*
- Patient education
  - *Apply heat to the breasts to increase circulation and comfort.*
  - *Encourage the woman to wear a supportive bra.*
  - *Instruct the woman to examine nipples before feedings for signs of irritation.*
  - *Instruct the woman to feed her infant or express milk if she is experiencing breast engorgement.*
- Document findings and interventions.
  - *Sample charting: The breasts are soft and nontender. There are no signs of nipple irritation. The patient is wearing a supportive bra.*

Nursing Actions for the Non-breastfeeding Woman

- Assess the breasts for primary engorgement.
  - *Inspect the breasts for signs of engorgement: Tenderness, firmness, warmth, and/or enlargement.*
  - *Expected assessment findings*

  - During the first 24 hours postpartum, the breasts are soft and nontender.
  - On postpartum day 2, the breasts are slightly firm and nontender.
  - On postpartum day 3, the breasts are firm and tender.
- Patient education
  - *Instruct the woman to wear a supportive bra 24 hours a day until her breasts become soft.*
  - *Instruct the woman who is experiencing engorgement to:*
    - Apply ice to the breasts.
    - Not express milk because this stimulates milk production.
    - Avoid heat to the breast because this can stimulate milk production.
    - Take an analgesic for pain.
  - *Inform the woman that breast engorgement will subside within 48 hours.*
- Document findings and interventions.
  - *Sample charting: Breasts are soft and nontender. The patient is wearing a supportive bra.*

Evidence-Based Practice: Breast Binding

Swift, K., & Janke, J. (2003). Breast binding … is it all that it's wrapped up to be. *JOGNN, 32,* 332–339.

The purpose of this study was to compare the difference in breast symptoms in non-breastfeeding women who used continuous breast binding and those who used continuous support bra wearing during the first 10 days postpartum. The sample included 60 women who were randomly assigned to either the breast-binding group or the supportive bra-wearing group.

Results

- There was no significant difference related to symptoms of breast engorgement.
- The breast-binding group reported a greater degree of breast tenderness, breast leakage, and use of pain relief measures.

Recommendations

- The use of breast-binding should be discouraged.
- Wearing a supportive bra should be encouraged.
- Continued research to determine methods to reduce pain related to breast engorgement.

THE CARDIOVASCULAR SYSTEM

Women have an average blood loss of 400 to 500 mL related to the vaginal birthing experience. This has a minimal effect on a woman's system due to pregnancy-induced hypervolemia. There is an increase in cardiac output during the first few postpartum hours related to blood that was shunted through the uteroplacental unit returning to the maternal system. Cardiac output returns to pre-pregnant levels within 48 hours. White blood cell (WBC) levels may increase to 25,000/mm within a few hours of birth and returns to normal levels within 7 days.

Women are at risk for thrombosis related to the increase of circulating clotting factors during pregnancy. Clotting factors slowly decrease after the birth of the placenta and return to normal ranges within the first 2 postpartum weeks.

There is an increased risk of **orthostatic hypotension,** a sudden drop in the blood pressure when the woman stands up, which is due to decreased vascular resistance in the pelvis. Most women will experience an episode of feeling cold and shaking during the first few hours following birth. This phenomenon is referred to as **postpartum chills** and is related to vascular instability.

Nursing Actions

■ Assess pulse and blood pressure:
  ■ *Every 15 minutes for the first hour*
  ■ *Every 30 minutes for the second hour*
  ■ *Every 4 hours for the next 22 hours*
  ■ *Every shift after the first 24 hours (Scoggin, 2004)*
  ■ *Expected assessment findings:*
    ■ Pulse and blood pressure within normal ranges
■ Assess for orthostatic hypotension
  ■ *Expected assessment findings*
    ■ May experience orthostatic hypotension during the first few postpartum days when moving from a sitting or lying position to a standing position. During first 24 hours postpartum, women need assistance when ambulating.

CRITICAL COMPONENT

Orthostatic Hypotension

■ Women are at risk for orthostatic hypotension during the first postpartum week.
■ Explain cause and incidence of orthostatic hypotension.
■ Instruct the patient to rise slowly to a standing position.
■ Assist the woman when ambulating during the first few hours post birth.
■ Assist the woman to a sitting position if she becomes dizzy or faint.
■ Use an ammonia ampule if the woman faints.

■ Assess for excessive blood loss.
  ■ *An increase in pulse rate may be an indicator of excessive blood loss.*
  ■ *Expected assessment findings:*
    ■ Blood loss within normal ranges; pulse rate normal
    ■ Hemoglobin and hematocrit within normal ranges.
      ■ *Hemoglobin decreases by 1.0 to 1.5 g/dL and hematocrit decreases 3% to 4% per 500 mL of blood loss (AWHONN, 2006).*
■ Assess for venous thrombosis.
  ■ *Assess for Homans' sign each shift.*
  ■ *Assess the legs for calf tenderness and sensation of warmth each shift.*
  ■ *Expected assessment findings:*
    ■ Negative Homans' sign
    ■ No tenderness or sensation of warmth
■ Assess for postpartum chills.
  ■ *Assess temperature.*
    ■ Women who are experiencing chills with temperature within normal ranges should be offered a warm blanket and reassurance that it is normal.
    ■ Women who are experiencing chills with elevated temperature need to be evaluated further for possible infection, and the physician or midwife needs to be notified.
■ Patient education
  ■ *Instruct the woman on ways to reduce risk of orthostatic hypotension.*
  ■ *Instruct the woman to take temperature if she experiences chills and report temperature elevations to her physician or midwife.*
■ Document findings and nursing interventions.

■ *Sample charting: The patient states that she is cold and shaking. Temperature is 98.6°F (37°C). A warm blanket is placed over the patient. Teaching is provided regarding postpartum chills.*

THE RESPIRATORY SYSTEM

There is a return of chest wall compliance after the birth of the infant due to reduction of pressure on the diaphragm. The respiratory system returns to a pre-pregnant state by the end of the postpartum period.

Nursing Actions

■ Assess the respiratory rate:
  ■ *Every 15 minutes for the first hour*
  ■ *Every 30 minutes for the second hour*
  ■ *Every 4 hours for the next 22 hours*
  ■ *Every shift after the first 24 hours (Scoggin, 2004)*
■ Expected assessment findings:
  ■ *Within normal limits*
■ Document findings and intervention.

THE IMMUNE SYSTEM

■ Temperature
  ■ *It is common for the postpartum woman to experience mild temperature elevations during the first 24 hours post-birth related to muscular exertion, exhaustion, dehydration, or hormonal changes.*
  ■ *A temperature greater than 100.4°F (38°C) after the first 24 hours on two occasions may be indicative of postpartum infection and requires further evaluation.*
■ Rubella
  ■ *Women who are rubella-nonimmune should be immunized for rubella before discharge.*

CRITICAL COMPONENT

Rubella Immunization

■ Women who contract rubella during the first trimester have a 90% chance of transmitting the virus to their fetuses.
■ Fetuses exposed to rubella during the first trimester are at risk for birth defects that include deafness, blindness, heart defects, and mental retardation.
■ Postpartum women who are rubella-nonimmune should be immunized for rubella before discharge.
■ Women who are immunized should avoid pregnancy for 3 months,, although the risk of the fetus developing birth defects from the vaccine is extremely low.

(World Health Organization, 2007)

■ Rh isoimmunization
  ■ *Rh isoimmunization occurs when an Rh-negative woman develops antibodies to Rh-positive blood related to exposure to Rh-positive blood either by blood transfusion or during pregnancy with an Rh-positive fetus.*

■ *Women who are sensitized produce IgG anti–D (antibody) which crosses the placenta and attacks the fetal red blood cells, causing hemolysis.*
■ *Rh isoimmunization is preventable.*

CRITICAL COMPONENT

Prevention of Rh Isoimmunization

■ Rho immune globulin given to Rh-negative women at 28 weeks' gestation.
■ Rh-negative women who gave birth to an Rh-positive neonate, are screened for anti-Rh antibodies (Coombs' test).
■ A second injection of Rho immune globulin is given to the woman if she is Coombs' negative.

$Rh_o(D)$ Immune Globulin (Rh_oGAM):

■ Indication: Administered to Rh-negative women who have given birth to an Rh-positive neonate
■ Action: Prevents production of anti-Rh (D) antibodies
■ Adverse reactions: Pain at the injection site
■ Route and dose: 300 mcg IM within 72 hours post-birth

(Deglin and Vallerand, 2009)

Nursing Actions

■ Assess temperature:
  ■ *Every 15 minutes for the first hour*
  ■ *Every 30 minutes for the second hour*
  ■ *Every 4 hours for the next 22 hours*
  ■ *Every shift after the first 24 hours (Scoggin, 2004)*
■ Temperature elevations less than 100.4°F (38°C) during the first 24 hours post-birth:
  ■ *Hydrate the woman.*
  ■ *Promote relaxation and rest.*
  ■ *Reassess in 1 hour after interventions.*
■ Temperature elevation 100.4°F (38°C) or higher after 24 hours post-birth:
  ■ *Hydrate the woman.*
  ■ *Notify the physician or midwife for further evaluation.*
■ Administer rubella vaccine as indicated.
■ Administer Rho(D) immune globulin (RhoGAM) as indicated.
■ Document findings and interventions.

THE URINARY SYSTEM

Bladder distention, incomplete emptying of the bladder and inability to void are common during the first few days post-birth. These are related to a decreased sensation of the urge to void and/or edema around the urethra. Diuresis, caused by decreased estrogen and oxytocin levels, occurs within 12 hours post-birth and aids in the elimination of excess tissue fluids. Primary complications are bladder distention and cystitis.

CRITICAL COMPONENT

Cystitis

■ Bladder inflammation/infection
■ Symptoms: Frequency, urgency, pain/burning on urination, and malaise
■ Treatment: Antibiotic therapy, increased hydration, rest

Nursing Actions

■ Assess for urinary disturbances.
  ■ *Measure voidings during the first 24 hours post-birth.*
    ■ If voiding is less than 150 mL, the nurse needs to palpate for bladder distention.
      ■ *This may indicate incomplete emptying of the bladder and the woman may need to be catheterized.*
    ■ If unable to void within 12 hours post-birth the woman may need to be catheterized.
      ■ *A Foley catheter is recommended when inability to void is related to edema.*
    ■ An alternative method to use when a woman is unable to void is the use of peppermint oil.
      ■ *Saturate a cotton ball with peppermint oil.*
      ■ *Place the saturated cotton ball in the "hat" (urine collection container) with a small amount of water.*
      ■ *Place the "hat" on the toilet.*
      ■ *Instruct the woman to sit on the toilet.*
      ■ *The vapors of the peppermint oil have a relaxing effect on the urinary sphincter.*
  ■ *Assess for frequency, urgency, and burning on urination.*
    ■ Notify the physician or midwife if the patient reports frequency, urgency and/or burning on urination. These are signs of possible cystitis.
  ■ *Expected assessment findings:*
    ■ The woman spontaneously voids within 6 to 8 hours post-birth.
    ■ Each voiding is a minimum of 150 mL.
    ■ The woman does not experience frequency, urgency, and burning on urination.
■ Assist the woman to the bathroom and encourage her to void within 6 hours post-birth.
  ■ *Early voiding decreases the risk of cystitis.*
■ Instruct the woman to increase fluid intake to a minimum of 8 glasses per day.
■ Document findings and interventions.
  ■ *Sample charting: The patient spontaneously voided 250 mL. The patient states no burning on urination.*

THE ENDOCRINE SYSTEM

Abrupt changes occur in the endocrine system after the delivery of the placenta. Estrogen, progesterone, and prolactin levels decrease. Estrogen levels begin to rise after the first week of postpartum.

■ Nonlactating women: Prolactin levels continue to decline throughout the first 3 postpartum weeks. Menses begins 6 to 10 weeks post-birth. The first menses is usually anovulatory. Ovulation usually occurs by the fourth cycle.
■ Lactating women: Prolactin levels increase in response to the infant's suckling. Lactation suppresses menses. Return of menses depends on the length and amount of breastfeeding. Ovulation is suppressed longer for lactating women than for nonlactating women.

CRITICAL COMPONENT

Contraception

■ All women, nonlactating and lactating, are advised to use a form of contraception when they resume sexual intercourse as ovulation can precede their first menses.
■ Breastfeeding is not an effective means of contraception.

Diaphoresis

Diaphoresis occurs during the first few postpartum weeks in response to the decreased estrogen levels. This profuse sweating, which often occurs at night, assists the body in excreting the increased fluid accumulating during pregnancy.

Nursing Actions

- Assess for diaphoresis.
  - *If present, assess for infection by taking the patient's temperature.*
  - *Expected assessment findings:*
    - Diaphoresis with temperature within normal ranges
- Patient education
  - *Instruct the patient regarding the cause of diaphoresis.*
  - *Discuss comfort measures such as wearing cotton nightwear.*
  - *Instruct the woman to check the temperature and notify the physician or midwife if elevated.*
  - *Provide information regarding return of menses and ovulation.*
  - *Encourage the couple to use contraception when they resume sexual intercourse.*
- Document findings and interventions.
  - *Sample charting: The patient reports that she is feeling hot and is sweating. The patient's temperature is 98.2°F (36.8°C). Patient education is provided on hormonal changes during the postpartum period.*

THE MUSCULAR AND NERVOUS SYSTEMS

After birth, the abdominal muscles have a reduction in tone and the abdomen appears soft and flabby. Some women experience a separation of the rectus muscle, which is noted as **diastasis recti abdominis** (Fig. 12-4). This separation becomes less apparent as the body returns to a pre-pregnant state.

- Women may experience muscular soreness related to the labor and birth experience.
- Lower body nerve sensation may be diminished for women who have received an epidural during labor.
  - *Delay ambulation until full sensation returns.*

Nursing Actions

- Assess for diastasis recti abdominis.
  - *The nurse can feel the separation of the rectus muscle when assessing the fundus.*
  - *Reassure the woman that this is normal and will diminish over time.*
- Assess for muscle tenderness.
  - *Expected assessment findings:*
    - None to mild muscle soreness
- Comfort measures for muscle soreness:
  - *Ice pack to area for 20 minutes*
  - *Heat to area*
  - *Warm shower*
  - *Analgesia*
- Assess for decreased nerve sensation.
  - *Expected assessment findings:*
    - Full sensation of lower extremities for women who did not receive an epidural during labor
    - Diminished lower body sensation for women who received an epidural during labor with full sensation returning within a few hours post-birth

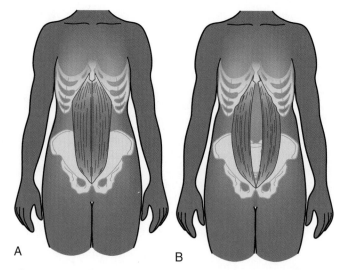

Figure 12-4   Diastasis recti abdominis. *A.* Normal location of rectus muscles of the abdomen. *B.* Diastasis recti. There is separation of the rectus muscles.

- *Delay ambulation or assist the woman when ambulating until full sensation has returned.*
- Document findings and interventions.
  - *Sample charting: The patient ambulates in the room without difficulty.*

THE GASTROINTESTINAL SYSTEM

There is a decrease in gastrointestinal muscle tone and motility post-birth with a return to normal bowel function by the end of the second postpartum week.

- Constipation
  - *Women are at risk for constipation due to:*
    - Decreased GI motility
    - Decreased physical activity
    - Dehydration and fluid loss from labor
    - Perineal pain and trauma
- Hemorrhoids
  - *It is common for women to develop hemorrhoids during pregnancy and/or the birthing process.*
  - *Hemorrhoids will slowly resolve, but can be painful.*
- Appetite
  - *Women are hungry after the birthing experience and can be given a regular diet, unless they are on a prescribed diet such as for diabetes.*
  - *Women are exceptionally hungry during the first few postpartum days and may require snacks.*
- Weight loss
  - *Most women will experience a significant weight loss during the first 2 to 3 weeks postpartum.*
  - *The average American woman at the end of 6 months postpartum is approximately 3 to 4 pounds above her pre-pregnancy weight (Olson et al., 2003).*

Nursing Actions

- Assess bowel sounds at each shift.
  - *Notify the physician or midwife if bowel sounds are faint or absent.*
- Assess for constipation.
  - *Ask the woman if and when she had a bowel movement.*

Evidence-Based Practice: Weight Changes in the First Six Weeks Postpartum

Walker, L., Sterling, B., Kim, M., Arheart, K. L., & Timmerman, G. (2006). Trajectory of weight changes in the first six weeks postpartum. *JOGNN*, 35, 472-481.

The purposes of this research study were to determine the weight changes of women during the first 6 weeks postpartum and variables that influence weight changes. Body mass index (BMI) was measured weekly. The sample included 26 low-income women who experienced an uncomplicated pregnancy.

There was a significant BMI decrease during the first 3 weeks postpartum among white women and a significant BMI decrease during the first 2 weeks among Black and Hispanic women. Plateaus were experienced by all subjects after the 2nd to 3rd decline in BMI. There was a significant positive effect of pre-pregnancy BMI and gestational weight gain on the postpartum BMI.

The small sample size limits the generalizability of the findings. This is the first research study focused on weight changes during the first 6 weeks of postpartum. Additional research that replicates this study is needed to expand the knowledge of weight changes during the postpartum period.

■ *Ask the woman what she did for constipation during pregnancy or in the past and implement these strategies.*
■ Administer a stool softener as per orders.

Medication

Docusate (Colace)

■ Indication: Prevention of constipation
■ Action: Promotes incorporation of water into the stool
■ Common side effects: Mild abdominal cramps
■ Route and dose: PO; 100 mg twice a day

(Data from Deglin and Vallerand, 2009)

■ Assess for hemorrhoids.
  ■ *Instruct the woman to lie on her side, then separate the buttocks to expose the anus.*
■ If hemorrhoids are present:
  ■ *Instruct the woman to increase fluid intake and increase fiber and roughage in diet to decrease risk of constipation.*
  ■ *Encourage the woman to avoid sitting for long periods of time by lying on her side.*
  ■ *Instruct the woman to take Sitz baths, which are helpful in promoting circulation and reducing pain.*
■ Assess appetite.
  ■ *Assess the amount of food eaten during meals.*
  ■ *Ask the woman if she is hungry.*
  ■ *Ask the woman if she is nauseous or has vomited.*
■ Patient education
  ■ *Instruct the woman to increase fluid intake, and increase fiber and roughage in diet to decrease risk of constipation.*
  ■ *Provide nutritional education. This is especially important for lactating women.*
  ■ *Encourage the woman to ambulate to increase GI motility and decrease risk of gas pains.*
  ■ *Instruct the woman to increase fluid intake to a minimum of 8 glasses per day.*
■ Document findings and interventions.
  ■ *Sample charting: Bowel sounds are present in all quadrants.*

CULTURAL AWARENESS: Food Preferences Across Cultures

■ Foods and how they are prepared can be significant to women of different cultures.
■ Ask women of different cultures if there are foods that they prefer to eat based on their cultural beliefs; if not available in the hospital, encourage patients to have family members bring them to the patient.
■ Ask women of Japanese or Chinese cultures if they prefer hot water versus ice water at the bedside.
■ In-service training should be provided to staff about cultures that are common to that unit.

DISCHARGE TEACHING

Discharge teaching for the woman and her partner focuses on:

■ Signs of complications that need to be reported to the physician or midwife:
  ■ *Excessive lochia indicates possible late postpartum hemorrhage.*
  ■ *Foul smelling lochia indicates possible infection*
  ■ *Increased temperature (100.4°F [38°C] or higher) indicates possible infection.*
  ■ *Pelvic or abdominal tenderness/pain is possible sign of infection*
  ■ *Frequency, urgency, or burning on urination indicates possible cystitis*
  ■ *Breast tender, warm, and reddened indicates possible mastitis (AWHONN, 2006)*
■ Health promotion
  ■ *Nutrition and fluids*
    ■ Instruct the woman about nutritional needs for lactating and nonlactating women.
      ■ *Lactating women should increase their caloric intake by 500 calories per day and have a fluid intake of approximately 2 liters per day.*
      ■ *Explain the food pyramid and how this can assist the woman in meeting her nutritional needs.*
  ■ *Activity and exercise*
    ■ Explain the importance of activity to decrease risk of constipation and to promote circulation and a sense of well-being.
    ■ Instruct the woman about appropriate exercises in the postpartum.
  ■ *Rest and comfort*
    ■ Teach the woman the importance of rest in promoting healing and lactation.
    ■ Problem solve with the woman ways to increase rest time (e.g., nap when the baby is napping).
    ■ Encourage the woman to take pain medication as ordered by the physician or midwife.
  ■ *Routine health check-ups*
    ■ Stress the importance of following through with follow-up visits to her physician or midwife.
■ Contraception
  ■ *Assess the couple's desire for future pregnancies.*
  ■ *Assess satisfaction with previous method of contraception.*
  ■ *Provide information on various methods of contraception (Table 12-2).*

TABLE 12–2   METHODS OF CONTRACEPTION

METHOD	FAILURE RATE	AVAILABILITY	ADVANTAGES	DISADVANTAGES
NATURAL METHOD				
Abstinence	0%	Handouts and information from care provider	Readily available	Must have knowledge and be willing to frequently monitor body functions: Temperature, vaginal mucus production and consistency
Natural family planning	20%–25%	Internet access of information	Personal	
Withdrawal	19%		No cost	
BARRIER METHODS				
Condoms (male and female)	14%–22%	OTC purchase	Readily available	Allergic reactions
			One time use	Higher rate of protection when combined with spermicides
Vaginal sponges	20% if no prior births	OTC available	May be placed before intercourse	Must be left in place for at least 6 hours post-intercourse (IC)
	40% if previous births	Most have spermicide added	May leave in for up to 30 hours	Irritation and allergic reaction
			Protects repeated acts of IC	May be difficult to insert and remove
				Need additional doses of spermicide for repeated IC
Cervical caps	20%–40%	Prescription	Fits snugly over cervix	May be difficult to insert and remove
Diaphragms	20%	Must be fitted by provider	Can remain in place >24 hours for repeated IC	Irritation
		If birth or large weight change needs to be refitted		Allergic reaction
Spermicidal-gels, cream suppository, or foam	25%–50%	OTC	Readily available	Irritation
			Use at time of IC	Allergic reaction

Method	Failure Rate	Administration	Action/Use	Side Effects/Risks
HORMONAL METHODS				
Combination estrogen/progesterone oral contraception	5%	Prescription only / 91-day option available; 12-week pill cycle with menses only 4 times per year	Suppresses ovulation / Take one pill a day	May have multiple side effects / Increase risks for blood clots, heart disease, and strokes
Emergency contraceptives (Not to be used as regular form of birth control)	20%	Postcoital ingestion of hormones / Must take within 72 hours of incident	Reduces risk of pregnancy for one time unprotected IC	Due to high dose of hormones, may have headache, nausea, vomiting, or abdominal pain
Progestin only	5%	Prescription only	Take one pill at same time every day	Irregular bleeding / Weight gain
Depo-Provera	3%	Prescription only / Injectable every 3 months	One injection 4 times a year	Irregular bleeding / Weight gain
Contraceptive patch	2%	Prescription only	Place patch for 3 weeks, then remove for one week	Risk same as for oral contraceptives / Possibly less effective for larger women / Possible skin irritation
Hormone implants	>1%	Two rods implanted in the arm / Office procedure	Once in place, there is minimal discomfort / Last for several years	Side effects similar to oral contraceptives / Skin irritation at site
Vaginal ring	2%	Prescription	Flexible hormone-filled ring inserted and left in the vagina for 3 weeks, then removed for 1 week	Side effects similar to oral contraceptives / Vaginal irritation and discharge / If ring falls out, need to use alternate protection for at least 1 week
INTRAUTERINE DEVICES (IUDS)				
Copper material or hormone releasing	0.8%	Prescription / Office procedure to insert	Long-term contraceptive method; good for 1–10 years	Risk of uterine perforation / Risk of pelvic inflammatory disease (PID) / Increase of cramping and bleeding in the first few cycles

Continued

TABLE 12–2   METHODS OF CONTRACEPTION—CONT'D

METHOD	FAILURE RATE	AVAILABILITY	ADVANTAGES	DISADVANTAGES
STERILIZATION				
Vasectomy	0.15%–1%	Surgical procedure done under local anesthesia in the office or clinic	Discomfort for 2–3 days Difficult to reverse High rate of effectiveness	Discomfort for 2–3 days Difficult to reverse Need to use alternative contraceptive method until two post-surgery sperm tests indicate procedure is effective. Bleeding or pain at incision site
Tubal ligation	0.5%	Surgical procedure done under general anesthesia	High rate of effectiveness	Difficult to reverse
Sterilization implant	0.5%–1%	Office procedure	Metallic implants placed in the fallopian tubes, which causes scar tissue that eventually block the tubes	Another contraceptive method needs to be used until blockage is confirmed, usually 3 months

- Sexual activity
  - *Instruct the couple to discuss with the physician or midwife when they can resume sexual intercourse.*
    - General guidelines are to resume sexual intercourse when the lochia has stopped, perineum has healed, and the woman is physically and emotionally ready.
  - *Explain that an artificial vaginal lubricant might be needed to increase comfort during intercourse.*

- *Explain the importance of using contraception when the couple resumes sexual activity.*
- Prescribed medications
  - *Explain all discharge medications including dose, frequency, action and side effects.*

Clinical Pathway for Uncomplicated Vaginal Delivery

Focus of Care	Postpartum: Admission	Postpartum: First 4 hours	Postpartum: Greater than 4 hours After Discharge	Expected Outcomes/ Discharge Criteria
Diagnostic Tests	RPR, HBSag, rubella, blood type and Rh status documented or drawn if no prenatal record available GBS status documented with appropriate interventions Urine toxicology screening as per policy	Fetal Rh study as indicated (woman Rh-negative and neonate Rh-positive)	Hemogram as ordered Notify CNM/MD of abnormal results or if the woman is symptomatic.	Rubella status known and vaccine given if indicated Rh status known – Rh$_o$ immune globulin given if indicated Hemogram within normal ranges
Activity and Safety	Moves legs Lifts bottom off bed Needs assistance with initial ambulation Infant security and safety reviewed	Women who received an epidural for labor and/or birth will need assistance with ambulation until return of sensory and motor sensation.	Able to stand and walk with minimal assistance.	Ambulates without assistance
Treatments and Patient Care	Assess vital signs Assess level of consciousness Assess fundus, lochia, and perineum Ice to perineum Assess for Homans' sign Assess Foley catheter if in place ·Assess IV site and fluids if in place Assess breast for potential breastfeeding problems	Vital signs as per orders Postpartum physical assessment as per orders Peri care with each voiding Ice to perineum Input & output while Foley catheter or IV in place Measure first 2 voidings; notify CNM/MD if urine output <30 mL/hr	Vital signs as per orders Postpartum physical assessment as per orders Peri care with each voiding ·Ice to perineum for first 24 hours Assess breast for signs of engorgement and nipple irritation	Vital signs stable and within normal limits Fundus firm, midline, and descending by 1 cm per day Lochia moderate to scant Perineum healing without signs of infection Breasts exhibit physiological changes of lactation. Breastfeeding without difficulty Bowel and bladder function within normal limits

Clinical Pathway for Uncomplicated Vaginal Delivery—cont'd

Focus of Care	Postpartum: Admission	Postpartum: First 4 hours	Postpartum: Greater than 4 hours After Discharge	Expected Outcomes/ Discharge Criteria
Medications	Maintain IV patency if indicated Oxytocin as indicated to reducing risk of or treat postpartum hemorrhage Analgesics and/or comfort measure as indicated for pain management	IV discontinued if fundus firm and lochia within normal limits Oxytocin discontinued if fundus firm and lochia within normal limits Analgesics and/or comfort measure as indicated for pain management	Analgesics and/or comfort measure as indicated for pain management Rubella vaccine administered, if indicated, at least 30 minutes before discharge $Rh_o(D)$ immune globulin administered as indicated Stool softener as ordered	Mild to moderate pain relieved with comfort measures and/or PO analgesia Rubella vaccine administered when indicated $Rh_o(D)$ immune globulin administered as indicated Discharge medication teaching provided
Nutrition	Regular diet as tolerated PO fluids	Regular diet as tolerated PO fluids	Regular diet as tolerated PO fluids	Maintains adequate diet and fluid intake
Discharge Planning/ Evaluation of Social Support	Evaluate need for referrals such as social worker, lactation specialist, and dietitian	Continue to evaluate need for referrals. Initiate referrals as indicated.	Review discharge preparation with the woman and her family.	The woman and her family have appropriate support on discharge. The woman and her family verbalize the importance of follow-up care for both the woman and infant.
Patient/Family Education	Initiate discharge teaching by assessing immediate learning needs Assist with breastfeeding	Continue discharge teaching based on the woman's/family's learning needs.	Complete discharge teaching.	The woman and her family verbalize understanding of infant needs and the woman's needs. The woman and her family demonstrate basic well baby care skills. The woman and her family verbalize understanding of signs and symptoms that warrant contact with the health care provider.

Nursing Care Plan

Problem (Check appropriate line)	Actual or Potential	Action (Initial care provided)	Expected Outcome/ Discharge Criteria (Initial outcomes obtained)
Potential or actual postpartum hemorrhage related to: _____ Uterine atony _____ Retained placenta _____ Laceration _____ Hematoma _____ Full bladder _____ Other_____	Initiated by: RN: _____ Date/Time _____ ☐ Actual ☐ Potential Change in status Date/Time _____ RN: _____ ☐ Actual ☐ Potential Resolved: Date/Time _____ RN: _____	_____ Monitor and assess vital signs including blood pressure and woman's mental status, lochia flow, and uterine tone per policy. _____ Encourage voiding every 2–3 hours. _____ Massage fundus as needed and instruct the woman on self-assessment. _____ Notify CNM/MD for heavy bleeding/ saturation of one pad in < 1 hour. _____ Give medications such as oxytocin, Methergine, or Hemabate per CNM/MD order. _____ Assist with activity PRN. _____ Notify the provider if the woman has continued excessive bleeding and/or dizziness.	_____ Lochia scant to moderate rubra _____ Fundus firm and at midline _____ No signs or symptoms of postpartum hemorrhage
Potential or actual alteration in comfort related to: _____ Uterine cramping _____ Incision _____ Perineal/rectal pain _____ Breast discomfort _____ Other _____	Initiated by: RN: _____ Date/Time _____ ☐ Actual ☐ Potential Change in status Date/Time _____ RN: _____ ☐ Actual ☐ Potential Resolved: Date/Time _____ RN: _____	_____ Pain assessment _____ Provide or assist with nonpharmacological comfort measures for relief. _____ Provide analgesics as ordered.	_____ Pain will be adequately controlled by analgesics and nonpharmacological comfort measures.

Nursing Care Plan—cont'd

Problem (Check appropriate line)	Actual or Potential	Action (Initial care provided)	Expected Outcome/ Discharge Criteria (Initial outcomes obtained)
Potential or actual postpartum infection related to: _____ Perineum _____ Uterus _____ Breast _____ GBS _____ Other _____	Initiated by: _____ Date/Time _____ ☐ Actual ☐ Potential Change in status Date/Time _____ RN: _____ ☐ Actual ☐ Potential Resolved: Date/Time _____ RN: _____	_____ Vital signs monitored per policy _____ CNM/MD notified immediately if any signs or symptoms of infection are present _____ Woman instructed in self-care including peri care, incisional care, and breast care _____ Woman instructed in signs and symptoms of infection	_____ Woman will exhibit no signs or symptoms of infection (i.e., temperature < 100.4°F (38°C), no abnormal discharge, incision clean and dry if present, breasts without redness) _____ Woman will verbalize understanding of signs and symptoms of infection and aware of when to notify CNM/MD
Potential or actual alteration in elimination related to: _____ Loss of bladder and/or bowel sensation/function following childbirth _____ Other _____	Initiated by: _____ Date/Time _____ ☐ Actual ☐ Potential Change in status Date/Time _____ RN: _____ ☐ Actual ☐ Potential Resolved: Date/Time _____ RN: _____	_____ Assess and monitor for bladder distention as needed. _____ Assess and document initial voidings after delivery to ensure >30 mL/hr without retention in first 6–12 hours. _____ If unable to void catheterize per CNM/MD order. _____ Provide instructions on Kegel exercises. _____ Encourage early ambulation, adequate fluid intake, diet with roughage to prevent constipation. _____ Provide stool softener as ordered.	_____ Woman is voiding without difficulty _____ Fundus is firm and midline _____ Woman is able to verbalize methods of avoiding constipation and to notify CNM/MD if no stool in 4 days

TYING IT ALL TOGETHER

As the nurse, you admit Margarite Sanchez to the postpartum unit at 1050 and receive the transfer report from Labor and Delivery stating the following:

■ Patient is a 28-year-old G3 P2 Hispanic woman who gave birth at 0839, vaginal delivery with a second-degree laceration.
■ She received two doses of Nubain in labor at 0215 and 0440 for pain relief in active labor.
■ Both mother and baby are stable.
■ The mother's bleeding in labor and delivery was moderate.
■ V.S. 120/68-72-20-98.2
■ Ms. Sanchez did not void in labor and delivery.
■ Ms. Sanchez nursed her baby for 15 minutes on each breast after the birth.

José, her husband, has accompanied her to the unit.

Detail the aspects of your initial assessment.

As part of the physical assessment you discover her fundus is 2 cm above the umbilicus and deviated to the left, her lochia is moderate, saturating one third of the pad during transfer, her perineum is swollen.

What are your immediate priorities in nursing care for Margarite Sanchez?
Discuss the rationale for the priorities.
Initial teaching would include the following:

At 5 hours postpartum Margarite rates her perineal pain at 6 on a scale of 0 to 10.

State the nursing diagnosis, expected outcome, and interventions related to this problem.

The next day you are assigned to care for the Sanchez family. Your report from the previous shift indicated that:

■ Her vital signs were within normal limits.
■ She had voided once during the night.
■ Her fundus was 1 below the umbilicus.
■ Lochia was scant to moderate.
■ She breastfed her infant twice.

Margarite informs you that she experienced night sweats.

Discuss your nursing actions including rationales.

You are anticipating that she will be discharged in the afternoon.

Discuss your plan for discharge teaching indicating the priority needs with rationales.

■ ■ ■ Review Questions ■ ■ ■

1. Your patient, who gave birth to a 7-pound baby boy 24 hours ago, is complaining of uterine cramping (afterpains). This is her second baby and she is breastfeeding. Your assessment reveals a firm fundus at midline at 1 cm below the umbilicus. Select all of your initial nursing actions.
   A. Instruct the patient to bottle feed for 36 hours or until the cramping has stopped.
   B. Place a warm blanket on her abdomen.
   C. Explain that these are normal for second-time mothers to experience.
   D. Offer the patient acetaminophen with codeine so she can continue to breastfeed.

2. Your patient gave birth to a 6-pound baby girl 6 hours ago. It was a spontaneous delivery. You note on your assessment of her perineum that there is some edema and slight bruising. She stated that her pain was at 1 on the pain scale. Your nursing action would be to:
   A. Continue applying ice to the perineum.
   B. Assist her with a Sitz bath.
   C. Encourage her to keep her bladder empty.
   D. Administer ibuprofen 800 mg.

3. To decrease the risk of orthostatic hypotension during the first few hours after the birth, the nurse should:
   A. Assist patient to the bathroom by using a wheelchair.
   B. Break open an ammonia ampule and have the patient take a deep breath before getting up.
   C. Have the patient sit on the side of the bed for a few minutes before standing.
   D. Check the patient blood pressure before assisting her to the bathroom.

4. Select the statements that are true regarding primary engorgement.
   A. Only women who are lactating will experience primary engorgement.
   B. It is caused by an increase in the vascular and lymphatic system of the breast.
   C. The breasts become large, firm, and warm to touch.
   D. It subsides within 24 to 36 hours.

5. During your discharge teaching, you are evaluating if your patient needs information on contraception. Select the responses that indicate she needs additional information.
   A. "I will be breastfeeding for the next 6 months. We will start using a condom after I have my first period."
   B. "My husband is getting a vasectomy. We will be using condoms until his second semen analysis is negative for sperm."
   C. "I plan to have an IUD. We will be using condoms until I get an IUD."
   D. "I used a diaphragm prior to this pregnancy and plan to use my old one."

References

Association of Women's Health, Obstetric and Neonatal Nurses (AWHONN). (2006). *The compendium of postpartum care.* Washington, DC: Author

Deglin, J., & Vallerand, A. (2009). *Davis's drug guide for nurses* (11th ed). Philadelphia: F. A. Davis.

Olson, C., Strawderman, M., Hinton, P., & Pearson, T. (2003). Gestational weight gain and postpartum behaviors associated with change from early pregnancy to 1 year postpartum. *International Journal of Obesity, 27,* 7–127.

Scoggin, J. (2004). Physical and psychological changes. In S. Mattson & J. Smith (Eds.), *Core curriculum for maternal-newborn nursing* (3rd ed). Philadelphia: Elsevier.

Swift, K., & Janke, J. (2003). Breast binding ... is it all that it's wrapped up to be? *JOGNN, 32,* 332–339.

Walker, L., Sterling, B., Kim, M., Arheart, K. L., & Timmerman, G. (2006). Trajectory of weight changes in the first six weeks postpartum. *JOGNN, 35,* 472–481.

World Health Organization (2007). *Immunization, vaccines, and biologicals.* Retrieved from www.who.int/immunization/topics/rubella/en/index1 (Accessed September 1, 2009).

The Transition to Parenthood

OBJECTIVES

On completion of this chapter, the student will be able to:

☐ Define key terms.

☐ Describe the process of "becoming a mother."

☐ Identify factors that influence women and men in their role transitions to mother or father.

☐ Discuss bonding and attachment.

☐ Identify factors that affect the family dynamics.

☐ Describe nursing actions that support couples during their transition to parenthood.

Nursing Diagnoses

■ Knowledge deficit related to role of parent due to being a first-time parent.

■ At risk for situational self-esteem disturbance due to new parenting role.

■ At risk for altered family processes related to incorporation of a new family member.

■ At risk for altered parent–infant attachment related to anxiety of being a new parent.

Nursing Outcomes

■ Parents will verbalize an understanding of parental role expectations and responsibilities.

■ Parents will verbalize stressors of new role.

■ Parents will demonstrate positive comments and actions when interacting with family members.

■ Parents will hold the newborn close to the body, attend to the newborn's needs, and interact with the newborn.

INTRODUCTION

The postpartum period is a time of both physiological and psychological adjustments. As the woman is adjusting to the numerous physiological changes within her body, she and her partner are adjusting to their new roles as parents and the effect these new roles have on the couple relationship and the family unit (Fig. 13-1). This chapter focuses on the psychological, emotional, and developmental changes that take place during the transition to parenthood.

TRANSITION TO PARENTHOOD

The **transition to parenthood** is a dynamic developmental process that begins with the knowledge of pregnancy and continues throughout the postpartum period as the couple takes on their new or expanded roles of mother and father. Whether this is the first child or tenth child, this transition is a major life event that is both exciting and stressful, and produces developmental challenges for the individual, the couple's relationship, and family members. Each individual deals with the growth, realization, and preparation of becoming a parent in different ways, and cultural beliefs have an effect on how the individual takes the role of parent (Table 13-1).

The transition to parenthood is fostered or hampered by many factors, some of which include:

■ Previous life experiences: Previous experiences with caring for infants and children can foster a smoother transition to parenthood.

■ Length and strength of the relationship between partners: A strong relationship between the couple can foster a smoother transition to parenthood.

■ Financial considerations: Financial concerns can hamper the transition to parenting.

■ Educational levels: Decreased ability to read and comprehend information regarding child care may hamper the couple's ability to gain knowledge in the care of the infant.

■ Support systems: A lack of positive support in the care of the woman and infant may hamper the transition to parenting.

■ Desire to be a parent: A lack of desire to be a parent can hamper the transition to parenting.

■ Age of parents: Adolescent parents may have a more difficult transition to parenting.

The transition to parenthood involves taking on the role of mother or father, viewing the child as an individual with his or her own personality, and incorporating the new child into the family system.

Want to reinforce your reading? Need to review for a test? Listen to this chapter on your accompanying CD.

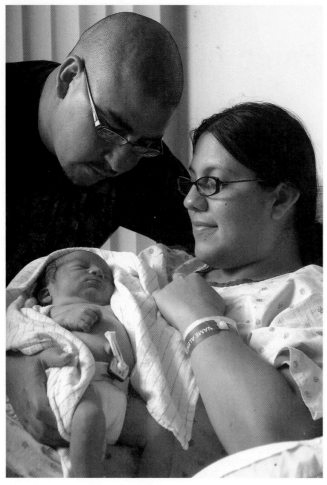

Figure 13-1   Mom and dad getting acquainted with their new son.

Evidence-Based Practice: Maternal Adaptation During the Early Postpartum Period

In the 1960s, Reba Rubin conducted qualitative research studies focusing on maternal adaptation during the early postpartum weeks. Her research is the foundation of our understanding of the psychosocial experience of women during the postpartum period. Two concepts identified through her research are "maternal phases" and "maternal touch." Rubin (1984) refined and modified the process as more evidence was linked to maternal adjustments and behaviors and identified areas of development that women progress through to "becoming a mother."

Ramona Mercer, a student and colleague of Rubin, added to and expanded this body of nursing knowledge through numerous research studies that focused on the maternal role. Based on these studies, Mercer (1995) developed the theory of "maternal role attainment" that describes and explains the process women progress through as they become a mother. Based on her previous research and the research of others, Mercer (2004) supports replacing the term of "maternal role attainment" with "becoming a mother." The term "becoming a mother" reflects that the process is not stagnant, but is continually evolving as the woman and her child are changing and growing.

The theories generated by Rubin's and Mercer's research agendas are the cornerstone of evidence-based knowledge used in establishing nursing guidelines for the care of postpartum women and families.

Parental Roles

Individuals have many roles throughout their lifetimes. As a child, the individual has the roles of son or daughter, sister or brother, grandchild, and student. Additional roles are acquired as the individual ages. Roles change over time as the individual matures and new roles are added. The role of mother or father evolves and changes over time as the child grows and additional children are added to the family. Each new role has expectations and responsibilities that the individual must learn in order to be successful in the role.

Couples are given the title of mother and father with the birth of their child, but must learn the expectations and responsibilities of these roles.

- Examples of parental role expectations are that others will acknowledge the person as being a parent or that the child will obey the parents.
- Examples of responsibilities are that the parents will love and protect their child.

Knowledge of these expectations and responsibilities is acquired through intentional learning (formal instructions) and incidental learning (observing others in the role). Most individuals have little intentional/instructional learning regarding the role of mother or father. The majority of learning of the expectations and responsibilities for these roles occurs through incidental learning. Examples of incidental learning of the parental role are:

- Observing other individuals who are mothers and fathers
- Recalling how they were parented
- Watching movies or television programs that have mothers and/or fathers as characters

The process of learning and developing parental roles should start during the pregnancy. Partners who learn together during the pregnancy have better outcomes when they take on the role of parents. Providing couples with written information regarding different styles of parenting roles allows the expectant couple to learn about parenting behaviors. The expectant couple can then discuss parenting issues and mutually agree on expectations and responsibilities for their new roles.

Expected Findings

- Parents identify changing roles and are willing to make lifestyle changes to accommodate the changes.
- Parents identify with the parental roles.
- Parents discuss what the roles mean to them.
- Couples incorporate a third person, the newborn, into their relationship.
- Couples support each other in mutual care giving tasks.

Nursing Actions

- Encourage, through active listening, the parents to talk about their birth experience and feelings regarding becoming parents.
- Provide an environment that is conducive to rest, such as uninterrupted periods of time so that parents can sleep.
- Provide culturally sensitive care.
- Provide a safe environment for parents to talk about concerns and fears about this new transition, and assist them to find ways to work together in resolving their fears and concerns.
- Discuss the process of transitioning to parenthood.
- Demonstrate positive behaviors and provide positive feedback when appropriate.

TABLE 13–1   CULTURAL BELIEFS AND THE POSTPARTUM FAMILY

CULTURE	BELIEFS AND PRACTICES
ARAB HERITAGE	Children are dearly loved and indulged. Care of the newborn includes wrapping the infant's abdomen at birth to prevent cold or wind from entering the body. The call to pray is recited in the newborn's ear. Male circumcision is a religious requirement of Muslims Breastfeeding is delayed 2–3 days based on the belief that the woman requires rest, and that nursing immediately after birth causes "colic" pain for the mother.
CHINESE HERITAGE	Pregnancy and childbirth are viewed as women's business. Postpartum care includes 1 month of recovery and women eat specific foods and avoid exposure to cold air to decrease the yin (cold) energy. Female relatives care for the newborn so that the woman can rest. Women, during the postpartum period, avoid drinking and touching cold water to decrease the yin (cold) energy.
FILIPINO HERITAGE	The mother often is the major decision maker regarding health, children, and finances. Older relatives such as grandparents share in the responsibility for the care and discipline of younger family members. The woman and her infant remain at home for the first 4 weeks except to go to the doctor.
HINDU HERITAGE	Older female relatives are considered to have expert knowledge in the use of home remedies during pregnancy and the postpartum period. The birth of a son is a blessing because he will carry the family name and take care of aging parents. The birth of a daughter may be cause of concern because of the traditions associated with a dowry. Exposure to cold air is considered dangerous. The mother and infant undergo purification rites on the 11th day after the birth. The baby is officially named on the 11th day. There are prescribed foods to eat and to avoid when the woman is breastfeeding.
JAPANESE HERITAGE	The primary relationship within the family is the mother–child relationship. It is customary for a mother to sleep with the youngest child until that child is 10 years old. Babies are not allowed to cry. Women constantly hold their babies. Women often return to their mother's home during the last 2 months of pregnancy and stay there for the first 2 months after birth. Female relatives assist with the care of the newborn so that the woman can rest. Maternal rest is viewed as important for successful breastfeeding. Women do not bathe, shower, or wash their hair for the first month after birth.
MEXICAN HERITAGE	Women care for the children and the home. Cutting the baby's hair or nails during the first 3 months is believed to cause blindness or deafness. Women are discouraged from taking baths or washing their hair for 6 weeks post-birth.
NAVAJO INDIAN HERITAGE	Grandmothers and mothers are at the center of Navajo society. Children may be named at birth, but the name is not revealed until their first laugh, when they are considered to officially have a soul. Infants are often kept in cradleboards until they can walk. It is taboo to purchase clothes for the baby before he or she is born. The placenta is buried soon after the birth as a symbol of the child being tied to the land. The newborn is given a mixture of juniper bark to cleanse his or her insides and dispel mucus.

Adapted from Purnell & Paulanka (2005).

- Provide parental education on care of the newborn by using a variety of educational strategies such as handouts, videos, and demonstrations of procedures (burping, swaddling, entertaining, and stimulating the infant).
- Provide information on community parenting classes and support groups.

BECOMING A MOTHER

Becoming a mother is a relatively new term used to describe and explain the process that women undergo in their transition to motherhood and establishment of their maternal identity (Mercer, 2004).

Evidence-Based Practice: Transition to Motherhood

Nelson, A. (2003). Transition to motherhood, *JOGNN*, 32, 465–477.

In a meta-synthesis of nine qualitative studies that focused on the transition to motherhood, Nelson (2003) identified actions of women that facilitate the transition to motherhood:

■ The woman's commitment to mothering: The higher the woman's commitment to being a mother, the smoother the transition

■ Prenatal discussion of realistic expectations for the transition to motherhood: The more realistic the woman's expectations of motherhood, the smoother the transition

■ The woman being actively involved in caring for her infant: Early and continuous involvement in infant care facilitates the transition.

■ Support during the first 6 postpartum months: The greater the perceived support, the smoother a smoother transition

■ The use of role models: The availability of positive motherhood role models facilitates a smoother transition.

Nursing care during the postpartum period that facilitates the transition to motherhood is based on a knowledge of these identified maternal actions.

Mercer describes four stages through which women progress in "becoming a mother":

■ Commitment, attachment, and preparation for an infant during pregnancy

■ Acquaintance with and increasing attachment to the infant, learning how to care for the infant, and physical restoration during the early weeks after birth

■ Moving toward a new normal during the first 4 months

■ Achievement of a maternal identity around 4 months (Mercer, 2006, p. 649)

The process of becoming a mother begins during pregnancy, but can occur before pregnancy. Some women begin preparing for this role as children when they fantasize about being mothers and role play being mothers with dolls. Others, before pregnancy, actively improve their health in preparation for the pregnancy (Mercer, 2006). The process of "becoming a mother" is influenced by:

■ How the woman was parented
■ Her life experiences
■ Her unique characteristics
■ The pregnancy experience
■ The birth experience
■ Support from partner, family, and friends
■ The woman's willingness to assume the role of mother
■ The infant's characteristics such as appearance and temperament (Mercer, 1995, 2006).

Nursing Actions

■ Review prenatal and labor records for risk factors such as complications during pregnancy and labor and birth.
■ Assess the stages of "becoming a mother."
  ■ *Expected assessment findings:*
    ■ Positive feelings toward being pregnant
    ■ Positive health behaviors
    ■ Nurturing behaviors toward the infant
    ■ Protective feelings toward infant

    ■ Increasing confidence in knowing and caring for the infant
    ■ Establishment of new family routines (Mercer, 2006)
■ Provide rooming-in or couplet care to facilitate bonding and attachment.
■ Provide private time for the parents to interact with their newborn.
■ Provide comfort measures for the woman to promote rest and healing.
■ Listen to the woman's concerns in order for her to process the incorporation of the newborn into her life.
■ Provide teaching on the care of newborns.
■ Praise the woman for the care she provides to her newborn.

Evidence-Based Practice: Nursing Process for the New Mother

Mercer, R. (2006). Nursing support of the process of becoming a mother. *JOGNN*, 35, 649–651.

Mercer summarizes the four stages in the process of becoming a mother and provides two major recommendations for supporting women during the process of becoming mothers:

■ Empathic listening: Listening to and understanding how the woman is affected by the process of becoming a mother.

■ Providing feedback to the woman regarding her infant caretaking skills and the way the woman interacts with her infant.

MATERNAL PHASES

Maternal phases, as defined by Rubin (1963, 1967), is a three-phase process that occurs during the first few weeks of the postpartum period (Table 13-2). A delay in transitioning through the phases may indicate that the woman is experiencing difficulty in becoming a mother. Factors that can affect the woman's transition through the maternal phases are:

■ Medications (e.g., magnesium sulfate or analgesics) that depress the central nervous system (CNS), leading to a sense of tiredness and a slow response to stimuli.
■ Complications during pregnancy, labor and birth, and/or postpartum (e.g., preterm labor, chronic illness, difficult birth, or cesarean birth) can cause the woman's focus to shift to her health and well-being, and/or to resolving feelings of disappointment.
■ Cesarean births can cause increased discomfort that interferes with the woman's ability to care for her infant.
■ Pain causes a shift of maternal attention from focusing on caring for baby to seeking pain relief for self.
■ Preterm infants or infants who experience complications can cause additional stresses on the woman and delay her transition through the phases.
■ Mood disorders, such as depression, cause the woman's focus to be more on self and less on the infant.
■ Lack of support from the partner and/or support system may lead to maternal exhaustion.
■ Adolescent mothers are more focused inwardly and on peer relationships than on care of the newborn.
■ The lack of financial resources forces the woman to focus on obtaining basic needs rather than on her infant.

TABLE 13–2   MATERNAL PHASES

TAKING-IN PHASE	TAKING-HOLD PHASE	LETTING-GO PHASE
The **taking–in phase,** a period of dependent behaviors, occurs during the first 24–48 hours after birth and includes the following maternal behaviors: ■ The woman is focused on her personal comfort and physical changes ■ The woman relives and speaks of the birth experience ■ The woman adjusts to psychological changes. ■ The woman is dependent on others for her and her infant's immediate needs ■ The woman has a decreased ability to make decisions. ■ The woman concentrates on personal physical healing (Rubin, 1963, 1967).	The **taking-hold phase**, the movement between dependent and independent behaviors, follows the taking-in phase and can last up to weeks and includes the following maternal behaviors: ■ The focus moves from self to the infant. ■ The woman begins to be independent. ■ The woman has an increased ability to make decisions. ■ The woman is interested in the newborn's cues and needs. ■ The woman gives up the pregnancy role and initiates taking on the maternal role. ■ The woman is eager to learn; it is an excellent time to initiate postpartum teaching. ■ The woman begins to like the role of "mother." ■ The woman may have feelings of inadequacy and being overwhelmed. ■ The woman needs verbal reassurance that she is meeting her newborn's needs. ■ The woman may show signs and symptoms of baby blues and fatigue. ■ The woman begins to let more of the outside world in (Rubin, 1963, 1967).	In the **letting-go phase**, the movement from independence to the new role of mother is fluid and interchangeable with the taking-hold phase. Maternal characteristics during this phase are: ■ Grieving and letting go of old relationship behaviors in favor of new ones ■ Incorporating the newborn into her life whereby the baby becomes a separate entity from her ■ Accepting the newborn as he or she really is ■ Giving up the fantasy of what it would/could have been ■ Independence returning; may go back to work or school ■ May have feelings of grief, guilt, or anxiety ■ Reconnection/growth in relationship with partner (Rubin, 1963, 1967)

■ Cultural beliefs can have an effect on the behaviors the woman takes on and the amount of time the woman spends in each phase. In some cultures, such as traditional Asian cultures, it is an expectation that the woman rest and not be actively involved in the care of her infant or in decision making during the first few months following the birth of her infant.

Nursing Actions

■ Review prenatal and labor records for factors that might delay progression through the maternal phases.
■ Assess for maternal phases.
  ■ *Expected assessment findings:*
    ■ Taking-in behaviors during the first 24 to 48 hours
    ■ Taking-hold behaviors from 24 to 48 hours through the first few weeks after birth
■ Nursing care during the taking-in phase is directed by the nurse because the woman is more dependent during this phase and has difficulty making decisions.
■ Nursing care during the taking-hold phase is directed more by the woman as she is becoming more independent and has an increased ability to make decisions.
■ Provide comfort measures such as backrubs, uninterrupted periods of rest, and analgesics.
■ Adapt teaching to reflect the maternal phase.

■ *During the taking-in phase, teaching is directed to immediate learning needs and provided in short sessions as the woman's focus is on self versus learning about the care of the newborn.*
■ *During the taking-hold phase, praise the woman for her learning as she is eager to learn but can become frustrated with not being able to master a new task quickly.*

*F*ATHERHOOD

Men's preparation for the role of father is vastly different from that of women. In general, men do not fantasize about being a father, nor do they role play being a father during childhood. During pregnancy, men mentally evaluate how they were fathered and how they want to father, but the reality of becoming a father may not occur until the child is born (May, 1982). Men are less likely than women to read about infant care and parenting during and after the pregnancy; yet during the postpartum period they report that they do not feel they have the knowledge, skills, and support for this new role (Jordan, 1990).

The meaning of father varies based on the man's interpretation of the role and its expectations and responsibilities. This is influenced by:

■ How he was fathered
■ How his culture defines the role
  ■ *In some cultures, men are not expected to be involved in the birthing process and/or care of the newborn.*

■ By friends and family, and by his partner.

The man's partner/wife has a major influence in the degree of the man's involvement in infant and child care. For the man to be an involved father, his partner/wife needs to share this desire and to be supportive.

Becoming a father evolves over time as the man has increasing contact with his infant, increasing knowledge of infant and infant care, and increasing experiences in infant care. Factors that influence the man's transition to fatherhood are:

■ Developmental and emotional age
■ Cultural expectations
■ Relationship with his partner/wife
■ Knowledge and understanding of fatherhood
■ Previous experiences as a father
■ The manner in which he was fathered
■ Financial concerns
■ Support from partner/wife, friends, and family

Nursing Actions that Assist Men in Their Transition to Fatherhood

■ Providing information on infant care and infant behavior
■ Providing opportunities for fathers to talk about the meaning of fathering
■ Demonstrating infant care such as diapering, feeding, and holding
■ Praising fathers for their interactions with their infants
■ Facilitating a discussion with fathers and their partners to identify mutual expectations of the fathering role

BONDING AND ATTACHMENT

Bonding and attachment are two phenomena that parents encounter during their transition to parenting and parental role attainment. **Bonding** is defined as the emotional feelings that begin during pregnancy or shortly after birth between the parent and the newborn (Klaus & Kennell, 1982). Bonding is unidirectional from parent to newborn. **Attachment** is an emotional connection that forms between the infant and his or her parents (Bowlby, 1969). It is bidirectional from parent to infant and infant to parent. Attachment has a lifelong impact on the developing individual. The quality of this attachment influences the person's physical and emotional development and is the foundation for the formation of future relationships. With each interaction, the parent and infant become more acquainted with each other, recognizing and becoming sensitive to each other's behaviors. This leads to reciprocal behaviors and emotional bonds between parent and newborn over time (Table 13-3).

Bonding and Attachment Behaviors

Bonding and attachment are affected by time, proximity of parent and infant, whether the pregnancy is planned/wanted, and the ability of the parents to process through the necessary development tasks of parenting. Other factors that influence bonding and attachment behaviors are:

■ The knowledge base of the couple
■ Past experience with children
■ Maturity and educational levels of the couple
■ Type of extended support system.
■ Maternal/paternal expectations from this pregnancy
■ Maternal/paternal expectations of the infant
■ Cultural expectations

Risk Factors for Delayed Bonding and/or Attachment

■ Maternal illness during pregnancy and/or the postpartum period that interferes with the woman's ability to interact with her infant
■ Neonatal illness such as prematurity that necessitates separation of the infant from the parents
■ Prolonged or complicated labor and birth that leads to exhaustion for both the woman and her partner
■ Fatigue during the postpartum period related to lack of rest and sleep
■ Physical discomfort experienced by women post-birth
■ Age and developmental age of the woman such as adolescent or developmentally challenged
■ Outside stressors not related to pregnancy or childbirth (e.g., concerns with finances, poor social support system, or need to return to work soon after the birth)

Nursing Actions

■ Review the prenatal and labor record for risk factors.
■ Assess for risk factors that would delay bonding and attachment.
■ Monitor at-risk parents more frequently and begin early interventions to promote bonding and attachment.
■ Assess for bonding and attachment by observation of parent–infant interaction.
  ■ *Expected assessment findings:*
    ▪ Parents hold the infant close.
    ▪ Parents refer to the infant by name or proper sex.
    ▪ Parents respond to the infant's needs.
    ▪ Parents speak positively about the infant.
    ▪ Parents appear interested in learning about the infant.
    ▪ Parents ask appropriate questions about infant care.
    ▪ Parents appear comfortable holding and caring for the infant.

TABLE 13–3 BONDING AND ATTACHMENT BEHAVIORS	
BONDING BEHAVIORS UNIDIRECTIONAL: PARENT → INFANT	**ATTACHMENT BEHAVIORS BIDIRECTIONAL: PARENT ←→ INFANT**
En face Calls baby by name Cuddles baby close to chest Talks/sings to baby Kisses the baby Breastfeeds the baby or holds the baby close when bottle-feeding	Parents respond to the infant's cry. The infant responds to the parents' comforting measures. Parents stimulate and entertain the infant while awake. Parents become "cue sensitive" to the infant's behavior.

- *Maladaptive assessment findings*
  - Parents call the infant "it."
  - Parents avoid eye contact with the infant (this can be viewed as adaptive based on culture).
  - Parents do not respond to the infant's cries.
  - Parents are emotionally unavailable to the infant.
  - Parents allow others to care for the infant, showing no interest (this can be viewed as adaptive based on culture).
  - Parents demonstrate poor feeding techniques such as propping bottles, not burping the infant, or seeming to be uncomfortable and/or irritated when nursing.
- Teach parents about bonding and attachment and the importance of these to the child's development of future relationships.
- Encourage women to breastfeed their infants by explaining how this naturally brings the infant close to their bodies in a very comforting and nurturing position.
- Instruct parents regarding the need for infants to have parents respond to their cues such as crying, cooing, and movement.
- Promote bonding and attachment by:
  - *Initiating early and prolonged contact between the parent and infant*
  - *Initiating rooming-in or couplet care*
  - *Providing positive comments to parents regarding their interactions with the infant*
  - *Encouraging the woman and her partner to talk about their birth experience and feelings regarding becoming parents*
- Promote attachment between mothers and infants separated due to either maternal illness or neonatal complications:
  - *Recommend that family members take pictures of the newborn and bring to the mother to keep in her room.*
  - *Assist parents to the NICU or nursery so that they can see and touch their infant.*
  - *Provide opportunities for parents to care for the infant in the NICU or nursery.*
  - *Instruct the woman on breast milk pumping and encourage her to bring breast milk to the NICU for use with her infant.*
  - *Inform parents that they can call the NICU or nursery any time of the day or night and talk with the nurse caring for their infant.*

PARENT-INFANT CONTACT

Early contact between the parents and their infant fosters the development of attachment of parents and infant and integration of the newborn into the maternal and paternal relationship. Continued contact and interaction provide the avenue for the parents and infant to learn more about each other. As they interact and perform for each other, they find themselves becoming more aware of the cues that make them respond to each other. This interaction cycle of behavior is called **reciprocity**. It is a **biorhythmic** or inherent rhythm that exists between the parents and newborn that becomes stronger with each interaction and the passing of time. This sequence of events strengthens the bonding and attachment processes that are the foundation for all other relationships the infant will establish throughout his or her life.

Maternal Touch

Maternal touch is a process that new mothers transition through beginning with the first physical contact with their newborns (Rubin, 1963). Most mothers do not instantly feel close to their newborns.

Feeling comfortable holding her newborn close to her body occurs over time with a progression through three stages. These stages, as described by Rubin, are:

- Initial stage: The woman touches her newborn tentatively with her fingertips.
- Second stage: The woman, as she becomes more comfortable with herself as a mother, uses her hand to stroke her newborn's head or body.
- Final stage: The mother holds her newborn in her arms and brings her newborn close to her body.

Rubin's maternal touch is a component of the acquaintance process through which mothers and newborns transition. Mothers go through multiple stages of awareness during early contacts with their newborns. The first time the new mother touches and meets her newborn, she is excited about her infant's features and verbally responds to sounds and expressions the baby makes. Later, after the new mother enters the final stage of maternal touch, she will hold her newborn **en face**, a position in which the mother and newborn are face-to-face with eye contact (Fig. 13-2). The en face position provides a positive connection that facilitates the bonding process. Some cultures believe that you should not gaze into the newborn's eyes.

Paternal-Infant Contact

In the 1980s, studies provided data that promoted and supported fathers' involvement in the birth of their infants. When expectant fathers participated in the labor and birth of their children in roles that were comfortable for them, they had a greater sense of belonging, which led to them being more engaged in the father role (Chapman, 1991). Reinforcement of this type of involvement has had positive benefits to the family unit and has strengthened early and positive parental involvement in the bonding and attachment process. Early physical contact with the newborn provides an opportunity for the new father to become comfortable touching and holding, which fosters a more active role in caring for his infant.

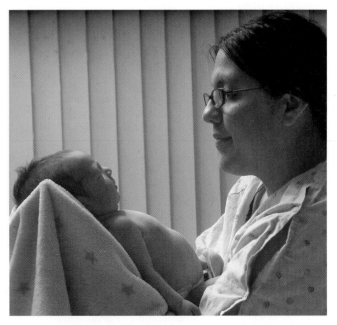

Figure 13-2 Mother and son in en face position.

CRITICAL COMPONENT

Paternal–Infant Contact

The new father, when holding his child for the first time, may feel awkward and uncomfortable and have a fear of injuring the baby. These feelings will decrease over time with continued contact with the newborn.

New fathers experience an intense preoccupation about and interest in their newborn. Greenberg and Morris (1974) identified these behaviors as **engrossment** (Fig. 13-3). They can vary based on the cultural beliefs of the couple.

Evidence-Based Practice: The Newborn's Impact on the Father

Greenberg, M., & Morris, N. (1974). Engrossment: The newborn's impact upon the father. *American Journal of Orthopyschiatry, 44*, 520–531.

In their research of new fathers, Greenberg and Morris identified the concept of engrossment that new fathers experience during the postpartum period in relationship to their newborns. They defined engrossment as an absorption, preoccupation, and interest with their newborns. New fathers can be observed gazing at their newborns for prolonged periods of time as if they are in a hypnotic trance. Greenberg and Morris described seven characteristics of engrossment:

- A visual awareness of the newborn: Seeing their newborn as being attractive
- A tactile awareness of the newborn: Having a desire to touch the newborn
- An awareness of their newborn's distinct features: Positive comments about their newborn's features
- A perception that their newborn is perfect
- A strong attraction to their newborn
- A feeling of strong elation
- An increase of self-esteem

Nursing Actions

- Assess for stages of maternal touch.
  - *Expected findings*
    - Tentatively touching her infant's extremities with her fingertips
    - Progressing to fuller touch and examination of the infant
    - Verbalizing positive comments about the infant
    - Snuggling and providing comfort to the infant
    - En face positioning to interact with the infant (varies based on cultural beliefs)
- Assess paternal–newborn interactions.
  - *Expected findings (varies based on cultural beliefs)*
    - Spends prolonged periods of time gazing at the newborn
    - Assists with infant care
    - Holds the newborn close to the body
    - Expresses delight in his infant's features
    - Verbally and physically expresses love and joy for both his newborn and his partner
  - *Maladaptive findings (may be viewed as adaptive based on cultural beliefs)*
    - Displays little or no interest in the infant
    - Makes negative comments about or to the infant
    - Ignores the infant's needs and cues

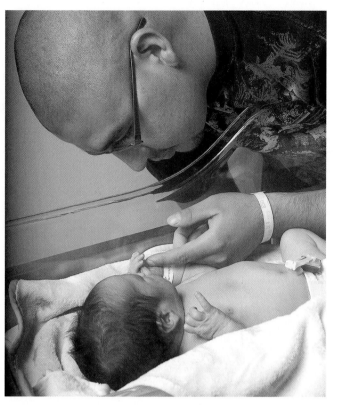

Figure 13-3   Father exhibiting sign of engrossment by gazing at his newborn son.

- Displays sadness or anger to the partner or infant
- Does not spend time with the infant or is emotionally absent
- Experiences mood swings
- Has conflict between family members over the infant
- Provide early and continuous periods of time for parents to see, hold, and interact with their newborn.
- Provide uninterrupted time for the mother to get acquainted with her newborn.
- Promote parental interaction with the newborn by delaying unnecessary procedures.
- Provide adequate rest periods (2–4 hours every 12 hours) for the parents. This ensures they have the stamina and rest to take care of and provide emotional support to each other.
- Facilitate rooming-in, which provides the opportunity for the newborn and father to stay in the mother's room throughout the hospital stay.
- Provide comfort measures to assist the parents in feeling rested and relaxed.
- Explain to new parents that they may not feel comfortable holding the newborn close and that these feelings will decrease with increasing contact with their newborn.
- Role model en face positioning.
- Role model appropriate behaviors by calling the infant by name and identifying normal infant behaviors.
- Provide therapeutic listening and positive feedback to parents when they are verbalizing their feelings about their newborn.
- Educate parents about newborn's unique behaviors and temperament.
- Educate and give information to both parents using multiple models of learning.
- Provide culturally sensitive care to the family unit.

CULTURAL AWARENESS: Cultural Beliefs Influence Parents

Cultural beliefs influence the ways parents relate and care for their newborns, and the role of fathers during the postpartum period and care of infants. An awareness of variations across cultural practices is an important component in providing appropriate care. Cultural beliefs can influence:

- The degree of father involvement in infant care
- The role extended family members have in the care of the infant and new mother
- The method of infant feeding
- Foods that are eaten and foods that are avoided during the postpartum period
- When a woman can bathe and wash her hair
- When the baby is named and who names the baby

COMMUNICATION BETWEEN PARENT AND CHILD

Communication is a bidirectional process that involves a sender and a receiver. People communicate through the use of verbal and written words, and through the use of their eyes, ears, faces, and body gestures. Newborns have the ability to see, hear, and smell; to respond to their environment; and to display displeasure. They rely on vocal noises such as crying and cooing, as well as facial expressions and body movements, to participate actively in relationship-building with other human beings. The challenge to parents and care providers is to learn the cues newborns and infants use to communicate their needs and pleasures.

Nurses are in the unique position to provide information about the newborn's ability to communicate. Nurses can help parents identify infant behaviors and offer appropriate interventions to promote positive interactions. Examples of newborn and infant communication styles and cues are:

- Crying
- Cooing
- Facial expressions
- Eye movements
- Smelling
- Cuddling
- Arm and leg movements
- **Entrainment**: A phenomenon in which the newborn and infant moves his or her arms and legs in rhythm with speech patterns of an adult.

Responding to and encouraging newborn and infant communication assists the infant in developing communication and language skills. The parents' ability to recognize their infant's positive response cues fosters the parents' confidence in their parenting skills. Teaching parents how to identify their newborn's unique cues and behaviors promotes a positive relationship that empowers the dyad to continue to grow and learn as the newborn matures and adds new skills and insights into the relationship.

Parents who are aware of and start to understand infant behaviors by becoming cue-sensitive will be able to identify:

- The best time to communicate with their newborn
- Ways to comfort
- Methods to assist infant to self-comfort

- When the infant is overstimulated and how to provide quiet times during these periods of fussiness (White, Simon, & Bryan, 2002)

Newborns have very acute senses when interacting with their parents. Newborns who are placed on their mothers' abdomens will crawl to the breast. Newborns also interact with their parents by responding to voices and touch. They look en face and root when stimulated. These initial interactions and ongoing interactions lead to **synchrony** events, which are reciprocal actions between parents and infants that show mutual expressions of contentment. These interactions are very pleasurable for parents and infants. Examples of synchrony events are:

- The mother holds the infant in an en face position. The response to this action is that they gaze into each other's eyes and talk, coo, or smile at each other.
- The father places his finger in the infant's hand. The infant grabs the father's finger and they gaze at each other.

CRITICAL COMPONENT

Positive Interactions between Parents and Newborns

Newborns have the ability to communicate, to interact, and to be stimulated by early interactions. Depending on the state of awareness, newborns have the ability to respond positively by becoming more alert, or negatively by crying. Nurses who understand newborn behaviors, infant state of awareness, and communication cues can identify and promote positive interactions between parents/caregivers and their newborns through role modeling and parent education (Table 13-4).

Nursing Actions

- Review prenatal, labor and birth, and postpartum records for factors that might delay or hinder parent–infant communication and provide early interventions.
- Assess parent–infant interactions.
  - *Expected findings*
    - Parents gently touch their newborn and hold the newborn close to the body.
    - Parents talk to or sing to their newborn.
    - Parents, when culturally acceptable, hold their newborn en face.
    - Parents respond to their newborn's cues for interaction and care.
    - The newborn response to his or her parents' touch and voice.
  - *Role model communication with infant.*
  - *Praise parents for their interactions with their infant.*
  - *Provide teaching on infant communication:*
    - The infant's ability and need to communicate
    - Eye contact, when culturally appropriate
    - Synchronized interactions
    - Recognizing and interpreting the infant's cues
    - Entrainment
    - Infant alertness states

FAMILY DYNAMICS

Family dynamics are unique ways in which family members interact and participate within the family. Adaptation to these dynamics determines the cohesiveness, or lack of such, in the family unit.

TABLE 13–4   INFANT STATES

STATES	BEHAVIORS	ACTIONS
DEEP SLEEP	Minimal body twitches and eye movement. Cycles between deep and light sleep	Do not try to wake up or feed infant.
LIGHT SLEEP	More active body movement; may smile	More easily aroused and stimulated
DROWSY	Awakens easily; can be rocked back to sleep or made more awake	May enjoy being held and cuddled Responds to gentle stimuli May self-comfort by sucking
QUIET ALERT	Eyes open; quiet and attentive	Best time for interacting
ACTIVE ALERT	More sensitive to stimuli, active body movement; may be tired or hunger or need changing	Decrease stimuli. Provide a quiet environment. Provide comfort measures. The infant may attempt to self-comfort.
CRYING	Grimaces, cries, or whimpers	The infant may self-comfort. Meet infant needs.

There are several types of relationships and family compositions. The family structure can be as small as the mother and newborn, or as large as two or more generations plus extended family members. Each has its own unique dynamics and structure that presents challenges and offers rewarding experiences to nurses who come into contact with these various family compositions. Examples of family compositions include:

- Married or non-married male–female couples
- Same-sex couples
- Adoptive couples
- Adolescent women with partner, mother, and/or grandmother as support system
- Adolescent women without support system
- Single adult women with no partner
- Blended families

The time immediately after childbirth is filled with many emotional changes for the partners and family members. Family members are redefining who they are as individuals and their roles within the family. Adjustments within the couple's relationship and family unit occur as the couple and family members incorporate and make room for the newest family member. Couples make adjustments within their relationship and learn how to support each other in their roles as parents. They reprioritize their responsibilities and roles to fit their new roles and responsibilities. Siblings take on the role of older brother or sister and adjust to the decreased amount of time the parents have available to interact with and care for them.

The family unit is affected and influenced by changes both within the family and outside the family. Outside influences, such as friends and relatives, may have positive or negative effects on the family. The couple needs to determine which resources are helpful and which are stressful, and whom they can seek for positive assistance. Nursing care is directed at assisting families in identifying their needs and adjustment during this period of transition.

Multiparas

The maternal role changes and becomes more complex with each additional child. Multiparas may have more knowledge and practice regarding the care of newborns, but they usually experience more exhaustion and have less help than with their first child. In a classic 1979 article Ramona Mercer described the unique concerns of multiparas:

- Concerns for her other children.
  - *Will her other children feel abandoned?*
- Concerns about being able to love the new child.
  - *Does she have the capacity to love this new child as she does her other children?*
- Concerns for her ability to care for more than one child.
  - *Does she have the time and energy to care for an additional child?*
- Concerns about her ability to get rest and sleep.
  - *Will she be able to find time for sleep and rest?*
- Concerns about having help at home to care for her and her expanding family.
  - *Will family members and friends be willing to help her with a second child?*

It is important that nurses who care for multiparous women provide the women with opportunities to express their concerns, fears, and doubts in caring for and loving another child. Nurses can facilitate this transition by providing reassurance and suggesting strategies in caring for an additional child.

Sibling Rivalry

The addition of a new family member can be a stressful life event for siblings within the family unit. They will need to make adjustments in their young lives in response to the incorporation of the newborn within the family. Depending on the age of the siblings and birth order, they have varying degrees of feeling displaced. Younger children experience a sense of loss over no longer being the "baby" of the family. Older children may have a sense of increased responsibility due to their parents' expectation that they assist in the care of younger children.

Preparing for the new family addition should begin during pregnancy as the parents talk about the expected new baby (see Chapter 5). Providing opportunities for the children to feel the fetus move and hear the fetal heartbeat are concrete ways to assist the children in understanding the upcoming event. Discussion on what it will mean to have a new baby in the family can also help in their adjustments.

Siblings should be introduced to their new brother or sister as soon as possible and spend time with mother and baby during the postpartum hospitalization. They should be allowed to hold and touch their new baby with supervision (Fig. 13-4).

CRITICAL COMPONENT

Sibling Adjustment

The addition of a new member to the family can be stressful for siblings. Actions that can facilitate their adjustment are:

- Spending time during the prenatal period talking about the upcoming arrival of a new baby
- Providing opportunities for siblings to feel the baby move and hear the heartbeat during the pregnancy
- Providing opportunities for siblings to spend time with their new brother or sister during the hospital stay
- Encouraging siblings to lie in bed with their mother during hospital visits
- Giving siblings a present that is from their new brother or sister
- Explaining to parents the importance of quality time with other children, such as sitting and readings books with them, playing games, and listening to them
- Taking siblings on a special outing while the newborn stays at home with a babysitter
- Explaining why babies cry and how they communicate

Nursing Actions

- Review the records for relationship issues, pregnancy history, and delivery summary.
- Assess for prior experiences with a newborn.
- Monitor adaptation behaviors of partners and siblings.
- Assess for maladaptive behaviors and make referrals to social services or the community health nurse as indicated.
- Keep an open mind and be culturally sensitive.
- Have a flexible plan of care for the postpartum family.
- Provide information of the potential adjustments parents, couples, and siblings will encounter as they incorporate the newborn into the family.
- Assist parents in identifying ways to assist their other children in their adjustments to the new family member.

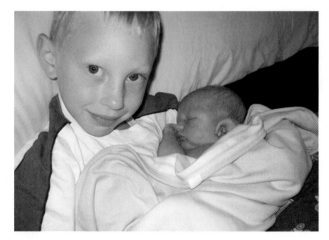

Figure 13-4 Big brother meets the new family member.

- Provide positive verbal reinforcement for their family interactions.
- Provide opportunities for family members to talk about the adjustments within the family.
- Provide opportunities for couples to talk about the adjustments within their couple relationship and ways to enhance their relationship.
- Respect cultural beliefs and incorporate them in the nursing care.

PARENTS WITH SENSORY OR PHYSICAL IMPAIRMENTS

Parents with sensory impairments such as visual loss or diminished hearing, or those with physical impairments such as decreased mobility, present challenges to nurses and other health care professionals. These challenges can turn into opportunities to be creative in ways to adapt nursing care to meet the needs of these parents. It is important that health care professionals be aware of the rights of disabled individuals, provide information in ways they can understand, and provide care that is sensitive to their needs.

There are ranges in the degree of visual impairment, auditory impairment, and physical impairment. Visual impairment/blindness ranges from visual loss, where the person can read large print, to complete blindness, where the person has no usable vision. Auditory impairment ranges from mild to profound hearing loss. Those with mild hearing loss have enough hearing to carry on a conversation under ideal conditions. People with profound hearing losses usually rely on sign language as their form of communication and will not be able to converse orally with hearing people. Physical impairment can range from a person being dependent on a cane, to people who do not have motor control of their arms and/or legs.

CRITICAL COMPONENT

Working with Parents with a Sensory or Physical Impairment

It is important to treat parents with sensory or physical impairments as people and not as disabilities.

Nursing Actions

Visually Impaired Parents

- When reporting, use the person's name. Do not refer to her as the "blind woman in room 211."
- When entering a room, address the person by name and introduce yourself and anyone else who is in the room.
- When leaving a room, announce your departure and indicate if others are staying or leaving.
- Speak directly to the person in a clear manner. Do not exaggerate word pronunciation or speak in a loud voice.
- Keep doors, cabinets, and closets closed to prevent injury.
- Use sighted-guide when assisting with ambulation (the visually impaired person holds the elbow of the sighted person when walking). Avoid shoving, pushing, or grabbing unless in an emergency.
- Do not pull on the person's cane to direct her.
- Do not play with a seeing-eye dog while it is in harness. Ask permission to touch the dog.

- Orient the person to the area of the room or new location after you have guided her to this new area.
- At a given point (the door or bed), orient the room by describing its contents in logical sequence of progressive order (e.g., "To the right as you lie in the bed is the nightstand with the phone and call button; beside that is the bed curtain and then a chair. Next to the chair is the door to the bathroom").
- Describe the location of food on a plate according to the clock face (e.g., "Potatoes are at 2:00, meat is at 5:00"). Ask the woman if she needs assistance.
- Offer to read printed material or ask for the preferred manner for receiving information that is in printed form.
- Provide space for Braillers and other special equipment used by the woman.
- Provide teaching in a manner the parents can understand. Example of teaching instructions:
  - *Instruct the parents in diapering by having them diaper their child while you explain the steps.*
- Provide discharge teaching and instructions in Braille or on audiotape.

Hearing Impaired Parents

- Face the parents when speaking to them.
- Be articulate, but do not exaggerate pronunciation.
- Speak in a normal voice volume.
- Be within 6 to 8 feet of the parents when speaking to them. Make sure that light from windows is behind the parents.
- Avoid putting your hand over your mouth or turning your back to the parents when you are speaking.
- When communicating information with the use of illustrations, provide time for parents to study the illustrations.
- If there is more than one speaker, take turns speaking with clear indications as to who is speaking.
- Minimize background noises (e.g., turn off volume of TV, close the door to the room).
- If there is misunderstanding, do not repeat words louder; instead use synonyms or other words that mean the same thing.
- Provide discharge teaching and information in written form that parents can easily understand.
- Use graphics and visuals when available.
- Ensure a registered interpreter for the deaf person is present when discussing medical information and teaching. When using an interpreter:
  - *Allow sufficient time for the interpreter to complete a thought.*
  - *Speak directly to the patient and not to the interpreter.*
  - *Avoid saying, "Tell him/her..."*
  - *Check the parent for understanding or if he or she are getting too much information.*
  - *Allow time for questions and concerns.*
- A head nod by the parent may have different meanings, such as "yes" or "continue"; it may not mean that the parent understands.
- Flick lights on and off to get the attention of the parent. Do not shout, wave, or touch for the purpose of getting attention.
- Be aware that hearing aids amplify sound 6 to 10 times, so shouting and loud noises can be uncomfortable.
- Provide closed captioned TV, TDD/TTY (telephone device for deaf), writing pad, and implements.
- Discuss with the parents how they have adapted their home for the newborn.
- Some parents will use a device that causes a light to flash in response to the infant's cry, thus alerting parents to check on their infant.

- Some parents might use closed-circuit TV to monitor the infant while in another room.

Parents with Physical Impairments

- Provide standard ADA-required facilities, such as raised toilets, wheelchair accessible rooms and hallways, and easy-to-use call buttons.
- Keep the environment free of clutter.
- Assess the type of assistance needed by asking him or her.
- Discuss the type of assistance parents will need in caring for their newborn at home.
- Assist parents in infant care.
- Assist parents in developing strategies to adapt infant care to their limitations.
- Make referrals to social services when indicated for additional assistance.

CRITICAL COMPONENT

Assisting Parents with an Impairment

Nurses can best assist parents who have sensory or physical impairments by exploring, identifying, and implementing techniques, tools, and alternative ways to:

- Facilitate bonding and attachment.
- Teach parents about infant care.
- Promote a safe environment for the newborn.
- Enhance the family dynamics.

POSTPARTUM BLUES

Postpartum blues, also known as baby blues, occur during the first few postpartum weeks, last for a few days, and affect a majority of women. During this period of time, the woman feels sad and cries easily, but she is able to take care of herself and her infant. Possible causes of postpartum blues are:

- Changes in hormonal levels
- Fatigue
- Stress from taking on the new role of mother

Signs and symptoms of postpartum blues are:

- Anger
- Anxiety
- Mood swings
- Sadness
- Weeping
- Difficulty sleeping
- Difficulty eating

Nursing Actions

- Provide information to the couple regarding postpartum blues.
- Explain that this occurs in the majority of postpartum woman.
- Explain the importance of rest in reducing stress.
- Explain to the woman's partner the importance of emotional and physical support during this period of time.
- Explain that the woman or family should seek assistance from the health care provider if the symptoms persist beyond 4 weeks or if it is of concern for her or her family, as she may be experiencing postpartum depression.

Clinical Pathway for Transition to Parenthood

Focus of Care	Postpartum Admission	Postpartum 4–24 Hours	Postpartum 24–48 Hours	Discharge Criteria
Emotional status	Taking-in phase	Progressing toward the taking-hold phase	Taking-hold phase. The woman shows more independence in managing her own and the infant's care	The woman is able to provide self-care. The woman demonstrates increased confidence in infant care.
Nursing action	Provide care and comfort to the woman. Provide positive reinforcement of appropriate behaviors. Discuss the infant's unique capabilities. Provide early and consistent contact with the infant to facilitate bonding.	Encourage the woman and her family to participate in self- and infant care. Encourage extended infant contact. Observe for bonding and attachment behaviors. Begin discharge education.	Observe for bonding and attachment behaviors, noting any signs of maladaptive behaviors. Provide written/visual information on infant behaviors and characteristics. Teach methods for comforting the infant	Positive bonding and attachment behaviors noted. Parents express understanding of infant behaviors and cues. Parents express positive understanding of how to care for the infant Provide resources for parents to call as needed.
Family dynamics	Parents demonstrate beginning bonding behaviors. Begins introducing the infant to the extended family	Parents demonstrate positive bonding and attachment behaviors Extended family demonstrate positive/supportive behaviors toward the newborn.	Parents continue to demonstrate bonding and attachment behaviors Extended family demonstrates positive behaviors towards newborn and parents	Parents demonstrate positive adaptive behaviors

TYING IT ALL TOGETHER

As the nurse in the postpartum unit you are caring for the Sanchez family. Margarite gave birth to a healthy boy 5 hours ago. Both she and her son are stable. She breastfed her son for 15 minutes after the birth.

You notice that she is lightly touching the top of her newborn's head with her fingertips. She comments that she does not feel comfortable holding her baby close to her body for breastfeeding.

Discuss your nursing actions that are based on your knowledge of maternal touch.

List the maternal phase and expected maternal behaviors for this period of time.

List five expected bonding behaviors for this period of time.

The next day you are again assigned to care for the Sanchez family. Mom and baby are stable. José, Margarite's husband, is present during the shift. Margarite and José voice concern about integrating their newborn into the family.

Discuss your nursing actions that reflect an understanding of the couple's transition to parenthood.

Discuss specific strategies to decrease sibling rivalry.

Margarite tells you that she thinks she experienced postpartum depression with her first baby. She tells you that she cried a lot during the first week at home, but was able to care for herself and her newborn.

Discuss the appropriate nursing actions in response to her concerns.

■ ■ ■ Review Questions ■ ■ ■

1. Your postpartum patient is 10 hours post-birth. She experienced an uncomplicated labor and birth and her newborn is full term with Apgar scores of 9 at 1 minute and 9 at 5 minutes. During your assessment, you note that she was hungry and very interested in telling you about her birth experience. You had to remind her to change her baby's diaper and to feed her baby. Based on this assessment you determine that she is:
   A. Having difficulty bonding with her baby
   B. Not concerned about her baby's needs
   C. In the taking-in phase
   D. In the taking-hold phase

2. Your postpartum patient is a 25 years old, white, single woman who gave birth to a healthy infant. She is 36 hours post-birth. You note that she holds her infant at a distance and refers to her infant as "it." Based on this assessment your initial nursing actions include:
   A. Obtain referral for a social worker.
   B. Ask the woman to tell you about her pregnancy and childbirth experience.
   C. Teach her the importance of holding her baby close to her body.
   D. Take her baby to the nursery so she can have some uninterrupted sleep.

3. Which 2-day postpartum woman has an abnormal finding that requires intervention?
   A. A 23-year-old Arabic woman who plans to breastfeed, but wants to bottle feed her newborn until her milk comes in
   B. A 28-year-old Chinese woman who refuses to take a shower
   C. A 20-year-old Japanese woman who has her mother care for her baby
   D. A 19-year-old Caucasian woman who requests that her baby stay in the nursery so she can sleep

4. You are providing discharge teaching to your patient. In addition to her newborn son, she has a 2-year-old daughter. Which of the following will you include in your teaching? Select all that apply.
   A. Stressing the importance of quality time with her 2-year-old daughter
   B. Instructing the woman to include the 2-year-old in the care of her baby brother
   C. Explaining that all children experience some degree of sibling rivalry
   D. Instructing the woman to explain to her daughter the reasons babies cry

5. Factors that can hamper a couple's transition to parenthood include which of the following? Select all that apply.
   A. First experience with newborns
   B. Change of employment
   C. Adolescent father
   D. Recent move to a new state

References

Bowlby, J. (1969). *Attachment and loss. Vol. 1. Attachment.* New York: Basic Books.

Chapman, L. (1991). Searching: Expectant fathers' experiences during labor and birth. *Journal of Perinatal Neonatal Nursing, 4*, 21–29.

Greenberg, M., & Morris, N. (1974). Engrossment: The newborn's impact upon the father. *American Journal of Orthopychiatry, 44*, 520–531.

Klaus, M., & Kennell, J. (1982). *Parent–infant bonding.* St. Louis, MO: C. V. Mosby.

May, K. (1982). Three phases of father involvement in pregnancy. *Nursing Research, 31*, 337–342.

Mercer, R. (1986). *First-time motherhood.* New York: Springer Publishing.

Mercer, R. (1995). *Becoming a mother: Research from Rubin to the present.* New York: Springer Publishers.

Mercer, R. (1997). Having another child: "She's a multip....she knows the ropes." *Journal of Maternal Child Nursing, 4*, 301–304.

Mercer, R. (2004). Becoming a mother versus maternal role attainment. *Journal of Nursing Scholarship, 36*, 226–232.

Mercer, R. (2006). Nursing support of the process of becoming a mother. *Journal of Obstetric, Gynecologic and Neonatal Nursing, 35*, 649–651.

Rubin, R. (1963a). Maternal touch. *Nursing Outlook, 11*, 828–831.

Rubin, R. (1963b). Puerperal change. *Nursing Outlook, 9*, 753–755.

Rubin, R. (1967). Attainment of the maternal role. Part 1. Processes. *Nursing Research, 16*, 237–346.

Rubin, R. (1984). *Maternal identity and the maternal experience.* New York: Springer Publishing.

White, C., Simon, M., & Bryan, A. (2002). Using evidence to educate birthing center nursing staff about infant states, cues, and behaviors. *Maternal Child Nursing, 27*, 294–298.

High-Risk Postpartum Nursing Care

OBJECTIVES

On completion of this chapter, the student will be able to:

- ☐ Define key terms.
- ☐ Describe the primary causes of postpartum hemorrhage and the related nursing actions and medical care.
- ☐ Describe the primary postpartum infections and the related nursing actions and medical care.
- ☐ Identify potential complications/disorders in later life related to childbirth trauma.
- ☐ Describe the primary postpartum psychological complications and the related nursing actions and medical care.

Nursing Diagnoses

- ■ At risk for hemorrhage related to uterine atony, lacerations, retained placental tissue, or hematoma
- ■ At risk for infection related to tissue trauma or prolonged rupture of membranes
- ■ At risk for mood disorders related to stress, hormonal changes, lack of rest, or lack of social support

Nursing Outcomes

- ■ The woman's fundus will remain firm and lochia within normal ranges.
- ■ The woman will remain free from symptoms of infection.
- ■ The woman will indicate that she feels supported by her family and is getting adequate rest.

INTRODUCTION

Most women do not experience a complication during the postpartum period, but when they do it can be life threatening and disruptive to the family unit. A majority of complications occur after discharge and may require readmission to the hospital. Most hospitals do not allow the infant to be readmitted with the mother. Thus, readmission to the hospital for treatment of complications can interfere with the attachment process and increase stress within the family unit.

A focus of postpartum nursing care is to reduce women's risks for complications related to childbirth and to identify complications early for prompt interventions. The woman needs to be evaluated by her health care provider when a complication is suspected.

Hemorrhage, coagulation disorders, and infections are the primary physiological complications. Women may also experience problems later in life due to tissue and reproductive organ trauma related to the childbirth. Postpartum depression and postpartum psychosis are the main psychological complications.

HEMORRHAGE

Postpartum hemorrhage (PPH) is classified into early and late hemorrhage.

Early PPH occurs within the first 24 hours after childbirth. Late PPH occurs after 24 hours post-birth. It is estimated that 10% of

CRITICAL COMPONENT

Risk Reduction for Postpartum Complications

Reducing a woman's risk for postpartum complications is a major component of postpartum nursing care. Nursing actions to reduce risk are:

- ■ Reviewing the prenatal and intrapartal records for risk factors such as anemia, long labor, and operative vaginal delivery and address these risk factors in planning care.
- ■ Assessing for early signs of a postpartum complication and intervening appropriately.
- ■ Using good hand washing techniques by health care workers, patients, and visitors.
- ■ Promoting health with appropriate diet, fluids, activity, and rest.
- ■ Providing emotional support for the parents and families.

postpartum women will experience a PPH (Wainscott, 2006). A major complication of PPH is hemorrhagic shock related to hypovolemia.

- ■ Early PPH is defined as a blood loss of greater than 500 mL within the first 24 hours, but in clinical practice it is diagnosed when the health care provider determines that the blood loss is greater than normal (You & Zahn, 2006).

Want to reinforce your reading? Need to review for a test? Listen to this chapter on your accompanying CD.

■ Causes of early PPH are uterine atony, lacerations, and hematomas.
■ Causes of late PPH are hematomas, subinvolution, and retained placental tissue.

CRITICAL COMPONENT

Risk Factors for PPH

■ Neonatal macrosomia: Birth weight greater than 4000 grams
■ Polyhydramnios
■ Operative vaginal delivery: Use of forceps or vacuum extractor
■ Augmented or induced labor
■ Ineffective uterine contractions during labor: Prolonged first or second stage of labor
■ Precipitous labor and/or birth
■ General anesthesia

CRITICAL COMPONENT

Indications of Possible Early PPH

■ A 10% decrease in the hematocrit post birth
■ Saturation of the peripad within 15 minutes
■ A fundus that remains boggy after fundal massage
■ Tachycardia
■ Decrease in blood pressure

Uterine Atony

Uterine atony, a decreased tone of the uterine muscle, is the primary cause of early PPH (Association of Women's Health, Obstetric and Neonatal Nursing [AWHONN], 2006). Uterine contractions constrict the open vessels at the placental site and assist in decreasing the amount of blood loss. When the uterus is relaxed the vessels are less constricted and the woman experiences an increase of blood loss.

Assessment Findings

■ Soft (boggy) fundus versus firm fundus
■ Saturation of the peripad within 15 minutes
■ Bleeding is slow and steady or sudden and massive
■ Blood clots may be present
■ Pale color and clammy skin
■ Anxiety and confusion
■ Tachycardia
■ Hypotension (Higgins, 2004)

Medical Management

■ Medications: Oxytocin, methergine, and hemabate to stimulate uterine contractions
■ IV therapy to reduce risk of hypovolemia
■ Blood replacement to reduce risk for hemorrhagic shock
■ Surgical interventions such as hysterectomy may be indicated when all other treatments have failed to contract the uterus.

Nursing Actions

■ Review prenatal and intrapartal records for risk factor for PPH and monitor more frequently women who are at risk for uterine atony.

■ Assess for a displaced uterus. An overdistention of the bladder can displace the uterus and cause it to relax.
  ■ *Assist the woman to the bathroom to void if the uterus is not midline and then re-assess the location and firmness of the fundus and the amount and characteristics of the lochia.*
  ■ *Catheterize the woman if she is unable to void and the uterus is displaced by the overdistention of the bladder.*
■ Assess the fundus for degree of firmness.
  ■ *Massage the boggy uterus and reassess (Critical Component: Management of Uterine Atony).*
■ Assess lochia for amount and for clots.
  ■ *Express clots: Clots can interfere with uterine contraction (MacMullen, 2005).*
■ Review laboratory tests such as hemoglobin and hematocrit (H & H).
■ Notify physician or midwife of assessment findings and abnormal test results.
■ Administer oxytocin, methergine, and/or hemabate as per orders.
■ Start and monitor blood transfusions as per orders and protocol.
■ Provide emotional support and teaching to both the woman and her support system, as PPH increases the anxiety and stress levels of the woman and her family.

CRITICAL COMPONENT

Management of Uterine Atony

■ Fundal massage is the first action to initiate when the uterus is midline and boggy (Fig. 14-1).
■ The physician or midwife is notified when the fundus does not respond to fundal massage.
■ Oxytocin therapy is initiated as per orders.
  ■ An IV is started with 1000 mL of Ringer's lactate solution with 20–40 units of oxytocin added as per orders; and
  ■ The IV infusion rate is started at 10 mL/min (200 mU/min) and regulated by the firmness of the fundus (You & Zahn, 2006).
■ If bleeding continues, Methergine or Hemabate is administered as per order.

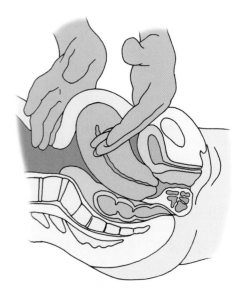

Figure 14-1 Fundal massage.

Medication

Methylergonovine (Methergine)

- Indication: PPH due to uterine atony or subinvolution
- Action: Stimulates contraction of the uterine smooth muscle
- Common side effects: Nausea, vomiting, and cramps.
- Route and dose: IM or IV; 200 mcg every 2–4 hours (only one IV dose)
- Precaution: Check blood pressure before injection; if elevated do not give until the physician or midwife has been notified. Use with caution with women who have PIH. This medication can increase the blood pressure.

(Data from Deglin & Vallerand, 2009)

Medication

Carboprost Tromethamine (Hemabate)

- Indication: PPH that has not responded to oxytocin or methergine therapy.
- Action: Uterine contractions
- Common side effects: Diarrhea, nausea, vomiting, and fever.
- Route and dosage: IM; 250 mcg which can be repeated every 15 to 90 minutes. Total dose should not exceed 2 mg.

(Data from Deglin & Vallerand, 2009)

Lacerations

Lacerations, which are the second most common cause of early PPH, can occur during childbirth. Common sites are the cervix, vagina, labia, and perineum.

Risk Factors

- Fetal macrosomia
- Operative vaginal delivery: Use of forceps or vacuum extraction
- Precipitous labor and/or birth

Assessment Findings

- A firm uterus that is midline with heavier than normal bleeding
- Bleeding is usually a steady stream without clots.
- Tachycardia
- Hypotension (Higgins, 2004)

Medical Management

- Visual inspection of cervix, vagina, perineum, and labia
- Suturing of laceration
- Prescribe IV medication for pain management

Nursing Actions

- Review labor and birth records for possible risk factors and monitor more frequently women who are at higher risk for lacerations.
- Monitor vital signs.
- Monitor blood loss.
- Notify the physician or midwife of increased bleeding with a firm fundus.
- Administer medications for pain management as per order.
- Prepare the woman for a pelvic examination.
- Provide emotional support to the woman and her family.

Hematomas

Hematomas occur when blood collects within the connective tissues of the vagina or perineal areas related to a vessel that ruptures and continues to bleed (Fig. 14-2). It is difficult to determine the degree of blood loss since the blood is retained within the tissue; thus, PPH may not be diagnosed until the woman is in hypovolemic shock.

Risk Factors

- Episiotomy is the major risk factor (You & Zahn, 2006)
- Use of forceps
- Prolonged second stage

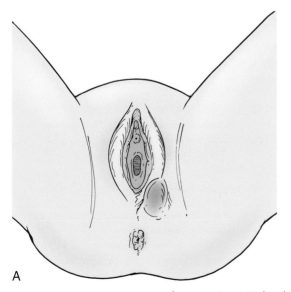
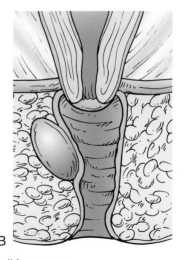

Figure 14-2 *A.* Vulvar hematoma. *B.* Vaginal wall hematoma.

Assessment Findings

- Women express severe pain in the vagina/perineal area and the intensity of pain cannot be controlled by standard postpartum pain management.
- Presence of tachycardia and hypotension.
- Hematomas that are located in the vagina cannot be visualized by the nurse. When located in the vaginal area women will express severe pain, a heaviness or fullness in the vagina, and/or rectal pressure.
- Hematomas in the perineal area present with swelling, discoloration, and tenderness.
- Hematomas with an accumulation of 200 to 500 mL can become large enough to displace the uterus and cause uterine atony which can increase the degree of blood loss.

Medical Management

- Small hematomas are evaluated and monitored without surgical intervention.
- Large hematomas are surgically excised and the blood evacuated. The open vessel is identified and ligated.
  - *Women experience immediate relief from pain once the blood has been evacuated.*

Nursing Actions

- Review the chart for risk factors and monitor more frequently women who are at risk for a hematoma.
- Apply ice to the perineum for the first 24 hours to decrease the risk of hematoma.
- Assess the degree of pain by use of a pain scale.
- Ask women who indicate either verbally or nonverbally an increase of pain if they are experiencing any heaviness or fullness in their vaginal or rectal areas.
- Monitor for decrease in blood pressure and an increase in pulse rate.
- Administer prescribed analgesia for pain management.
- Review laboratory reports such as H & H: A decrease in H & H may be an indication of blood loss.
- Notify the physician or midwife of nursing assessment findings for further evaluation.

Subinvolution of the Uterus

Subinvolution of the uterus is a term used when the uterus does not decrease in size and does not descend into the pelvis. This usually occurs later in the postpartum period. Before the diagnosis of subinvolution the uterus and lochia had been undergoing normal involution.

Risk Factors

- Fibroids
- Endometritis
- Retained placental tissue

Assessment Findings

- The uterus is soft and larger than normal for the days postpartum.
- Lochia returns to the rubra stage and can be heavy.
- Back pain is present.

Medical Management

- Medical intervention depends on the cause of the subinvolution.
  - *A dilation and curettage (D&C) is performed for retained placental tissue.*
  - *Methergine PO is prescribed for fibroids.*
  - *Antibiotic therapy is initiated for endometritis.*

Nursing Actions

- Review prenatal and labor records for risk factors.
- Monitor women who are at risk for subinvolution of the uterus more frequently.
- Patient education is the primary action, as PPH from subinvolution usually occurs after discharge.
  - *Provide education on involution and signs to report such as increased bleeding, clots, or a change in the lochia to bright red bleeding.*
  - *Provide education on ways to reduce risk for infection such as changing peripads frequently, hand washing, nutrition, adequate fluid intake, and adequate rest.*
  - *Explain to women who have fibroids that they are at risk for subinvolution. Provide instruction on the proper use of discharge medication, since these women are usually discharged with an order for Methergine PO.*

Retained Placental Tissue

Retained placental tissue is the most common cause of LPH. It occurs when small portions of the placenta, referred to as cotyledons, remain attached to the uterus during the third stage of labor. The retained placental tissue can interfere with involution of the uterus and can lead to endometritis.

Risk Factor

- Manual removal of the placenta

Assessment Findings

- Profuse bleeding that suddenly occurs after the first postpartum week
- Subinvolution of the uterus
- Elevated temperature and uterine tenderness if endometritis is present
- Pale skin color
- Tachycardia
- Hypotension

Medical Management

- D&C is performed to remove retained placental tissue.
- IV antibiotic therapy may be prescribed because there is an increased risk for endometritis.

Nursing Actions

- Review the labor record for risk factors.
- Monitor more frequently women who are at risk.
- Review laboratory reports such as H&H. A decrease in H&H may be an indication of blood loss.
- Patient education is a primary intervention, as PPH from retained placental fragment usually occurs after discharge.
  - *Instruct women to report to their health care provider any sudden increase in lochia, bright red bleeding, elevated temperature, or uterine tenderness.*

Nursing Actions Following a PPH

- Assess the fundus and lochia every hour for first four hours after hemorrhage.
- Teach how to assess the fundus and how to do fundal massage, and the signs of PPH that should be reported to the health care provider.
- Increase oral and IV fluid intake to decrease risk of hypovolemia.
- Explain the importance of preventing an overdistended bladder to reduce the risk for further PPH.
- Assist with ambulation since there is an increase of orthostatic hypotension related to blood loss.
- Explain the importance of rest to decrease the risk of fatigue related to blood loss.
- Provide uninterrupted rest periods while in the hospital.
- Provide an opportunity for the woman and her support system to talk about their feelings and experiences with PPH, as this experience can cause feelings of fear, anxiety, and stress.
- Provide information on foods high in iron and the importance of eating a high-iron diet to decrease the risk of anemia.
- Review the H&H laboratory report. Notify the physician or CNM of abnormal results.

COAGULATION DISORDERS

A variety of complications can occur during the postpartum period related to alterations in the clotting mechanisms. Three of these complications are disseminated intravascular coagulation, amniotic fluid embolism, and thrombosis.

Disseminated Intravascular Coagulation

Disseminated intravascular coagulation (DIC) is a syndrome in which the coagulation pathways are hyperstimulated (Venes, 2009). When this occurs the woman's body breaks down blood clots faster than it can form them, thus quickly depleting the body of clotting factors and leading to hemorrhage. This complication can rapidly lead to maternal death. Women who experience DIC are transferred to critical care units and a perinatologist, when available, manages the care.

Risk Factors

- Abruptio placenta
- Pregnancy induced hypertension
- HELLP syndrome
- Prolonged PPH
- Amniotic fluid embolism
- Sepsis

Assessment Findings

- Prolonged, uncontrolled uterine bleeding
- Bleeding from the IV site, incision site, gums, and bladder
- Increased anxiety
- Signs and symptoms of shock related to blood loss:
  - *Pale and clammy skin*
  - *Tachycardia*
  - *Tachypnea*
  - *Hypotension*

Medical Management

- Laboratory tests (e.g., fibrinogen levels, prothrombin time [PT], partial thromboplastin time [PTT], and platelet count) to assess for abnormal clotting.
- IV therapy
- Blood replacement
- Identification of the primary cause of bleeding and intervention based on this knowledge
- Oxygen therapy
- Consult with the perinatologist
- Transfer of the woman to the critical care unit

Nursing Actions

- Review prenatal and labor records for risk factors.
- Monitor women more frequently who are at risk for DIC.
- Assess for PPH and intervene appropriately. Early intervention can decrease the risk of DIC.
- Monitor vital signs and immediately report to the MD or CNM abnormal findings, such as an increase in heart rate, a decrease in blood pressure, and a change in quality of respirations.
- Start IV as per orders.
- Administer oxygen as per orders.
- Obtain laboratory specimens as per orders.
- Transfer the woman to the critical care unit as per orders.
- Start a blood transfusion as per orders.
- Review laboratory results and notify the physician of results.

Amniotic Fluid Embolism

Amniotic fluid embolism (AFE) is a rare but often fatal complication that occurs during pregnancy, labor and birth, and the first 24 hours post-birth. Amniotic fluid that contains fetal cells, lanugo, and vernix enters the maternal vascular system and initiates a cascading process that leads to cardiorespiratory collapse and disseminated intravascular coagulation (DIC). It is estimated that there is one case per 8,000 to 30,000 pregnancies (Moore, 2007).

Risk Factors

- Induction of labor, which increases the risk to two times greater than that of women not induced
- Maternal age of 35 years or older
- Cesarean birth, forceps-assisted delivery, and vacuum-assisted delivery
- Placenta previa
- Abruptio placenta
- Polyhydramnios
- Eclampsia
- Fetal intolerance of labor
- Cervical and/or uterine lacerations (Kramer, Rouleau, Baskett, & Joseph, 2006)

Assessment Findings

- Hypotension
- Dyspnea
- Cyanosis
- Pulmonary edema identified on x-ray exam
- Uterine atony that causes massive hemorrhage and leads to disseminated intravascular coagulation (DIC)
- Cardiac and respiratory arrest

Evidence-Based Practice: Amniotic Fluid Embolism

Schoening, A. (2006). Amniotic fluid embolism: Historical perspective and new possibilities. *MCN, 31,* 78-83.

Schoening provided a review of the literature focusing on amniotic fluid embolism (AFE). Based on her review, AFE is described as a two-stage process.

Stage I: Amniotic fluid and fetal cells enter the maternal circulation → release of endogenous mediators → pulmonary artery vasospasm and pulmonary hypotension → elevated right ventricular pressure and hypoxia → myocardial and pulmonary capillary damage → left heart failure and acute respiratory distress.

Those who survive the first stage will enter the second stage.

Stage II: Hemorrhage and DIC.

Nursing actions identified are: Prepare for respiratory and/or cardiac arrest and call code team as indicated, assess for signs of seizure, administer oxygen by mask, collect lab work as per orders, prepare to administer blood products and coagulation factors, have pressor agents such as dopamine available to use when ordered, monitor vaginal blood loss, prepare to transfer to the critical care unit, and provide the family with emotional support and information regarding the plan of care.

Medical Management

- The focus is on maintaining cardiac and respiratory function, stopping the hemorrhage, and correcting blood loss.
- Complete blood count (CBC), platelet count, arterial blood gases, fibrinogen, and PT are a few of the laboratory tests that might be ordered.
- Blood type and screen for possible transfusion.
- Chest x-ray exam
- Blood replacement, packed red blood cells, and platelets.
- Transfer the woman to the critical care unit.
- A heart–lung bypass machine, when available, may be used to help stabilize the woman.

Nursing Actions

- Review prenatal and labor records for risk factors.
- Monitor more frequently women who are at risk for AFE.
- Notify the physician of assessment findings that indicate possible AFE. The physician needs to be notified immediately.
- Administer oxygen at 8 L/min. Start an IV when assessments indicate a possible AFE.
- Obtain laboratory specimens as per orders.
- Administer blood replacement as per order.
- Provide emotional support to the woman and her support system.
- Call code and initiate CPR when indicated (Kramer, Rouleau, Baskett, & Joseph, 2006; Schoening, 2006).

Thrombosis

Thrombosis is a blood clot within the vascular system. During pregnancy and the first 6 weeks post-birth, women are at risk for forming blood clots. This is related to the normal physiological changes that occur during pregnancy. During pregnancy, there is an increase in clotting factors I, II, VII, IX, X, and XII, as well as an increase in

fibrinogen. These components of clotting remain elevated during the postpartum period. Thrombosis during pregnancy and/or the postpartum period usually occurs in a vein of the legs and is referred to as a deep veinous thrombosis (DVT). A major concern is that the clot will detach, becoming an embolism, and travel to a vital organ; an example is a pulmonary embolism. Nursing actions focus on decreasing the risk for formation of thrombosis and risk of embolism.

Risk Factors

- Normal physiological changes in coagulation related to pregnancy
- Cesarean birth, which has a risk five times greater than vaginal birth
- Endometritis, which can spread to the vascular system causing thrombophlebitis and can lead to thrombosis
- Decreased mobility, which increases the risk for venous stasis
- Obesity, which places extra pressure on pelvic vessels, causing venous stasis
- Increased parity

Assessment Findings

- Positive Homans' sign
- Tenderness and heat over the affected area
- Leg pain with walking
- Swelling in the affected leg

Medical Management

- Doppler ultrasonography to confirm the diagnosis
- Compression stockings, which reduce venous stasis and risk of DVT
- Coagulation therapy of IV heparin
- Antibiotic therapy if thrombosis is related to infection
- Bed rest with the affected leg elevated

Nursing Actions

- Review prenatal and labor records for risk factors.
- Monitor women who are at greater risk for thrombosis more frequently.
- Apply compression stockings as per orders.
- Assist with ambulation. Early ambulation increases circulation and decreases the risk of venous stasis.
- Report assessment finding of possible signs of thrombosis to the physician or CNM for further evaluation.
- Administer medications as per orders, which include analgesia for pain and anticoagulants.

INFECTIONS

It is estimated that 1% to 8% of postpartum women will experience a postpartum infection (Kennedy, 2007). It is also estimated that 0.6 maternal deaths per 100,000 live births are attributed to postpartum infections (Kennedy, 2007). The most common sites for infections during the postpartum period are the uterus, bladder, breast, and incisional site. Most infections that occur during the postpartum period can be easily treated when identified at an early stage. Infections that are not identified and treated at an early stage can lead to serious complications such as abscess formation, cellulitis, thrombophlebitis, and septic shock.

Endometritis

Endometritis is the most common postpartum infection. It is an infection of the endometrium that usually starts at the placental site and spreads to encompass the entire endometrium (AWHONN, 2006). Approximately 2% of women who experience a vaginal birth and 15% of women who experience a cesarean birth develop endometritis.

Risk Factors

■ Prolonged rupture of membranes
■ Prolonged labor
■ Cesarean birth
■ Internal fetal and uterine monitoring
■ Anemia
■ Malnutrition
■ PPH
■ Diabetes

Assessment Findings

■ Elevated temperature of 39.5°C (101°F) or greater with or without chills
■ Tachycardia
■ Uterine tenderness
■ Subinvolution
■ Malaise
■ Lower abdominal pain or discomfort
■ Lochia heavy and foul smelling when anaerobic organisms are present
  ■ *Foul smelling lochia is a later sign that occurs when the entire endometrium is involved.*
■ Lochia is scant and odorless when beta-hemolytic *Streptococcus* is present.

Medical Management

■ CBC to assess for leukocytosis (white blood cell [WBC] count >20,000/mm³).
■ Endometrial cultures
■ Blood cultures
■ Urinalysis to rule out urinary tract infection which can present with similar symptoms
■ Antibiotic therapy
  ■ *A broad-spectrum cephalosporin or penicillin is frequently used in mild to moderate cases.*
  ■ *Antibiotics are given by IV; the route of administration is changed to PO 24 hours after there has been no temperature elevation.*

Nursing Actions

■ Review prenatal and labor records for risk factors.
■ Monitor more frequently women who are at risk for endometritis.
■ Review laboratory reports such as WBC count and notify physician and/or midwife of abnormal results.

■ Encourage intake of fluids to rehydrate by explaining to the woman that maintaining adequate hydration can decrease the risk for infection. Women should have a minimum fluid intake of 3000 mL/day (AWHONN, 2006).
■ Instruct the woman in proper pericare and to wipe the perineum from front to back.
■ Instruct the woman to change her peripads after each voiding or defecation because lochia is a medium for bacterial growth.
■ Educate the woman regarding proper hand washing technique to reduce the spread of bacteria.
■ Encourage early ambulation by explaining how ambulation reduces the risk for infection by promoting uterine drainage (AWHONN, 2006).
■ Educate the woman on a diet high in protein and vitamin C, which helps with tissue healing.
■ Report assessment findings that indicate a possible endometritis to the physician or midwife for further evaluation.
■ Administer antibiotics as per orders.
■ Provide pain management measures.
■ Provide emotional support to the woman and her family.

Cystitis

Cystitis, an infection of the bladder, is a common occurrence in the postpartum period. Cystitis is easily treated, but if left untreated or if there is a delay in treatment the woman is at risk for pyelonephritis.

Risk Factors

■ Epidural anesthesia, which decreases the woman's ability to feel the urge to void, leading to an increased risk for an overdistended bladder
■ Overdistended bladder or incomplete emptying of the bladder, which can cause an increase of bacterial growth in the bladder
■ A Foley catheter inserted during the labor process
■ Neonatal macrosomia, which can cause edema around the urethra
■ Operative vaginal deliveries, forceps, or vacuum extractor, which can cause edema around the urethra
■ Intrapartal vaginal exams and the birth process, which can contaminate the urethra with bacteria

Assessment Findings

■ Low-grade fever (< 38.5°C/101°F)
■ Burning on urination
■ Suprapubic pain
■ Urgency to void
■ Small, frequent voidings—less than 150 mL per voiding

Medical Management

■ Antibiotics (usually PO) started before culture results
■ Urinalysis, CBC, and urine culture and sensitivity

Nursing Actions

■ Review prenatal and labor records for risk factors.
■ Monitor more frequently women who are at risk for cystitis.
■ Assist the woman to the bathroom to void within a few hours after birth. This will flush bacteria out of the urethra.
■ Catheterize the woman if she is unable to void within 12 hours post-birth as per orders.
■ Remind the woman to void every 3 to 4 hours.

■ Measure voidings for the first 24 hours, assessing for complete emptying of the bladder. Each voiding should be equal to or greater than 150 mL.

■ Change peripads at least every 3 to 4 hours. Soiled peripads can encourage growth of bacteria that can enter the urethra.

■ Remind postpartum women to drink a minimum of 3000 mL/day (AWHONN, 2006).

■ Encourage foods that increase acidity in urine such as cranberry juice, apricots, and plums (AWHONN, 2006).

■ Report findings of possible urinary tract infection (UTI) to the physician or CNM for further evaluation.

■ Obtain laboratory specimens as per orders.

■ Administer antibiotics as per orders.

■ Provide information on proper use of discharge medications.

■ Review laboratory reports such as urinalysis, CBC, and culture and sensitivity. Notify the physician or midwife of abnormal findings.

■ Provide information on signs and symptoms of cystitis to report to the health care provider.

Mastitis

Mastitis is an inflammation/infection of the breast that is common among lactating women. It usually occurs in just one of the breasts and within the first 2 postpartum weeks after milk flow has been established. Infection resolves within 24 to 48 hours of antibiotic therapy. Abscess formation can occur when there is a delay in treatment.

Risk Factors

■ History of mastitis with a previous infant

■ Cracked and/or sore nipples

■ Use of antifungal nipple cream, which is often applied when the newborn has thrush (Foxman, D'Arcy, Gillespie, Bobo, & Schwartz, 2002)

Assessment Findings

■ A hard, tender palpable mass

■ Redness in the area around the mass

■ Acute pain in affected breast

■ Temperature elevation

■ Tachycardia

■ Malaise

■ Purulent drainage

Medical Management

■ Administer oral antibiotics that are safe to use with lactating women

Nursing Actions

■ Palpate and inspect the breasts for signs of mastitis.

■ Teach the woman methods to decrease nipple irritation and tissue breakdown, such as correct infant latch on and removal from the breast, and air-drying nipples after feedings (refer to Chapter 16 for additional information).

■ Explain to the woman the importance of washing her hands before feeding to decrease spread of bacteria.

■ Instruct the woman to wear a supportive bra for comfort.

■ Administer analgesia as per orders.

■ Teach the woman signs of mastitis before hospital discharge because mastitis usually occurs after discharge.

■ Explain to the woman that it is very common for lactating women to experience mastitis and that it is easily treated when identified early.

■ Teach the woman the importance of a healthy diet and adequate fluids to decrease risk for any infection.

■ Report findings of possible mastitis to the physician or CNM.

■ Apply warm compresses to the affected area for comfort and promotion of circulation.

■ Administer antibiotics as per orders.

■ Instruct the woman to continue to breastfeed or to massage and express milk from the affected breast to promote continuation of milk flow.

Wound Infections

Wound infections can occur at the episiotomy site, cesarean incision site, and laceration site.

Risk Factors

■ Obesity

■ Diabetes

■ Malnutrition

■ Long labor

■ Premature rupture of membranes

■ Preexisting infection

■ Immunodeficiency disorders

■ Corticosteroid therapy

■ Poor suturing technique

Assessment Findings

■ Erythema

■ Redness

■ Heat

■ Swelling

■ Tenderness

■ Purulent drainage

■ Low-grade fever

■ Increased pain at incision or laceration site

Medical Management

■ Obtain a culture specimen from the wound or laceration.

■ For mild to moderate wound infections that do not have purulent drainage:
  ■ *Administer oral antibiotic therapy.*
  ■ *Apply warm compresses to area.*

■ Wound infections with purulent drainage:
  ■ *Open and drain the wound.*
  ■ *Begin IV antibiotic therapy.*

Nursing Actions

■ Review prenatal and labor records for risk factors.

■ Monitor women more frequently who are at risk for wound infection. Notify the physician or midwife of abnormal assessment findings.

■ Use proper hand washing technique before and after contact with the wound.

■ Provide education on proper diet, fluids, and rest that can decrease the risk for infection and assist in the healing process.

■ Use hot packs for abdominal wounds or sitz baths for perineal wounds to promote comfort and circulation as per orders.

■ Obtain laboratory specimens such as cultures as per orders.

■ Review laboratory reports such as CBC. Report abnormal findings to the physician or midwife.

■ Administer antibiotics as per orders.

■ Administer analgesia for fever and discomfort as per order.
■ Provide information on proper use of discharge medications.

POSTPARTUM PSYCHOLOGICAL COMPLICATIONS

A women's psychological state is affected during the postpartum period by hormonal changes, lack of sleep, and stress of integrating a new person within the woman's life and within the family unit. A majority of women will experience postpartum blues, which are short term and require no medical intervention (see Chapter 13). A small percentage of women, 6.5% to 12.9%, will experience major mood disorders that have a profound effect on their ability to care for themselves and/or their infants (AWHONN, 2006). Mood disorders during the first year after childbirth have a negative effect on the mother–infant relationship (AWHONN, 2006). Two major mood disorders are postpartum depression and postpartum psychosis. These disorders require management by mental health care professionals. The primary role of the perinatal nurse is assessing for early signs of potential mood disorders and reporting these findings to the woman's health care provider for further evaluation and treatment.

Postpartum Depression

Postpartum depression (PPD) is a mood disorder characterized by severe depression that occurs within the first 6 to 12 months postpartum. It is estimated that this occurs in 6.5% to 12.9% of postpartum women (AWHONN, 2006). PPD has an effect on the woman, her partner, and other children within the family unit. A major difference between postpartum blues and PPD is that PPD is disabling; the woman is unable to safely care for herself and/or her baby (Table 14-1). Women who receive proper treatment will recover from PPD, but they grieve over the lost time with their infants (AWHONN, 2006).

Risk Factors

■ History of depression before pregnancy
■ Depression or anxiety during pregnancy
■ Inadequate social support
■ Poor quality relationship with partner
■ Life and child care stresses (Horowitz & Goodman, 2005)

Assessment Findings

■ Sleep and appetite disturbance
■ Despondency

■ Uncontrolled crying
■ Anxiety, fear, and/or panic
■ Inability to concentrate
■ Feelings of guilt, inadequacy, and/or worthlessness
■ Inability to care for self and/or baby
■ Decreased affectionate contact with the infant
■ Decreased responsiveness to the infant
■ Thoughts of harming baby
■ Thoughts of suicide (AWHONN, 2006; Higgins, 2004; Horowitz & Goodman, 2005; Miller, 2002)

Medical/Psychiatric Management

■ Mild to moderate PPD
  ■ *Antidepressant medications*
  ■ *Interpersonal psychotherapy*
  ■ *Cognitive therapy (Miller, 2002)*
■ Severe PPD and suicidal ideation
  ■ *Intense psychiatric care*
  ■ *Crisis interventions*
  ■ *Pharmacotherapy (Miller, 2002)*

Nursing Actions

■ Review prenatal record for risk factors.
■ Monitor mother–infant interactions more closely for women at risk for PPD.
■ Teach the woman and her partner signs of PPD that should be reported to her health care provider.
■ Be supportive and encouraging in interactions.
■ Provide the woman with information regarding postpartum support groups and other community resources to assist her with parenting issues and to provide support.

Evidence-Based Practice: Postpartum Depression

Beck, C., Records, K., & Rice, M. (2006). Further development of the postpartum depression predictors inventory-revised. *JOGNN, 35*, 735-745.

A purpose of this longitudinal study of 139 women was to test the sensitivity and specificity of the Postpartum Depression Predictors Inventory-Revised (PDPI-R) as an instrument used to screen for risk of postpartum depression.

The PDPI-R is an interview tool that can be used by clinicians during the prenatal period. The prenatal version has 10 predictor items. These are marital status, socioeconomic status, self-esteem, prenatal depression, prenatal anxiety, unplanned/unwanted pregnancy, history of depression, social support, marital/partner satisfaction, and life stress. Each item is assigned a score based on the evaluation by the clinician. There are a possible 32 points for the prenatal version of the PDPI-R. This research study indicated that a cut-off score of 10.5 has a sensitivity of .76 and a specificity of .54 in predicting depression in the postpartum period.

Women who have a score of 10.5 or higher should be referred to a mental health professional during pregnancy for further evaluation and possible treatment. It is recommended that women who score 7.5 or higher be closely followed during the postpartum period for signs and symptoms of PPD.

It is recommended that women be screened for depression during the antepartum and postpartum periods (AWHONN, 2006).

TABLE 14–1	MAJOR DIFFERENCES BETWEEN POSTPARTUM BLUES AND POSTPARTUM DEPRESSION
POSTPARTUM BLUES	**POSTPARTUM DEPRESSION**
Symptoms disappear without medical intervention.	Requires psychiatric interventions.
Occur within the first 2 weeks postpartum.	Occurs within the first 6 months postpartum.
Able to safely care for self and baby.	Unable to safely care for self and/or baby.

Postpartum Psychosis

Postpartum psychosis (PPP) is a variant of bipolar disorder and is the most serious form of postpartum mood disorders. This is a rare postpartum mood disorder that occurs in 1 to 2 women per 1,000 births (AWHONN, 2006). Onset of symptoms can be as early as the third postpartum day. Women with PPP require immediate hospitalization and evaluation, as they are at risk for injuring themselves or their infants.

Risk Factors

■ Women with known bipolar disorder
■ Personal or family history of bipolar disorder (Sit, Rotherschild, & Wisner, 2006)

Assessment Findings

■ Delusions, paranoia, hallucinations
■ Mood swings
■ Extreme agitation
■ Depressed or elated moods
■ Distraught feelings about ability to enjoy infant
■ Confused thinking
■ Strange beliefs, such as that she or her infant must die
■ Disorganized behavior (AWHONN, 2006; Sit, Rotherschild, & Wisner, 2006)

Medical/Psychiatric Management

■ Hospitalization to the psychiatric unit
■ Psychiatric evaluation
■ Antidepressant and antipsychotic drug treatment
■ Psychotherapy
■ Electroconvulsive therapy

Nursing Actions

■ Review the prenatal record for risk factors.
■ Educate women who are at risk and their support system of early signs of PPP such as mood swings, hallucinations, and strange beliefs, and instruct them to contact the health care provider if symptoms are present.

DISORDERS LATER IN LIFE RELATED TO CHILDBIRTH TRAUMA

Childbirth causes trauma to the woman's body that places her at risk for reproductive disorders later in life. The risk factors for reproductive disorders later in life related to childbirth trauma are high parity, large babies, forceps deliveries, vacuum extraction delivery, advancing maternal age, and poor suturing technique of physician or midwife with repair of episiotomies or lacerations. Common disorders are uterine prolapse, genital fistula, cystocele, rectocele, and urinary incontinence (Fig. 14-3).

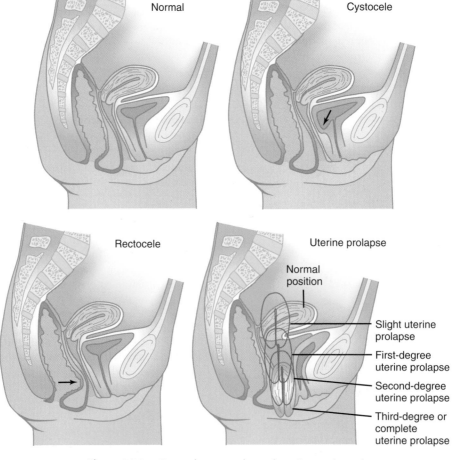

Figure 14-3   Cystocele, rectocele, and uterine prolapsed.

Uterine Prolapse

Uterine prolapse occurs when there is a weakening of the pelvic connective tissue, pubococcygeus muscle, and uterine ligaments, allowing the uterus to descend into the vagina.

Risk Factors

■ Aging
■ Obesity
■ Low estrogen levels, which weaken the pelvic floor muscles

Assessment Findings

■ Protrusion of uterus into the vaginal area
■ Low backache
■ Sensation of heaviness in the pelvis or vagina
■ Difficult or painful intercourse

Medical Management

■ Vaginal pessary, which is placed in the vagina and supports the uterus, is used in a mild degree of prolapse.
■ Surgery, which may include hysterectomy

Nursing Actions

■ Reduce risk by providing information regarding the importance of Kegel exercises and on how to do these exercises. This is the major nursing action during the postpartum period.
■ Explain that excess weight can increase the risk for uterine prolapse and provide information on healthy eating.

Genital Fistulas

Genital fistulas are abnormal connections between the vagina and bladder, rectum, and/or urethra. The fistula provides a pathway for fecal material and/or urine to enter the vagina.

Risk Factors

■ Trauma of tissues during childbirth
■ Vaginal surgery
■ Radiotherapy

Assessment Findings

■ Leakage of urine and/or fecal material from the vagina
■ Foul vaginal odor
■ Irritation of the vaginal mucosa

Medical Management

■ Obtain a fistulogram to determine the location and severity of fistulas.
■ Small fistulas may resolve on their own if tissue is allowed to rest.
■ Larger fistulas may require surgical repair.

Nursing Actions

■ Nurses working in a woman's clinic will reinforce teaching and clarify information provided by the primary health care provider.

Cystocele

Cystocele is the bulging of the bladder into the vagina, which occurs when the wall between the vagina and bladder weakens and stretches.

Risk Factors

■ Excessive straining during childbirth, with chronic constipation and heavy lifting
■ High parity
■ Obesity
■ Aging, which leads to a decrease in estrogen and a weakening of the pelvic floor muscles
■ Hysterectomy, which can weaken the pelvic floor muscles

Assessment Findings

■ Sense of fullness or pressure in the vagina or pelvis
■ Discomfort when straining, coughing, bearing down, or lifting
■ Stress incontinence
■ Bladder infections
■ Pain or urine leakage during intercourse

Medical Management

■ Pessary
■ Hormone replacement therapy
■ Surgery

Nursing Actions

■ Instruct the woman on the importance of Kegel exercises to maintain her muscle strength and teach her how to do Kegel exercises.
■ Instruct the woman on the treatment and prevention of constipation, such as a high-fiber diet and increased fluid intake.
■ Instruct the woman to avoid heavy lifting.
■ Explain the relationship between increased weight and increased risk of cystoceles and discuss weight reduction strategies.

Rectoceles

Rectoceles occur when the front wall of the rectum bulges into the vagina.

Risk Factors

■ Excessive straining during childbirth, with chronic constipation and with heavy lifting
■ High parity
■ Chronic constipation
■ Chronic cough or bronchitis
■ Obesity
■ Aging, which leads to a decrease in estrogen and a weakening of the pelvic floor muscles
■ Hysterectomy, which can weaken the pelvic floor muscles

Assessment Findings

■ Sense of fullness or pressure in the vagina or pelvis
■ Low back pain that is relieved by lying down
■ Constipation or difficulty having a bowel movement
■ Difficulty in controlling passage of stool

Medical Management

■ Pessary
■ Hormone replacement therapy
■ Surgery

Nursing Actions

- Instruct women on the importance of Kegel exercises to maintain muscle strength and teach how to do Kegel exercises.
- Instruct women on the treatment and prevention of constipation such as increased fiber in diet and increased fluid intake.
- Instruct women to avoid heavy lifting.
- Explain the relationship between increased weight and increased risk of rectoceles and discuss weight reduction strategies.

Urinary Incontinence

Urinary incontinence is the loss of bladder control.

Risk Factors

- Childbirth
- Aging, which leads to a decrease in estrogen and a weakening of muscles which decreases the ability of the urethra to remain closed
- Hysterectomy
- Obesity
- Smoking, which causes chronic coughing and places stress on the urinary sphincters
- Diabetes

Assessment Findings

- Stress incontinence, which is the leakage of urine when coughing, sneezing, laughing, or lifting
- Sudden and intense urge to void followed by uncontrolled voiding

Medical Management

- Medications such as anticholinergic drugs (Detrol)
- Estrogen cream applied to the genital tissues
- Pessary
- Surgery

Nursing Actions

- Instruct the woman on the importance of Kegel exercises to maintain muscle strength and teach her how to do Kegel exercises.
- Instruct the woman on the treatment and prevention of constipation by increasing fiber in the diet and increasing fluid intake.
- Instruct her to avoid heavy lifting.
- Explain the relationship between increased weight and increased risk of urinary incontinence and discuss weight reduction strategies.
- Maintain skin integrity by instructing the woman to keep the area clean and dry.
- Encourage the woman to decrease alcohol and caffeine intake, as both cause an increase in urination.
- Provide strategies for retraining the bladder such as scheduling toileting times and gradually increasing the wait time after she feels the urge to void.

Medication

Tolterodine (Detrol)

- Action: Inhibits cholinergic mediated bladder contractions.
- Common side effects: Dry mouth, headache, and dizziness.
- Route and dosage: PO; 2 mg twice daily

(Data from Deglin & Vallerand, 2009)

CONCEPT MAP

Postpartum Hemorrhage

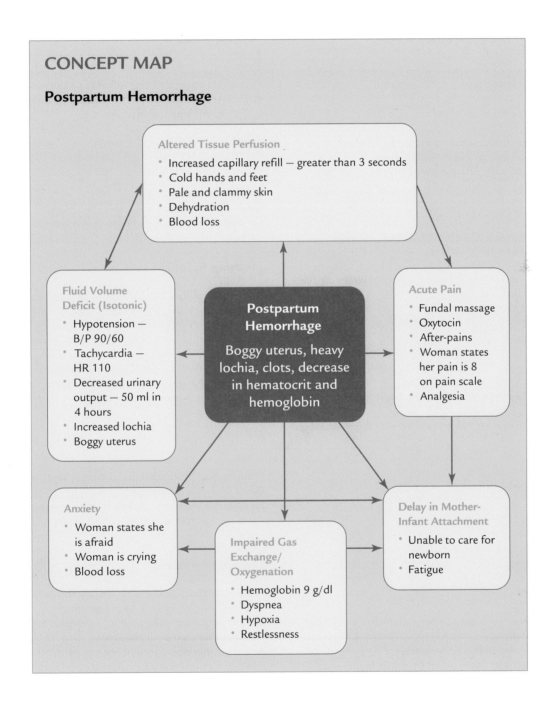

Altered Tissue Perfusion
- Increased capillary refill — greater than 3 seconds
- Cold hands and feet
- Pale and clammy skin
- Dehydration
- Blood loss

Fluid Volume Deficit (Isotonic)
- Hypotension — B/P 90/60
- Tachycardia — HR 110
- Decreased urinary output — 50 ml in 4 hours
- Increased lochia
- Boggy uterus

Postpartum Hemorrhage
Boggy uterus, heavy lochia, clots, decrease in hematocrit and hemoglobin

Acute Pain
- Fundal massage
- Oxytocin
- After-pains
- Woman states her pain is 8 on pain scale
- Analgesia

Anxiety
- Woman states she is afraid
- Woman is crying
- Blood loss

Impaired Gas Exchange/ Oxygenation
- Hemoglobin 9 g/dl
- Dyspnea
- Hypoxia
- Restlessness

Delay in Mother-Infant Attachment
- Unable to care for newborn
- Fatigue

Problem No. 1: Fluid volume deficit (isotonic)
Goal: Increase fluid volume
Outcome: Patient's blood pressure and heart rate will be within normal ranges, and intake and output will be within 200 mL of each other by the end of the shift.

Nursing Actions

1. Assess fundus for firmness: Massage if boggy.
2. Assess lochia for amount, color, and clots.
3. Instruct and remind the woman to drink a minimum of one glass of fluid per hour.
4. Initiate IV therapy as per orders.
5. Initiate oxytocin therapy as per orders.
6. Assess intake and output.
7. Assist the woman to the bathroom every 3 to 4 hours.
8. Monitor blood pressure and pulse every 2 hours.
9. Assess skin turgor and mucus membrane every 4 hours.

Problem No. 2: Altered tissue perfusion
Goal: Normal tissue profusion
Outcome: Blood pressure and pulse within normal limits; capillary fill less than 3 seconds

Nursing Actions

1. Every 2 hours, monitor vital signs, capillary refill, and motor and sensory status.
2. Compare post-hemorrhage Hb/Hct with results on admission to labor.
3. Administer oxygen as per orders and monitor oxygen saturation levels.

Problem No. 3: Anxiety
Goal: Decreased anxiety
Outcome: Patient verbalizes that she feels less anxious.

Nursing Actions

1. Be calm and reassuring in interactions with patient and family.
2. Explain all procedures.
3. Teach patient relaxation breathing techniques.
4. Encourage patient and family to verbalize their feelings regarding recent hemorrhage by asking open-ended questions.

Problem No. 4: Delay in mother–infant attachment
Goal: Positive mother–infant attachment
Outcome: Patient will hold the infant close and respond to the infant's needs and will state she enjoys her baby.

Nursing Actions

1. When the patient is stable, have the infant remain in the patient's room.
2. Assist the patient with infant care as needed.
3. Encourage infant holding by assisting the patient in a comfortable position and placing infant in patient's arms.
4. Praise the patient for positive mother–infant interactions.
5. Provide information on infant care.

Problem No. 5: Acute pain
Goal: Decreased pain
Outcome: Patient will state that pain is less than 3 on pain scale.

Nursing Actions

1. Assess level, location, and type of pain.
2. Prevent overdistention of the bladder by reminding the patient to void every 3–4 hours.
3. Administer pain medications based on assessment data as per orders.
4. Provide an environment that is conducive to relaxation, such as low lights, decreased noise, and uninterrupted rest periods.
5. Teach patient relaxation techniques.

Problem No. 6: Impaired gas exchange/oxygenation
Goal: Maintain oxygenation
Outcome: Oxygen saturation is 98% and respiratory rate and pattern are within normal limits.

Nursing Actions

1. Monitor respirations, breath sounds, and oxygen saturation.
2. Provide oxygen by mask as per orders.
3. Instruct and assist the patient with deep breathing and coughing to decrease the risk of pneumonia
4. Initiate iron replacement therapy as per orders.
5. Provide nutritional information on food high in iron such as green leafy vegetables.

TYING IT ALL TOGETHER

You are a nurse working in the postpartum unit. You are assigned Ms. Mallory, a 42-year-old African American woman. (Refer to Tying It All Together in Chapters 7 and 10 for antepartum and intrapartum data.)

Summary of Labor and Delivery Record

Ms. Mallory was admitted 2 days ago at 32 weeks' gestation and managed in the birthing unit for preterm labor with magnesium sulfate and antibiotics. She received betamethasone. The magnesium sulfate was discontinued 3 hours before delivery. Her labor was augmented during the transitional phase. She spontaneously delivered a 1559-g (3 lb. 7 oz.) boy with Apgar scores of 5 and 7 at 1 and 5 minutes. Her baby is experiencing mild signs of respiratory distress and is in the NICU.

Postpartum Report

Ms. Mallory is 4 hours post-birth and has an IV of D5 lactated Ringer's solution with 10 units of oxytocin running in her left arm. She voided in the recovery unit 2 hours post-birth.

Assessment Findings

Vitals signs: Temperature 37°C; pulse 98 bpm; respirations 14 breaths/min; blood pressure 110/70 mm Hg
   Fundus is at the umbilicus and boggy.
   Lochia is heavy.
Based on your assessment findings and Ms. Mallory's history, what are your immediate nursing actions?
Discuss the rationale for your nursing actions.

You reevaluate Ms. Mallory 10 minutes after your initial nursing actions. Her fundus is firm, midline, and 1 finger breadth below the umbilicus with scant lochia. You continue to monitor Ms. Mallory and 15 minutes later her fundus is boggy with heavy lochia. The fundus becomes firm after massage. Her pulse is 100 bpm and blood pressure is 100/60 mm Hg. You notify her CNM and report your findings.

Detail the aspects of your assessment findings that you will report to the CNM.

The CNM orders 20 units of oxytocin in 1000 mL of lactated Ringer's solution. The ordered infusion rate is 10 mL/min, to be regulated by firmness of the uterus.

Discuss your nursing actions and rationale for actions.
Discuss the assessment data needed to determine effectiveness of medical and nursing actions.

You note that in her prenatal chart she has a diagnosis of fibroids.

Discuss the implications of the diagnosis as it relates to your nursing care and discharge teaching plan.

■ ■ ■ Review Questions ■ ■ ■

1. Your patient is a 25-year-old gravid 1 woman who is 2 hours postpartum. You note on assessment that her fundus is firm and midline. She is experiencing a steady stream of blood. The bed linen under her is soaked in blood. Based on these findings and observations you suspect that she is exhibiting early signs/symptoms of a postpartum hemorrhage related to:
   A. Uterine atony
   B. Laceration of the cervical or vaginal area
   C. Retained placental tissue
   D. Fibroids

2. Mrs. Fischer is 4 days post-birth. She calls the clinic and tells the triage nurse that she has a temperature and does not feel well. What additional assessment findings does the triage nurse need to obtain to assist in her nursing assessment? Select all that apply.
   A. When did she notice an increase in temperature and what is her temperate?
   B. Is she experiencing pain, and if so, where is it located?
   C. What is the amount of her fluid intake within the past 24 hours?
   D. What is the color and amount of her bleeding?

3. Foul smelling lochia occurs:
   A. When beta-hemolytic *Streptococcus* is the primary organism associated with endometritis
   B. Within the first 24 hours post-birth related to endometritis
   C. When the entire endometrium is infected
   D. During the normal involution process

4. Women who experience mastitis should be instructed to:
   A. Stop breast feeding until 48 hours after the start of antibiotic treatment
   B. Continue to breast feed or massage and express milk from the affected breast
   C. Wash nipples with antibiotic soap before each feeding session
   D. Apply cream to nipples after each feeding until mastitis has resolved.

5. Signs and symptoms of postpartum depression include which of the following? Select all that apply.
   A. Sleep and appetite disturbance
   B. Uncontrolled crying
   C. Delusions
   D. Feelings of guilt and/or worthlessness

References

Association of Women's Health, Obstetric and Neonatal Nursing (AWHONN). (2006). *The compendium of postpartum care*. Philadelphia: Medical Broadcasting Company.

Beck, C., Records, K., & Rice, M. (2006). Further development of the postpartum depression predictors inventory-revised. *JOGNN, 35*, 735–745.

Deglin, J., & Vallerand, A. (2009). *Davis's drug guide for nurses* (11th ed.). Philadelphia: F. A. Davis.

Foxman, B., D'Arcy, H., Gillespie, B., Bobo, J., & Schwartz, K. (2002). Lactation mastitis: Occurrence and medical management among 946 breastfeeding women in the United States. *American Journal of Epidemiology, 155*, 103–114.

Higgins, P. (2004). Postpartum complications. In S. Mattson & J. Smith (Eds.), *Core curriculum for maternal-newborn nursing* (3rd ed., pp. 850–870). St. Louis, MO: W. B. Saunders.

Horowitz, J., & Goodman, J. (2005). Identifying and treating postpartum depression. *JOGNN, 34*, 264–273.

Kennedy, E. (2007). Pregnancy, postpartum infections. *eMedicine*. [Online] Retrieved from: http://www.emedicine.medscape.com/article/796892-overview (Accessed September 2, 2009).

Kramer, M., Rouleau, J., Baskett, M., & Joseph, K. (2006). Amniotic fluid embolism and medical induction of labour: A retrospective, population cohort study. *The Lancet, 368*, 1444–1448.

MacMullen, N., Dulski, L., & Meagher, B. (2005). Red alert: Perinatal hemorrhage. *MCN, The American Journal of Maternal Child Nursing, 30*, 46–51.

Miller, L. (2002). Postpartum depression. *JAMA, 287*, 762–765.

Moore, L. (2007). Amniotic fluid embolism. *eMedicine*. [Online] Retrieved from http://www.emedicine.medscape.com/article/2553068-overview (Accessed September 2, 2009).

Schoening, A. (2006). Amniotic fluid embolism: Historical perspective and new possibilities. *MCN, The American Journal of Maternal Child Nursing, 31*, 78–83.

Sit, K., Rotherschild, A., & Wisner, K. (2006). A review of postpartum psychosis. *Journal of Women's Health, 15*, 352–368.

Venes, D. (2009). *Taber's cyclopedic medical dictionary* (21st ed.). Philadelphia: F. A. Davis.

Wainscott, M. (2006). Pregnancy, postpartum hemorrhage. *eMedicine*. [Online] Retrieved from: http://www.emedicine.medscape.com/article/275038-overview (Accessed September 2, 2009).

You, W., & Zahn, C. (2006). Postpartum hemorrhage: abnormally adherent placenta, uterine inversion, and puerperal hematomas. *Clinical Obstetrics and Gynecology, 49*, 184–197.

The Neonatal Period

Physiological and Behavioral Responses of the Neonate

15

OBJECTIVES

On completion of this chapter, the student will be able to:

☐ Define key terms.
☐ Identify the changes that occur during the transition from intrauterine to extrauterine life and the related nursing actions.
☐ List the critical elements of neonatal assessment.
☐ List the critical elements of neonatal gestational age assessments.
☐ Discuss methods used in neonatal pain management.
☐ Describe the nursing care for neonates during the first week of life.
☐ Describe the common laboratory and diagnostic tests for neonates.
☐ Discuss the nursing actions that support parents in the care of their newborn.
☐ Describe the most common therapeutic and surgical procedures used for neonates and the related nursing care.

Nursing Diagnoses

■ At risk for altered body temperature related to decreased amounts of subcutaneous fat and/or large body surface
■ At risk for infections related to tissue trauma and/or poor hand washing techniques by health care providers and parents
■ At risk for impaired gas exchange related to transitioning from fetal to neonatal circulation, cold stress, and/or excessive mucus production
■ At risk for fluid volume deficit related to limited oral intake
■ At risk for knowledge deficit related to first-time parenting and/or limited learning resources

Nursing Outcomes

■ The neonate's temperature will be within normal limits, and the skin will be pink and feel warm to touch.
■ The neonate will not exhibit signs or symptoms of an infection.
■ The neonate's respiratory rate and heart rate will be within normal ranges; the skin will be pink and the airway will remain clear.
■ The neonate will void six times daily.
■ Parents will respond to their newborn's needs.

INTRODUCTION

The **neonatal period** is from birth through the first 28 days of life. During these few weeks, the neonate transitions from intrauterine to extrauterine life and adapts to a new environment. Most neonates who are term and whose mothers experienced a healthy pregnancy and low-risk labor and birth, accomplish this transition with relative ease.

Want to reinforce your reading? Need to review for a test? Listen to this chapter on your accompanying CD.

The focus of nursing care during this time is to protect and support the neonate as he undergoes numerous physiological changes and adapts to extrauterine life (Verklan & Padhye, 2004). This is accomplished by:

■ Maintaining body heat
■ Maintaining respiratory function
■ Decreasing risk for infection

- Assisting parents in providing appropriate nutrition and hydration
- Assisting parents in learning to care for their newborn

TRANSITION TO EXTRAUTERINE LIFE

The transition to extrauterine life begins at birth when the umbilical cord is clamped and the neonate takes his first breath. This initiates various changes within the neonate's physiological systems. Each system needs to adapt to the changes that occur during this transition. The most critical and dynamic changes occur in the respiratory and cardiovascular systems. Thermoregulatory, metabolic, hepatic, gastrointestinal, and immune systems also undergo significant changes.

The Respiratory System

The establishment of extrauterine respirations is the most critical and immediate physiological change that occurs in the transition from fetus to neonate. This change is initiated by compression of the thorax, lung expansion, increase in alveolar oxygen concentration, and vasodilatation of the pulmonary vessels.

- Mechanical and chemical stimuli are the primary factors that initiate extrauterine respirations (Figs. 15-1 and 15-2).
- Sensory stimuli such as exposure to temperature changes, sounds, lights, and touch also influence respirations by stimulating the respiratory center of the medulla.
- In utero, the lungs are filled with amniotic fluid. Approximately 30 mL of amniotic fluid is forced out of the lungs during the delivery process.
- The presence of surfactant, a phospholipid, within the alveoli assists in the establishment of functional residual capacity. This residual capacity assists in keeping the alveolar sacs partially open at the end of exhalation, which decreases the amount of pressure and energy required on inspiration (see Chapter 17).
- The initiation of respiration has an effect on the pulmonary circulation and gas exchange:
  - *First breath → ↑ alveolar oxygen tension (PaO₂) and ↓ arterial pH → dilation of pulmonary arteries → ↓ pulmonary vascular resistance → ↑ blood flow through pulmonary vessels → ↑ oxygen and carbon dioxide exchange within the lungs*
- Two factors that negatively affect the transition extrauterine respirations are:
  - *Decreased surfactant levels related to immature lungs*
  - *Persistent hypoxemia and acidosis that leads to constriction of the pulmonary arteries*
- Approximately 10% of neonates require some degree of assistance with respirations at the time of delivery and 1% require extensive resuscitation.

CRITICAL COMPONENT

Signs of Respiratory Distress

- Cyanosis
- Abnormal respiratory pattern such as apnea and tachypnea
- Retractions of the chest wall
- Grunting
- Flaring of nostrils
- Hypotonia

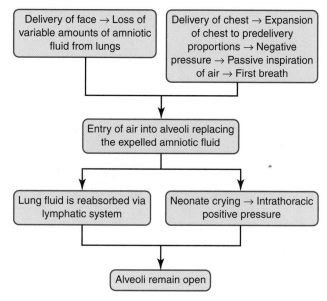

Figure 15-1   Transition to extrauterine pulmonary function: Mechanical stimuli.

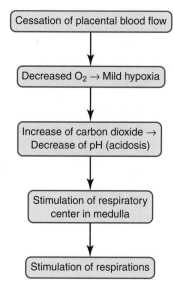

Figure 15-2   Transition to extrauterine pulmonary function: Chemical stimuli.

The Circulatory System

The transition from fetal circulation to neonatal circulation begins rapidly within seconds of the clamping of the umbilical cord and the initiation of the first breath. The transition to neonatal circulation is strongly influenced by the changes within the respiratory system. Fetal circulation is discussed in Chapter 3.

- The decrease in pulmonary vascular resistance causes an increase in pulmonary blood flow and the increase in systemic vascular resistance influences the cardiovascular changes (Fig. 15-3).

The three major fetal circulatory structures that undergo changes are the ductus venosus, foramen ovale, and the ductus arteriosus.

- The **ductus venosus**, which connects the umbilical vein to the inferior vena cava, closes by day 3 of life and becomes a ligament. Blood flow through the umbilical vein stops once the cord is clamped.

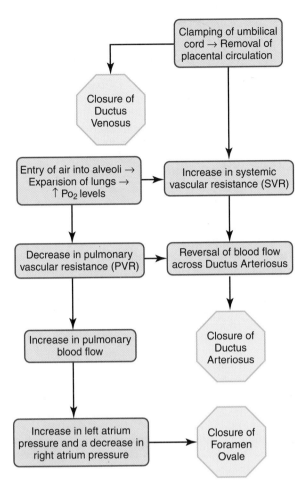

Figure 15-3 Transition to neonatal circulation.

■ The **foramen ovale**, which is an opening between the right atrium and the left atrium, closes when the left atrial pressure is higher than the right atrial pressure. This closure occurs when:
  ■ *Increased PaO₂ → decreased pulmonary pressure → increased pulmonary blood flow → increased pressure in left atrium → closure of foramen ovale*
  ■ *Significant neonatal hypoxia can cause a reopening of the foramen ovale*
■ The **ductus arteriosus**, which connects the pulmonary artery with the descending aorta, usually closes within 15 hours post-birth.
  ■ *This closure occurs when the pulmonary vascular resistance becomes less than system vascular resistance → left to right shunt → closure of ductus arteriosus.*
  ■ *It will remain open if lungs fail to expand or PaO₂ levels drop.*

The Thermoregulatory System

The fetus is surrounded in amniotic fluid that maintains a fairly constant environmental temperature based on the maternal body temperature. Once the neonate enters the extrauterine world, he must adapt to changes in the environmental temperatures. The neonate's responses to extrauterine temperature changes during the first few weeks are delayed and place the neonate at risk for cold stress. The neonate responds to cold by an increase in metabolic rate, an increase of muscle activity, peripheral vascular constriction, and metabolism of brown fat. A neutral thermal environment (NTE) decreases

possible complications related to the delayed response to environmental temperature changes.

■ A **neutral thermal environment (NTE)** is an environment that maintains body temperature with minimal metabolic changes and/or oxygen consumption.
■ **Brown fat,** also referred to as brown adipose tissue or nonshivering thermogenesis, is a highly dense and vascular adipose tissue that is unique to neonates.
  ■ *It is located in the neck, thorax, axillary area, intrascapular areas, and around the adrenal glands and kidneys.*
  ■ *Heat is produced by intense lipid metabolic metabolism of the brown fat.*
  ■ *Brown fat reserves are rapidly depleted during periods of cold stress.*
  ■ *Preterm neonates have limited brown fat.*
■ Neonates are at higher risk for thermoregulatory problems related to:
  ■ *Higher body surface-area-to-body-mass ratio*
  ■ *Higher metabolic rate*
  ■ *Limited and immature thermoregulatory abilities*
■ Factors that negatively affect thermoregulation are:
  ■ *Decreased subcutaneous fat*
  ■ *Decreased brown fat in preterm neonates*
  ■ *Large body surface*
  ■ *Loss of body heat from convection, radiation, conduction, and/or evaporation*
    ■ **Convection**: Loss of heat from the neonate's warm body surface to cooler air currents such as air conditioners or oxygen masks
    ■ **Radiation**: Transfer of heat from the neonate to cooler objects that are not in direct contact with the neonate such as cold walls of the isolette or cold equipment near the neonate
    ■ **Conduction**: Transfer of heat to cooler surface by direct skin contact such as cold hands of caregivers or cold equipment
    ■ **Evaporation**: Loss of heat that occurs when water on the neonate's skin is converted to vapors such as during bathing or directly after birth

Cold Stress

Cold stress is a term that describes excessive heat loss that leads to hypothermia and results in the utilization of compensatory mechanisms to maintain the neonate's body temperature (Fig. 15-4). Neonates function at close to maximal capacity and have little reserve to respond to physiological stresses. Cold stress occurs when there is:

■ A decrease in environmental temperatures → a decrease in the neonate's body temperature → an increase in respiratory rate, heart rate → an increase on oxygen consumption, a depletion of glucose, and a decrease in surfactant → respiratory distress

Risk Factors

■ Prematurity
■ Small for gestational age
■ Hypoglycemia
■ Prolonged resuscitation efforts
■ Sepsis
■ Neurological, endocrine, or cardiorespiratory problems

Signs and Symptoms

■ Axillary temperature at or below 36.5°C (97.6°F)
■ Cool skin

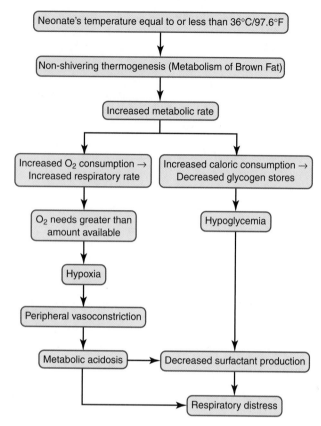

Figure 15-4   Cold stress.

- Lethargy
- Pallor
- Tachypnea
- Grunting
- Hypoglycemia
- Hypotonia
- Jitteriness
- Weak suck

Nursing Actions

- Preventative actions
    - *Dry the neonate thoroughly immediately after birth to decrease heat loss due to evaporation.*
    - *Remove wet blankets from the neonate's direct environment to decrease heat loss due to radiation and conduction.*
    - *Place a stocking cap on the neonate's head to decrease heat loss due to radiation and convection*
    - *Skin-to-skin contact with the mother with a warm blanket over the mother and neonate decreases heat loss due to radiation and conduction.*
    - *Swaddle in warm blankets to decrease heat loss due to convection and radiation.*
    - *Maintain a NTE to decrease heat loss due to convection and radiation.*
- Action when the neonate displays signs/symptoms of cold stress
    - *Skin-to-skin contact with the mother with a warm blanket over both the mother and neonate when there is a mild decrease in temperature; reassess temperature as per institutional protocol.*
    - *Swaddle in warm blankets; reassess temperature as per institutional protocol, which is generally every 30 minutes until stable.*
    - *Place a stocking cap on the neonate's head.*

- *Place the naked neonate under a preheated radiant warmer.*
    - Attach the servo-controlled probe on the neonate's abdomen or other body surface (avoid bony areas or brown fat areas) that is closest to the radiant source.
    - Set the control to 36.5°C.
    - Monitor the neonate's temperature, respiratory rate, and heart rate every 5 minutes when rewarming.
    - Assess and adjust the neonate's fluid requirement; fluids may need to be increased to compensate for insatiable water loss.
- *Monitor temperature as per institutional protocol.*
- *Obtain a heel stick to assess for hypoglycemia (glucose <40 mg/dL).*
    - Treat hypoglycemia.

The Metabolic System

Large quantities of glycogen are stored by the fetus during pregnancy in preparation for meeting energy requirements when transitioning from intrauterine to extrauterine life. Immediately after birth, the neonate becomes independent of his mother's metabolism and must balance the amount of insulin production with glucose availability.

- Hypoglycemia (blood glucose level under 40 mg/dL in the neonate) is common during this transitional time, especially in neonates of diabetic mothers.
    - *During intrauterine life, neonates of diabetic mothers produce high levels of insulin in response to the high levels of circulating maternal glucose. During the first few hours of extrauterine life the neonate's insulin level remains higher than normal, leading to hypoglycemia.*

CRITICAL COMPONENT

Hypoglycemia

Hypoglycemia is defined as a blood glucose level <40 mg/dL in the neonate.

Risks for Hypoglycemia

- Neonates of diabetic mothers
- Neonates weighing >4000 grams or large for gestational age
- Post-term neonates
- Preterm neonates
- Small for gestational age neonates
- Hypothermia
- Neonatal infection
- Respiratory distress
- Neonatal resuscitation
- Birth trauma

Signs and Symptoms

- Jitteriness
- Hypotonia
- Irritability
- Apnea
- Lethargy
- Temperature instability

Nursing Actions

- Monitor for signs and symptoms of hypoglycemia.
- Assess blood glucose level with use of glucose monitor.
- Assist the woman with breastfeeding.
- Feed the neonate either formula or dextrose water when the glucose level is <40 mg/dL as per institutional protocol, generally 5 mL/kg.
- Maintain NTE to decrease risk of cold stress.

The Hepatic System

The neonate's liver is immature, but is capable of carbohydrate metabolism and blood coagulation.

■ Bilirubin conjugation is limited.
  ■ *Indirect bilirubin (unconjugated bilirubin), a fat-soluble substance, is produced from the breakdown of red blood cells (RBCs). It is converted to direct bilirubin (conjugated bilirubin), a water-soluble substance, by liver enzymes. Direct bilirubin is in a form that can be excreted in the urine and stool.*
  ■ *Hyperbilirubinemia, is a condition in which there is a high level of unconjugated bilirubin in the neonate's blood related to the immature liver function, high RBC count that is common in neonates, and an increased hemolysis caused by the shorter life span of fetal RBCs (see Chapter 17 for information on hyperbilirubinemia/jaundice).*
■ Blood coagulation
  ■ *Coagulation factors II, VII, IX, and X are synthesized in the liver.*
  ■ *Vitamin K influences the activation of these factors. During intrauterine life, the fetus receives vitamin K from his mother. After birth, the neonate experiences a decrease in vitamin K and is at risk for delayed clotting and for hemorrhage.*
  ■ *Vitamin K is synthesized in the intestinal flora, which is absent in the newborn. The intestinal flora develops after the introduction of microorganisms, which usually occurs with the first feedings.*
  ■ *A vitamin K injection is given as a prophylaxis to decrease the risk of bleeding related to vitamin K deficiency.*
    ▪ The decline of maternally acquired vitamin K levels is greater in breastfed neonates, neonates with a history of perinatal asphyxia, and neonates of mothers who are on warfarin (Blackburn, 2007).

Medication

Phytonadione (Vitamin K, AquaMEPHYTON)

■ Indication: Prevention of hemorrhagic disease in neonate
■ Action: Vitamin K is required for the hepatic synthesis of blood coagulation factors II, VII, IX, and X
■ Common side effects: Erythema, pain, and swelling at injection site
■ Route and dose: IM; 0.5-1 mg within 1 hour of birth
(Data from Deglin & Vallerand, 2009)

The Gastrointestinal System

The neonate's gastrointestinal system is functionally immature, but rapidly adapts to demands for growth and development through ingestion, digestion, and absorption of nutrients, as well as eliminations of waste.

■ Gastric capacity for the first few days is approximately 40 to 60 mL and increases to 90 mL around day 3 or 4.
■ Neonates should feed at least every 4 hours, but may need to be fed more frequently as stomach emptying time is 2 to 4 hours.
■ During the first few days, neonates may appear uninterested in feeding, which may be related to a quiet sleep state.
■ The characteristics of stools and stool pattern vary depending on the type, frequency, and amount of feeding and the age of the neonate. The types of stools are:
  ■ *Meconium stool begins to form during the 4th gestational month and is the first stool eliminated by the neonate. It is sticky, thick, black, and odorless. It is first passed within 24 to 48 hours.*
  ■ *Transitional stool begins around the 3rd day and can continue for 3 or 4 days. The stool transitions from black to greenish black,*

to greenish brown, to greenish yellow. This phase of stool characteristics occurs in both breastfed and formula-fed neonates.
  ■ *Breastfeed stool is yellow and semiformed. Later it becomes a golden yellow with a pasty consistency, and has a sour odor.*
  ■ *Formula-feed stool is drier and more formed than breastfeed stools. It is a paler yellow or brownish yellow and has an unpleasant odor.*
  ■ *Diarrheal stool is loose and green.*
■ Breastfed neonates tend to have more stools per day than do formula-fed neonates. It is not uncommon for the neonate to pass 4 to 8 stools per day.
■ Constipation usually does not occur in breastfed neonates.
■ Constipation can occur in bottle-fed infants when formula is not properly diluted.

The Immune System

The immune system protects the body from invasion by foreign materials such as bacteria and viruses (Scanlon & Sanders, 2007). Before rupture of membranes, the fetus lives in the sterile environment of the maternal uterus and relies on the maternal immune system to protect him from pathogenic organisms. During the transition from intrauterine to extrauterine life, the neonate begins the process of developing normal microbial flora and must respond to colonization by potential pathogenic bacteria (Blackburn, 2007). The immune system is complex.

■ Major components of the immune system:
  ■ *Active humoral immunity is the process in which B cells detect antigens and produce antibodies against them. Active humoral immunity is further classified as:*
    ▪ Acquired immunity that develops from vaccination
    ▪ Natural immunity that develops from exposure to antigens, after which the individual produces antibodies
  ■ *Passive immunity, which is not permanent, is acquired either naturally or artificially.*
    ▪ An example of natural passive immunity is the placental transmission of antibiotics from the mother to the fetus. This provides protection for the neonate during the first few months of life from the pathogens to which the mother has been exposed.
    ▪ An example of artificial passive immunity is gamma globulin, which provides immediate protection for a short time.
  ■ *Lymphocytes are white blood cells that are primarily composed of T cells and B cells.*
    ▪ The number of T cells within the neonate's system is comparable to that in adults, but their functional abilities are decreased, which delays the response to microorganisms (Blackburn, 2007).
    ▪ The functional abilities of B cells are also hyporesponsive (Blackburn, 2007).
  ■ *Immunoglobulins are classified as IgG, IgA, IgM, IgD, and IgE (Table 15-1).*
    ▪ Maternal IgGs are the primary antibodies that cross the placenta and enter the fetal system and provide passive immunity for the neonate (Blackburn, 2007).
    ▪ The maternal transfer of IgG antibodies protects the neonate from bacterial and viral infections for which the mother has developed antibodies, such as rubella, tetanus, and diphtheria (Blackburn, 2007).
■ Neonates are at risk for infection related to:
  ■ *Immature defense mechanism*
  ■ *Lack of experience with and exposure to organisms, which leads to a delayed response to antigens*

TABLE 15–1   CLASSES OF IMMUNOGLOBULINS

NAME	LOCATION	FUNCTION
IgG	Blood Extracellular fluid	Crosses the placenta to provide passive immunity for newborns Provides long-term immunity after recovery or a vaccine
IgA	External secretions (tears, salvia, etc.)	Present in breast milk to provide passive immunity for breast-fed infants Found in secretions of all mucus membranes
IgM	Blood	Produced first by the maturing immune system of infants Produced first during an infection (IgG production follows) Part of the ABO blood group
IgD	B lymphocytes	Receptors on B lymphocytes
IgE	Mast cells or basophils	Important in allergic reaction (mast cells release histamine)

Source: Scanlon & Sanders (2007).

■ *Breakdown of skin and mucus membranes that provides a portal of entry for bacteria (Blackburn, 2007)*

■ During the transitional period, the neonate's immune system begins to:

■ *Develop normal microbial flora of the skin, respiratory tract, and gastrointestinal tract*

■ *Respond to bacterial colonization of potential pathogens (Blackburn, 2007)*

■ Neonates are first exposed to organisms from the maternal genital tract during the birthing process.

■ *The maternal genital tract may contain group B Streptococcus and E. coli, which can result in neonatal sepsis (see Chapter 17).*

NEONATAL ASSESSMENT

A neonatal assessment should be done within 2 hours after birth. This initial assessment provides the baseline data for the neonate and assists in determining the course of nursing and medical care.

CRITICAL COMPONENT

Methods of Reducing Heat Loss

The thermoregulatory systems of neonates respond more slowly to external temperature changes than those of adults. Prevention of heat loss is critical when doing assessments. Methods to reduce heat loss during assessments are:

■ Ensure that the room is warm and free of air drafts.

■ Place the infant under a warming unit to help maintain a NTE **or** assess the neonate in the mother's arms. Skin-to-skin contact between the mother and neonate can decrease the amount of heat loss.

■ When doing assessments in an open crib or in a parent's arms, keep the neonate wrapped and expose only the body area that is being assessed.

Preparation for Assessment

■ Gather the equipment needed for the assessment: Latex gloves, measuring tape, infant stethoscope, thermometer, scale for weighing, and documentation records.

■ Ensure that assessment is done in a NTE (i.e., close doors to prevent drafts and regulate room temperature).

■ Inform the parents of the assessment and invite them to watch. This is especially helpful for new fathers when the initial assessment is done in the labor/delivery/recovery room.

General Survey

■ Review the prenatal record and birth record for factors that could place the neonate at risk for complications. Examples of risk factors are:

■ *Maternal malnutrition prior to and/or during pregnancy*
■ *Maternal age younger than 16 and older than 35 years*
■ *Chronic maternal illnesses such as diabetes and hypertension*
■ *Hypertensive disorders of pregnancy*
■ *Labor and birth before 38 weeks of gestation*
■ *Long labor: Greater than 24 hours*
■ *Operative delivery: Use of forceps or vacuum extractor*
■ *Medications during labor that have an effect on the central nervous system (CNS; e.g., magnesium sulfate and analgesia/anesthesia)*
■ *Prolonged rupture of membranes (longer than 24 hours)*
■ *Meconium-stained amniotic fluid*
■ *Placental abnormalities*
■ *Apgar score 7 or below at 5 minutes*

■ Complete a general survey of the neonate before the head-to-toe assessment.

■ *Observe the respiratory pattern and assess respirations and breath sounds.*

■ It will become more difficult to assess respiratory rate once the neonate responds (cries) to being handled during the assessment.

■ *Observe posture.*
■ *Assess the skin for color, birth trauma, and birthmarks.*
■ *Observe the level of alertness/activity.*
■ *Assess muscle tone and posture.*

■ The complete assessment begins after this initial overall observation.

Neonatal Assessment by Area/System

See Tables 15-2, 15-3, and 15-4.

TABLE 15–2   NEONATAL ASSESSMENT BY AREA/SYSTEM

AREA OR SYSTEM	TECHNIQUE AND ASSESSMENT	EXPECTED FINDINGS FOR TERM NEONATES	DEVIATIONS FROM NORMAL
POSTURE	Unwrap the newborn and observe posture when the neonate is quiet.	Extremities are flexed.	Extension of extremities often related to prematurity; effects of medications given to mother during labor such as magnesium sulfate and analgesics/anesthesia; birth injuries; hypothermia; or hypoglycemia
HEAD CIRCUMFERENCE	Measure by placing tape around the head just above the ears and eyebrows. Measurement is usually recorded in centimeters.	33–35.5 cm (13–14 inches)	**Microcephaly:** Head circumference is below the 10th percentile of normal for newborns gestational age. This is often related to congenital malformation, maternal drug or alcohol ingestion, or maternal infection during pregnancy. **Macrocephaly:** Head circumference is >90th percentile. This can be related to hydrocephalus.
CHEST CIRCUMFERENCE	Measure by placing tape around the chest over the nipple line.	30.5–33 cm (12–13 inches) or 2–3 cm less than head circumference	
LENGTH	Measure the length of body by securing tape on a flat surface. Place the top of neonate's head at the top of the tape. Extend the body and one leg. Measurement is taken from the top of the head to the bottom of the heel	45–53 cm (19–21 inches)	Molding may interfere with accurate assessment of length. Neonates whose length is <45 cm should be further assessed for causes such as intrauterine growth restriction or prematurity.
WEIGHT	Clean scale before use. Place clean paper on the scale. Set the scale at zero. Place the naked neonate on the scale. Record the neonate's weight. Do not leave the neonate unattended while weighing.	2,500–4,000 g (5 lbs. 8 oz.–8 lbs. 13 oz.) Weight loss of 5%–10% of birth weight during the first week is normal. This is due to water loss through urine, stools, and lungs and an increase in metabolic rate. It is also related to limited fluid intake. The neonate will regain birth weight within 10 days	Weights above the 90th percentile are common in neonates of diabetic mothers. Weight below the 10th percentile is due to prematurity, intrauterine growth restriction, malnutrition during the pregnancy.

Continued

TABLE 15–2   NEONATAL ASSESSMENT BY AREA/SYSTEM—CONT'D

AREA OR SYSTEM	TECHNIQUE AND ASSESSMENT	EXPECTED FINDINGS FOR TERM NEONATES	DEVIATIONS FROM NORMAL
TEMPERATURE	Place a clean temperature probe in the axillary area. Axillary temperatures are preferred because of the risks of tissue trauma, perforation, and cross-contamination associated with the rectal temperature method (Blackburn, 2007).	36.4°–37.2°C (97.5°–99°F)	Hypothermia or hyperthermia is related to infection, environmental extremes, and/or neurological disorders.
RESPIRATIONS	Assess respiratory rate by observing the rise and fall of the chest and abdomen for one full minute.	30–60 breaths per minute Slightly irregular Diaphragmatic and abdominal breathing Rate increases when crying and decreases when sleeping.	Periods of apnea >15 seconds Tachypnea that may be related to sepsis, hypothermia, hypoglycemia, or respiratory distress syndrome Respirations <30; may be related to maternal analgesia and/or anesthesia during labor
PULSE	Assess apical pulse rate by auscultating for one full minute. Assess rate and rhythm. Use of a stethoscope designed for neonates is recommended.	120–160 bpm Rate increases (to 180 bpm) with crying and decreases (to 100 bpm) when asleep. Murmurs may be heard; most are not pathological and disappear by 6 months.	Tachycardia (> 160 bpm) indicates possible sepsis, respiratory distress, congenital heart abnormality. Bradycardia (<100 bpm) indicates possible sepsis, increased intracranial pressure, or hypoxemia.
BLOOD PRESSURE	Blood pressure is not a routine part of neonatal assessment. Requires the use of specially designed equipment for neonates. The blood pressure is obtained from both the arm and the leg of the neonate.	50–75/30–45 mm Hg	

TABLE 15–2   NEONATAL ASSESSMENT BY AREA/SYSTEM—CONT'D

AREA OR SYSTEM	TECHNIQUE AND ASSESSMENT	EXPECTED FINDINGS FOR TERM NEONATES	DEVIATIONS FROM NORMAL
INTEGUMENTARY/SKIN	Inspect the skin for color, intactness, bruising, birth marks, dryness, rashes, warmth, texture, and turgor. Inspect nails.	Skin is pink with **acrocyanosis** (cyanosis of hands and feet). Milia is present on the bridge of the nose and chin (see Table 15-3). Lanugo is present on the back, shoulders, and forehead, which decreases with advancing gestation (see Table 15-3). Peeling or cracking is often noted on infants >40 weeks' gestation. Mongolian spots (see Table 15-3) Hemangiomas such as salmon-colored patch (stork bites), nevus flammeus (port-wine stain), and strawberry hemangiomas which are developmental vascular abnormalities. Stork bites are found at the nape of the neck, on the eyelid, between the eyes, or on the upper lip. They deepen in color when the neonate cries. They disappear within the first year of life. Nevus flammeus are purple- to red-colored flat areas that can be located on various portions of the body. These do not disappear. Strawberry hemangiomas are raised bright red lesions that develop during the neonatal period. They spontaneously resolve during early childhood. Erythema toxicum, newborn rash (see Table 15-3).	Jaundice within the first 24 hours is pathological (see Chapter 17). Pallor indicates anemia, hypothermia, shock, or sepsis. Greenish/yellowish vernix indicates passage of meconium during pregnancy and/or labor. Persistent ecchymosis or petechiae indicates thrombocytopenia, sepsis, or congenital infection. Abundant lanugo indicates prematurity. Thin and translucent skin, and increased amounts of vernix caseosa are common in preterm neonates. Nails are longer in neonates >40 weeks' gestation. **Pilonidal dimple:** A small pit or sinus in the sacral area at top of crease between the buttocks; the sinus can become infected later in life.
HEAD	Note the shape of the head. Inspect and palpate fontanels and suture lines. Inspect and palpate the head for caput succedaneum and/or cephalohematoma (see Table 15-3).	Molding present (see Table 15-3). Fontanels are open, soft, intact, and slightly depressed. They may bulge with crying. The anterior fontanel is diamond shaped, approximately 2.5–4 cm (closes by 18 months of age). The posterior fontanel is a triangle shape that is approximately 0.5–1 cm (closes between 2 and 4 months). May be difficult to palpate due to excessive molding. There are overriding sutures when there is increased molding.	Fontanels are firm and bulging that is not related to crying is an indication of increased intracranial pressure. Depressed fontanels indicate dehydration. Bruising and laceration at the site of the fetal scalp electrode or vacuum extractor Presence of caput succedaneum and/or cephalohematoma (see Table 15-3).

Continued

TABLE 15–2   NEONATAL ASSESSMENT BY AREA/SYSTEM—CONT'D

AREA OR SYSTEM	TECHNIQUE AND ASSESSMENT	EXPECTED FINDINGS FOR TERM NEONATES	DEVIATIONS FROM NORMAL
NECK	Lift the chin to assess the neck area. 	The neck is short with skin folds. Positive tonic neck reflex (see Table 15-4).	Webbing indicates genetic disorders. Absent tonic neck reflex indicates nerve injury.
EYES	Assess the position of the eyes. Open the eyelids and assess color of sclera and pupil size. Assess for blink reflex, red light reflex, and pupil reaction to light. 	Eyes are equal and symmetrical in size and placement. The neonate is able to follow objects within 12 inches of the visual field. Edema may be present due to pressure during labor and birth and/or reaction to eye prophylaxes. The iris is blue-gray or brown. The sclera is white or bluish-white. Subconjunctival hemorrhages related to birth trauma. Pupils are equally reactive to light. Positive red light reflex and blink reflex. No tear production (tear production begins at 2 months). Strabismus and nystagmus related to immature muscular control	Absent red light reflex indicates cataracts. Unequal pupil reactions indicate neurological trauma. Blue sclera indicates osteogenesis imperfecta.
EARS 	Inspect the ears for position, shape, and drainage. Hearing test is done before discharge.	Top of the pinna is aligned with external cantus of the eye. Pinna without deformities, well formed and flexible. The neonate responds to noises with positive startle signs. Hearing becomes more acute as Eustachian tubes clear. Neonates respond more readily to high-pitched vocal sounds.	Low-set ears indicate genetic disorders such as Down's syndrome. Absent startle reflex indicates possible hearing loss.

TABLE 15–2   NEONATAL ASSESSMENT BY AREA/SYSTEM—CONT'D

AREA OR SYSTEM	TECHNIQUE AND ASSESSMENT	EXPECTED FINDINGS FOR TERM NEONATES	DEVIATIONS FROM NORMAL
NOSE	Observe the shape of the nose. Inspect the opening of the nares. Assess patency of the nares by inserting a small soft catheter (This may not be done on all infants. Check hospital policy and procedure manual.)	The nose may be flattened or bruised related to the birth process. Nares should be patent. Small amount of mucus. Neonates primarily breathe through their noses.	Large amounts of mucus drainage can lead to respiratory distress. A flat nasal bridge is seen with Down's syndrome. Nasal flaring is a sign of respiratory distress.
MOUTH	Inspect lips, gums, tongue, palate, and mucus membranes. Open the mouth by placing gentle pressure on the lower lip. Test for rooting, sucking, swallowing, and gag reflexes (see Table 15-4).	Lips, gums, tongue, palate, and mucus membranes are intact, pink, and moist. Reflexes are positive. Epstein's pearls are present (see Table 15-3). Thrush	Natal teeth, which can be benign or related to congenital abnormality (see Table 15-3). Thrush, a fungal infection, can be contracted during vaginal birth. It appears as white patches on the mucus membranes of the mouth. Cleft lip and/or palate, which is a congenital abnormality in which the lip and/or palate does not completely fuse (see Chapter 17).
CHEST/LUNGS	Inspect shape, symmetry, and chest excursion. Inspect the breast for size and drainage. Auscultate breath sounds.	The chest is barrel-shaped and symmetrical. Breast engorgement is present in both male and female neonates related to the influence of maternal hormones. This resolves within a few weeks. Clear or milky fluid from nipples related to maternal hormones. Lung sounds are clear and equal. Scattered crackles may be detected during the first few hours after birth. This is due to retained amniotic fluid which will be absorbed through the lymphatics.	Funnel chest is a congenital abnormality. Pigeon chest can obstruct respirations. Chest retractions are a sign of respiratory distress. Persistent crackles, wheezes, stridor, grunting, paradoxical breathing, decreased breath sounds, and/or prolonged periods of apnea (>15–20 seconds) are signs of respiratory distress. Decreased or absent breath sounds are often related to meconium aspiration or pneumothorax.

Continued

TABLE 15–2   NEONATAL ASSESSMENT BY AREA/SYSTEM—CONT'D

AREA OR SYSTEM	TECHNIQUE AND ASSESSMENT	EXPECTED FINDINGS FOR TERM NEONATES	DEVIATIONS FROM NORMAL
CARDIAC	Auscultate heart sounds; listen for at least one full minute. Palpate peripheral pulses.	Point of maximal impulse (PMI) at the 3rd or 4th intercostal space. S_1 and S_2 are present. Normal rhythm with variation related to respiratory changes. Murmurs in 30% of neonates which disappear within 2 days of birth. Peripheral pulses are present and equal. The femoral pulse may be difficult to palpate.	Dextrocardia: Heart on the right side of the chest. Displaced PMI occurs with cardiomegaly. Persistent murmurs indicate persistent fetal circulation or congenital heart defects.
ABDOMEN	Inspect size and shape of the abdomen. Palpate the abdomen, assessing for tone, hernias, and diastasis recti. Auscultate for bowel sounds. Inspect the umbilical cord.	The abdomen is soft, round, protuberant, and symmetrical. Bowel sounds are present, but may be hypoactive for the first few days. Passage of meconium stool within 48 hours post-birth. The cord is opaque or whitish-blue with two arteries and one vein, and covered with Wharton's jelly. The cord becomes dry and darker in color within 24 hours post-birth and detaches from the body within 2 weeks.	Asymmetrical abdomen indicates a possible abdominal mass. Hernias or diastasis recti are more common in African-American neonates and usually resolve on their own within the first year. One umbilical artery and vein is often associated with heart or kidney malformation. Failure to pass meconium stool is often associated with imperforated anus or meconium ileus.
RECTUM	Inspect the anus.	The anus is patent. Passage of stool within 24 hours.	Imperforated anus requires immediate surgery. Anal fissures or fistulas.
GENITOURINARY FEMALE	Place thumbs on either side of the labia and gently separate tissue to visually inspect the genitalia. Assess for the presence and position of clitoris, vagina, and urinary meatus.	Labia majora covers labia minora and clitoris. Labia majora and minora may be edematous. Blood-tinged vaginal discharge related to the abrupt decrease of maternal hormones (pseudomenstruation). Whitish vaginal discharge in response to maternal hormones. The neonate urinates within 24 hours. The urinary meatus is midline and an uninterrupted stream is noted on voiding.	Prominent clitoris and small labia minora are often present in preterm neonates. Ambiguous genitalia; may require genetic testing to determine sex. No urination in 24 hours may indicate a possible urinary tract obstruction, polycystic disease, or renal failure.

TABLE 15–2 NEONATAL ASSESSMENT BY AREA/SYSTEM—CONT'D

AREA OR SYSTEM	TECHNIQUE AND ASSESSMENT	EXPECTED FINDINGS FOR TERM NEONATES	DEVIATIONS FROM NORMAL
GENITOURINARY MALE	Inspect the penis, noting the position of the urinary meatus. Inspect and palpate the scrotum to assess for testicles. With the thumb and forefinger of one hand, palpate each testis while the other thumb and forefinger are placed over the inguinal canal to prevent the ascent of testes during assessment. Start at the upper aspect of the scrotum and move away from the body.	The urinary meatus is at the tip of the penis. The scrotum is large, pendulous, and edematous with rugae (ridges/creases) present. Both testes are palpated in the scrotum. The neonate urinates within 24 hours with an uninterrupted stream.	**Hypospadias:** the urethral opening is on the ventral surface of penis. **Epispadias:** the urethral opening is on the dorsal side of penis. **Undescended testes** are testes not palpated in the scrotum. **Hydrocele** is enlarged scrotum due to excess fluid. No urination in 24 hours may indicate possible urinary tract obstruction, polycystic disease, or renal failure. Ambiguous genitalia may require genetic testing to determine sex. Inguinal hernia.
MUSCULOSKELETAL	Inspect extremities, spine, and gluteal folds. Palpate the clavicles. Perform the Barlow–Ortolani maneuver.	Arms are symmetrical in length and equal in strength. Legs are symmetrical in length and equal in strength. 10 fingers and 10 toes. Full range of motion of all extremities No clicks at joints. Equal gluteal folds. C curve of spine with no dimpling.	**Polydactyly:** Extra digits may indicate a genetic disorder. **Syndactyly:** Webbed digits may indicate a genetic disorder. Unequal gluteal folds and/or positive Barlow-Ortolani maneuver are associated with congenital hip dislocation. Decreased range of motion and/or muscle tone indicates possible birth injury, neurological disorder, or prematurity. Swelling, crepitus, and/or neck tenderness indicates possible broken clavicle which can occur during the birthing process in neonates with large shoulders. Simian creases, short fingers, wide space between big toe and second toe are common with Down's syndrome.

Continued

TABLE 15–2   NEONATAL ASSESSMENT BY AREA/SYSTEM—CONT'D

AREA OR SYSTEM	TECHNIQUE AND ASSESSMENT	EXPECTED FINDINGS FOR TERM NEONATES	DEVIATIONS FROM NORMAL
NEUROLOGICAL	Assess posture. Assess tone. Test newborn reflexes (see Table 15-4).	Flexed position Rapid recoil of extremities to the flexed position Positive newborn reflexes	**Hypotonia:** Floppy, limp extremities indicate possible nerve injury related to birth, depression of CNS related to maternal medication received during labor or to fetal hypoxia during labor, prematurity, or spinal cord injury. **Hypertonia:** Tightly flexed arms and stiffly extended legs with quivering indicate possible drug withdrawal. Paralysis indicates possible birth trauma or spinal injury. Tremors are possibly due to hypoglycemia, drug withdrawal, cold stress.

Adapted from Dillon, P. (2007). *Nursing health assessment,* chapter 24, an F.A. Davis publication with expected findings supported by AWOHNN sponsored publication, Matterson, S., & Smith, J. (2004). *Core curriculum for maternal-newborn nursing.*

TABLE 15–3   COMMON NEWBORN CHARACTERISTICS

CHARACTERISTIC	APPEARANCE	SIGNIFICANCE
ACROCYANOSIS	Hands and/or feet are blue.	Response to cold environment Immature peripheral circulation
CIRCUMORAL CYANOSIS	A benign localized transient cyanosis around the mouth	Observed during the transitional period; if it persists it may be related to a cardiac anomaly.
MOTTLING	A benign transient pattern of pink and white blotches on the skin	Response to cold environment
HARLEQUIN SIGN	One side of body is pink and the other side is white.	Related to vasomotor instability
MONGOLIAN SPOTS	Flat bluish discolored area on the lower back and/or buttock. Seen more often in African American, Asian, Latin, and Native American infants.	Might be mistaken for bruising. Need to document size and location. Resolves on own by school age.

TABLE 15–3   COMMON NEWBORN CHARACTERISTICS—CONT'D

CHARACTERISTIC	APPEARANCE	SIGNIFICANCE
ERYTHEMA TOXICUM	A rash with red macules and papules (white to yellowish-white papule in center surrounded by reddened skin) that appear in different areas of the body, usually the trunk area Can appear within 24 hours of birth and up to 2 weeks.	Benign Disappears without treatment.
MILIA 	White papules on the face; more frequently seen on the bridge of the nose and chin	Exposed sebaceous glands that resolve without treatment. Parents might mistake these for "whiteheads." Inform parents to leave them alone and let them resolve on own.
LANUGO 	Fine, downy hair that develops after 16 weeks of gestation. The amount of lanugo decreases as the fetus ages. Often seen on the neonate's back, shoulders, and forehead.	Gradually falls out. The presence and amount of lanugo assist in estimating gestational age. Abundant lanugo may be a sign of prematurity or genetic disorder.
VERNIX CASEOSA 	A protective substance secreted from sebaceous glands that covered the fetus during pregnancy It looks like a whitish cheesy substance. May be noted in auxiliary areas and genital areas of full-term neonates.	The presence and amount of vernix assist in estimating gestational age. Full-term neonates usually have none or small amounts of vernix.

Continued

TABLE 15–3   COMMON NEWBORN CHARACTERISTICS—CONT'D

CHARACTERISTIC	APPEARANCE	SIGNIFICANCE
JAUNCDICE	Yellow coloring of skin. First appears on the face and extends to the trunk and eventually the entire body. Best assessed in natural lighting. When jaundice is suspected the nurse can apply gentle pressure to the skin over a firm surface such as nose, forehead, or sternum. The skin blanches to a yellowish hue.	Jaundice within the first 24 hours is pathological; usually related to problem of the liver (see Chapter 17). Jaundice occurring after 24 hours is referred to as physiological jaundice and is related to increased amount of unconjugated bilirubin in the system (see Chapter 17).
MOLDING	Elongation of the fetal head as it adapts to the birth canal	Resolves within 1 week.
CAPUT SUCCEDANEUM Suture line Scalp Edema Periosteum Skull Brain	A localized soft tissue edema of the scalp It feels "spongy" and can cross suture lines.	Results from prolonged pressure of the head against the maternal cervix during labor. Resolves within the first week of life.
CEPHALHEMATOMA Suture line Scalp Periosteum Blood Skull Brain	Hematoma formation between the periosteum and skull with unilateral swelling. It appears within a few hours of birth and can increase in size over the next few days. It has a well-defined outline. It does not cross suture lines.	Related trauma to the head due to prolonged labor, forceps delivery, or use of vacuum extractor Can contribute to jaundice due to the large amounts of red blood cells being hemolyzed. Resolves within 3 months.

Abnormal if stays

abnormal if stays

TABLE 15–3   COMMON NEWBORN CHARACTERISTICS—CONT'D

CHARACTERISTIC	APPEARANCE	SIGNIFICANCE
EPSTEIN'S PEARLS	White, pearl-like epithelial cysts on gum margins and palate.	Benign and usually disappears within a few weeks
NATAL TEETH	Immature caps of enamel and dentin with poorly developed roots Usually only one or two teeth are present.	They are usually benign, but can be associated with congenital defects. Natal teeth are often loose and need to be removed to decrease the risk of aspiration.

Adapted from Dillon, P. (2007). *Nursing assessment* (pp. 855–867). Philadelphia: F. A. Davis.

TABLE 15–4   NEWBORN REFLEXES

REFLEX	HOW ELICITED	EXPECTED RESPONSE	ABNORMAL RESPONSE
MORO Present at birth; disappears by 6 months.	Jar the crib or hold the baby in a semisitting position and let the head slightly drop back.	Symmetrical abduction and extension of arms and legs, and legs flex up against trunk. The neonate makes a "C" shape with thumb and index finger.	A slow response might occur with preterm infants or sleepy neonates. An asymmetrical response may be related to temporary or permanent birth injury to clavicle, humerus, or brachial plexus.
STARTLE Present at birth; disappears by 4 months	Make a loud sound near the neonate.	Same as Moro response	Slow response when sleeping Possible deafness Possible neurological deficit

Continued

TABLE 15–4   NEWBORN REFLEXES—CONT'D

REFLEX	HOW ELICITED	EXPECTED RESPONSE	ABNORMAL RESPONSE
TONIC NECK Present between birth and 6 weeks; disappears by 4 to 6 months	With the neonate in a supine position, turn the head to the side so that the chin is over the shoulder.	The neonate assumes a "fencing" position with arms and legs extended in the direction in which the head was turned.	Response after 6 months may indicate cerebral palsy.
ROOTING Present at birth; disappears between 3 and 6 months	Brush the side of a cheek near the corner of the mouth.	The neonate turns his head toward the direction of the stimulus and opens his mouth. Instruct mothers who are lactating to touch the corner of the neonate's mouth with a nipple and the infant will turn toward the nipple for feeding.	May not respond if recently fed. Prematurity or neurological defects may cause weak or absent response.
SUCKING Present at birth; disappears at 10–12 months	Place a gloved finger or nipple of a bottle in the neonate's mouth.	Sucking motion occurs.	May not respond if recently fed. Prematurity or neurological defects may cause weak or absent response.
PALMER GRASP Present at birth; disappears at 3–4 months	The examiner places a finger in the palm of the neonate's hand.	The neonate grasps fingers tightly. If the neonate grasps the examiner's fingers with both hands, the neonate can be pulled to a sitting position.	Absent or weak response indicates a possible CNS defect; or nerve or muscle injury.
PLANTAR GRASP Present at birth; disappears at 3–4 months	Place a thumb firmly against the ball of the infant's foot.	Toes flex tightly down in a grasping motion	Weak or absent may indicate possible spinal cord injury.

TABLE 15–4   NEWBORN REFLEXES—CONT'D

REFLEX	HOW ELICITED	EXPECTED RESPONSE	ABNORMAL RESPONSE
BABINSKI Present at birth; disappears at 1 year	Stroke the lateral surface of the sole in an upward motion. 	Hyperextension and fanning of toes	Absent or weak may indicate a possible neurological defect.
STEPPING OR DANCING Present at birth; disappears at 3–4 weeks	Hold the neonate upright with feet touching a flat surface.	The neonate steps up and down in place. 	Diminished response may indicate hypotonia.

Adapted from Dillon, P. (2007). *Nursing assessment* (pp. 868–873). Philadelphia: F. A. Davis.

Gestational Age Assessment

Gestational age assessment of the newborn is based on the mother's menstrual history, prenatal ultrasonography, and/or neonatal maturational examination. The calculation of gestational age, either by Dubowitz neurological exam or Ballard scale of physical and neuromuscular maturity, assists in predicting potential problems and establishing plan of care based on gestational age.

■ Most hospital nurseries have written policies on which neonates should routinely be assessed for gestational age. Gestational age assessment is commonly completed on:
  ■ *Neonates who, based on the maternal menstrual history, are* **preterm***, born before 37 weeks; or* **postterm***, born after 42 weeks by dates*
  ■ *Neonates who weigh less than 2500 grams or more than 4000 grams*
  ■ *Neonates of diabetic mothers*
■ Neonates whose condition requires admission to a neonatal intensive care unit (NICU). The **Dubowitz neurological exam** is a standardized tool that assesses 33 responses in four areas:
  ■ *Habituation (the response to repetitive light and sound stimuli)*
  ■ *Movement and muscle tone*
  ■ *Reflexes*
  ■ *Neurobehavioral items*
■ The **Ballard Maturational Score (BMS)** is calculated by assessing the physical and neuromuscular maturity of the neonate. It can be completed in less time than the Dubowitz neurological exam. It consists of six evaluation areas for neuromuscular maturity and six items of observed physical maturity (Table 15-5). The examination

determines weeks of gestation and classifies the neonate as preterm (<37 weeks), term (37–42 weeks), or postterm (>42 weeks).
■ The scores from these exams provide a gestational age that is graphed based on weight, length, and head circumference to determine if the neonate is average for gestational age (AGA), small for gestational age (SGA), or large for gestational age (LGA) (Fig. 15-5).
  ■ *SGA is a term used for neonates whose weight is below the 10th percentile for gestational age.*
  ■ *LGA is a term used for neonates whose weight is above the 90th percentile for gestational age.*

Pain Assessment

Neonates are subjected to a variety of painful stimuli during their transition to extrauterine life (e.g., injections, heel sticks for blood samples, and circumcision). In the past, health care providers believed that neonates did not experience the sensation of pain, so little attention was given to assessing and reducing pain in the neonate. In the 1990s, researchers began to address this lack of knowledge by gaining a better understanding of neonatal pain, developing tools that assess for neonatal pain, and determining appropriate and safe pain management for neonates.

■ The 1995 National Association of Neonatal Nurses (NANN) position statement on pain management in infants states that all health care professionals who care for neonates/infants need ongoing education in the assessment and management of neonatal pain and that neonates/infants be protected from the adverse effects of pain (NANN, 1995).

TABLE 15–5   BALLARD MATURATIONAL ASSESSMENT

NEUROMUSCULAR MATURITY	PHYSICAL MATURITY
POSTURE Assess the position the neonate assumes while lying quietly on his back. The more mature, the greater degree of flexion in legs and arms	**SKIN** The examiner inspects the neonate's chest and abdominal skin areas for texture, transparency, thickness, and for peeling and/or cracking. A preterm neonate's skin is smooth, thin, and translucent (numerous veins visible). A full-term neonate's skin is thicker and more opaque with some degree of peeling.
SQUARE WINDOW Assess the degree of the angle created when the examiner flexes the neonate's hand toward the forearm. The more mature, the greater the flexion.	**LANUGO** The examiner assesses the amount of lanugo on the neonate's back. Lanugo begins to form around the 24th week of gestation. It is abundant in preterm neonates and decreases in amount as the neonate matures.
ARM RECOIL With the neonate in a supine position, the examiner fully flexes the forearm against the neonate's chest for 5 seconds. The examiner extends the arms and releases them. The more mature, the faster the arms return to the flexed position (recoil).	**PLANTAR CREASES** The examiner inspects the bottom of the feet for location of creases. The more creases over the greater proportion of the foot, the more mature the neonate
POPLITEAL ANGLE With the neonate in a supine position and pelvis flat, the examiner flexes the neonate's thigh to the abdomen. The leg is then extended. The angle at the knee is estimated. The lesser the angle, the greater the maturity.	**BREAST TISSUE** The examiner assesses the degree of nipple formation. The size of the breast bud is measured by gently grasping the tissue with thumb and forefinger and measuring the distance between thumb and forefinger. The greater the degree of nipple formation and size of the breast bud, the greater the maturity
SCARF SIGN With the neonate in a supine position, the examiner takes the neonate's hand and moves the arm across the chest toward the opposite shoulder. The examiner notes where the elbow is in relationship to the midline of the chest. The more preterm, the more the elbow crosses the midline.	**EAR FORMATION** The examiner assesses the ear for form and firmness. The more defined the ear is and the firmer it is, the more mature the neonate
HEEL TO EAR With the neonate in a supine position, the examiner takes the neonate's foot and moves it toward the ear. The lesser the flexion (the further the heel is from the ear), the greater the maturity.	**GENITALIA** Male: The examiner palpates the scrotum for the presence of testis and inspects the scrotum for appearance. The greater the descent of the testis and the greater degree of rugae (creases), the greater the maturity Female: The examiner moves the neonate's hip one half abduction and visually inspects the genitalia. The more the labia majora covers the labia minora and clitoris, the greater the maturity

■ The 2001 Joint Commission on Accreditation of Healthcare Organizations (JCAHO) pain management standards states that "every patient has a right to have his or her pain assessed and treated" (JCAHO, 2001), including neonates.

■ Several pain scales, such as Premature Infant Pain Profile (PIPP) and Neonatal Infant Pain Scale (NIPS), have been developed to assess for neonatal pain. Pain assessment tools commonly look at state of arousal, cry, motor activity, respiratory pattern, and facial expressions. Some tools may also include blood pressure and oxygen saturation level.

■ Pain assessment is part of the nursing care of neonates, and the tool used for assessment varies based on hospital policies and procedures.

BEHAVIORAL CHARACTERISTICS

The neonate is a biosocial being with very unique behavioral characteristics that affect parent–infant attachment (see Chapter 13). Temperament can vary from a neonate being an "easy" baby to a

Neuromuscular Maturity

	-1	0	1	2	3	4	5
Posture							
Square Window (Wrist)	-90°	90°	60°	45°	30°	0°	
Arm Recoil		180°	140°-180°	110°-140°	90°-110°	<90°	
Popliteal Angle	180°	160°	140°	120°	100°	90°	<90°
Scarf Sign							
Heel To Ear							

Physical Maturity

Skin	sticky friable transparent	gelantinous red translucent	smooth pink visible veins	superficial peeling or rash, few veins	cracking pale areas rare veins	parchment deep cracking no vessels	leathery cracked wrinkled
Lanugo	none	sparse	abundant	thinning	bald areas	mostly bald	
Plantar Surface	heel-toe 40–50 mm:-1 <40 mm:-2	>50 mm no crease	faint red marks	anterior transverse crease only	creases ant. 2/3	creases over entire sole	
Breast	imperceptible	barely perceptible	flat areola no bud	stippled areola 1–2 mm bud	raised areola 3–4 mm bud	full areola 5–10 mm bud	
Eye/ear	lids fused loosely:-1 tightly:-2	lids open pinna flat stays folded	sl. curved pinna; soft; slow recoil	well-curved pinna; soft but ready recoil	formed and firm instant recoil	thick cartilage ear stiff	
Genitals (Male)	scrotum flat, smooth	scrotum empty faint rugae	testes in upper canal rare rugae	testes descending few rugae	testes down good rugae	testes pendulous deep rugae	
Genitals (Female)	clitoris prominent labia flat	prominent clitoris small labia minora	prominent clitoris enlarging minora	majora and minora equally prominent	majora large minora small	majora cover clitoris and minora	

Maturity Rating

Score	Weeks
-10	20
-5	22
0	24
5	26
10	28
15	30
20	32
25	34
30	36
35	38
40	40
45	42
50	44

Figure 15-5 Ballard Gestational Age Assessment Tool.

Evidence-Based Practice: Neonatal Infant Pain Scale

Gallo, A. (2003). The fifth vital sign: Implementation of the neonatal infant pain scale. *JOGNN, 32*, 199–206.

In this article the author describes the steps taken in the implementation of the neonatal pain scale in the labor and delivery room unit of a southern California hospital with a birth rate of approximately 7,000 infants/year.

Step 1: Review of the literature to select a pain assessment tool for neonatal pain. The neonatal infant pain scale (NIPS) was selected based on (1) the literature review and (2) no requirement for additional assessment skills or equipment.

Step 2: Education of core RN staff on (1) the physiological aspects of neonatal pain, (2) how to assess for pain, (3) non-pharmacological pain interventions, and (4) documentation of pain. A 30-minute video was used as part of the education/training step. The video showed three different neonates. The nurses assessed each infant for pain using the NIPS. The core staff then became part of the training and mentoring of the nursing staff.

Step 3: Education and training of the nursing staff was provided by the core staff. This was accomplished through in-service classes, teaching at the neonate's bedside, and viewing the video.

Step 4: This was the evaluation step assessing the staff's adherence to using the NIPS. It was accomplished by auditing medical records. The audit checked to see if a pain assessment was completed and findings documented.

Conclusions

The hospital successfully implemented the use of the NIPS and incorporated infant assessment as a component of neonatal care.

"fussy" baby. Most neonates vacillate between the two extremes of temperament. The neonate experiences predictable periods referred to as periods of reactivity.

Periods of Reactivity

During the first 6 to 8 hours of extrauterine life, the neonate transitions between periods of activity and inactivity. This is often referred to "periods of reactivity." Each of the periods has predictable neonatal behaviors.

Initial Period of Reactivity

- Occurs in the first 15 to 30 minutes post-birth
- The neonate is alert and active.
- The neonate vigorously responds to external stimuli.
- Respirations are irregular and rapid (can be as high as 90 breaths per minute)
- The neonate may exhibit momentary grunting, flaring, and retractions.
- Brief periods of apnea may occur.
- The heart rate is rapid and can be as high as 180 beats per minute.
- Brief period of cyanosis can occur.
- The amount of oral mucus increases.

Period of Relative Inactivity

- Begins approximately 30 minutes after birth and lasts 2 hours
- Sleep state
- The neonate is unresponsive to external stimuli.

- The respiratory rate decreases and can fall slightly below normal range.
- The heart rate decreases and is within normal limits.
- Oral mucus production decreases.

Second Period of Reactivity

- Follows the period of relative inactivity and lasts 2 to 8 hours
- Varies between active alert and quiet alert state
- Periods of rapid respiration in response to stimuli and activity
- Heart rate varies related to activity level and response to stimuli.
- Increased bowel activity and may pass meconium stool
- The neonate responds to external stimuli.

The initial period of activity provides an opportunity for the parents and neonate to respond to each other. It is an ideal time to initiate breastfeeding. The neonate is not responsive during the period of inactivity and will not be interested in feeding/sucking. During the second period of reactivity, the neonate is interested in feeding/sucking and this is another ideal time for breastfeeding.

Brazelton Neonatal Behavioral Assessment Scale

The Brazelton Neonatal Behavioral Assessment Scale (BNBAS) is used to assess the neonate's neurobehavioral system. The BNBAS was originally developed as a research tool and has been adapted for use in the clinical setting. The BNBAS is not routinely preformed on healthy neonates. It is composed of 28 behavior items and 18 reflex items. These behaviors/reflex items are divided into six categories:

- **Habituation**: The development of decreased sensitivity to a repeated stimulus such as light, sound, or heel stick. It is a protective mechanism against overstimulation. Habituation may not be fully developed in premature neonates or in neonates with CNS abnormalities or injuries.
- **Orientation**: The ability of the neonate to focus on visual and/or auditory stimuli. The neonate will turn his or her head in the direction of sound or will follow a visual stimulus. This response is diminished in premature neonates.
- **Motor maturity**: The ability of the neonate to control and coordinate motor activity. Normal findings are smooth, free movement with occasional tremors. Movement is jerky in premature neonates and/or in neonates with CNS abnormalities or injuries.
- **Self-quieting ability:** The neonate's ability to quiet and comfort self. It is accomplished by sucking on the fist/hand or attending to external stimuli. The ability is diminished in neonates with neurological injuries or in neonates exposed to drugs in utero.
- **Social behaviors:** The ability of the neonate to respond to cuddling and holding. These behaviors are diminished or absent in neonates with neurological injuries or in neonates exposed to drugs in utero.
- **Sleep/awake states**: These are also referred to as infant states or behavior states. There are two sleep states and four awake states.
  - *Deep sleep: During this state, there is no body movement except for an occasional startle reflex. The startle reflex is delayed in response to external stimuli. External stimuli are less likely to cause a change in state. The eyes are closed and there are no eye movements. Breathing is smooth and even.*
  - *Light sleep: During this state, there is random body movement. Rapid eye movement (REM) is present. The neonate responds to external stimuli with a startle reflex and with a possible change of state. Breathing is irregular.*
  - *Drowsy: During this state, there is intermittent body movement. Eyes open and close, and have a dull and heavy-lidded appearance.*

Breathing is irregular. Response to sensory stimuli is delayed. External stimuli will most likely cause a change in state. Breathing is irregular.
  - *Alert: During this state the neonate's eyes are wide open with a bright look and focus on the sources of stimuli. There is a delay in response to stimuli and minimal body movement. Respirations are regular.*
  - *Eyes open: During this state, there is considerable body movement with periods of fussiness. The eyes are open. The neonate responds to external stimuli with increased startle reflexes and motor activity. Breathing is irregular.*
  - *Crying: During this state, there is a high motor activity and intense crying. It is difficult to calm the neonate. The eyes are opened or tightly closed. Breathing is irregular (Brazelton & Nugent, 1995).*

NURSING CARE OF THE NEONATE

Nursing care of the neonate during hospitalization is divided into two time frames. The first is the 4th stage of labor, which is from birth through the first 4 hours of extrauterine life. The second is from 4 hours of age to discharge.

Nursing Actions during the 4th Stage of Labor

The major changes that occur in the neonate's body during the transition to extrauterine life require frequent assessments and monitoring to identify early signs of physiological compromise. Early identification of complications or difficulty with transition allows for earlier initiation of nursing and medical actions to support the neonate in a healthy transition. The following are nursing actions that may occur in the labor/delivery/recovery room and/or nursery depending on hospital policies and health state of the neonate. These actions are supported by the Association of Women's Health, Obstetric and Neonatal Nurses (AWHONN) in their 2004 publication, *Core curriculum for maternal-newborn nursing*.

- Review prenatal and intrapartal records for factors that place the neonate at risk, such as prolonged rupture of membranes (risk of infection), meconium-stained fluid (risk of respiratory distress), and gestational diabetes (risk of hypoglycemia).
- Note the time of delivery.
- Use universal precautions and wear gloves until after the neonate has been bathed.
- Dry the neonate immediately after birth to prevent excessive heat loss through evaporation.
- Discard wet blankets and place the neonate on dry, warm blankets or sheets.
- Place the neonate under a preheated radiate warmer or in the mother's arms with skin-to-skin contact and a warm blanket over both.
- Place a stocking cap on the neonate's head to decrease the risk of heat loss through convection.
- Support respirations by clearing the mouth and nose of excessive mucus with a bulb syringe when indicated.
- Obtain the Apgar score at 1 and 5 minutes and initiate appropriate actions based on the score (see Chapter 8).
- Assess vital signs.
  - *This is usually done within 30 minutes of birth, 1 hour after birth, and then every hour for the remainder of the recovery period. The frequency of assessments may vary based on institutional policies.*

■ *Assessment of vital signs varies based on the health of the neonate.*

■ *Vital signs are assessed every 5 to 15 minutes for neonates with signs of distress.*

■ *Administer O₂ per institutional protocol, if the heart rate is below 100 beats per minute, cyanosis is present, and/or apnea occurs. Before administration of O₂ the nurse should:*

   ■ Check the airway and apply suction if indicated.

   ■ Stimulate the neonate by rubbing his back.

■ Inspect the clamped cord for number of vessels and for bleeding.

■ Complete and place identifying bands on the neonate and parents before the neonate is separated from parents (e.g., taken to the nursery or NICU).

■ Weigh and measure the neonate.

■ Complete a neonatal assessment within 2 hours of birth.

■ Complete a gestational age assessment as per hospital policies.

■ Obtain blood glucose levels by using a glucose monitor.

   ■ *This is done on all neonates who exhibit symptoms of hypoglycemia as well as neonates who are at risk for hypoglycemia.*

■ Administer erythromycin ophthalmic ointment to each eye.

   ■ *The American Academy of Pediatrics (AAP) and Centers for Disease Control and Prevention (CDC) recommend that ophthalmic neonatorum prophylaxis be administered to all newborns within a few hours of birth.*

   ■ *Refer to intuitional policies for timing of the application of ointment.*

■ Administer phytonadione IM.

■ Bathe the neonate with neutral pH soap. The initial bath is delayed until 2 hours post-birth and until the neonate's temperature is stable and within normal limits.

■ Explain to the parents the assessments and procedures performed on the newborn.

■ Promote parent–infant attachment as soon as possible.

■ Notify the neonate's physician or nurse practitioner of the neonate's date and time of birth, and assessment findings.

Medication

Erythromycin Ophthalmic Ointment (0.5%)

■ Indication: Prophylaxis treatment for gonococcal or chlamydial eye infections

■ Action: Prevents bacterial growth by inhibiting folic acid synthesis

■ Common side effects: Edema and inflammation of eyelids

■ Route and dose: Apply a ¼-inch bead of ointment to lower eyelid of each eye

■ Precaution: Prevent the applicator tip from directly touching the eye by holding the application tube ½ inch from the eye.

Nursing Actions from 4 Hours of Age to Discharge

The second stage of neonatal care focuses on monitoring the neonate's adaptation to extrauterine life and assisting parents in learning about their newborn and how to care for her. The nursing actions listed are for neonates who do not exhibit signs of distress or potential complications.

■ Assess vital signs as per hospital policy.

   ■ *Vital signs for stable neonates are assessed at a minimum of once a shift.*

      ■ The neonate may continue to have difficulty in regulating her body temperature.

      ■ Notify the physician or nurse practitioner if temperature decrease persists.

CRITICAL COMPONENT

Promoting Parent–Infant Attachment

The promotion of parent–infant attachment is a critical component of nursing care, and needs to occur as soon as possible after birth. Often nurses allow other nursing actions to take priority over parent–infant attachment or find it is easier to do assessments under the warming unit. Assessments and monitoring of vital signs can be performed in the parent's arms when the neonate is full term, the Apgar score is 8 or higher, and there were no signs of fetal distress during labor or at the time of birth.

Nursing Actions

■ Skin-to-skin contact with a warm blanket over the neonate and parent.

■ Point out and explain expected neonatal characteristics such as molding, milia, and lanugo.

■ Provide alone time for the couple and their newborn by organizing care that allows for uninterrupted time.

■ Delay administration of eye ointment until parents have had an opportunity to hold the baby. Once ointment is administered, the neonate is less likely to open his or her eyes and make eye contact with parents.

CRITICAL COMPONENT

Danger Signs

The following signs may be an indication of an abnormality or complication. Document these signs in the neonatal record and report them to the physician or nurse practitioner:

■ Tachypnea (>60 breaths per minute)
■ Retractions of chest wall
■ Grunting
■ Nasal flaring
■ Abdominal distention
■ Failure to pass meconium stool within 48 hours of birth
■ Failure to void within 24 hours of birth
■ Convulsions
■ Lethargy
■ Jaundice within first 24 hours of birth
■ Abnormal temperature either abnormally high or low
■ Jitteriness
■ Persistent hypoglycemia
■ Persistent temperature instability

■ Complete neonatal assessment once per shift. The type of assessment varies based on institutional policies.

■ Promote parent–infant attachment by providing uninterrupted times with the infant.

■ Promote sibling attachment by providing opportunities for interactions with the newborn such as having older siblings assist with newborn care or listen to the newborn's heart.

■ Prevent infant abduction from the hospital. Each hospital has policies and procedures addressing methods to prevent infant abduction. Common steps that are taken are:

   ■ *Footprints and photo of infant for identification purposes.*

   ■ *Arm bands on the mother, father, and neonate that contain the same identification number. The bands of the neonate should be checked with the bands of the parents at the being of each shift and when taking or returning the neonate from or to the mother's room.*

■ *Personnel working in the maternal–newborn units should have name tags that are specific to that unit. Name tags should have a photo and name of the person.*

■ *Instruct parents and family members to not allow people to take their newborn if the person does not possess the appropriate identification that is specific to the maternity unit.*

■ *Encourage parents to accompany any person who removes their infant from the mother's room.*

■ *Place the neonate's crib on the far side of the room away from the door leading to the hallway.*

■ *Instruct parents not to leave their newborn in the mother's room unattended. This includes when she is taking a shower.*

■ *The maternal–newborn units should be secure and only visitors with identification allowed to enter.*

■ Assist parents with infant feeding (see Chapter 16).

■ Provide information to parents on newborn care (see Chapter 16).

■ Teach parents about normal newborn characteristics (see Table 15-3).

■ Instruct parents to place their newborn on his back or side to decrease the risk of sudden infant death syndrome (see Chapter 16).

CRITICAL COMPONENT

Hypothermia

Neonates with temperatures below 36.4°C (97.6°F) are at risk for hypothermia.

Nursing actions:

■ Parent–infant skin-to-skin contact with a warm blanket over both the neonate and the parent.

■ Wrap the neonate in warm blankets.

■ If the temperature remains below 36.4°C (97.6°F), place the neonate under a preheated warmer. Unwrap the neonate so that the skin is exposed to the radiant heat. Attach the electronic skin probe. The warmer is set at 1.5°C above the neonate's temperature. Continue to adjust the radiant temperature in relationship to the neonate's temperature.

■ Monitor the blood glucose level as per institutional policies, as hypothermia can lead to hypoglycemia.

■ Notify the physician or nurse practitioner if the neonate's temperature does not return to normal ranges.

■ Document the temperature and actions taken.

SKIN CARE

The skin of a term neonate is smooth, soft, slightly transparent, and has less pigmentation than that of an older child (Blackburn, 2007). The neonate's skin at birth is immature. The natural drying out and flaking of the skin during the first few weeks of life is a natural process in the skin's transition from fetal to neonatal skin. The neonate's skin is subjected to a variety of stresses related to the birthing process and transition to extrauterine life. Causes of potential threats to skin integrity are:

■ Pressure exerted on the presenting part of the fetus during the labor and birthing process from maternal structures such as the pelvis, causing edema and hematomas

■ Abrasions, bruising, and edema of the skin related to use of vacuum extractors, forceps, and internal fetal monitoring

■ Exposure to bacteria from the maternal genital tract

CULTURAL AWARENESS: Cultural and Ethical Variations in Infants

African American: Mongolian spots and other birthmarks are more prevalent than in other ethnic groups.

Amish: Babies are seen as gifts from God. Have high birth rates, large families

Appalachian: Newborns wear bands around the abdomen to prevent umbilical hernias and asafetida bags around the neck to prevent contagious diseases

Arab American: Children are "dearly loved."

Chinese American: Male circumcision is a religious requirement; children are highly valued; Mongolian spots occur in about 80% of infants; bilirubin levels are higher in Chinese newborns than in others, with the highest levels seen on post-birth day 5 or 6.

Cuban American: Childbirth is a celebration; the family takes care of both the mother and infant for the first 4 weeks; tend to bottle feed rather than breastfeed; if breastfeeding, weaning is early, around 3 months; if bottle feeding, weaning is late, around 4 years

Egyptian American: Children are very important

Filipino American: Eyes are almond shaped, low to flat nose bridge with mildly flared nostrils; Mongolian spots common

French Canadian: Five mutations account for 90% of phenylketonuria (PKU); high incidence of cystic fibrosis and muscular dystrophy

Greek American: High incidence of two genetic conditions: thalassemia and glucose-6-phosphate dehydrogenase (G6PD) deficiency

Iranian American: Believe in hot/cold influences, with baby boys "hotter" than baby girls; infants may be confined to the home for the first 40 days; ritual bath between the 10th and 40th post-birth day.

Jewish American: Children are seen as valued treasures; high incidence of Tay-Sachs disease; male circumcision is a religious ritual

Mexican American: Wear stomach belt (*ombliguero*) to prevent umbilicus from popping out when the infant cries

Navajo Native American: Infants are kept in cradle boards until they can walk; Mongolian spots are common.

Vietnamese American: Mongolian spots are common.

(Purnell & Paulanka, 2008)

■ Use of adhesives

■ Diaper dermatitis

Because intact and healthy skin is a first line defense against infection, the neonate's skin needs to be assessed at each shift and with each diaper change and care provided to maintain health skin. The AWHONN has developed an evidence-based practice guideline for the care of neonatal skin. AWHONN's (2001) *Quick Care Guide for Neonatal Skin Care is provided in Appendix A.*

LABORATORY AND DIAGNOSTIC TESTS

Newborn Screening

Newborn screening is a blood test that screens for infections, genetic diseases, and inherited and metabolic disorders and is performed on all babies born in the United States (ACOG, 2003).

■ Routine newborn screening began in the 1960s when all babies were screened for **phenylketonuria** (PKU), and over the years technologies advanced and can now screen for approximately 30 disorders.
  ■ *PKU is an inborn error of metabolism. Neonates with PKU are unable to metabolize phenylalanine, which is an amino acid commonly found in many foods such as breast milk and formula. This leads to a buildup of phenylpyruvic and phenylacetic acids, which are abnormal metabolites of phenylalanine. The buildup of abnormal metabolites can cause permanent brain damage and death, which can be prevented by early detection and dietary management.*
■ Each state has statutes or regulations on newborn screening, and the degree of screening varies from state to state.
■ The National Newborn Screening and Genetics Resource Center provides a current status report as to which tests are required for each state. The list can be accessed at http://genes-r-us.uthscsa.edu/nbsdisorders.pdf.
■ Disorders that most states include in the newborn screening are:
  ■ *PKU*
  ■ *Congenital hypothyroidism*
  ■ *Galactosemia*
  ■ *Sickle cell disease*
  ■ *Biotinidase deficiency*
  ■ *Congenital adrenal hyperplasia*
  ■ *Maple syrup urine disease*
  ■ *Toxoplasmosis (ACOG, 2003; Spahis & Bowers, 2006).*
■ Some states screen for human immunodeficiency virus (HIV).
■ Obtaining blood sample:
  ■ *The blood is obtained from a heel stick and may be collected by nursing or laboratory personnel.*
  ■ *The ideal time of collection is at 2 to 5 days of age, which provides time for the neonate to ingest breast milk or formula. Most are done within the first 24 to 48 hours because of discharges occurring during that time period. Neonates are usually retested later at a routine newborn check-up.*
  ■ *Provide parents with information regarding the screening test. Some states require the parents' written consent.*

Newborn Hearing Screening

The National Institute on Deafness and Other Communication disorders (NIDCD) reports that 2 to 3 out of every 1,000 infants in the United States are born with a hearing impairment (NIDCD, 2006). The 2007 U.S. screening status report lists 31 states and Washington, DC that have laws requiring hearing screening of all newborns (NNSGRC, 2007). The hearing screening test is usually done in the hospital before discharge by a member of the nursing staff who has completed special training and education in conducting the test (Fig. 15-6).

■ There are two types of screening tests that may be used either alone or together. The screening tests rely on physiological measures versus behavioral response (Widen, Warren, & Folsom, 2003). The screening tests do not provide information on the type or degree of hearing impairment. These screening tests are:
  ■ *Otoacoustic emissions (OAE) is a painless test that is conducted when the neonate is sleeping. A tiny, flexible ear plug that contains a microphone is inserted into the neonate's ear. It records responses of the outer hairs cells of the cochlea to clicking sounds coming from the microphone (Marlowe, 2003). A referral is made to a hearing specialist when there is no recorded response from the cochlear hair cells.*

CRITICAL COMPONENT

Heel Stick

■ The heel stick is a common procedure performed on neonates.
■ Blood is collected to assess blood glucose and hematocrit and for newborn screening.

Procedure

1. Provide parents with information on the test that has been ordered for their child.
2. Obtain required consents.
3. Don gloves.
4. Warm the neonate's foot for 10 minutes by wrapping in a warm, moist washcloth. This will help facilitate circulation to the peripheral area.
5. With the nondominant hand, hold the neonate's foot in a dorsiflexed position. The nurse or technician should have a firm grasp of the foot, but the foot should not be squeezed.
6. Clean the heel with alcohol.
7. Puncture the skin in the lateral or medial aspect of the heel to decrease the risk of nerve damage.

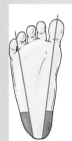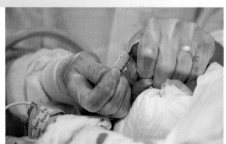

8. Wipe off the first few drops of blood.
9. Allow large drops of blood to form and to fall on the testing material.
10. Clean the puncture area and place a small dressing over it.

Document that blood was collected, type of test, site of puncture, and response of the neonate.

  ■ *Auditory brain stem response (ABR) is a painless test conducted when the neonate is sleeping. Electrodes are attached with adhesive to the neonate's scalp. This screening test assesses electrical activity of the cochlea, auditory nerve, and brain stem in response to sound (Marlowe, 2003). A referral to a hearing specialist is recommended for neonates who do not have a positive response to the sound stimuli.*
■ Both tests need to be conducted in a quiet room.
■ Vernix, blood, and amniotic fluid in the ear can interfere with accurate screening.

THERAPEUTIC AND SURGICAL PROCEDURES

Immunizations

Hepatitis B is a disease that is spread through contact with blood of an infected person or by sexual contact with an infected person and causes inflammation of the liver.

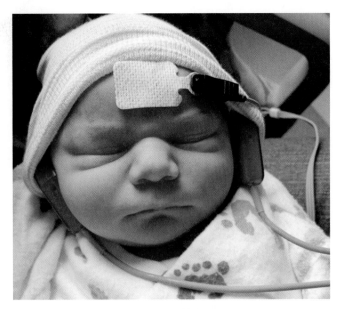

Figure 15-6   Neonatal hearing screening.

■ The CDC recommends that all neonates be vaccinated for hepatitis B before hospital discharge.
■ CDC also recommends that neonates who have been or possibly have been exposed to hepatitis B during birth be given both hepatitis B vaccine and hepatitis B immune globulin (HBIG) within 12 hours of birth.
■ The second dose of hepatitis B vaccine is given 4 weeks to 4 months after the first dose. The third dose is given 6 to 18 months after the first dose.

Circumcision

Male circumcision is an elective surgery to remove the foreskin of the penis. Approximately 1.2 million newborn males are circumcised each year in the United States (Box 15-1; AAP, 1999). The decision to circumcise the neonate is made by the parents and is based on their cultural, religious, and personal beliefs.

■ Contraindications for circumcision include:
  ■ *Preterm neonates*
  ■ *Neonates with a genitourinary defect*
  ■ *Neonates at risk for bleeding problems*
  ■ *Neonates with compromising disorders such as respiratory distress syndrome*
■ Risks related to circumcision:
  ■ *Hemorrhage*
  ■ *Infection*
  ■ *Adhesions*
  ■ *Pain*
■ Benefits related to circumcision:
  ■ *Decreased incidence of urinary tract infections*
  ■ *Decreased incidence of sexually transmitted infections*

Procedure

■ The surgical procedure is commonly performed by the physician before discharge or at the first well-child check-up.

CRITICAL COMPONENT

Intramuscular Injections

Procedure

1. Review the written orders for the newborn.
2. Inform the parents of the reason for the medication or vaccine.
3. Obtain written consent when required.
4. Follow the five rights of medication administration.
5. Draw up medication or vaccine in a 1-mL syringe with a 25-gauge 5/8 needle.
6. Invite the parents to comfort their infant by stroking the infant's head or hands.
7. Put on gloves.
8. Undo the diaper for full exposure of the leg.
9. Identify the injection site. The preferred site is the vastus lateralis.
10. Clean the area with an alcohol swab and let the area dry. It is extremely important to remove all maternal blood and amniotic fluid from the injection site to prevent transmission of blood-borne pathogens.
11. Stabilize the knee with the heel of hand. Grasp the tissue of the injection site with your thumb and forefinger.
12. Insert the needle at a 90-degree angle and aspirate. If no blood is aspirated, slowly inject medication or a vaccine to decrease the amount of discomfort.

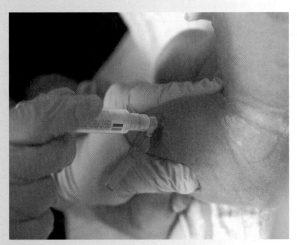

13. Withdraw the needle and rub the site to promote absorption.
14. Place a small dressing over the site.
15. Properly dispose of the needle and syringe
16. Document date, time, and location of injection.

■ There are two commonly used devices, Gomco clamp and Plastibell (Fig. 15-7).
■ Educate parents on the benefits and risk of circumcisions, and the procedure.
■ Obtain written consent.
■ The neonate should not eat 2 to 3 hours before the procedure to decrease risk of vomiting and aspiration during the procedure.
■ Verify that the neonate has voided.

BOX 15–1 STANDARD OF PRACTICE:
CIRCUMCISION

The American Academy of Pediatrics conducted an analysis of medical research on circumcisions. The following is a summary of their findings and recommendations:

"Existing scientific evidence demonstrates potential medical benefits of newborn circumcision; however, these data are not sufficient to recommend routine neonatal circumcision. In the case of circumcision, in which there are potential benefits and risks, yet the procedure is not essential to the child's current well-being, parents should determine what is in the best interest of their child. To make an informed choice, parents of all male infants should be given accurate and unbiased information and be provided the opportunity to discuss their decision. It is legitimate for parents to take into account cultural, religious, and ethnic traditions, in addition to the medical factors, when making this decision. Analgesia is safe and effective in reducing procedural pain associated with circumcision; therefore, if a decision for circumcision is made, procedural analgesia should be provided. If circumcision is performed in the newborn period, it should be done on infants who are stable and healthy."

Source: American Academy of Pediatrics (1999).

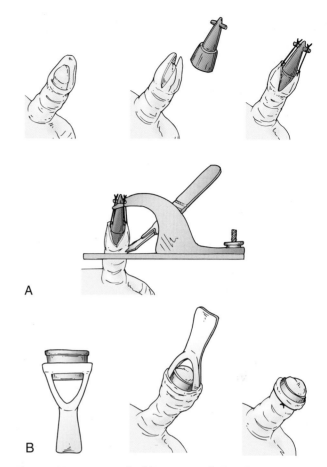

Figure 15-7 Removal of the prepuce during circumcision. *A.* Gomco clamp. *B.* Plastibell.

■ Administer acetaminophen 1 hour before procedure per the physician's order (Geyer et al., 2002).
■ An ear bulb should be near the neonate to use if there is vomiting or increased mucus.
■ The neonate is positioned and secured on a specially designed plastic board, often referred to as a circumcision board. The upper part of the neonate is kept covered to prevent loss of body heat.
■ The penis is cleansed and a sterile drape specially designed for circumcision is placed over the trunk.
■ A penile nerve block is administered by the physician (AWHONN, 2006).
■ The Gomco clamp or Plastibell is properly placed by the physician (see Fig. 15-7).
■ The foreskin is surgically removed with a scalpel by the physician.
■ Petroleum-impregnated gauze is wrapped around the end of the penis (AWHONN, 2006). This reduces the amount of irritation from the diaper.
■ The penis should be assessed every 15 minutes for the first hour for signs of bleeding, then every 2 to 3 hours according to hospital policies.
■ The neonate should void within 24 hours after the procedure.
■ Instruct parents to watch for bleeding and signs of infection, and to note when their child voids.
■ The physician needs to be notified if:
  ■ *Bleeding is present (larger than the size of a quarter),*
  ■ *Signs of infection are present, or*
  ■ *The neonate has not voided within 24 hours.*
■ Inform parents that the gauze will fall off on its own and they should not pull it off.
■ Instruct parents to fasten diapers loosely.
■ Acetaminophen PO may be ordered every 4 to 6 hours as needed for pain.

Evidence-Based Practice: Multidisciplinary Protocol for Neonatal Circumcision Pain Management

Geyer, J., Ellsbury, D., Kleiber, C., Litwiller, D., Hilton, A., & Yankowitz, J. (2002). An evidence-based multidisciplinary protocol for neonatal circumcision pain management. *JOGNN, 32,* 403–410.

A multidisciplinary team from the University of Iowa Hospitals and Clinics reviewed the literature for pain management that focused on neonatal circumcision. Seven areas for pain management were identified and evaluated. Based on the review and critique of the literature the multidisciplinary team developed a protocol for pain management for circumcision-related pain. The protocol includes:

■ Administration of acetaminophen 1 hour before the procedure and then every 4 to 6 hours for 24 hours post procedure.
■ Administration of a dorsal penile nerve block.
■ Offering a sucrose-dipped pacifier during the block and procedure.
■ Swaddling the upper body of the neonate during the procedure.
■ Padding the circumcision board with blankets.
■ Modifying the environment with soft music and dim lights.

Clinical Pathway for Full-Term Low-Risk Neonate

Delivery Date and Time

Focus of Care	Birth to First Hour	1 to 4 Hours of Age	4 to 24 Hours of Age	24 Hours of Age to Discharge
Assessments	Obtain Apgar score at 1 and 5 minutes. Inspect the skin for abrasions or bruises.	Complete neonatal assessment by 2 hours of age Complete gestational assessment as per hospital policy. Weigh and measure the head, chest, and length.	Assess at the beginning of each shift or per hospital policies. Weigh the newborn each day per hospital policy.	Assess at the beginning of each shift or per hospital policies and before discharge. Weigh the newborn each day per hospital policy.
Thermoregulation	Close the doors to the birthing room to prevent heat loss from convection. Dry the neonate thoroughly and place in a prewarmed crib or skin-to-skin on the mother's chest with a warm blanket over them. Place a stocking cap over the top of the neonate's head. Assess axillary temperature every 30 minutes or per hospital policy.	Prevent heat loss by maintaining a NTE. Encourage skin-to-skin contact with either the mother or father and with a warm blanket over both the neonate and parent. Wrap the neonate in blankets when in an open crib. Place a stocking cap on the head.	Prevent heat loss by maintaining a NTE. Wrap the neonate in blankets when in an open crib. Place a stocking cap on the neonate's head.	Prevent heat loss by maintaining a NTE. Assist the mother in dressing her infant for discharge in clothing and blankets that help maintain the neonate's normal body temperature.
Respiratory	Clear the nose and mouth of mucus with use of an ear bulb. Assess respirations every 30 minutes. Assess lung sounds. Monitor for signs of respiratory distress: grunting, flaring, retractions.	Keep the nose and mouth free of mucus with use of an ear bulb. Assess respirations every hour. Assess lung sounds. Monitor for signs of respiratory distress: grunting, flaring, retractions.	Assess respirations once per shift. Assess lung sounds once per shift. Monitor for signs of respiratory distress: grunting, flaring, retractions.	Assess respirations once per shift. Assess lung sounds once per shift and before discharge.
Cardiovascular	Assess skin color for cyanosis. Assess heart rate every 30 minutes.	Assess skin color for cyanosis. Assess heart rate every hour.	Assess the heart rate once per shift.	Assess heart rate once per shift and before discharge.

Clinical Pathway for Full-Term Low-Risk Neonate—cont'd

Delivery Date and Time

Focus of Care	Birth to First Hour	1 to 4 Hours of Age	4 to 24 Hours of Age	24 Hours of Age to Discharge
Activity	Assess the level of activity and compare to periods of reactivity. Monitor for signs of hypoglycemia, i.e., jitteriness.	Assess the level of activity and compare to periods of reactivity. Monitor for signs of hypoglycemia, i.e., jitteriness.	Assess the level of activity and compare to periods of reactivity. Monitor for signs of hypoglycemia, i.e., jitteriness.	Assess the level of activity.
Nutrition	Ideal time to introduce breastfeeding if the neonate is in the first period of reactivity. May need to feed the neonate glucose water or formula if hypoglycemic.	Breastfeed on demand. May need to feed the neonate glucose water or formula if hypoglycemic.	The ideal time for feeding is when the neonate is in the second period of reactivity. Breastfeed or bottle feed on demand; feeding should be every 3 to 4 hours.	Breastfeed or bottle feed on demand; feeding should be every 3 to 4 hours.
Elimination	The neonate may or may not void or pass meconium stool.	The neonate may or may not void or pass meconium stool.	The neonate voids within 24 hours. The neonate may or may not pass meconium stool.	The neonate voids a minimum of 6 times per day. The neonate passes meconium or transitional stools several times a day.
Medications Immunizations	Inform the parents which medications are being administered and why. Administer vitamin K injection and instill eye ointment as per physician's order.	Inform parents which medications are being administered and why. Administer vitamin K injection and instill eye ointment if not done during first hour as per physician order.	Provide parents with information on hepatitis B vaccine and obtain written consent if required. Administer hepatitis B vaccine as per physician order. Administer hepatitis B immune globulin vaccine when indicated per physician order.	
Special Procedures	Heel stick to assess glucose levels as indicated, i.e., jitteriness, LGA, and SGA.	Heel stick to assess glucose levels as indicated, i.e., jitteriness, LGA, and SGA.		Newborn screening tests: ☐ Blood sample collected. ☐ Newborn hearing screening conducted. Circumcision might be done several hours before discharge.

Continued

Clinical Pathway for Full-Term Low-Risk Neonate—cont'd

Delivery Date and Time

Focus of Care	Birth to First Hour	1 to 4 Hours of Age	4 to 24 Hours of Age	24 Hours of Age to Discharge
Family attachment	Delay eye ointment until parents have had the opportunity to hold their newborn. Provide time for parents to see and touch and/or hold the newborn. Explain to the new father that he can stay with his newborn while assessments are being completed.	Complete necessary assessments as quickly as possible in order to provide uninterrupted time for parents to hold and be with their newborn Complete assessments at bedside when possible.	Arrange nursing care to provide uninterrupted time for parents and their newborn. Teach parents about normal newborn characteristics and behavior.	Arrange nursing care to provide uninterrupted time for parents and their newborn.
Education	Point out normal newborn characteristics such as molding, lanugo, and vernix. Begin education on breastfeeding (e.g., positioning, latching on, releasing suction).	Teaching is kept to a minimum since parents are usually tired during this period of time or want to call family members to announce the birth.	Ideal time for teaching. Provide information on caring for a newborn (see Chapter 16).	Continue teaching parents about the care of their newborn (see Chapter 16). Complete the appropriate hospital discharge teaching forms. Give parents a copy of written discharge instructions. Explain the importance of follow-up well-child check ups and the importance of scheduling their first appointment as recommend by their pediatrician or PNP.
Safety	Place completed ID bands on the neonate, mother, and father. Keep the side of warmer up when not at crib side. Teach parents how to support the head and neck of their neonate. Use the five rights when administering medications. Wear gloves until after the first bath.	Teach parents abduction prevention protocol. Place the neonate on his back. Instruct parents not to leave the newborn unattended on a flat surface such as the mother's bed. Teach parents the importance of placing the neonate on his back. Wear gloves if there is the possibility of exposure to body fluids.	Provide education on infant safety (see Chapter 16). Follow hospital policies to prevent infant abduction. Wear gloves if there is the possibility of exposure to body fluids.	Review infant safety before discharge. Follow hospital policies to prevent infant abduction. Wear gloves if there is the possibility of exposure to body fluids. Inform parents that a federally approved car seat will be needed to transport the infant home, and that it will need to be properly placed in the car.

Nursing Care Plan

Problem (Check appropriate line)	Actual or Potential	Action (Initial care provided)	Expected Outcome/ Discharge Criteria (Initial outcomes obtained)
Altered body temperature related to: _____ Decreased subcutaneous fat _____ Large body surface _____ Heat loss due to radiation, convection, conduction, and/or evaporation	Initiate by: RN _____ Date/Time _____ ☐ Actual ☐ Potential Change in status: Date/Time _____ RN _____ ☐ Actual ☐ Potential Resolved: Date/Time _____ RN _____	_____ Maintain NTE by keeping doors closed and adjusting environmental temperature. _____ Keep the neonate dry. _____ Wrap the neonate in warm, dry blankets. _____ Place a stocking cap on the neonate's head. _____ Place the neonate in skin-to-skin contact with the parent and a warm blanket over both. _____ Monitor temperature per institutional protocol. _____ Place in a preheated warmer with a skin probe attached. _____ Notify the physician or nurse practitioner if the neonate's temperature remains low or is elevated.	_____ Neonate's temperature within normal ranges _____ No signs of cold stress _____ No sign of respiratory distress
Infection related to: _____ Breakdown of skin _____ Poor hand washing techniques by health care providers, parents, and/or visitors _____ Prematurity	Initiate by: RN _____ Date/Time _____ ☐ Actual ☐ Potential Change in status: Date/Time _____ RN _____ ☐ Actual ☐ Potential Resolved: Date/Time _____ RN _____	_____ Monitor skin for tissue breakdown. _____ Monitor temperature per institutional protocol. _____ Keep the skin clean and dry. _____ Instruct parents and visitors in proper hand washing before touching the neonate. _____ Instruct parents to wash hands after changing diapers. _____ Notify the physician or nurse practitioner if the neonate is lethargic, has elevated temperature or skin lesions, is eating poorly, and/or has signs of respiratory distress.	_____ Temperature within normal ranges _____ Skin intact with no signs of irritation _____ No signs or symptoms of infection

Continued

Nursing Care Plan—cont'd

Problem (Check appropriate line)	Actual or Potential	Action (Initial care provided)	Expected Outcome/ Discharge Criteria (Initial outcomes obtained)
Impaired gas exchange related to: _____ Transition from intrauterine to extrauterine live _____ Cold stress _____ Excessive mucus	Initiate by: RN _____ Date/Time _____ ☐ Actual ☐ Potential Change in status: Date/Time _____ RN _____ ☐ Actual ☐ Potential Resolved: Date/Time _____ RN _____	_____ Monitor respiratory and cardiac function as per institutional protocol. _____ Auscultate breath sounds. _____ Assess for the presence and location of cyanosis. _____ Maintain NTE. _____ Suction the mouth and nose PRN. _____ Position the neonate on his back. _____ Administer oxygen per protocol/orders. _____ Report signs of respiratory distress to the physician or nurse practitioner.	_____ Respiratory rate within normal limits _____ Breath sounds clear _____ Heart rate and rhythm within normal limits _____ Skin pink and warm to touch _____ Airway is clear _____ No signs of respiratory distress
Fluid volume deficit related to: _____ Limited oral intake _____ Insensible water loss	Initiate by: RN _____ Date/Time _____ ☐ Actual ☐ Potential Change in status: Date/Time _____ RN _____ ☐ Actual ☐ Potential Resolved: Date/Time _____ RN _____	_____ Monitor intake and output. _____ Monitor for signs of dehydration, i.e., sunken fontanels, poor skin turgor, dry mucus membranes. _____ Initiate oral feedings. _____ Maintain NTE.	_____ Feeds every 3 to 4 hours _____ 6 to 8 wet diapers per day _____ Vital signs within normal limits

Nursing Care Plan—cont'd

Problem (Check appropriate line)	Actual or Potential	Action (Initial care provided)	Expected Outcome/ Discharge Criteria (Initial outcomes obtained)
Knowledge deficit related to: _____ First time parenting _____ Limited learning resources	Initiate by: RN _____ Date/Time _____ ☐ Actual ☐ Potential Change in status: Date/Time _____ RN _____ ☐ Actual ☐ Potential Resolved: Date/Time _____ RN _____	_____ Assess level of parents' knowledge. _____ Provide information on newborn characteristics and behavior. _____ Provide information on newborn care (see Chapter 16). _____ Assist parents with care of their newborn. _____ Praise parents for their care of their newborn.	_____ Parents feed newborn without difficulty _____ Parents change newborns diapers without difficulty _____ Parents verbalize understanding of newborn characteristics, behaviors and care

TYING IT ALL TOGETHER

You are assigned to the mother–baby couplet unit. Your assignment for the day includes the Sanchez family. Margarite is a 28-year-old G3 P2 Hispanic woman who gave birth to a healthy boy, Manuel, at 0839. Margarite experienced an uncomplicated labor of 12 hours. Membranes ruptured 7 hours before delivery. She received 2 doses of Nubain during labor. The last dose was given at 0440.

Manuel weighs 3800 grams and is 50 cm in length. His 1- and 5-minute Apgar scores were 8 and 9. Manuel is 2 hours old. The Ballard score indicate that Manuel is 39 weeks. Margarite breastfed her son for 15 minutes on each breast immediately after the birth.

Your initial shift assessment findings are:

Vital signs: Axillary temperature, 36.2°C; apical pulse, 100 beats per minute; respirations, 30 breaths per minute.
Skin is warm and pink with acrocyanosis.
Fontanels are soft and flat.

Molding is present.
Lung sounds are clear.
There is mild nasal flaring.
Manuel is in a sleep state and unresponsive to external stimuli.

Based on the above information, discuss the primary nursing diagnoses for baby Manuel.

Discuss the immediate nursing actions for baby Manuel. Provide rationales for your nursing actions.

Thirty minutes later you note that Manuel is jittery and exhibits signs of hypoglycemia.

List the signs and symptoms of hypoglycemia and related nursing actions.

Several hours later, Manuel's father is present and holding Manuel.

List signs of parent–infant bonding.
Discuss nursing actions that will support parent–infant attachment.

■ ■ ■ Review Questions ■ ■ ■

1. The most critical physiological change required of neonates during the transition from intrauterine to extrauterine life is:
   A. Initiation and maintenance of cardiac function
   B. Initiation and maintenance of respiratory function
   C. Initiation and maintenance of metabolic function
   D. Initiation and maintenance of hepatic function

2. You are caring for a newborn girl who weighs 3,800 grams with an estimated gestational age of 41 weeks. During your assessment at 1 hour of age, you note that the newborn is jittery and irritable. Your first nursing action is:
   A. Increase the temperature of the warmer
   B. Feed the infant formula
   C. Transfer the infant to the NICU
   D. Assess the blood glucose level

3. Heat loss through evaporation can be reduced by:
   A. Closing the door to the room
   B. Using warming equipment on the neonate
   C. Drying the neonate
   D. Placing the crib near a warm wall

4. The nurse would expect the stools of a 3-day-old breastfed newborn to be:
   A. Sticky, thick, and black
   B. Greenish-brown to greenish-yellow
   C. Golden yellow and pasty
   D. Loose and green

5. In the birth suite during the initial newborn assessment, the new father seems concerned and asked why his baby girl is so hairy. The best response is:
   A. "Over the next few months the hair on the back will fall out."
   B. "This is a normal characteristic of newborns, so no need to be concerned."
   C. "This is called lanugo which covered the baby while inside the mother. It will fall out in a few months."
   D. "You seem overly concerned about this. Do you want to talk about your feelings?"

References

American Academy of Pediatrics (AAP). (1999). Circumcision policy statement. *Pediatrics, 103,* 686–701.

American College of Obstetricians and Gynecologists (ACOG). (2003). Newborn screening: ACOG committee opinion No. 287. *Obstetrics and Gynecology, 102,* 887–889.

Association of Women's Health, Obstetric and Neonatal Nurses (AWHONN). (2006). *The compendium of postpartum care* (2nd ed.). Philadelphia: Medical Broadcasting Company.

Ballard, J., Khoury, J., Wedig, K., Wang, L., Eilers-Walsman, B., & Lipp, R. (1991). New Ballard Score, expanded to include extremely premature infants. *Journal of Pediatrics, 119,* 417–423.

Blackburn, S. (2007). *Maternal, fetal, and neonatal physiology* (3rd ed). St. Louis, MO: W. B. Saunders.

Brazelton, T., & Nugent, J. (1995). *Neonatal behavioral assessment scale.* London: MacKeith Press.

Deglin, J., & Vallerand, A. (2009). *Davis's drug guide for nurses* (11th ed.). Philadelphia: F. A. Davis.

Dillon, P. (2007). *Nursing health assessment* (2nd ed.). Philadelphia: F. A. Davis.

Gallo, A. (2003). The fifth vital sign: Implementation of the neonatal infant pain scale. *JOGNN, 32,* 199–206.

Geyer, J., Ellsbury, D., Kleiber, C., Litwiller, D., Hilton, A., & Yankowitz, J. (2002). An evidence-based multidisciplinary protocol for neonatal circumcision pain management. *JOGNN, 32,* 403–410.

Joint Commission on Accreditation of Healthcare Organizations (JCAHO). (2001). Pain management standard [online]. Retrieved from www.jcaho.org (Accessed September 3, 2009).

Marlowe, J. (2003). *Newborn hearing screening: Testing, follow-up and communication with families.* Washington, DC: Association of Women's Health, Obstetric and Neonatal Nurses.

Matterson, S., & Smith, J. (2004). *Core curriculum for maternal-newborn nursing.* St. Louis, MO: Elsevier Saunders.

National Association of Neonatal Nursing (NANN). (1995). Position statement on pain management in infants. *Neonatal Network, 14,* 54–55.

National Institute on Deafness and Other Communication Disorders. (2006). Has your baby's hearing been screened [online]. Retrieved from www.nidcd.nih.gov (Accessed September 3, 2009).

National Newborn Screening and Genetics Resource Center (NNSGRCU). (2007). National newborn screening status report [online]. Retrieved from http:/genes-r-us.uthscsa.edu/nbsdisorders.pdf (Accessed September 3, 2009).

Scanlon, V., & Sanders, T. (2007). *Essentials of anatomy and physiology* (5th ed). Philadelphia: F. A. Davis.

Spahis, J., & Bowers, N. (2006). Navigating the maze of newborn screening. *MCM, 31,* 190–196.

Verklan, M., & Padhye, N. (2004). Spectral analysis of heart rate variability: An emerging tool for assessing stability during transition to extrauterine life. *JOGNN, 33,* 256–265.

Widen, J., Warren, B., & Folsom, R. (2003). Newborn hearing screening: What it means for providers of early intervention services. *Infants and Young Children Nursing, 16,* 249–257.

Discharge Planning and Teaching

OBJECTIVES

On completion of this chapter, the student will be able to:

☐ Define key terms.

☐ Incorporate principles of teaching and learning when providing newborn care information to parents.

☐ Discuss the nutritional needs of newborns and infants.

☐ Demonstrate awareness of cultural values in care of newborns.

☐ Describe the stages of human milk.

☐ Describe the process of human milk production.

☐ Develop a teaching plan for breastfeeding.

☐ Develop a teaching plan for formula feeding.

☐ Provide information regarding newborn care to parents that reflects the assessed learning needs of parents.

Nursing Diagnoses

■ Knowledge deficit related to infant feeding due to lack of experience and/or information

■ Knowledge deficit related to newborn care due to lack of experience and/or information

■ Knowledge deficit related to signs of newborn/infant illness related to lack of information

Nursing Outcomes

■ The woman will effectively feed her newborn.

■ The parents will demonstrate proper care of their newborn.

■ The parents will convey they are comfortable with caring for their newborn.

■ The parents will list signs of potential newborn/infant illness that need to be reported to the health care provider.

INTRODUCTION

Caring for a newborn and raising a child is a major responsibility couples take on with minimal formal educational preparation; yet, it is one of the most important roles a person assumes in his or her lifetime. Couples' knowledge pertaining to newborn care varies based on their past experiences with children, their cultural beliefs, information gained from friends and relatives, and what they have read or classes they have attended.

Discharge planning and teaching begins during pregnancy, when couples are encouraged to read about infant care and attend infant care classes in preparation for their emerging role of parent, and as they receive information from their health care provider. Throughout the postpartum hospital stay, teaching is provided in short sessions to the woman, her partner, and other significant people who will be assisting the woman in the care of the newborn. Topics of instruction are reviewed on the day of discharge to ensure that all teaching topics have been covered and parents feel ready to care for their newborn. Most hospital or birthing centers have standard discharge teaching forms that are completed and signed by the woman and the discharge

nurse. A written copy of key points of infant care is given to parents on discharge, so that they can refer back to the information provided.

PRINCIPLES OF TEACHING AND LEARNING

Teaching plans need to be individualized and reflect the needs of the parents. This is accomplished by incorporating teaching–learning principles in the parents' education regarding the care of their newborn. The five rights of teaching should be included in teaching plans for parents (Box 16-1).

NEWBORN NUTRITION AND FEEDING

Breastfeeding and bottle feeding are the two basic methods of infant feeding. Neonates who are unable to suck and/or swallow are gavage fed (see Chapter 17). The choice between breastfeeding and bottle feeding is influenced by past infant feeding experiences, cultural beliefs, friends and family, health of the woman and baby, support of the partner, perceived health effects, and discussion during pregnancy with a health care provider.

Want to reinforce your reading? Need to review for a test? Listen to this chapter on your accompanying CD.

BOX 16–1   THE FIVE RIGHTS OF TEACHING

When you are making a teaching plan, you can use this as a checklist to ensure that you consider each of the five "rights" of teaching in the plan.

Right Time
- Is the learner ready, free from pain and anxiety, and motivated?
- Do you and the learner have a trusting relationship?
- Have you set aside sufficient time for the teaching session?

Right Context
- Is the environment quiet, free of distractions, and private?
- Is the environment soothing or stimulating, depending on the desired effect?

Right Goal
- Is the learner actively involved in planning the learning objectives?
- Are you and your client both committed to reaching mutually set goals of learning that achieve the desired behavioral changes?
- Are family and friends included in planning so that they can help follow through on behavioral changes?
- Are the learning objectives realistic and valued by the client; do they reflect the client's lifestyle?

Right Content
- Is the content appropriate for the client's needs?
- Is the information new or a reinforcement of information that has already been provided?
- Is the content presented at the learner's level?
- Does the content relate to the learner's life experiences or is it otherwise relevant to the learner?

Right Method
- Do the teaching strategies fit the learning style of the client?
- Do the strategies fit the client's learning ability?
- Are the teaching strategies varied?

Source: Wilkinson & Van Leuven (2007), p. 530, Box 24-1.

BOX 16–2   POSITION STATEMENTS ON BREASTFEEDING

"AWHONN supports breastfeeding as the optimal method of infant nutrition. AWHONN believes that women should be encouraged to breastfeed and receive instruction and support from the entire health care team to successfully initiate and sustain breastfeeding. Discussions with the woman and her significant others concerning breastfeeding should begin during the preconception period and continue through the first year of life or longer" (AWHONN, 2007).

"Breastfeeding is the ideal way of providing young infants with the nutrients they need for healthy growth and development. Virtually all mothers can breastfeed, provided they have accurate information, and the support of their family and health care system" (www.who.int/topics/breastfeeding).

"The U.S. Surgeon General recommends that babies be fed with breast milk only – no formula – for the first 6 months of life. It is better to breastfeed for 6 months and best to breastfeed for 12 months, or longer ..." (www.womenshealth.gov/breastfeeding).

"From its inception, the American Academy of Pediatrics (AAP) has been a staunch advocate of breastfeeding as the optimal form of nutrition for infants. Although economic, cultural, and political pressures often confound decisions about infant feeding, the AAP firmly adheres to the position that breastfeeding ensures the best possible health as well as development and physiological outcomes of the infant" (www.aap.org/breastfeeding).

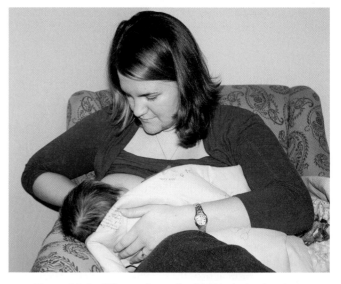

Figure 16-1   Woman breastfeeding her baby daughter.

Breastfeeding

Breastfeeding is the method of infant feeding recommended by the Association of Women's Health, Obstetric and Neonatal Nurses (AWHONN), the American College of Nurse-Midwives (ACNM), American Academy of Pediatrics (AAP), and the American College of Obstetricians and Gynecologist (ACOG) (Box 16-2 and Fig. 16-1). A goal of *Healthy People 2010* is an increase in the number of women who breastfeed their infants. Target goals are that by 2010 there will be increases in:

- Breastfeeding in the early postpartum period from 64% to 75%
- Breastfeeding at 6 months from 29% to 50%
- Breastfeeding at 12 months from 16% to 25% (DHHS, 2000b)

The decision to breastfeed is influenced by the woman's age, educational level, previous infant feeding method, career obligations, support from her partner, and cultural beliefs.

Immigrants to the United States are often eager to assimilate into the new culture and are more likely to choose bottle feeding the longer they live in the United States.

- The woman's partner plays a significant role in the woman's choice to breastfeed and to continue breastfeeding.
  - *The partner's knowledge and attitudes regarding breastfeeding are influenced by the partner's culture, past experiences, age, and family and friends.*
  - *The woman's feelings and success at breastfeeding are enhanced when her partner supports breastfeeding, assists in the care of the newborn, and does household tasks, which facilitate the woman's ability to rest and conserve energy.*

CULTURAL AWARENESS: Breastfeeding Beliefs	
Cultural Heritage	**Beliefs Regarding Breastfeeding**
Arab	Breastfeeding is delayed until the 2nd or 3rd postpartum day so that the mother can rest.
Chinese	May use formula until milk comes in.
Filipino	Women from rural areas are more likely to breastfeed for longer periods of time than are women from urban areas. Start supplementing with other fluids as early as 2 months.
Greek	Believe that taking showers in the first few days of breastfeeding can cause diarrhea and milk allergy in the infant.
Hindu	Some believe that colostrum is not suitable for newborns and feed sugar water or formula until milk comes in. Breastfeeding is often supplemented with cow's milk that is diluted with sugar water.
Japanese	The grandmother will feed the infant formula if the mother is sleeping to provide the rest needed for successful breastfeeding.
Mexican	May use a mixture of cornstarch and cow's milk when weaning from the breast.
Navajo Indian	Soon after birth, the newborn is given a mixture with juniper bark to cleanse her insides and remove the mucus. A ceremonial food of corn pollen and water is given.
Vietnamese	Some women will not feed newborn colostrum and will feed the newborn a rice paste or boiled water until milk comes in.

(Purnell & Paulanka, 2008)

Advantages of Breastfeeding

■ Decreased risk (200%) of infant diarrhea
■ Decreased risk of respiratory infections (200% decreased risk of being hospitalized for respiratory syncytial virus)
■ Decreased risk (300%) of otitis media (ear infection)
■ Decreased risk of childhood obesity
■ Decreased cost (DHHS, 2000a; Owen, Martin, Whinsup, Smith, & Cook, 2005)

Contraindications for Breastfeeding

■ Women who are using illicit drugs
■ Women with active and untreated tuberculosis
■ Women who are receiving diagnostic or therapeutic radioactive isotopes

■ Women who are receiving antimetabolites or chemotherapeutic agents
■ Women who have herpes simplex lesions on a breast
■ Women who are HIV positive (AAP, 2005a; DHHS, 2000a)
  ■ *In the developing world, the risks of artificial feedings outweigh the risks of acquiring HIV through breast milk; therefore, women are encouraged to breastfeed (AAP, 2005a).*

Composition of Human Milk

■ Contains proteins, carbohydrates, and fats that are synthesized in alveolar glands of the breast
  ■ *Protein in human milk is easier to digest than protein in prepared formulas. Proteins account for approximately 6% of the calories in human milk.*
  ■ *Lactose is the main carbohydrate. Carbohydrates account for approximately 42% of the calories in human milk.*
  ■ *Cholesterol, which is essential for brain development, is higher in human milk. Fats account for approximately 52% of the calories in human milk.*
■ Contains vitamins and minerals that are transferred to the human milk from the maternal plasma
■ Contains antibodies from the maternal system, which decreases the risk for neonatal infections

Stages of Human Milk

There are three stages of human milk as the body establishes the lactation process.

■ Stage 1: **Colostrum** is a yellowish breast fluid that is present for 2 to 3 days after birth. Colostrum is also excreted during the later part of pregnancy.
  ■ *It has higher levels of protein and lower levels of fats, carbohydrates, and calories than mature human milk.*
  ■ *It is high in immunoglobulins G and A.*
  ■ *It acts as a laxative and assists in the passage of meconium.*
■ Stage 2: Transitional milk consists of colostrum and milk.
  ■ *This stage lasts from day 3 to day 10.*
■ Stage 3: Mature milk is composed of 20% solids and 80% water.
  ■ *It contains approximately 22 to 23 calories per ounce.*
  ■ ***Foremilk*** *is the milk that is produced and stored between feedings and released at the beginning of the feeding session. It has a higher water content.*
  ■ ***Hind milk*** *is the milk produced during the feeding session and released at the end of the session. It has a higher fat content.*

Overview of Milk Production

■ **Lactation** is the production of breast milk.
■ The woman's body prepares for lactation as the breasts develop during puberty and undergo further changes during pregnancy.
■ Milk is produced in the alveolar glands and is transported to the nipple through the lactiferous ducts (Fig. 16-2).
■ Milk production is influenced by hormones and suckling.
■ **Prolactin**, the primary hormone responsible for lactation, is produced during pregnancy, but high levels of estrogen and progesterone suppress lactation.
  ■ *Estrogen and progesterone levels decrease after childbirth and prolactin levels increase, which results in the stimulation of milk production.*
■ Suckling increases prolactin levels and volume of milk production.
  ■ *Milk production can be viewed as a supply–demand effect. The more milk the infant takes in, the more milk is produced.*
■ Extreme malnutrition can lower the fatty acid content of breast milk.

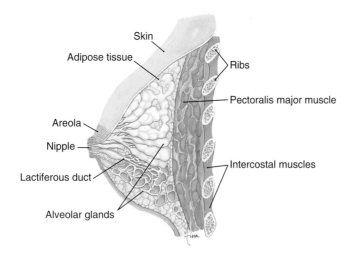

Figure 16-2 Mammary gland shown in midsagittal section.

Let-down Reflex

The **let-down reflex** or milk ejection reflex results in milk being ejected into and through the lactiferous duct system.

- Oxytocin causes the myoepithelial cells of the alveoli to contract and force the milk into the duct system.
- Oxytocin is released in response to suckling and/or maternal emotional response to hearing a baby cry or thinking of her baby.
- The let-down reflex can occur during sexual arousal or activity due to the natural release of oxytocin in response to an orgasm.
- The let-down reflex can be inhibited by stress, anxiety, pain, and fatigue.
- Let-down occurs multiple times during each feeding.

Process of Breastfeeding

- Breastfeeding is a natural process, with its success dependent on the mother's desire to breastfeed, proper positioning, latching-on, suckling, and transferring of milk (Mulder, 2006).
- Newborns indicate hunger by being in an awake/alert state, making mouth and tongue movements, making hand-to-mouth movements, and rooting (AWHONN, 2006).

CRITICAL COMPONENT

Infant Crying

- Crying is a late sign of hunger.
- Newborns whose cry is strong and continuous have difficulty latching onto the breast.
- Newborns who are crying need to be calmed by holding or by other comfort measures before being put to the breast.

- The woman needs to be in a comfortable position. Sitting is recommended because it facilitates good body posture.
  - *Other positions are lying on the side or back or sitting in bed.*
  - *The newborn can be held in a cradle position, "football" position, or cross cradle position.*
- Pillows are used to support the newborn and/or the woman.
- The front of the newborn is completely facing the breast to prevent the newborn's head from being turned. Another way to describe this is that the newborn's ear, shoulder, and hip are aligned.

- The woman supports her breast by placing one hand around the breast several inches behind the areola.
  - *Supporting the breast takes the weight of the breast away from the newborn's chin and makes latching on easier (AWHONN, 2006).*
  - *The woman should avoid pushing down on the breast, which can tip the nipple upward and increase the risk for sore nipples.*
- The newborn is brought to the breast, and not the breast to the newborn.
  - *The woman brings the newborn to her breast when the newborn's mouth is open wide. This assists with latching on.*
    - To encourage the newborn to open wide, take advantage of the rooting reflex by touching the newborn's chin to the breast. This signals the newborn to open the mouth. The newborn then reaches up and over the nipple to achieve an asymmetrical latch with more areola visible at the top of the mouth than on the bottom.
  - ***Latching-on** refers to the newborn's ability to grasp the breast and to effectively suckle. The newborn's mouth is around the areola with the nipple in the back of the newborn's mouth. The lips create a firm seal around the areola.*

CRITICAL COMPONENT

Signs of Successful Breastfeeding

- The woman feels a tugging sensation when the newborn begins to suckle.
- Latch-on pain should last no longer than 10 seconds. Pain beyond this is a sign of poor latch.
- The newborn's tongue is between the lower gum and breast.
- Swallowing can be heard (AWHONN, 2006).

- Newborns rapidly suckle at the beginning of the feeding session. Suckling gradually decreases and the newborn relaxes.
- Signs that the newborn's hunger has been satisfied are that the newborn:
  - *Spontaneously releases suction from breast*
  - *Does not respond with a rooting reflex when stimulated*
  - *Is relaxed and calm (Mulder, 2006)*
- The newborn should feed completely from one side and then be offered the second breast. Many newborns and infants nurse only from one breast at each feeding. It is recommended to start feeding from the breast that the newborn finished on during the previous feeding. This promotes complete emptying of each breast every 6 to 8 hours and facilitates adequate milk supply in each breast.
- Newborns are burped at the end of the feeding session.

Removing the Newborn from the Breast

Proper removal of newborn from the breast is important in decreasing nipple irritation.

- Place a clean finger in the corner of the newborn's mouth and slide it into the mouth to break suction.
- Once suction is broken, leave the finger in while removing the newborn from the breast.

Teaching Topics

An increasing number of lactation consultants are employed by hospitals to assist women with breastfeeding. Lactation consultants are valuable members of the maternity nursing staff, but do not replace the nurse's responsibility in providing proper breastfeeding teaching and support. The nurse and lactation consultant work together to ensure a positive breastfeeding experience. Before discharge, the woman should be given information on lactation consultants and lactation groups she can contact if she has questions or problems.

A primary role of nurses caring for woman who are breastfeeding is to facilitate successful breastfeeding by providing information and assisting the woman in her breastfeeding techniques. It is recommended that at least three complete feeding sessions per day during hospitalization be observed by the nurse or lactation consultant to assess the woman's ability to assist her infant with correctly latching-on to the breast (AWHONN, 2007).

- AWHONN Quick Care Guide to Breastfeeding is a summary of AWHONN's evidence-based clinical guidelines for breastfeeding support that can be used to assist nurses in providing evidence-based nursing care (Appendix B).
- Maternal and newborn positions
  - *Lying down position: The woman lies in bed or on the sofa in a comfortable position. Pillows are used to provide proper support of her head and neck. The newborn lies next to the woman on his side so that his head is directly facing the nipple. A pillow or rolled blanket can be used to support the newborn in this position.*
  - *Sitting position: The woman sits in a chair or bed with shoulders and back straight to reduce strain on her back and shoulder. The newborn can be held in several different positions. Three of these positions are:*
    - Cross-cradle position: The newborn's head is supported by the woman's hand and the newborn's back is against the woman's forearm. The abdomen of the newborn is facing/touching the woman's abdomen. This is an ideal position to use when the woman is first learning to breastfeed and it facilitates good head control.
    - Cradle position: The newborn's head is cradled in the crook of the woman's arm. The woman supports the newborn's back with her arm and his buttock with her hand. The abdomen of the newborn is facing/touching the woman's abdomen (Fig. 16-3).
    - Football hold position: The newborn's head is cradled in the woman's hand and the body is supported between the mother's arm and her side. The newborn's head is directly facing the nipple (see Fig. 16-3).
- Determining effective feeding

- *The woman feels physically and emotionally comfortable when feeding her newborn.*
- *The newborn properly latches on, as indicated by no nipple pain or trauma.*
- *The newborn suckles and the woman can hear and/or see swallowing, which indicates the transfer of milk.*
- *The newborn spontaneously releases his grip on the breast when satiated.*
  - Limiting time is not necessary and can be harmful in the establishment of milk supply (Chantry, Howard, & McCoy, 2003).
- *Newborn is drowsy and arms and legs are relaxed at the end of the feeding session.*
- *There are at least eight wet diapers and several stools per day once breast milk has come in and breastfeeding is established.*
- *The newborn recovers his birth weight by 2 weeks of age.*
- *A common tool used to assess and document breastfeeding efforts is LATCH (Table 16-1).*
  - The tool assesses both the woman and her infant and assists in determining the level of support needed and the type of interventions required for the dyad.
  - The lower the score, the higher the need for support and education.
  - The score can vary from one feeding to the next feeding.
- Decreasing the risk of nipple tissue breakdown
  - *Nipple irritation can lead to tissue breakdown and mastitis.*
  - *Painful nipples are a major reason that women stop breastfeeding before the 8th week (Lewallen et al., 2006).*
  - *Interventions to decrease irritation include:*
    - Teach proper technique for latching-on and releasing suction. Problems with latching-on increase the risk for early cessation of breastfeeding (Lewallen et al., 2006).
    - Apply warm compresses to the breasts/nipples before feeding to enhance the let-down reflex (AWHONN, 2006).
    - Instruct the woman to express colostrum or milk and rub it on the nipple and areola at the end of the feeding session (AWHONN, 2007).
    - Teach the woman to inspect her nipples for signs of irritation: redness, bruising, and tissue breakdown.
    - Change holding positions when feeding (e.g., football to cradle hold) to reduce pressure areas that have signs of irritation, as the pressure exerted on the nipples by the newborn is not uniform.

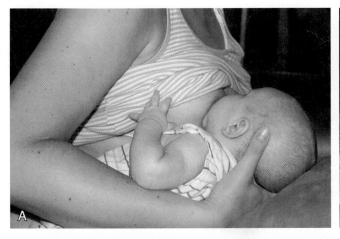
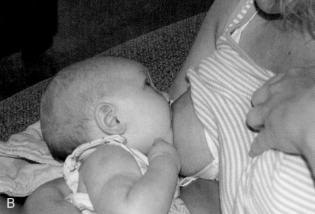

Figure 16-3 Positions for breastfeeding. *A.* Football hold. *B.* Cradle hold.

TABLE 16–1   LATCH SCORING SYSTEM

	0	1	2
L Latch	Too sleepy or reluctant No latch achieved	Repeated attempts Hold nipple in mouth Stimulate to suck	Grasps breast Tongue down Lips flanged Rhythmic sucking
A Audible swallowing	None	A few with stimulation	Spontaneous and intermittent < 24 hours old Spontaneous and frequent >24 hours old
T Type of nipple	Inverted	Flat	Everted (after stimulation)
C Comfort (Breast/nipple)	Engorged Cracked, bleeding, large blisters, or bruises Severe discomfort	Filling Reddened/small blisters or bruises Mild/moderate pain	Soft Tender
H Hold (Positioning)	Full assist (staff holds infant at breast)	Minimal assist (i.e., elevate head of bed; placed pillow for support) Teach one side; mother does the other side Staff holds and then mother takes over	No assist from staff Mother able to position/ hold infant

Source: Jensen, Wallace, & Kelsay (1994).

■ Begin the feeding session on the less sore breast because suck-ling is more vigorous at the beginning of the feeding session.

■ Instruct the woman to wash her breasts with water only. She should avoid use of soaps and alcohol, which cause excessive dryness of the breast/nipple.

■ Instruct the woman to contact her health care provider if she is experiencing cracked and/or bleeding nipples. The breasts then need to be assessed for signs of possible infection.

■ Comfort and relaxation

High levels of anxiety and discomfort interfere with successful breastfeeding by preventing or delaying the let-down reflex, which can cause a decrease in milk transfer and a decrease in milk supply (Mulder, 2006). Decreased milk supply is one reason women stop breastfeeding by or before the 8th week (Lewallen et al., 2006).

■ *Assist in lowering the maternal anxiety level by:*

■ Providing the woman/couple with easily understood breastfeeding information over several teaching sessions so she is not overwhelmed by too much information.

■ Being calm and patient in interactions with the woman/couple during breastfeeding sessions.

■ Explaining that it can take time for both the woman and newborn to become comfortable with breastfeeding.

■ Ensuring that the newborn is alert and ready to feed before bringing him or her to the breast. Newborns will not feed well when they are asleep/not ready to feed.

■ Praising the woman for her decision to breastfeed her infant.

■ *Provide instructions on methods to reduce pain and to promote comfort:*

■ Explain the relationship of rest, relaxation, and comfort on milk production.

■ Teach the proper use of analgesics that are recommended by the health care provider and are safe for lactating women.

■ Demonstrate the use of pillows to support both the mother's and newborn's body.

■ Teach breathing and relaxation techniques.

■ Nutrition and fluids

Decreased caloric intake and fluids can decrease milk volume. Lactating women need to consume an additional 500 calories/day over the recommended pre-pregnant requirements due to the increased energy requirement for milk production.

■ *Instruct women to develop a food plan based on the food pyramid.*

■ *Instruct women to have a glass of fluid next to them and drink it while they are nursing their infant since it is common to become thirsty while nursing.*

■ Expressing and storing breast milk

Teach women who breastfeed how to express milk and how to store milk properly, as most will need to skip a feeding or feedings when they are away from their infant for more than a few hours or when returning to work. Milk can be expressed by hand or with the use of an electric breast pump.

■ *For manual expression of milk, instruct the woman to:*

1. Wash her hands before touching her breasts.

2. Massage each quadrant of her breast.

3. Place her thumb and forefinger so they form the letter "C" with the thumb at the 12 o'clock position and the forefin-ger at the 6 o'clock position.

4. Push the thumb and finger toward the chest wall.
5. Lean over and direct the spray of milk into a clean container.
6. Repeat this several times.
7. Occasionally massage the distal area of the breast.
8. Reposition the thumb and forefinger to the 3 and 9 o'clock positions and repeat the above sequence (Biancuzza, 1999).

■ *Electric breast pumps*
  ■ A variety of electric and battery-operated breast pumps are available.
  ■ Electric pumps can be fitted with bilateral accessory kits so that both breasts can be pumped at the same time.
  ■ Electric pumps closely simulate the suckling of infants.
  ■ Instruct women to follow the directions provided with the electric pump of choice.

■ *Women can begin expressing and storing milk once they are comfortable with breastfeeding and the milk supply is established.*

■ *Women can express milk at the end of a feeding session and store it for use when they are not present to breastfeed.*

■ *Women's hands and nails should be washed and all equipment properly cleaned before expressing and storing milk.*

■ *Breast milk can be stored:*
  ■ At room temperature (77°F) for up to 6 to 8 hours
  ■ In the refrigerator for up to 5 days
  ■ In the freezer that is attached to a refrigerator for 3 to 6 months
  ■ In a deep freezer for 6 to 12 months (Academy of Breastfeeding Medicine [ABM], 2008; AWHONN, 2006)

■ *Glass or hard plastic containers should be used for milk being stored longer than 72 hours. Plastic bags designed for storage of breast milk can be used for storage of less than 72 hours.*

■ *Breast milk is thawed by placing it under lukewarm water.*

■ *Breast milk should not be heated in the microwave oven as it can cause uneven heating or overheating (AWHONN, 2006). Overheating either by microwave or stovetop can destroy antibodies within the breast milk (ABM, 2008).*

■ Medications
  ■ *Instruct the woman to check with her primary care provider and the infant's primary care provider before she takes prescribed and nonprescribed medications, including vitamins and herbal supplements (AWHONN, 2007).*

Bottle Feeding

Breast milk is the recommended form of newborn/infant nutrition, but owing to maternal or newborn health or personal reasons, not every woman breastfeeds (Fig. 16-4). Commercially prepared formulas are a nutritious alternative to breast milk.

Advantages of Formula Feeding

■ Provides a very pleasurable child caring experience for the partner, as either parent can feed the newborn/infant.
■ Provides the opportunity for the woman to leave the newborn/infant with other people while she goes out or returns to work without the need to pump her breast or plan activities around the newborn/infant's feeding schedule.
■ Decreases the frequency of feedings because digestion of formula is slower than that of human milk.

Disadvantages of Formulas Feeding

■ Need for increased time to prepare formula
■ Increased cost compared to breastfeeding

■ Increased risk of infection due to lack of antibodies that are naturally present in human milk.
■ Increased risk of childhood obesity and insulin-dependent diabetes.

Composition of Manufactured Formulas

■ Contains 50% more protein than human milk.
■ Uses vegetable oils which are easier to digest than animal fat, but are devoid of cholesterol.
  ■ *Cholesterol is essential for brain development.*

Teaching Topics

■ Formula preparation
  ■ *Formulas are available in powder, concentrated, and ready-to-use forms.*
  ■ *Instruct parents to follow the directions provided by the manufacturer when mixing powder or diluting concentrated forms of formulas. Prolonged overdilution of formulas can cause water intoxication and prolonged underdilution can cause dehydration.*
  ■ *Inform parents that once bottles of formula have been prepared they need to be kept refrigerated and used within 48 hours (Walker & Creehan, 2001).*
  ■ *Inform parents that opened cans or bottles of ready-to-use formula need to be kept refrigerated and used within 48 hours (Walker & Creehan, 2001).*
  ■ *Instruct parents to clean bottles, nipples, and can openers in a dishwasher or with hot soapy water.*

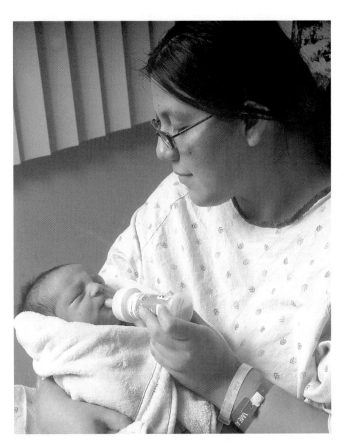

Figure 16-4 Bottle feeding is an alternate method of nourishing a newborn.

■ *Instruct parents to discard unused formula that remains in the bottle at the end of feeding.*
■ Frequency and amount of feedings
  ■ *Newborns take in ½ to 1 ounce (15–30 mL) per feeding during the first few days of life. This increases to 2 ½ to 3 ounces (75–90 mL) per feeding by day 4 and gradually increases to 32 ounces (950 mL) per day (AWHONN, 2006).*
  ■ *Newborns/infants can be fed on demand or at least every 3 to 4 hours.*
■ Feeding positions
  ■ *Newborns/infants should be held during feedings with the head slightly higher than the trunk of the body (AWHONN, 2006).*
  ■ *Newborns/infants are usually fed in a cradle holding position.*
■ Burping
  ■ *Burp the newborn/infant halfway through feeding and at end of feeding.*
  ■ *Tap the newborn/infant on the back for a few minutes.*
  ■ *Some newborns/infants may not need to burp with each feeding (AWHONN, 2006).*

CRITICAL COMPONENT

Bottle Feeding

■ Mix the formula as directed by the manufacturer.
■ Hold the newborn/infant close to the body, similar to breastfeeding.
■ Tilt the bottle so that the nipple is full of milk to decrease the amount of air swallowed by the newborn/infant.
■ Do not prop bottles, as propping bottles places infants at higher risk for chocking, otitis media, and tooth decay.
■ Discard unused formula from the bottle at the end of the feeding.

Nutritional Needs

During the first year of life, the infant experiences rapid growth. The infant will double his birth weight by 5 months and triple his or weight by its first birthday. Caloric needs vary based on size of infant, rate of growth, activity, and metabolic rate.

■ Infants experience growth spurts at 3 to 5 days, 1 week, 6 weeks, 3 months, and 6 months and require more frequent feedings during these periods of time (AWHONN, 2006).
■ Adequate nutritional intake is determined by plotting the weight and length of the infant at each well-child check-up.

Birth to 4 Months

■ The nutritional requirements for infants are ideally met by breast milk. Iron-fortified infant formula is substituted when the woman is not breastfeeding.
  ■ *Breastfeeding is on demand. Newborns usually feed 8 to 12 times per day during the first few weeks, gradually decreasing to 6 to 10 feedings per day. Women produce 500 to 600 mL of breast milk per day during the first few weeks and 700 to 800 mL until semisolid foods are introduced. Milk production decreases once semisolid foods are introduced.*
  ■ *Formula feeding is either on demand or every 3 to 4 hours. Newborns start with ½ to 1 ounce (15–30 mL) per feeding and gradually increase to 32 ounces (960 mL) per day.*

4 to 6 Months

■ Feeding breast milk or formula is continued.
■ Rice cereal is the first semisolid food that is introduced during this time frame, followed by oats and barley.
■ Cereals need to be given by spoon.
  ■ *Cereal should not be given in bottles because there is an increased risk of choking and aspiration when cereal is given by bottle.*
■ Introduction of solid foods is determined by the physician or nurse practitioner in collaboration with parents. American Academy of Pediatrics (AAP) and World Health Organization (WHO) guidelines recommend waiting to start solids until 6 months of age to reduce allergy risks.
■ Parents should not introduce solid foods until recommended by the health care provider.
■ Infants are ready for semisolid foods when they:
  ■ *Can sit independently*
  ■ *Can draw in the lower lip as a spoon is removed*
  ■ *Indicate hunger by opening the mouth*
  ■ *Refuse food by closing the mouth and turning away*
■ Before 4 to 6 months, the sucking reflex forces semisolid food out of the mouth versus to the back of the mouth.

NEWBORN CARE

It is the responsibility of the nursing staff in the postpartum unit to ensure that couples have an adequate knowledge of newborn care to safely care for their child. A teaching plan is developed for all couples based on assessment of their knowledge level. Some couples require a minimal amount of teaching while others require intensive amounts of teaching. The following information on infant care is in alphabetical order for easier reference.

Bathing

■ The first few bathing experiences can be stressful for the parents, but over time become a very pleasurable experience for both the parents and their child.
■ Daily bathing with soap is not necessary and can cause skin irritation (AWHONN, 2006). Cleansing of genital and rectal areas at each diaper change and washing face and neck areas after feedings with plain water is adequate.
■ Mild soap that has neutral pH and is preservative free is recommended to decrease the risk of skin irritation.
■ Use of soap on the face is not recommended.
■ Bathing is done in a warm room that is free from drafts.
■ Do not leave the newborn/infant unattended in bath water.
■ Gather all items required for bathing (e.g., soap, towels, washcloth, clean clothing, diapers, blankets) before the bath.
■ Bathing is best done before a feeding to decrease the risk of emeses related to jostling during bathing.
■ Use warm water for bathing (100.4°F [38°C]; AWHONN, 2006).
■ Immerse the newborn/infant in warm water deep enough to cover the shoulders (AWHONN, 2006). There is controversy regarding when an infant can be immersed in water. Some believe that it needs to be delayed until the cord has fallen off and the cord site is healed, whereas others do not. Follow the institution's policy on newborn bathing.
■ The newborn/infant's head and neck is supported by the parent's forearm (Fig. 16-5).
■ Start from the cleanest area (eyes) and end with the dirtiest area (buttock).

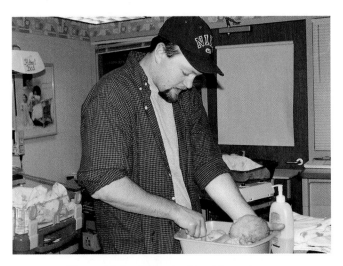

Figure 16-5 Father bathing his newborn.

■ Cleanse eyes from the inner to outer aspects using a clean corner of the washcloth per eye. This helps to reduce the risk of transfer of infection from one eye to the other.

■ Wash hair and massage the scalp.

■ Lift the chin to clean neck folds, where milk often collects.

■ Cleanse the upper body

■ Cleanse the lower body.

■ Clean female genitals by washing from front to back to decrease the risk of cystitis.

■ Elevate the scrotum and cleanse the area.

■ Dry the newborn/infant and put on a clean diaper and clothes.

Evidence-Based Practice: Tub Bathing versus Sponge Bathing for Newborns

Bryanton, J., Walsh, D., Barrett, M., & Gaudet, D. (2004). Tub bathing versus traditional sponge bathing for newborns. *JOGGN, 33,* 704–712.

Sponge bathing newborns until the cord site has healed has been a common recommended practice taught to parents. It was based on the belief that immersing newborns in water before the cord fell off and the site healed increased the risk for infection and delayed drying of cord and healing of the cord site.

Bryanton et al. conducted a randomized control study to compare the effects of tub bathing to sponge bathing. Fifty-one mother–newborn couplets were in the infant tub bathing group and 51 mother–newborn couplets were in the sponge bath group. Newborn temperature, umbilical cord healing, infant contentment, and maternal pleasure and confidence were measured.

There was significantly less temperature loss, more infant contentment, and higher maternal pleasure for couplets in the tub-bathing group. There was no significant difference in umbilical cord healing or maternal confidence.

Based on their research data they concluded that tub-bathing is safe and pleasurable.

Bulb Syringe

■ Instruct parents in the proper use of a bulb syringe for clearing mucus from the newborn/infant's mouth and nose.
  ■ *Each newborn should have his or her own bulb syringe and it should be cleaned with soapy water and rinsed after each use.*

■ *Compress the syringe and insert it into either the nose or the mouth.*
  ■ When using in the mouth, the syringe is placed in each side of the mouth, the roof of the mouth, and the back of the mouth (Fig. 16-6).
  ■ When using in the nose, the syringe is placed in each nostril.
■ *Release pressure from the syringe and allow it to slowly expand.*
■ *Remove the syringe from the area.*
■ *Remove drainage from the syringe and into a tissue by compressing it.*

Clothing

■ The amount of clothing varies based on whether the newborn/infant is inside or outside and on the temperature of the environment.

■ Newborns/infants are usually comfortable wearing a diaper, t-shirt, and loose-fitting outfit when inside. A blanket is placed over the newborn/infant when sleeping.

■ More clothing or heavier blankets are used when the newborn/infant is outside in cooler weather.

■ A hat should be used when the newborn/infant is outside during colder weather.

■ The newborn/infant's skin needs to be protected from the sun. Newborns/infants can become overheated with too many clothes or blankets.

Circumcision Care

■ Gomco procedure:
  ■ *Petroleum-impregnated gauze is placed by the physician on the tip of the penis immediately after the circumcision.*
  ■ *Instruct parents to leave the gauze in place until it naturally falls off.*
  ■ *The circumcised area heals within 2 weeks.*
■ Plastibell method:
  ■ *Applying lubricants on the penis when a Plastibell has been used is not recommended because lubricants can increase the risk of displacement of the plastic ring (AWHONN, 2006).*
  ■ *The plastic ring falls off in 7 to 10 days. Parents should not pull it off.*
■ The **glans penis** (tip of the penis) appears red and forms yellow crusted areas as it heals. Parents should not wash off these areas.

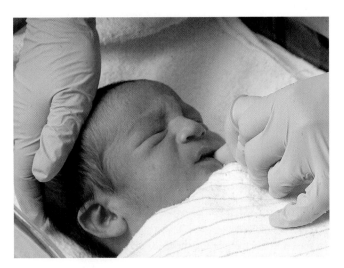

Figure 16-6 A bulb syringe in used to remove mucus.

■ Instruct parents to notify the health care provider if the newborn has not voided within 24 hours.
■ Instruct parents to check for bleeding every 4 hours for the first 24 hours and to notify the health care provider if there is bleeding at the circumcised area.

Colic

■ **Colic** is uncontrollable crying in healthy infants younger than the age of 5 months. The cause of colic is unknown.
  ■ *It is common for newborns to have a steady increase in crying until age 6 weeks, when it gradually decreases. This type of pattern is not necessarily colic.*
■ Healthy infants who cry for 3 hours for 3 or more days a week and for at least 3 weeks are considered to be colicky.
■ Infants can cry at any time of the day, but crying usually occurs in the evening.
■ The infant may also extend and flex his legs during crying periods.
■ Parents of colicky infants become frustrated as it becomes increasingly difficult to calm/comfort their infant. Parents should give each other "breaks" so the partner can rest and "regroup."
■ Methods for soothing colicky infants:
  ■ *Hold the infant and sway from side to side or walk around with the infant.*
  ■ *Give the infant a pacifier.*
  ■ *Swaddle the infant.*
  ■ *Place the infant (abdomen facing down) over the knees and gently rub or pat the infant's back.*
  ■ *Place the infant in a baby bouncer.*
  ■ *Place the infant in a car seat and take him or her for a ride in the car.*
  ■ *Place the infant in a car seat and put on top of a running clothes dryer. Do not leave the infant unattended on the dryer.*
  ■ *Place the infant in a stroller and go for a walk.*

Cord Care

■ The umbilical cord begins to dry once the cord is clamped and cut.
■ The cord clamp is removed after 24 hours of life. At this point, the cord is dry, hard, and black.
■ The cord falls off and the site heals within 2 weeks.
■ The cord is cleaned at each diaper change with water or alcohol based on institutional policy.
■ Place diapers below the cord to facilitate keeping the area dry (Fig. 16-7).
■ Instruct parents to contact the health care provider if there is bleeding from the cord site, foul-smelling drainage, redness in the surrounding skin, or fever.

Diapering

■ Most parents use disposable diapers that come in various sizes based on the weight of the infant.
■ Change a diaper when it becomes wet or soiled to prevent skin irritation. Parents need to check diapers every few hours to see if they need changing.
■ Gather supplies (e.g., clean diaper, clean clothing, and wet washcloth) before placing the newborn/infant on a flat surface such as a changing table.
■ Unfasten diaper tabs and lower the front of the diaper.

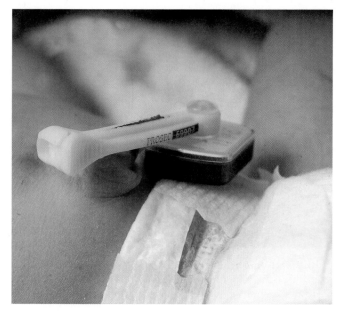

Figure 16-7   When diapering, the cord is left exposed.

■ Lift the newborn/infant's bottom using an ankle hold and fold the soiled diaper under the bottom.
■ Use water to clean genital and rectal areas, wiping from front to back.
■ Lift the bottom of the newborn/infant with use of an ankle hold, remove the soiled diaper, and then place a clean diaper under the newborn/infant.
■ Fasten both sides of the diaper so that there is a snug fit.
■ Dress the newborn.
■ Properly dispose of the diaper.
■ Wash hands.

Elimination

■ Instruct parents on the stages of newborn stools (see Chapter 15).
■ Explain that newborns/infants pass several stools per day. At 1 month of age, breastfed infants may pass only a stool every other day due to breast milk being more easily digested, while bottle-fed infants continue to pass one or two stools per day.
■ Inform parents that newborns/infants should have at least six wet diapers per day once breastfeeding or bottle feeding has been established.
■ Inform parents that newborn diapers may have a pink stain related to urates, which is a normal occurrence.
  ■ *Urates persisting in more than two diapers may suggest dehydration and weight loss. Parents need to report a continued presence of urates to the physician or nurse practitioner for further evaluation.*
■ Inform parents that blood may occur on the diaper of newborn girls related to a withdrawal of maternal hormones. This is referred to as **pseudomenstruation**.
■ Instruct parents to notify the health care provider if stools are runny and green and/or if newborn/infant has less than six wet diapers per day.
■ Instruct parents to notify the health care provider if the newborn/infant becomes constipated. Constipation can be a sign of inadequate intake and needs to be evaluated by the health care provider.

Feeding

Refer to information provided earlier in this chapter.

Follow-up Care

Routine follow-up care of the newborn is an important component of health promotion. The well-child check-ups provide an opportunity to:

- Assess the infant's growth
- Assess feeding pattern
- Assess the developmental level
- Assess for jaundice
- Provide the appropriate immunizations
- Do follow-up metabolic screening
- Continue teaching parents about the care of their child and what to expect at each developmental milestone.

Parents need to understand the importance of the check-ups and how they can promote wellness. The American Academy of Pediatrics recommends the following:

- First visit within 3 to 4 days after hospital discharge
- The second visit is 2 weeks later
- Subsequent visits are at 1, 2, 4, 6, 9, and 12 months of age

Nonnutritive Sucking

Sucking is a pleasurable experience for newborns and infants. There is both nutritive sucking (sucking during breastfeeding or bottle feeding) and nonnutritive sucking. Nonnutritive sucking, using a pacifier or the infant's fist and fingers, is used to soothe or calm an infant.

- The parents' choice to use a pacifier is influenced by cultural, societal, and community norms.
- A pacifier should not be used with breastfed infants until 1 month of age. This provides the time needed for infants to establish breastfeeding.
  - *Pacifiers have been linked to shorter breastfeeding duration.*
  - *The mouth motions a newborn uses when breastfeeding, referred to as suckling, are different from the mouth motions (sucking) used with bottle feeding or use of pacifier.*
- A pacifier should not be used to delay feedings or substitute for parental attention.
- Do not tie the pacifier around the newborn/infant's neck. A cord around the neck places the infant at risk for strangulation.
- Wash pacifiers with warm soapy water.

Potential Signs of Illness

AWHONN (2006) recommends that parents notify the infant's health care provider in the following situations:

- Increased axillary temperature (>99.3°F or 37.4°C).
- Loss of appetite
- Lethargy (infant is sleepy and not as active as usual)
- Watery green stools
- Vomiting
- Decrease in the number of wet diapers
- Skin rash
- Fontanels are sunken or bulging
- Bleeding from circumcision site and/or cord site
- Foul odor from the circumcision site and/or cord site

Prevention of Dental Decay

Infants' teeth are susceptible to "baby bottle tooth decay," a condition that occurs when sweetened liquids are given in bottles to infants and allowed to remain in the mouth for a period of time. Within 20 minutes, the sugar from the sweetened liquid responds to mouth bacteria and forms acids that cause dental decay (ADA, 2007). Infants who fall sleep with a bottle in her mouth or who receives several bottles of sweetened liquids during the day are at higher risk for tooth decay.

CRITICAL COMPONENT

Decreasing the Risk of Baby Bottle Tooth Decay

The American Dental Association (2007) recommends the following to decrease risk of baby bottle tooth decay:

- Do not put infants to bed with a bottle of milk, juice, or sugar water.
- Do not give infants bottles with sugar water or sodas.
- Clean the infant's gums with a clean gauze after each feeding.
- Brush teeth once the first tooth erupts.
- Consult a dentist regarding fluoride treatments if the water supply does not contain fluoride.
- Begin regular dental appointments by the first birthday.

Safety

Parents are responsible for the safety of their children. Newborns and infants are at risk for injury related to falls, ingestions of harmful products, and accidents.

- Infant car seats
  - *Infant car seats need to be used for all infants when traveling in a motor vehicle, including on the day of discharge from the hospital.*
  - *Infants are safest when secured in the back seat. Rear-facing car seats are used with infants until they are 1 year of age and weigh 20 pounds.*
  - *Parents need to select a car seat that best fits their vehicle and follow the instructions on how to secure the seat to the vehicle's seat and how to properly position and secure the infant into the car seat.*
  - *Parents can contact a certified Child Passenger Safety Technician (CPS) for assistance in the installation and use of infant car seats before bringing the newborn home. Instruct parents to visit www.seatcheck.org to locate a CPS near their home.*
  - *Each state has laws that govern the use of infant and children car seats. Laws for specific states can be viewed at www.seatcheck.org.*
  - *Instruct parents to never leave their child in a car unattended.*
- Prevention of falls
  - *Instruct parents not to leave their newborn/infant on an elevated flat surface without supervision.*
  - *Instruct parents not to leave their newborn/infant in a car seat on an elevated surface unattended.*
  - *Install gates at stairwells.*
  - *Select a highchair with a wide base to prevent tipping over.*
- Prevention of ingesting harmful substances
  - *Place all cleaning materials in upper cabinets out of the infant's reach.*
  - *Place all medications including vitamins in upper cabinets out of the infant's reach.*

- *Place safety latches on all lower cabinets and keep the cabinet doors closed.*
- *Remove lead paint from older cribs and infant furniture and walls.*
- *Never leave infants unattended in rooms or yards.*
- Preventions of accidents
  - *Keep small objects out of the reach of infants to prevent chocking.*
  - *Remove strings and ribbons from bedding, sleepwear, and pacifiers to prevent strangulation.*
  - *Keep plastic bags out of reach.*
  - *Keep all sharp objects in drawers or cabinets out of the infant's reach.*
  - *Check water temperature used for bathing. Water temperature should be 100.4°F (38°C) (AWHONN, 2006).*
    - Set the hot water heater thermostat at 120°F or lower.
  - *Do not leave the infant in the bathtub unsupervised.*
  - *Keep any guns unloaded and locked and out of the infant's reach.*
  - *Install safety devices around swimming pools.*
  - *Do not cook while holding the infant.*
  - *Supervise infants when pets are in the room.*
  - *Ensure crib slats are less than 2 3/8 inches apart to prevent the infant's head from becoming trapped between slats and to decrease the risk of strangulation.*
  - *Cover electrical outlets.*

Shaken Baby Syndrome

Shaken baby syndrome, also referred to as abusive head trauma, is a traumatic brain injury that occurs when an infant is violently shaken (NINDS, 2007). Approximately 20% of shaken baby syndrome cases are fatal (National Center on Shaken Baby Syndrome, 2008).

- Infants are at higher risk for injury related to violent shaking due to:
  - *Weak neck muscles*
  - *Large and heavy head*
- When the infant is violently shaken, his or her brain bounces back and forth against the skull, causing bruising, swelling, and bleeding within the brain tissue. Permanent and severe brain damage or death can occur as a result of the trauma (NINDS, 2007).
- Symptoms of shaken baby syndrome are extreme irritability, poor feeding, breathing problems, convulsions, vomiting, and pale or bluish skin (NINDS, 2007).
- Parents need to be educated regarding this syndrome and given resources they can seek when their frustrations levels are high and they need assistance in caring for their infant.

Sibling Rivalry

There will be some degree of sibling rivalry when a new baby is introduced into the family. Older children will feel the shift of attention from them to the new baby and may react to this change in a negative manner. Toddlers may begin wetting themselves or wanting to use diapers or crying to get attention. Others may want to drink from a bottle. Some children may hit or pinch their new sibling.

- Methods to decrease the degree of sibling rivalry:
  - *Start preparing older children during pregnancy for the new family addition by talking to them about becoming an older brother or sister; having them feel the baby kick; and having them around newborn infants (see Chapter 5).*
  - *Have older siblings attend sibling classes that are offered by some hospitals and agencies.*

- *Bring older children to the postpartum unit to meet their new sibling.*
- *Give the older children a gift and tell them it is from their new brother or sister.*
- *Spend quality time with older children such as reading or playing games.*
- *Take older children on special outings without the new sibling.*
- *Teach the older sibling about why babies cry and why mom or dad needs to attend to the baby's cry.*

Sudden Infant Death Syndrome

Sudden infant death syndrome (SIDS) is the sudden death of an infant younger than the age of 1 year (AWHONN, 2006). There has been a 50% reduction of deaths related to SIDS since parents have been instructed to place their infants on their backs when sleeping (AWHONN, 2006).

CRITICAL COMPONENT

Reducing the Risk of SIDS

To reduce the risk of SIDS, the American Academy of Pediatrics recommends:

- Placing newborns and infants on their backs when sleeping (Fig. 16-8)
- Placing newborns or infants on a firm mattress for sleeping
- Keeping pillows or stuffed animals out of the sleeping area
- Breastfeeding
- Maintaining a smoke-free environment
- Preventing overheating of the infant by controlling room temperature and using lightweight clothing (AAP, 2005b)

Skin Care

The newborn's skin is delicate and can be irritated easily. The skin should be inspected daily for signs of tissue irritation and breakdown (Appendix B).

- General skin care (Appendix A)
  - *Avoid daily bathing with soap.*
  - *Use cleansers that have neutral pH.*

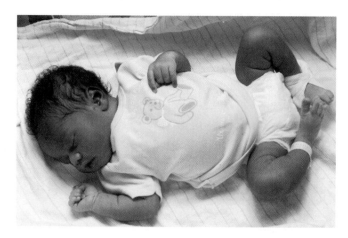

Figure 16-8   Place the baby on his back to sleep.

■ *Avoid use of adhesives because they can remove the epidermis layer of the skin and lead to a breakdown of the skin barrier.*
■ *Apply petroleum-based ointments sparingly to dry skin and avoid the head and face.*
■ *Avoid use of skin ointments with perfume, dyes, and preservatives (AWHONN, 2001).*
■ Diaper dermatitis is common. Methods to reduce risk of diaper dermatitis include:
■ *Changing diapers frequently*
■ *Using petroleum-based or zinc oxide ointments during diaper changes*
■ *Avoiding use of powders. Powders increase the risk of bacterial and candidal growth.*
■ *Avoiding use of antibiotic ointments, which can increase the risk of allergic skin reactions (AWHONN, 2001).*

Soothing Babies

Newborns and infants cry when they are hungry, uncomfortable, bored, or exposed to new experiences. There are various methods to soothe the newborn/infant:

■ Feed if crying is related to hunger.
■ Reposition the newborn/infant when it is sleep time.
■ Swaddle the newborn/infant.
■ Hold the newborn/infant close to the body so she can feel the warmth of the parent's body and hear the parent's heartbeat.
■ Hold the newborn/infant and rock back and forth or walk around the house or dance with the infant in the parent's arms.
■ Place the newborn/infant in a stroller and go for a walk.

Swaddling

Swaddling is wrapping the newborn's blanket snugly around him. This provides warmth and a sense of security for the newborn, which can have a calming effect.

1. Place the blanket on a flat surface.
2. Fold the top corner over (Fig. 16-9).
3. Place the newborn on the blanket with the neck at the fold line of the blanket.
4. Fold one corner across the newborn's body and tuck under his back (Fig. 16-10).
5. Bring the bottom corner up and fold under the neck (Fig. 16-11).
6. Pull the remaining corner across the newborn's body and tuck under the back (Fig. 16-12).

Temperature Taking

■ Instruct parents to take the newborn/infant's temperature before calling the health care provider if they feel that their child is sick.
■ Digital thermometers are recommended over mercury-filled thermometers.
■ The American Academy of Pediatrics (2007) recommends the following:
■ *Rectal temperatures for children 3 years of age and younger*
■ *Oral temperatures for children 4 years of age and older*
■ *Axillary temperature (although not as accurate) can also be used for children older than 3 months.*
■ Instruct parents to take an axillary temperature by placing thermometer in the axillary region and holding the newborn's arm against his side until the thermometer beeps (approximately 1 minute) (Fig. 16-13).
■ Teach parents how to take a rectal temperature:
1. Clean the end of the thermometer with alcohol or soapy water and rinse in cold water.
2. Lubricate the end of the thermometer with a lubricant such as petroleum jelly.
3. Place the infant on his or her back and hold the legs in a flexed position.
4. Insert the thermometer no further than 0.5 inches into the rectum.
5. Hold the thermometer in place until it beeps.
6. Remove the thermometer after it has beeped and check the digital reading.
■ Teach parents how to read a thermometer.
■ *An elevated temperature might be related to overheating from too many blankets or clothing. Instruct parents to decrease the amount of clothing and retake the temperature after 15 to 20 minutes.*
■ *Notify the health care provider if the temperature remains elevated (greater than 99.3°F [37.4°C]).*

Uncircumcised Male

■ Do not force the foreskin over the penis.
■ *The foreskin fully retracts on its own around 5 years of age.*
■ *Forcing the foreskin over the penis or using cotton swabs to clean under the foreskin can damage the inner layer of the foreskin, which can lead to adhesion formation.*
■ Gently cleanse the penis when bathing the infant and when changing the diaper.

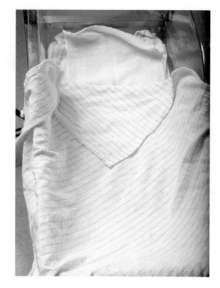

Figure 16-9   Top fold.

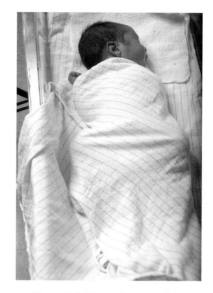

Figure 16-10   Left corner fold.

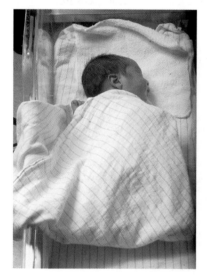

Figure 16-11   Bottom fold.

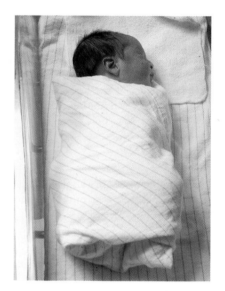

Figure 16-12   Right corner fold.

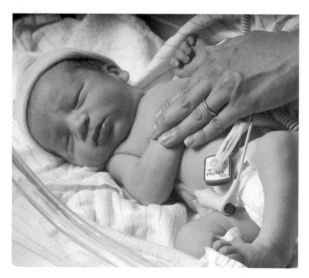

Figure 16-13   Placement of thermometer when taking an axillary temperature.

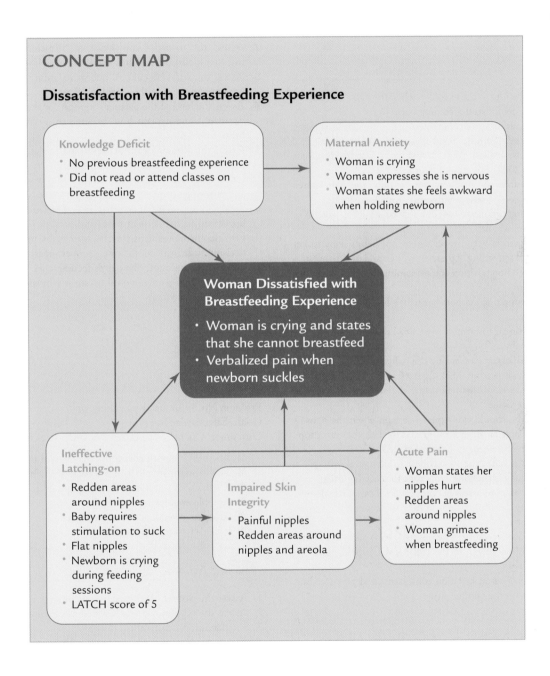

CONCEPT MAP

Dissatisfaction with Breastfeeding Experience

Knowledge Deficit
- No previous breastfeeding experience
- Did not read or attend classes on breastfeeding

Maternal Anxiety
- Woman is crying
- Woman expresses she is nervous
- Woman states she feels awkward when holding newborn

Woman Dissatisfied with Breastfeeding Experience
- Woman is crying and states that she cannot breastfeed
- Verbalized pain when newborn suckles

Ineffective Latching-on
- Redden areas around nipples
- Baby requires stimulation to suck
- Flat nipples
- Newborn is crying during feeding sessions
- LATCH score of 5

Impaired Skin Integrity
- Painful nipples
- Redden areas around nipples and areola

Acute Pain
- Woman states her nipples hurt
- Redden areas around nipples
- Woman grimaces when breastfeeding

Problem No. 1: Knowledge deficit

Goal: The woman will demonstrate proper breastfeeding techniques before discharge.

Outcome: Establishment of breastfeeding as evidenced by:

- Proper alignment of the baby and woman
- Proper latch-on
- LATCH score of 8 or greater
- Audible swallowing
- Absence of reddened areas or blisters
- The woman states she feels comfortable with breastfeeding

Nursing Actions

1. Explain that the ideal time to feed is when the baby is in a quiet alert state and demonstrates feeding cues.
2. Provide information on newborn feeding cues such as sucking movements and sounds, hand-to-mouth movements, and rooting reflects; explain that crying is a late feeding cue (AWHONN, 2007).
3. Demonstrate different positions for holding the baby when breastfeeding: cross cradle, cradle, and football positions.
4. Provide information on use of pillows in assisting the woman in a comfortable position.
5. Teach the woman how to properly align the baby's body to her body when breastfeeding, by assisting her and the baby in a proper breastfeeding position and explaining how this facilitates effective feeding.
6. Instruct the woman to support her baby's head and neck while the baby nurses.
7. Instruct the woman to bring the baby to her breast and not the breast to the baby.
8. Explain the importance of having the baby's mouth cover most of her areola with her nipple in the back of the baby's mouth.
9. Explain that the woman should feel a tugging sensation as the baby begins to suckle.
10. Explain that she should not experience pain when the baby is suckling. Pain may be an indication that the baby has not properly latched on and needs to be repositioned.
11. Teach the woman that she should hear audible swallowing as a sign that the baby is suckling properly and receiving milk.
12. Instruct the woman to assess her nipples for signs of nipple irritation and provide information on how to decrease the risk of nipple irritation.
13. Demonstrate how to properly remove the baby from her breast by placing a clean finger in the side of the baby's mouth to release the suction.
14. Provide information on lactation consultants and breastfeeding support groups in the community.

Problem No. 2: Maternal anxiety

Goal: Decrease of anxiety level

Outcome: The woman expresses that she feels comfortable with breastfeeding.

Nursing Actions

1. Assess the woman's beliefs, attitudes, concerns, and questions regarding breastfeeding to identify the source of anxiety to assist in identifying areas to address in action plan.
2. Assess the woman's knowledge of breastfeeding and provide information to increase her knowledge level.
3. Assess the woman's cultural beliefs regarding breastfeeding and incorporate these in the teaching plan.
4. Assess the level of the partner's support for the woman's desire to breastfeed and explain how he/she can assist the woman with breastfeeding.
5. Assess the woman's comfort level and initiate methods to promote comfort such as relaxation techniques, proper positioning for feeding, use of pillows to support the woman and her baby, and ensuring adequate rest and sleep for the woman.
6. Establish an environment that is conducive for the woman to breastfeed such as a quiet room and privacy.
7. Provide encouragement for the woman by praising her for her decision to breastfeed, for using proper breastfeeding techniques and for responding to the baby's feeding cues.
8. Reevaluate the woman's level of anxiety by assessing verbal and nonverbal behaviors.

Problem No. 3: Ineffective latching-on

Goal: Effective latching-on

Outcome: The baby will effectively latch-on as evidenced by:

- The baby's mouth covers the majority of the woman's areola.
- The woman's nipple is in the back of the baby's mouth.
- The baby's lips create a firm seal around the areola.
- Audible swallowing.
- Absence of reddened areas or blisters.
- LATCH score of 8 or greater

Nursing Actions

1. Assess the woman's breastfeeding technique.
2. Assess the nipples and areola for signs of irritation.
3. Provide information on latching-on.
4. Assist the woman and her baby with proper positioning that facilitates latching-on.
5. Instruct the woman to bring the baby to her breast when the baby's mouth is wide open.
6. Instruct the woman to delay use of a pacifier until the baby is able to latch-on and breastfeeding is established, which is usually 1 month (AWHONN, 2007).

Problem No. 4: Acute pain

Goal: Absence of pain

Outcome: The baby will properly latch-on and the woman will state that she is not experiencing pain in the breast area when feeding her baby.

Nursing Actions

1. Assess the level of pain using a pain scale.
2. Assess the breast for signs of irritation such as reddened areas, blisters, or cracking and provide information on methods to decrease irritation.
3. Assess the breastfeeding technique by observing the woman during a feeding session.
4. Provide information and assistance to facilitate latching-on.
5. Provide information on various positions for holding the baby during feeding sessions.
6. Explain that warm moist compresses may decrease nipple pain (AWHONN, 2007).
7. Medicate with analgesia PRN.

Problem No. 5: Impaired skin integrity

Goal: Skin will remain intact.

Outcome: The tissue of the nipples and areola will be intact with no redness or blisters.

Nursing Actions

1. Assess nipples and areolas for signs of irritation.
2. Instruct the woman to inspect her nipples and areolas after each feeding.
3. Assess the woman during feeding sessions for proper breastfeeding techniques.
4. Provide information on proper positioning of the baby for breastfeeding.
5. Provide information on latching-on.
6. Instruct the woman to gently rub breast milk around her nipples and areolas after each feeding session (AWHONN, 2007).

TYING IT ALL TOGETHER

As the nurse, you are caring for Margarite Sanchez, a 28-year-old G3 P2 Hispanic woman who delivered a healthy boy, Manuel. Margarite and her husband have a healthy 2½-year-old boy. Margarite informs you that she breastfed her older child, José, for 9 months without problems. Her older son was interested in the pregnancy and being a big brother, but he has been crying, and is restless and irritable during hospital visits. He also does not want to hold his baby brother and is demanding to be taken to the toy store.

Margarite's husband tells you that he was very involved in the care of his first child.

A circumcision is planned for Manuel the morning of discharge.

Based on your knowledge of the Sanchez family, list the priority learning needs and state the rationale for your selection of learning needs.

Describe your teaching plan based on the identified priority learning needs. The plan should include:

■ *Preparation of the learning environment*
■ *Methods to assess their learning needs*
■ *Information that will be shared with the couple*
■ *Method for evaluating effectiveness of teaching*

■ ■ ■ Review Questions ■ ■ ■

1. Teaching regarding the care of the newborn begins:
   A. During pregnancy.
   B. Within a few hours after delivery.
   C. Twelve hours after delivery.
   D. The day of discharge.

2. During a feeding session your 19-year-old primipara, who is 12 hours post-birth, asks you how she can tell if her baby girl is getting any milk when nursing. Your best response is:
   A. "Your baby is getting colostrum. Your milk will come in around 2 to 3 days."
   B. "When your baby falls asleep while nursing."
   C. "You will hear swallowing noises from your baby as she suckles."
   D. "Your baby will refuse to latch-on."

3. You are assigned to a 21-year-old primipara, who is 36 hours post-birth and breastfeeding her healthy newborn son. During your assessment, you note that there is a small reddened area on the right side of the left areola. Based on this assessment finding, which of the following is the priority nursing action?
   A. Instruct the woman to change feeding position from cradle hold to football hold
   B. Instruct the woman to air-dry her nipples for 15 minutes after each feeding
   C. Instruct the woman to apply a lanolin cream to the area after each feeding
   D. Instruct the woman to feed from only the right breast for 24 hours

4. You are assigned a 16-year-old primipara, who is bottle feeding her healthy full-term baby boy. She asks you why the other nurse told her to tilt the baby's bottle when feeding. Your best response is:
   A. "I will go and get the other nurse so she can clarify the instruction she gave you."
   B. "By tilting the bottle the nipple is in a more comfortable placement in your baby's mouth."
   C. By tilting the bottle you keep the nipple full of formula and decrease the amount of air your baby swallows."
   D. "The tilted position provides greater pressure coming from the bottle and makes it easier for your baby to take in the formula."

5. You are developing a discharge teaching plan for your patient. Their newborn is a girl and is full term and healthy. Both the woman and her partner are college educated and have one other healthy child, a boy who is 2 years old. The woman bottle-fed her son and plans to breastfeed her daughter. She plans to return to work when her daughter is 3 months old. Based on this information, the three primary learning needs for this couple are:
   A. Breastfeeding, sibling rivalry, and infant/child safety
   B. Breastfeeding, storage of breast milk, and bathing
   C. Safety, colic, and storage of breast milk
   D. Cord care, breastfeeding, and safety

References

American Academy of Breastfeeding Medicine (AABM). (2008). *Protocol #8: Human milk storage information for home use for healthy full-term infants.* Retrieved from www.bfmed.org

American Academy of Pediatrics (AAP). (2005a). Breastfeeding and use of human milk. *Pediatrics, 115,* 496–506.

American Academy of Pediatrics (AAP). (2005b). The changing concepts of sudden infant death syndrome: Diagnostic coding shifts, controversies regarding sleep environment and new variables to consider in reducing risk. *Pediatrics, 116,* 1245–1255.

American Academy of Pediatrics (AAP). (2007). What is the best way to take a child's temperature? Retrieved from www.aap.org/puliced/BR_Fevere.htm

American Academy of Pediatrics (AAP). (2008). Breastfeeding initiative. Retrieved from www.aap.org/breastfeeding (Accessed April 15, 2008).

American Dental Association (ADA). (2007). Early childhood tooth decay. www.ada.org

Association of Women's Health, Obstetric and Neonatal Nursing. (AWHONN) (2001). *Neonatal skin care.* Washington, DC: Association of Women's Health, Obstetrics and Neonatal Nursing.

Association of Women's Health, Obstetric and Neonatal Nursing. (AWHONN). (2006). *The compendium of postpartum care.* Philadelphia: Medical Broadcasting Company.

Association of Women's Health, Obstetric and Neonatal Nursing. (AWHONN). (2007). *Breastfeeding support: Prenatal care through the first year. evidence-based clinical practice guideline* (2nd ed). Washington, DC: Author.

Biancuzzo, M. (1999). *Breastfeeding the newborn.* St. Louis: C. V. Mosby.

Bryanton, J., Walsh, D., Barrett, M., & Gaudet, D. (2004). Tub bathing versus traditional sponge bathing for newborns. *JOGGN, 33,* 704–712.

Chantry, C., Howard, C., & McCoy, R. (2003). *Protocol #5: Peripartum breastfeeding management for the healthy mother and infant at term.* The Academy of Breastfeeding Medicine. Retrieved from www.bfmed.org

Lewallen, L., Dick, M., Flowers, J., Powell, W., Zickefoose, K., Wall, Y., & Price, Z. (2006). Breastfeeding support and early cessation. *JOGNN, 35,* 166–172.

Mulder, P. (2006). A concept analysis of effective breastfeeding. *JOGNN, 35,* 332–339.

National Center on Shaken Baby Syndrome. (2008). *What is shaken baby syndrome.* Retrieved from www.dontshake.com (Accessed April 5, 2008).

National Institute of Neurological Disorders and Strokes (NINDS). (2007). *NINDS shaken baby syndrome information page.* Retrieved from www.ninds.nih.gov/disorders/shakenbaby/shakenbaby.htm

Owen, C., Martin, R., Whinsup, P., Smith, G., & Cook, D. (2005). Effect of infant feeding on the risk of obesity across the life course: A quantitative review of published evidence. *Pediatrics, 115,* 1367–1377.

Purnell, L., & Paulanka, B. (2008). *Guide to culturally competent health care.* Philadelphia: F. A. Davis.

U.S. Department of Health and Human Services (DHHS). (2000a). *Breastfeeding: HHS blueprint for action on breastfeeding.* Retrieved from www.womanshealth.gov/breastfeeding/bluprntbk2.pdf

U.S. Department of Health and Human Services (DHHS). (2000b). *Healthy people 2010* [online]. Retrieved from www.healthypeople.gov/Document/HTML/Volume2/16MICH.htm

Walker, M., & Creehan, P. (2001). Newborn nutrition. In K. Simpson & P. Creehan. *AWHONN perinatal nursing* (2nd ed.). Philadelphia: Lippincott.

Wilkinson, J., & Van Leuven, K. (2007). *Fundamentals of nursing.* Philadelphia: F. A. Davis.

World Health Organization (WHO). (2008). *Breastfeeding.* Retrieved from www.who.int/topics/breastfeeding (Accessed April 15, 2008).

High-Risk Neonatal Nursing Care

17

OBJECTIVES

On completion of this chapter, the student will be able to:

☐ Define key terms.

☐ Describe the physiology and pathophysiology associated with selected complications of the neonatal period.

☐ Identify critical elements of assessment and nursing care of the high-risk neonate.

☐ Develop a discharge plan for high-risk neonates.

☐ Describe the loss and grief process experienced by parents whose infant has died.

Nursing Diagnoses

■ Impaired gas exchange related to inadequate surfactant and immature lung tissue

■ Risk for ineffective airway clearance related to meconium aspiration

■ Ineffective thermoregulation related to prematurity, lack of subcutaneous fat, and environmental temperature

■ Imbalanced nutrition related to prematurity; inability to absorb nutrients; decreased perfusion to gastrointestinal tract; postnatal change from high glucose exposure to low glucose exposure and hyperinsulinism; cleft lip/cleft palate

■ Risk for infection related to prematurity, exposure to infectious agents, and maternal chorioamnionitis

■ Pain related to procedures; birth trauma

■ Risk for injury related to lack of oxygen to the brain; prolonged ventilation and oxygen administration; effects of drugs on fetal/neonatal growth and development; birth trauma; hypoglycemia; asphyxia; meconium aspiration; kernicterus

■ Risk for ineffective parent/family coping related to infant illness or death

■ Grieving related to the infant with a high-risk condition; loss of the dream of the perfect infant, death of the infant

■ Risk for impaired parent–infant attachment related to separation

Nursing Outcomes

■ The infant exhibits a breathing pattern within normal limits with respiratory rate between 30 and 60 breaths per minute with no signs of respiratory distress.

■ The infant maintains temperature within normal limits.

■ The infant gains weight, consumes adequate nutritional intake, has adequate output, and is free of signs of hypoglycemia or malnutrition.

■ The infant remains free of signs of infection; the white blood cell count is within normal limits.

■ The infant exhibits decreased signs of pain after receiving nonpharmacological or pharmacological pain reduction interventions.

■ The infant is free of signs of injury.

■ Parents communicate needs, state ability to cope, identify a support system, and ask for help and information when needed.

■ Parents identify what to expect during the grieving process.

■ Parents visit the infant in the nursery, demonstrate caregiving behaviors, express interest in the newborn, and respond to the infant's behavioral cues.

INTRODUCTION

Infant mortality rates in the United States have significantly decreased from 47.0 per 1,000 live births in 1940 to 6.76 per 1,000 in 2004 (Kochanek & Holditch-Davis, 2004; Minino et al., 2006). Although this is a significant decrease, the infant mortality rate, which indicates that 27,838 infants died in 2004, is too high for a nation with the amount of available wealth and resources that the United States possesses. One of the primary causes of illness and death in the neonate is complications related to prematurity.

This chapter provides an overview of the critical components of care of the high-risk neonate, which is a subspecialty of maternity nursing. Nurses who elect to work in a neonatal intensive care nursery will need to gain an in-depth knowledge of high-risk neonates through additional readings and classes that focus on the unique needs of high-risk neonates and their parents.

PRETERM NEONATES

Period of gestation and birth weight are the two most important predictors of an infant's health and survival. Preterm neonates and neonates with low birth weights are at higher risk of death as well as long-term and short-term disabilities than neonates born at term or with a birth weight of 2500 grams or more (Matthews & MacDorman, 2008). Prematurity is classified as:

- **Very premature**: Neonates born at less than 32 weeks' gestation (Fig. 17-1)
- **Premature**: Neonates born between 32 and 34 weeks' gestation
- **Late premature**: Neonates born between 34 and 37 weeks' gestation

The number of premature births has risen from 10.6% of live births in 1990 to 12.7% in 2005 (Hamilton et al., 2006).

- The greatest increase is in late premature births, which increased by 1.8% between 1990 and 2005 (Table 17-1).
- The percentage of premature births based on the race of the mother are:
  - *Non-Hispanic black: 18.4%*
  - *American Indian or Alaska Native: 14.1%*
  - *Hispanic: 12.1%*
  - *Non-Hispanic white: 11.7%*
  - *Asian or Pacific Islander: 10.8% (Hamilton et al., 2006)*
- Prematurity is a primary reason for low birth weight. Classification of birth weight (regardless of gestational age) is as follows:
  - *Low birth weight: Less than 2500 grams at birth*
  - *Very low birth weight: Less than 1500 grams at birth*
  - *Extremely low birth weight: Less than 1000 grams at birth*

Multiple factors place a woman at risk for preterm labor and birth. Many are modifiable, and many are not (Table 17-2). Common complications related to prematurity are respiratory distress syndrome, retinopathy of prematurity, bronchopulmonary dysplasia, patent ductus arteriosus, periventricular–intraventricular hemorrhage, and necrotizing enterocolitis (NEC).

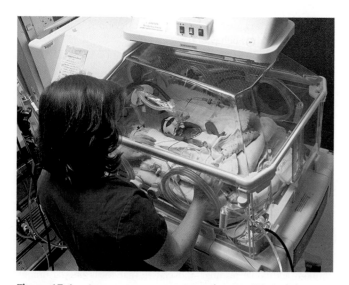

Figure 17-1 A very premature neonate born at 27 weeks' gestation.

TABLE 17–1	PERCENTAGE OF PRETERM BIRTHS	
	1990	2005
VERY PRETERM	1.9	2.0
PRETERM	1.4	1.6
LATE PRETERM	7.3	9.1

Source: Hamilton, Martin, & Ventura (2006).

Assessment Findings

- Gestational age by Ballard score is at or below 37 weeks.
- Physical characteristics vary based on gestational age (Fig. 17-2)
  - *Tone and flexion increase with greater gestational age. Early in gestation resting tone and posture are hypotonic and extended.*
  - *The skin is translucent, transparent, and red.*
  - *Subcutaneous fat is decreased.*
  - *Lanugo is present between 20 and 28 weeks' gestation. At 28 weeks' gestation, lanugo begins to disappear on the face and the front of the trunk.*
  - *Creases on the anterior part of the foot are not present until 28 to 30 weeks. As gestation increases, plantar creases increase and spread toward the heel of the foot.*
  - *Eyelids fused in very preterm neonates. Eyelids open between 26 and 30 weeks' gestation.*
  - *Overriding sutures are common among premature, low birth weight neonates.*
  - *The pinna of the ear is thin, soft, flat, and folded.*
  - *The testes are normally not descended, and are found in the inguinal canal.*
  - *Tremors and jittery movement may be noted.*
  - *The cry is weak.*
  - *Reflexes may be diminished or absent.*
  - *Immature suck, swallow, and breathing pattern is observed in very premature infants. These neonates may not be able to take adequate oral feedings.*
- **Apnea,** cessation of breathing for at least 10 to 15 seconds, and **bradycardia,** heart rate less than 100 beats per minute, are commonly observed (Goodwin, 2004).
- Hypotension may occur among extremely low birth weight infants.
- Heart murmur may be present related to patent ductus arteriosus.
- Anemia is common, especially among very low birth weight babies (Aher & Ohlsson, 2006).

Medical Management

- Determine lung maturity with lecithin/sphingomyelin (L/S) ratio or phosphatidylglycerol (PG) before elective induction or cesarean birth, and for women in preterm labor.
- Corticosteroids, betamethasone or dexamethasone, are administered to the pregnant woman, if the woman presents in preterm labor, or if preterm birth is anticipated. Evidence suggests that corticosteroid administration results in reduced respiratory distress syndrome, NEC, cerebroventricular hemorrhage, need for respiratory support, systemic infections, admission to the NICU, and neonatal death (Roberts & Dalziel, 2006).
- Continuous pulse oximetry

TABLE 17–2   RISK FACTORS FOR PRETERM LABOR AND BIRTH

NONMODIFIABLE RISK FACTORS	TREATABLE/MODIFIABLE RISK FACTORS

Previous preterm birth
Multiple abortions
Race/ethnic group
Uterine/cervical anomaly
Multiple gestation
Polyhydramnios
Oligohydramnios
Pregnancy induced hypertension
Placenta previa (after 22 weeks)
DES exposure
Short interval between pregnancies
Abruptio placenta
Parity (0 or >4)
Premature rupture of membranes
Bleeding in first trimester
	Age at pregnancy <17 or >34 years
	Unplanned pregnancy
	Single
	Low educational level
	Poverty, unsafe environment
	Domestic violence
	Life stress
	Number of implanted embryos in assisted
	  reproduction
	Low pre-pregnancy weight
	Obesity
	Health problems that can be treated: hyper-
	  tension, diabetes, clotting problems, anemia.
	Incompetent cervix
	Genitourinary infection
	Infection
	Periodontal disease
	Substance/alcohol use
	Cigarette smoking
	Long hours of employment/standing
	Late or no prenatal care
	Air pollution

Source: Moore (2003).

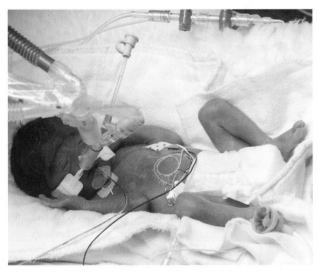

Figure 17-2   A 27 week gestation neonate.

- Cardiac monitoring, oxygen saturation, arterial blood gases, and end CO_2.
- Provide respiratory support.
  - *Nasal continuous positive airway pressure (NCPAP) or intubation*
- Order laboratory tests
  - *Bilirubin levels for neonates who are jaundiced*
  - *Blood cultures for neonates with signs of infection*
  - *Complete blood count with differential*
  - *Electrolytes*
  - *Blood glucose*
  - *Calcium, bicarbonate, blood urea nitrogen (BUN), creatinine, phosphorus, magnesium, triglycerides, albumin, protein, liver*

function, urine glucose, and ketones for neonates on total parenteral nutrition (Bakewell-Sachs & Brandes, 2004)
- Medications
  - *Sodium bicarbonate to treat metabolic acidosis if present*
  - *Dopamine or dobutamine for treatment of hypotension*
  - *Erythropoietin administration to stimulate production of red blood cells if indicated*
    - Evidence suggests that erythropoietin administration reduced the need for red blood cell transfusions among preterm/low birth weight infants (Aher & Ohlsson, 2006).
  - *Antibiotic therapy as indicated for decreasing risk of infection or treatment of infection*
  - *Opioids to treat pain associated with procedures that cause moderate to severe pain such as with surgical procedures*
- Blood transfusion if the neonate is anemic, or to replace blood loss due to laboratory tests, or blood loss during birth (Maguire, 2004)
- Intravenous fluids as indicated
- Parenteral (intravenous) nutrition if indicated by the neonate's gestational age and/or clinical condition
- Central line if long-term parenteral nutrition is required
- Umbilical artery and umbilical vein catheters
- Provide parents with information about their neonate's condition, treatment plan, and follow-up care.

Nursing Actions

- Review prenatal, intrapartal, and neonatal history.
- Participate in resuscitation of the neonate as indicated.
  - *The NICU nurse, neonatologist, and/or neonatal nurse practitioner should be present at high-risk births.*
- Transfer the neonate to the neonatal intensive care unit.
- Perform gestational assessment to determine age and size of neonate.

■ Perform a physical assessment, evaluating for problems associated with prematurity.
■ Assess for signs of respiratory distress.
■ Assess cardiovascular system:
  ■ *Signs of patent ductus arteriosus*
  ■ *Murmurs*
  ■ *Pulses*
  ■ *Assess capillary refill.*
■ Apply transcutaneous monitor or pulse oximeter to monitor O_2 levels.
■ Monitor vital signs, oxygen saturation, arterial blood gases, and end CO_2 as per orders.
■ Assess for signs of NEC such as abnormal vital signs, abdominal distention (increase in abdominal circumference), abdominal discoloration, bowel loops, feeding intolerance, emesis, residuals, bloody stools, and behavioral changes.
■ Assess response to interventions. These responses may be changes in breathing, oxygen saturation, vital signs, and neonatal behavior.
■ Assess for signs of jaundice.
■ Obtain laboratory test as per orders.
■ Provide respiratory support.
  ■ *Maintain a patent airway.*
  ■ *Administer oxygen as ordered.*
    ■ Short-term oxygen administration may be given using a mask.
    ■ Long-term oxygen administration may be given using nasal cannula, oxygen hood, NCPAP, or ventilator.
    ■ Oxygen is humidified and warmed.
  ■ *Suction airway as needed for removal of secretions.*
■ Maintain neutral thermal environment by:
  ■ *Drying the infant gently immediately after birth to prevent heat loss from evaporation*
  ■ *Keeping the head covered*
  ■ *Using plastic barriers made of polyethylene to cover preterm neonates after birth to prevent heat loss and transepidermal water loss*
    ■ Extremely low birth weight (ELBW) neonates are at high risk for cold stress during the period immediately after birth (Knobel & Holditich-Davis, 2007). Neonates placed in plastic barriers immediately after birth had higher admission temperatures compared to nonwrapped neonates (Cramer, Wiebe, Hartling, Crumley, & Vohra, 2005).
  ■ *Prewarming radiant warmers, incubators, and linens*
  ■ *Controlling environmental temperature with use of servo control. A temperature control probe should be placed on the neonate's abdomen, to assist in maintaining the neonate's temperature within the normal range (axillary 97.4°–98.4°F [36.3°–36.9°C] for premature neonates)*
  ■ *Placing the neonate in a double-walled incubator to prevent transepidermal water loss and heat loss*
  ■ *Encouraging kangaroo care (skin-to-skin care) in stable neonates*
  ■ *Weaning infants gradually from incubator to an open crib (AWHONN & NANN, 2001; Maguire, 2004; McCall, Alderdice, Halliday, Jenkins, & Vohra, 2005; Sinclair & Sinn, 2007).*
■ Administer medications as per order.
■ Provide skin care:
  ■ *The skin of the preterm neonate is predisposed to injury related to it being thin and fragile. It is important to carefully assess for skin breakdown and signs of infection (Fig. 17-3) (AWHONN & NANN, 2001).*
    ■ Refer to Figure 17-3, a skin assessment tool developed by Association of Women's Health, Obstetric and Neonatal Nurses (AWHONN).
  ■ *Quick Care Guide Neonatal Skin Care, an evidence-based document developed by Association of Women's Health, Obstetric and*

AWHONN/NANN RBP4 NEONATAL SKIN CONDITION SCORE (NSCS)
Dryness
1 = Normal, no sign of dry skin 2 = Dry skin, visible scaling 3 = Very dry skin, cracking/fissures
Erythema
1 = No evidence of erythema 2 = Visible erythema, <50% body surface 3 = Visible erythema, ≥50% body surface
Breakdown/excoriation
1 = None evident 2 = Small, localized areas 3 = Extensive
Note: Perfect score = 3, worst score = 9

This scoring system, developed for the AWHONN/NANN Neonatal Skin Care Project (RBP4) was adapted from a visual scoring system used in a previous study (Lane and Drost, 1993). It can facilitate assessment of neonatal skin condition. This tool continues to undergo reliability and validity testing.

Figure 17-3   Neonatal Skin Condition Score.

Neonatal Nurses, summarizes skin care for infants of all ages (see Appendix A).
■ Provide cardiovascular support.
  ■ *Monitor blood pressure, oxygen saturation, and arterial blood gases.*
  ■ *Obtain and monitor hemoglobin and hematocrit as per order.*
  ■ *Administer blood transfusion as per order.*
■ Maintain fluid and electrolyte balance.
  ■ *Monitor input and output carefully by:*
    ■ Weighing diapers to determine output
    ■ Assessing frequency, color, amount, and specific gravity of urine
    ■ Recording fluid intake and output: nasal and oral gastric tubes, chest tubes, Foley catheter, stomas
  ■ *Restrict fluid intake as per order. Fluid restriction is commonly ordered for neonates with bronchopulmonary dysplasia (BPD) and patent ductus arteriosus (PDA) or other complications that can lead to pulmonary edema.*
  ■ *Monitor electrolyte levels as per order.*
    ■ Hyperkalemia (elevated potassium levels), hyponatremia (low sodium level), and hypernatremia (high sodium level) may occur among low birth weight infants (Maguire, 2004).
  ■ *Administer intravenous fluids as per order.*
    ■ Closely monitor the site of intravenous access for signs of infection, skin breakdown, and infiltration.
  ■ *Add humidity to the neonate's environment to decrease water loss that can occur through the neonate's immature skin, known as* **transepidermal water loss (TEWL)**.
    ■ Humidity added to the environment prevents heat loss, improves skin integrity, decreases TEWL, and promotes electrolyte balance (Maguire, 2004; Sinclair & Sinn, 2007).
■ Meet the neonate's nutrition requirements.

■ *Obtain and monitor blood glucose levels as per order.*

■ *Administer parenteral nutrition (intravenous) if the neonate is unable to receive enteral (via gastrointestinal tract) feedings.*

■ Extremely low birth weight neonates (<1500 grams) or neonates less than 32 weeks' gestation:

■ *May lack the ability to digest and absorb feedings*

■ *May have an inability to suck, swallow, and breathe*

■ *Will most likely require parenteral nutrition (Maguire, 2004).*

■ The dextrose content is titrated based on the serum glucose level (Maguire, 2004).

■ *Administer **trophic feedings** (small volume enteral feedings) as per order. They are often given while neonates are receiving parenteral feedings to ease the transition to full enteral feedings, and enhance gastrointestinal functioning (Maguire, 2004; Tyson & Kennedy, 2005).*

■ *Administer enteral feedings orally or by gastric tube (gavage feedings) depending on the infant's gestational age and clinical condition. Most neonates who are older than 34 weeks' gestation usually receive oral feedings soon after birth.*

■ Human milk is preferred for enteral feeding.

■ Human milk requires fortification because it does not provide the calories, protein, calcium, sodium, and phosphorus that the premature infant needs (Bakewell-Sachs & Brandes, 2004).

■ Formulas developed specifically for preterm infants are available. These formulas are modified to promote absorption and digestion for babies with immature gastrointestinal functioning, and contain the extra calories, protein, minerals, and vitamins required by preterm babies (Bakewell-Sachs & Brandes, 2004).

■ Use proper technique for gavage feedings.

■ When feedings are initiated and before each feeding, assess for signs of feeding tolerance as follows (Bakewell-Sachs & Brandes, 2004):

■ *Check for the presence of bowel sounds.*

■ *Assess the abdomen for bowel loops.*

■ *Measure abdominal girth.*

■ *Check for gastric residuals by aspirating stomach contents with the syringe. Note the amount, color, and consistency of the contents.*

■ *Assess for emesis.*

■ *Check stools for occult blood as per order.*

■ *Check stools for reducing substances as per order.*

■ *Assess stools for consistency, amount, and frequency.*

■ Use nonnutritive sucking with a pacifier during gavage feedings (Pinelli & Symington, 2005). Nonnutritive sucking eases the transition from gavage feeding to bottle feeding, and results in decreased length of hospital stay for preterm neonates (Pinelli & Symington, 2005).

■ Monitor weight daily. Weight gain of 10 to 20 grams per kilogram per day indicates appropriate growth and caloric intake for a preterm neonate (Bakewell-Sachs & Brandes, 2004).

■ Monitor length and head circumference weekly.

■ Calculate and monitor intake of fluids, calories, and protein daily (Bakewell-Sachs & Brandes, 2004). Preterm infants require between 105 and 130 kcal/kg/day.

■ Transition the neonate from tube feedings to oral feedings.

■ *Transitioning to oral feedings occurs when the neonate is:*

■ Free of signs of respiratory distress

■ Able to coordinate suck, swallow, and breathe

■ Bowel sounds are present (Bakewell-Sachs & Brandes, 2004)

CRITICAL COMPONENT

Procedure for Gavage Feeding

Gavage feedings are appropriate for neonates who are <32 weeks' gestation or who cannot safely receive oral feedings.

1. Use a size 5 to 8 french feeding tube.

2. Measure the tube (used for orogastric route) from the mouth to the ear, and from the ear to the lower end of the sternum.

3. Check for proper placement of the tube after each insertion and before each feeding by:

■ Placing syringe on end of tube and pulling to remove stomach contents, and/or

■ Injecting a small amount of air into the tube with a syringe while listening for a whooshing/gurgling sound with a stethoscope placed on the neonate's abdomen.

4. Use tape to ensure that the tube is secured.

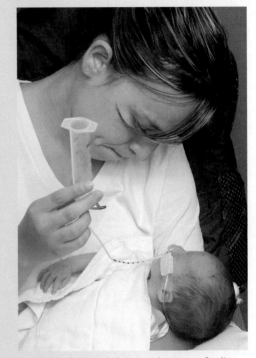

Mother feeding helping with gavage feeding

5. Check for residuals before starting the feeding by aspirating stomach contents with the syringe. Note the amount, color, and consistency of the contents.

6. Feedings may be given by gravity or pump over 15–30 minutes.

7. In some cases continuous tube feedings may be ordered.

8. To remove the tube after the feeding, pinch it closed and remove it swiftly.

9. Assess the neonate for feeding intolerance throughout feeding.

(Bakewell-Sachs & Brandes, 2004)

■ *Properly position the neonate for bottle feeding by holding the swaddled baby in a semiupright or upright position.*

■ *Observe the neonate closely for respiratory status, apnea, bradycardia, oxygenation, and feeding tolerance.*

■ *Pace feeding and allow for breathing breaks since preterm neonates may become fatigued during feedings.*

■ Support breastfeeding.
  ■ *Evidence suggests that breast milk decreases the incidence of NEC (Caplin, 2006; Cincinnati Children's Medical Center, 2005).*
  ■ *During the period of time that the neonate is unable to breastfeed, instruct the mother in the use of a breast pump and storage of breast milk.*
  ■ *Encourage the mother to bring breast milk to the NICU so that it can be used for enteral feedings for her infant.*
  ■ *Teach the mother about feeding cues, breastfeeding positions, correct latch, and evaluating the feeding.*
  ■ *Weigh the neonate before and after breastfeeding to monitor intake.*
  ■ *See Appendix B for additional nursing actions.*
■ Manage pain.
  ■ *Assess the neonate for signs of pain frequently, and especially during painful procedures. Instruments to measure neonatal pain among preterm neonates are available and should be integrated into routine care.*
  ■ *Administer sucrose and promote nonnutritive sucking during painful procedures.*
  ■ *Administer opioids as per orders to treat pain associated with procedures that cause moderate to severe pain.*
  ■ *Evaluate the effectiveness of nonpharmacological and pharmacological interventions.*

Evidence-Based Practice: Sucrose for Analgesia

Stevens, B., Yamada, J., & Ohlsson, A. (2007). Sucrose for analgesia in newborn infants undergoing painful procedures. *The Cochrane Database of Systematic Reviews, 3.*

A systematic review of the research literature was conducted to determine the effective use of sucrose for reducing neonatal pain during potentially painful procedures. Conclusion of the review is that nonnutritive sucking and sucrose administration diminish neonatal pain during procedures such as heel sticks and venipuncture.

■ Provide developmentally appropriate care to decrease stress on neonate by:
  ■ *Maintaining a quiet setting*
  ■ *Keeping lighting dim and changing lighting in NICU to simulate night and day*
  ■ *Clustering nursing activities to provide for extended periods of sleep*
  ■ *Avoiding clustering painful interventions together*
  ■ *Providing care when the neonate is awake*
  ■ *Providing individualized care based on the neonate's responses and needs*
  ■ *Allowing a break in care/stimulation if neonate becomes stressed*
  ■ *Minimizing handling for neonates who are in an unstable condition*
  ■ *Positioning and swaddling*
    ■ Change the neonate's position slowly and gently.
    ■ Reposition every 2 to 3 hours. Assess the infant's response to repositioning.
    ■ Position neonate in the side lying or prone position (enhances oxygenation, and gastric emptying).
    ■ The head of the bed may be elevated 15 degrees.
    ■ Swaddle in flexion with arms and hands placed toward the infant's midline.
    ■ Create a nest with blankets to enhance containment. Avoid swaddling or nesting that is overly restrictive to

neonatal movement (Carrier, 2004; Goodwin, 2004; Maguire, 2004).
■ Encourage kangaroo care (skin-to-skin care with the parents) for medically stable neonates. Benefits of kangaroo care are:
  ■ *Decreases risk of low body temperature (McCall, Alderdice, Halliday, Jenkins, & Vohra, 2005)*
  ■ *Reduces illness, infection, and breastfeeding difficulties (Anderson, Moore, Hepworth, & Bergman, 2003; Conde-Agudelo, Diaz-Rossello, & Belizan, 2003).*
  ■ *Improves daily weight gain and mother–infant attachment*
  ■ *Decreases the length of hospital stay (Conde-Agudelo, Diaz-Rossello, & Belizan, 2003)*
■ Provide emotional support to parents and family members.
■ Involve parents and family in all aspects of the infant's care.
  ■ *Teach parents what to expect from their preterm infant and how to interpret behavioral cues.*
  ■ *Teach parents how to provide care for their infant (Fig. 17-4).*
  ■ *Encourage parent-infant bonding by welcoming them to the NICU and praising them for their involvement with their infant.*
  ■ *Teach parents about the infant's condition and involve them in the plan of care.*
■ Prepare the family for the neonate's discharge by:
  ■ *Teaching parents about infant feeding*
  ■ *Teaching about use of any equipment such as apnea monitors that may be needed to care for their infant at home*
  ■ *Teaching parents how to perform treatments such as dressing changes, suctioning, and oxygen administration*
  ■ *Teaching parents about medication administration*
  ■ *Teaching parents about safety issues such as car seat use, and positioning the infant on his or her back during sleep*
  ■ *Encouraging parents to learn infant CPR*
  ■ *Teaching parents about basic newborn care*
  ■ *Educating parents on what to expect after discharge, such as sleep patterns, feeding, infant behavior, and developmental milestones*
  ■ *Discussing follow-up care such as physician's visits, immunization schedules, and appointments for developmental care*

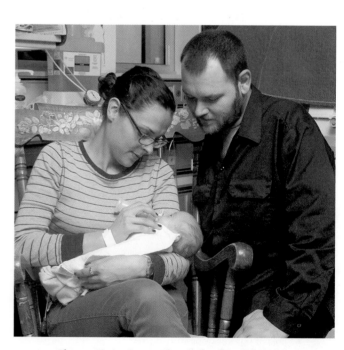

Figure 17-4   Parents bottle feeding their baby.

Respiratory Distress Syndrome

Respiratory distress syndrome (RDS) is a life-threatening lung disorder that results from underdeveloped and small alveoli and insufficient levels of pulmonary surfactant. It was the seventh leading cause of infant deaths with a mortality rate of 21.3 per 100,000 live births in 2004 (Minino, Heron, & Smith, 2006). These two combined factors can cause an alteration in alveoli surface tension that eventually results in atelectasis. The effects of atelectasis are:

■ Hypoxemia and hypercarbia
■ Pulmonary artery vasoconstriction.
■ Right-to-left shunting through the ductus arteriosus and foramen ovale as the neonate's body attempts to counteract the compromised pulmonary perfusion
■ Metabolic acidosis that occurs from a buildup of lactic acid that results from prolonged periods of hypoxemia
■ Respiratory acidosis that occurs from the collapsed alveoli being unable to rid the body of excess carbon dioxide

The risk of RDS decreases with increasing gestational age. It occurs in:

■ 60% of neonates born before 28 weeks' gestation
■ 30% born between 28 and 34 weeks' gestation
■ Less than 5% born after 34 weeks' gestation (American Lung Association, 2006)

Pulmonary surfactant is a substance that is composed of 90% phospholipids and 10% proteins.

■ It is produced by type II alveolar cells within the lungs.
■ The alveolar cells begin to produce pulmonary surfactant around 24 to 28 weeks and continue to term.
■ It reduces the surface tension within the lungs and increases the pulmonary compliance which prevents the alveoli from collapsing at the end of expiration. Surfactant replacement therapy is discussed later in this chapter.

Tests used to evaluate fetal lung maturity are:

■ Phosphatidylglycerol (PG):
  ■ *PG is synthesized from mature lung alveolar cells.*
  ■ *It is present in the amniotic fluid within 2 to 6 weeks of full-term gestation.*
  ■ *The presence of PG indicates lung maturity and a decreased risk of respiratory distress syndrome.*
■ Lecithin/sphingomyelin (L/S) ratio:
  ■ *Lecithin and sphingomyelin are two phospholipids that are detected in the amniotic fluid.*
  ■ *The ratio between the two phospholipids provides information on the level of surfactant.*
  ■ *A L/S ratio is greater than 2:1 in a nondiabetic woman, indicating the fetus's lungs are mature.*
  ■ *A L/S ratio of 3:1 in a diabetic woman indicates the fetus's lungs are mature.*

Complications of respiratory distress syndrome (RDS) include:

■ Patent ductus arteriosus
■ Pneumothorax
■ Bronchopulmonary hypertension
■ Pulmonary edema
■ Hypotension
■ Anemia
■ Oliguria
■ Hypoglycemia and altered calcium and sodium levels
■ Retinopathy of prematurity

■ Seizures
■ Intraventricular hemorrhage

Assessment Findings

■ Respiratory distress varies based on degree of prematurity.
■ Respiratory difficulty begins shortly after delivery and the neonate must work progressively harder at breathing to maintain open terminal airways (Zukowsky, 2004).
■ Tachypnea is present.
■ Intercostal retractions; seesaw breathing patterns occur.
■ Expiratory grunting.
■ Nasal flaring is present.
■ Increased oxygen requirements are increased to maintain a PaO_2 and $PaCO_2$ within normal limits.
  ■ *The normal range of PaO_2 is 60 to 70 mm Hg.*
  ■ *The normal range of $PaCO_2$ is 35 to 45 mm Hg.*
■ Skin color is gray or dusky.
■ Breath sounds on auscultation are decreased. Rales are present as RDS progresses.
■ The neonate is lethargic and hypotonic.
■ X-ray exam shows a reticulogranular pattern of the peripheral lung fields and air bronchograms (Ghodrat, 2006).
■ Hypoxemia may occur (PaO_2 <50 mm Hg).
■ Acidosis may result from sustained hypoxemia.

Medical Management

■ Continuous pulse oximetry
■ Cardiac monitoring, oxygen saturation, arterial blood gases, and end CO_2
■ Endotracheal tube when clinically indicated
■ Exogenous surfactant as indicated for neonates at risk for RDS or with RDS
■ Respiratory support as indicated. The mode of ventilation and settings are based on the neonate's condition and arterial blood gas results. The PaO_2 should be maintained in the normal range of 50 to 70 mm Hg and a pulse oximetry reading of 90% (Maguire, 2004). Methods of respiratory support include:
  ■ *Oxygen therapy by mask, hood, or cannula for neonates requiring short-term oxygen support*
  ■ *Continuous positive airway pressure (CPAP) used for neonates who are at risk for RDS or with RDS. It can be administered by mask, nasal prongs, endotracheal tube, or nasopharyngeal route.*
  ■ *Mechanical ventilation used when CPAP is not effective (use judiciously to avoid damage to lung tissue)*
  ■ *High-frequency oscillatory ventilation used when mechanical ventilation has proven unsuccessful*
    ■ Delivers small volumes of gas at a high rate (>300 breaths/minutes)
    ■ Less traumatic on fragile lung tissue
  ■ *Extracorporeal membrane oxygenation therapy (ECMO) is a cardiopulmonary bypass machine with a membrane oxygenator that is used when the neonate does not respond to conventional ventilator therapy. Blood shuts from the right atrium and returned to aorta, allowing time for lungs to heal and mature.*
■ Diagnostic tests
  ■ *Chest x-ray exam to assist in evaluation of RDS*
■ Laboratory tests
  ■ *Arterial blood gases*
  ■ *Blood cultures if infection is suspected*
■ Medications
  ■ *Antibiotics as indicated*

CRITICAL COMPONENT

Surfactant Replacement Therapy Administration

Natural Surfactant

- Composed of calf, pig or cow lung combined with lipids
- Examples: Survanta, Curosurf, Infasurf

Synthetic Surfactant

- Example: Exosurf

Action

- Reduces surface tension of the alveoli, thus preventing collapse during expiration
- Enhances lung compliance, allowing easier inflation which decreases the work of breathing

Indications: Respiratory distress, meconium aspiration syndrome, persistent pulmonary hypertension
Route: Administered via endotracheal tube
Dosing regimen (dose and technique vary by product):

- Prophylaxis: Initiated within 15 minutes of birth, based on risk factors of RDS such as gestational age less than 27-30 weeks. Multiple doses can be given if indicated.
- Rescue therapy: Treatment of confirmed RDS. Treatment is typically initiated within 8 hours of birth for infants who have increased oxygen demands and need mechanical ventilation.

Adverse Effects

- Bradycardia, decreased oxygen saturation, tachycardia, reflux, gagging, cyanosis, blockage of the endotracheal tube, hypotension

Benefits of Surfactant Therapy

- Prophylactic therapy decreases the occurrence of RDS and mortality in preterm neonates
- Decreased risk of pneumothorax
- Decreased risk of intraventricular hemorrhage
- Decreased risk of bronchopulmonary dysplasia
- Decreased risk of pulmonary interstitial emphysema

(Ghodrat, 2006)

Nursing Actions

Nursing actions for neonates with RDS are similar to actions for preterm neonates, with additional emphasis on the following:

- Provide respiratory support.
  - *Maintain a patent airway.*
  - *Assess for correct placement of endotracheal tube if in place.*
  - *Administer oxygen as ordered.*
    - Short-term oxygen administration may be given using a mask or tubing.
    - Long-term oxygen administration may be given using nasal cannula or oxygen hood.
    - Oxygen is humidified and warmed.
  - *Administer and monitor continuous positive airway pressure (CPAP), mechanical ventilation, high-frequency oscillatory ventilation, and/or ECMO as per order.*
  - *Minimize oxygen demand by maintaining a neutral thermal environment, clustering care to decrease stress, and treating acidosis as clinically indicated and ordered.*
  - *Suction airway as needed for removal of secretions.*

- Monitor vital signs, oxygen saturation, arterial blood gases, and end CO_2 as per orders.
- Maintain neutral thermal environment to decrease risk of cold stress.
- Monitor intake and output.
- Monitor daily weights.

Bronchopulmonary Dysplasia

Bronchopulmonary dysplasia (BPD) is a chronic lung problem that affects neonates who have been treated with mechanical ventilation and oxygen for problems such as RDS. Neonates who are dependent on oxygen beyond 28 days of life and/or have been on mechanical ventilation are at risk for BPD. BPD leads to decreased lung compliance and pulmonary function secondary to fibrosis, atelectasis, increased pulmonary resistance, and overdistention of the lungs (Bancalari, 2006; Zukowsky, 2004). Pulmonary edema results from the increased pulmonary vascular resistance (Martin, Sosenko, & Bancalari, 2001). Long-term outcomes may include prolonged hospitalization, long-term oxygen therapy that may be required after discharge, cerebral palsy, retinopathy of prematurity, and hearing loss. Roughly 10% to 15% of infants with BPD will die during the first year of life (Zukowsky, 2004).

- Risk factors for BPD
  - *Prematurity*
  - *RDS*
  - *Oxygen toxicity*
  - *Intubation*
  - *Assisted ventilation with positive pressure*
  - *Lower gestational age and birth weight (<32 weeks)*
  - *Infection*
  - *Pulmonary vascular damage secondary to excessive fluid administration, right-to-left shunting associated to patent ductus arteriosus, and increased airway resistance (Bancalari, 2006)*
- Complications of BPD:
  - *Pneumonia, upper respiratory infection*
  - *Ear infections*
  - *Congestive heart failure*
  - *Developmental delays*
  - *Cerebral palsy*
  - *Hearing loss*
  - *Retinopathy of prematurity*
  - *Sudden death*

Assessment Findings

- Chest retractions
- Audible wheezing, rales, and rhonchi
- Hypoxia
- Respiratory acidosis
- Bronchospasm
- Difficulty weaning from ventilator or increased requirements for ventilator
- Intolerance to fluids: edema, decreased urinary output, and weight gain
- Chest x-ray exam results exhibit cardiomegaly, lung hyperinflation, and tissue damage (Zukowsky, 2004)

Medical Management

- Diagnostic tests
  - *Chest x-ray exam to assess for cardiomegaly, lung hyperinflation, and tissue damage*
  - *Echocardiogram if cardiac complications are suspected*

- Laboratory tests
  - *Electrolytes*
  - *Arterial blood gases*
- Medications
  - *Bronchodilators: Administered to reduce bronchoconstriction*
  - *Corticosteroids: Administered to reduce bronchospasm, edema, and inflammation of pulmonary tissue*
  - *Diuretics: Administered to treat fluid retention and decrease risk for pulmonary edema*
- Prophylaxes against respiratory syncytial virus, as infants with BPD are predisposed to this infection
- Chest physiotherapy
- Determine the method of respiratory assistance and oxygen therapy.
- Determine amount of fluid intake.
- Determine the method of feeding to meet the neonate's nutritional and caloric needs.

Nursing Actions

Nursing actions for neonates with BPD are similar to actions for preterm neonates with additional emphasis on the following:

- Provide chest physiotherapy as per order.
- Provide mechanical ventilation and oxygen administration as per orders.
  - *Gradually wean neonate from mechanical ventilation as per orders.*
- Administer medications as per orders.
- Monitor intake and output.
- Restrict fluid intake as per orders.

Patent Ductus Arteriosus

Patent ductus arteriosus (PDA) occurs when the ductus arteriosus remains open after birth (Fig. 17-5). Normally the ductus arteriosus closes shortly after birth, but prematurity may lead to delayed closure. The incidence of PDA among term neonates is 1:2,000 live births (Sadowski, 2004).

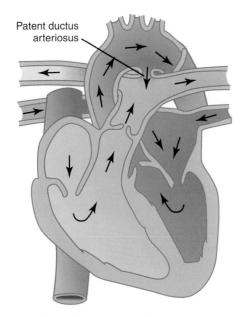

Patent ductus arteriosus

Figure 17-5   Patent ductus arteriosus.

- Risk factors for PDA
  - *Prematurity. The occurrence of PDA is greater among neonates of lower gestational age and birth weight.*
    - 45% of neonates who weigh less than 1750 grams
    - 80% of neonates who weigh less than 1200 grams at birth (Sadowski, 2004)
- Complications
  - *Congestive heart failure in preterm neonates*
  - *Chronic lung disease*
  - *Renal failure*
  - *NEC*
  - *Intraventricular hemorrhage (Malviya, Ohlsson, & Shah, 2003)*

Assessment Findings

- Heart murmur heard at the upper left sternal border (some neonates with PDA may not have an audible murmur)
- Apnea and bradycardia if the neonate is not on mechanical ventilation
- Bounding pulses
- Difficulty weaning from ventilator support
- Increased demand for oxygen or ventilation
- The presence of a patent ductus arteriosus confirmed by echocardiogram
- Chest x-ray exam may show increased pulmonary vasculature, pulmonary edema, and mild enlargement of the heart (Sadwoski, 2004).

Medical Management

- Diagnostic tests
  - *Echocardiogram to assist in evaluation of PDA*
- Medications
  - *Indomethacin, a prostaglandin inhibitor, is administered to facilitate the closure and reduces the risk for surgical intervention. It is also administered to decrease the risk of severe intraventricular hemorrhage (Fowlie & Davis, 2002).*
    - *Diuretics*
- Consultation with cardiologist to determine the method of treatment and need for surgical intervention
- Surgical ligation (suture, clip, or coil) of PDA is indicated for neonates with a hemodynamically significant PDA who do not respond to indomethacin.

Nursing Actions

Nursing actions for neonates with PDA are similar to actions for preterm neonates with additional emphasis on the following:

- Administer oxygen and mechanical ventilation as per orders.
- Monitor intake and output.
- Restrict fluids as per orders.
- Administer medications as per orders.
- Prepare the neonate and family for surgery.

Periventricular–Intraventricular Hemorrhage

Periventricular/Intraventricular hemorrhages (PVH/IVH) are common forms of intracranial hemorrhage in the neonate. They occur among premature neonates, neonates who experience RDS, and those who experience complications associated with ventilation such as pneumothorax, hypercarbia, and acidosis (Martin, Fanaroff, & Walsh, 2006). The incidence of PVH/IVH is:

- 30% among neonates born weighing less than 750 g
- 1% among neonates who weigh more than 1500 g (Badr & Purdy, 2006)

The occurrence of PVH/IVH is most common among neonates born between 24 and 28 weeks' gestation (Badr & Purdy, 2006). Very few full term neonates (2%–3%) have PVH/IVH (Lynam & Verklan, 2004). The majority of hemorrhages occur within the first week of life, with 90% occurring within 72 hours after birth (Lynam & Verklan, 2004; Martin, Fanaroff, & Walsh, 2006). There are four grades of intraventricular hemorrhage based on the extent of involvement; the higher the grade the higher the risk for long-term sequelae.

- Grade I: Hemorrhage in germinal matrix
- Grade II: Intraventricular hemorrhage without ventricular dilatation
- Grade III: Intraventricular hemorrhage with ventricular dilatation; clots fill more than 50% of the ventricle
- Grade IV: Extension of blood into cerebral tissue or parenchymal involvement
- Risk factors for PVH/IVH:
  - *Prematurity, birth at less than 34 weeks' gestation*
  - *Amniotic fluid infection*
  - *Perinatal asphyxia*
  - *RDS, or respiratory failure necessitating ventilatory support*
  - *Increased arterial pressure*
  - *Low 5-minute Apgar score*
  - *Maternal general anesthesia*
  - *Low birth weight*
  - *Alteration of blood pressure, either hypotension or hypertension*
  - *Acidosis, hypercarbia*
  - *Low hematocrit*
  - *Pneumothorax (Lynam & Verklan, 2006)*
- The long-term prognosis often depends on the severity of the hemorrhage and includes:
  - *A death rate of 5% for small hemorrhage, 15% for moderate hemorrhage, and 50% for severe hemorrhage*
  - *10% of neonates with a small hemorrhage, 40% with a moderate hemorrhage, and 80% with a severe hemorrhage will exhibit neurodevelopment problems such as cerebral palsy and delayed mental development.*
  - *Approximately 50% of premature infants do not experience neurological problems, and 25% to 30% of very low birth weight neonates who had PVH/IVH do not exhibit neurodevelopment problems (Lynam & Verklan, 2004).*

Assessment Findings

- Sudden change in condition
- Bradycardia
- Oxygen desaturation
- Hypotonia
- Metabolic acidosis
- Shock
- Decreased hematocrit
- Full and/or tense anterior fontanel
- Hyperglycemia (Lynam & Verklan, 2004)
- Signs that bleeding is worsening include:
  - *Apnea*
  - *Increased need for ventilator support*
  - *Drop in blood pressure*
  - *Acidosis*
  - *Seizures*
  - *Full and tense fontanels and rapid increase in head size*
  - *Diminished activity or level of consciousness (Lynam & Verlan, 2004)*

Medical Management

- Assess for signs of hemodynamic, neurological, and behavior changes.
- Diagnostic tests
  - *Cranial ultrasounds for all high-risk neonates within the first week of life to assess for PVH/IVH*
  - *Lumbar puncture to assist in evaluation of PVH/IVH. Cerebrospinal fluid is analyzed for red blood cells, xanthochromia, decreased glucose, and increased protein (Lynam & Verklan, 2004; Scher, 2001).*
  - *Electroencephalogram (EEG) to evaluate seizure activity*
- Laboratory tests
  - *Hemoglobin and hematocrit to evaluate extend of bleeding*
- Blood transfusions as indicated

Nursing Actions

Nursing actions for neonates with PVN/IVH are similar to actions for preterm neonates with additional emphasis on the following:

- Assess for changes in vital signs, behavior, and neurological status, which may indicate increase intracranial bleeding.
- Reduce stress to neonate by maintaining a quiet and dark environment.
- Administer fluid volume replacement slowly to minimize fluctuation in blood pressure.

Necrotizing Enterocolitis

Necrotizing enterocolitis (NEC) is a gastrointestinal disease that affects neonates. This disease results in inflammation and necrosis of the bowel, usually the proximal colon or terminal ileum (Watson, 2004). Preterm neonates are predisposed to NEC because of multiple factors including:

- Altered blood flow regulation, particularly to the intestines
- Impaired gastrointestinal host defense when faced with stress/injury to the intestinal tissue
- Alterations in the inflammatory response (Caplan, 2006)

The majority (90%) of NEC cases are among preterm neonates, 5% to 10% of cases occur in neonates who were born at 37 weeks or more gestation (Watson, 2004). In term neonates NEC is usually associated with a particular problem (e.g., asphyxia, intrauterine growth restriction) resulting in an ischemic episode in the bowel (Martin, Fanaroff, & Walsh, 2006). Causes of intestinal ischemia/asphyxia include hypotension, hypoxia, stress, low body temperature, hypovolemia, polycythemia, and patent ductus arteriosus (Watson, 2004).

- Risk factors for NEC
  - *Prematurity is the most common risk factor for NEC. Roughly 90% of cases occur among premature neonates.*
  - *Bacterial colonization can occur from contaminated nasogastric feeding tubes among premature neonates receiving formula.*
  - *Umbilical catheter placement (Martin, Fanaroff, & Walsh, 2006; Watson, 2004)*
- Long-term outcomes include:
  - *Approximately 30% of neonates with NEC will die.*
  - *30% will have mild NEC and recover with medical management.*
  - *An estimated 25% of neonates with NEC will develop bowel obstruction.*

- *Short bowel syndrome may occur in neonates who have had surgical treatment.*
- *Neurodevelopmental problems such as cerebral palsy may develop (Caplan, 2006).*

Assessment Findings

Symptoms typically begin between 3 and 10 days after birth.

- Apnea, bradycardia, and tachycardia
- Respiratory failure
- Hypoxemia
- Unstable temperature
- Hypotension, shock
- Abdominal distention, bloody stools, abdominal tenderness, vomiting, increased gastric residuals, discoloration of abdomen, visible bowel loops
- Lethargy
- Abnormally high or low white blood cell count, thrombocytopenia
- Abnormal electrolyte levels
- Metabolic acidosis
- Abdominal x-ray films of neonates of NEC may show distention of the intestines with gas; gas in one part of the intestine, and lack of gas in other parts; air in the wall of the intestine and/or the portal venous system; dilated loops of bowel; and air in abdomen (Watson, 2004).

Medical Management

- Diagnostic tests
    - *Abdominal x-ray exam to assist in evaluation of NEC*
- Laboratory tests
    - *Blood cultures to assess for infection related to perforation of bowel*
- Medications
    - *Antibiotics*
    - *Analgesia*
    - *Antihypertensives*
- Gastric decompression
- Intravenous fluids
- Surgical intervention for the removal of necrotic bowel, resection of bowel, or for perforation of bowel related to NEC. A temporary colostomy may be performed.

Nursing Actions

Nursing actions for neonates with NEC are similar to actions for preterm neonates with additional emphasis on the following:

- Assess for abdominal distention, emesis, and bloody stools.
- Monitor intake and output.
- Withhold feedings as per orders.
- Perform gastric decompression as per orders by placing an orogastric tube and connecting it to low suction.
- Prepare the neonate and family for surgery when indicated.

Retinopathy of Prematurity

Retinopathy of prematurity (ROP) occurs in premature neonates who are less than 28 weeks' gestation. Before this age, the retina is not completely vascularized and is susceptible to stress or injury (Phelps, 2006). If injury or exposure to a stressor occurs, the normal vascularization of the retina may be interrupted. Vasoproliferation, an abnormal growth of vasculature, occurs when tissue grows within the retina, or extends into the vitreous body. Ultimately, abnormal vascularization and associated bleeding, and fluid leakage, cause scar tissue that pulls and distorts the retina and displaces the macula (Phelps, 2006). It also causes retinal folds and can lead to retinal detachment (Phelps, 2006).

The incidence of ROP is related to gestational age and birth weight. The incidence of acute ROP is:

- 84% of neonates born at less than 28 weeks' gestation
- 90% of neonates weighing less than 750 g (Hendson, Phelps, & Anderson, 2002)

Long-term outcome for this disease depends on the extent of its progression, and ranges from full recovery to blindness (Phelps, 2006).

- Risk factors for ROP
    - *Prematurity and low birth weight are primary problems associated with ROP; the risk of ROP increases as gestational age and birth weight decrease.*
    - *Prolonged hyperoxia (exposure to high levels of oxygen), and duration of mechanical ventilation*
    - *Hypoxia, hypercapnia, hypocapnia, and acidosis*
    - *Shock; vitamin E deficiency*
    - *Infection/sepsis*
    - *Patent ductus arteriosus*
    - *Multiple gestation*
    - *Intraventricular hemorrhage*
    - *Blood transfusion*
    - *Maternal diabetes, bleeding, smoking, and hypertension (Askin & Deihl-Jones, 2004; Phelps, 2006)*

Manifestations of ROP are primarily observed during an eye examination performed by a pediatric ophthalmologist. The International Classification of Retinopathy of Prematurity provides a system of five stages to classify ROP based on the severity of the disease. Stage 4 is partial retinal detachment, and stage 5, the most severe, is complete retinal detachment. The progression of ROP is variable. An aggressive type of ROP, termed Rush disease, can manifest at 3 to 5 weeks post delivery and progress quickly to complete detachment of the retina. In many cases, ROP evolves slowly and may take a year to become stable (Phelps, 2006).

- Decreasing risk of ROP includes:
    - *Proper use of oxygen to maintain prescribed pulse oximetry parameters*
    - *Continuous monitoring and assessments of preterm neonates on continuous oxygen therapy*
    - *Careful use of oxygen during procedures such as suctioning*
    - *Use of equipment such as oxygen blenders to ensure the exact concentration of oxygen*
    - *Properly maintaining and calibrating oxygen systems (Askin & Diehl-Jones, 2004)*
- Long-term outcomes include:
    - *90% of neonates with ROP experience recovery with no or minimal loss of vision.*
    - *Treatment modalities such as cryotherapy and laser therapy have decreased the risk of complications leading to blindness.*
    - *Complications such as glaucoma, strabismus, cataracts, amblyopia, retinal detachment, and blindness may occur.*
    - *Corrective glasses may be needed to treat visual acuity deficits (Askin & Diehl-Jones, 2004; Phelps, 2006).*

Assessment Findings

- Retinal changes noted on ophthalmic examination

Medical Management

- Eye evaluation for possible ROP completed by the pediatric ophthalmologist for all neonates born before 29 weeks' gestation, or with a birth weight less than 1500 g at birth. Neonates who weigh between 1500 grams and 2000 grams at birth with medical complications should also receive an eye exam. The eye examination should occur at 4 to 6 weeks after birth (Phelps, 2006). Neonates with immature or abnormal vessel development should have repeated eye exams to monitor progression of the disease (Askin & Diehl-Jones, 2004).
- Treatment for ROP is determined by the extent of abnormal vessel development and may include (Askin & Diehl-Jones, 2004):
  - *Laser photocoagulation; laser is used to coagulate the avascular periphery of the retina to prevent vessel proliferation*
  - *Cryotherapy; a supercooled probe is used to prevent vessel proliferation by freezing the avascular retina.*
  - *Vitreoretinal surgery to reattach the retina if the retina becomes detached*

Nursing Actions

- Reduce the risk for ROP.
  - *Administer oxygen to maintain prescribed pulse oximetry parameters.*
  - *Use oxygen blenders and oxygen calibrating system to ensure exact concentration of oxygen.*
  - *Avoid bright lights by keeping lighting in the nursery at a low level.*

POSTMATURE NEONATES

A **postterm neonate** is a neonate who is delivered after the completion of 42 weeks' gestation. The incidence of postterm pregnancy is 7% (Gilbert, 2007). Postmaturity is related to a higher risk of morbidity and mortality (Furdon & Benjamin, 2004). The cause of postterm pregnancies is unknown. Placental insufficiency related to the aging of the placenta may result in **postmaturity syndrome**, in which the fetus begins to use its subcutaneous fat stores and glycemic stores (Gilbert, 2007). Placental function decreases, resulting in altered oxygenation and nutrient transport, which increases the risk for hypoxia and hypoglycemia at the onset of labor. If the placenta continues to function well after term, the result may be a newborn who is large for gestational age (LGA). The risk of **macrosomia**, or a birth weight above 4000 to 4500 grams, increases when pregnancy is prolonged.

- Risk factors
  - *Anencephaly*
  - *History of postterm pregnancies*
  - *First pregnancy*
  - *Grand multiparous women*
- Postmature neonates are at risk for:
  - *Meconium aspiration: The presence of meconium in the amniotic fluid related to fetal hypoxia places the neonate at risk for meconium aspiration syndrome (discussed later in this chapter).*
  - *Fetal hypoxia related to placental insufficiency and a decrease in amniotic fluid, which increases the risk of cord compression*
  - *Neurological complications such as seizures related to fetal asphyxia during labor and birth due to alteration in oxygenation*
  - *Hypoglycemia related to alteration in nutrient transport due to decreased placental functioning*

- *Hypothermia related to:*
  - A lack of development of subcutaneous fat
  - Loss of subcutaneous fat related to insufficient nutrient transport through the placenta
- *Polycythemia, a compensatory response, is caused by an alteration in oxygenation associated with placental insufficiency; hematocrit greater than 65% is considered polycythemia in a neonate (Gilbert, 2007; Kraus & Fanaroff, 2001; Zukowsky, 2004).*

Assessment Findings

- Dry, peeling, cracked skin
- Lack of vernix
- Profuse hair
- Long fingernails
- Thin, wasted appearance
- Meconium staining (green or yellow staining on the infant's skin, nail beds, or umbilical cord)
- Hypoglycemia

Medical Management

- Suctioning the oropharynx immediately after the delivery of the neonate's head to decrease risk of meconium aspiration
- Oxygen therapy administered for perinatal depression or respiratory distress
- Hematocrit to assess for polycythemia
- Blood glucose monitoring for hypoglycemia

Nursing Actions

- Assess the prenatal record and intrapartum history including Apgar scores for risk factors.
- Assess the neonate for:
  - *Gestational age with use of gestational age scoring system*
  - *Birth trauma if neonate is macrosomic*
  - *Respiratory distress (e.g., grunting, nasal flaring, chest retractions, tachypnea)*
  - *Cyanosis*
  - *Oxygen saturation if respiratory distress or cyanosis is present.*
  - *Signs of meconium staining*
  - *Blood glucose levels*
  - *Vital signs*
  - *Weight*
  - *Gross anomalies*
- Monitor for signs of hypoglycemia.
- Provide early and frequent feedings if respiratory status is stable.
- Monitor intake and output.

MECONIUM ASPIRATION SYNDROME

Meconium aspiration syndrome (MAS) results in significant respiratory morbidity and mortality among term infants in the United States (Ghodrat, 2006). The fetus may pass meconium stool into the amniotic fluid. This occurs when there is a relaxation of the fetal anal sphincter, usually due to fetal asphyxia in utero, but can also occur with breech presentations and in normal births without evidence of asphyxia (Blackburn, 2007). Meconium is released into the amniotic fluid in roughly 13% of deliveries and in 5% to 12% of these cases, meconium aspiration syndrome occurs (Zukowsky, 2004). There is a risk that the fetus can aspirate the meconium-stained fluid at the time of delivery.

The presence of meconium fluid in the neonate's lungs can cause a partial obstruction of the lower airways that leads to a trapping of air and a hyperinflation of the airway distal to the obstruction, causing uneven ventilation (Blackburn, 2007). The presence of meconium in the lungs can also cause a chemical pneumonitis and inhibit surfactant action (Blackburn, 2007). These changes place the neonate at risk for atelectasis.

- Complications related to meconium aspiration
  - *Obstruction of the airway*
  - *Hyperinflation of the alveoli due to the trapping of air*
  - *Chemical pneumonia*
  - *Decreased surfactant proteins*
  - *Hemorrhagic pulmonary edema that interferes with surfactant production (Zukowsky, 2004)*

Assessment Findings

- Meconium-stained amniotic fluid
- Meconium visualized below the vocal cords
- Greenish or yellowish discoloration of the skin, nail beds, and umbilical cord
- Respiratory depression at the time of birth or within a few hours after birth
- Low Apgar scores
- Need for resuscitation after delivery due to perinatal depression
- Signs of respiratory distress such as nasal flaring, grunting, chest retractions
- Chest may appear barrel shaped and overdistended.
- The expiration phase of breathing may be extended
- Diminished air movement, and the presence of rales and rhonchi assessed on auscultation
- Atelectasis and hyperinflated areas through the lungs noted on chest x-ray film
- Arterial blood gas findings may include low PaO_2 despite administration of 100% oxygen, and respiratory and metabolic acidosis in serious cases (Zukowsky, 2004).

Medical Management

- Suctioning of the oropharynx and the nasopharynx to remove meconium immediately after the delivery of the neonate's head and before the first breath is a common practice. Evidence does not support this practice as effective in preventing meconium aspiration (Mercer, Erickson-Owens, Braves, & Haley, 2007).
- Direct tracheal suctioning using a tracheal tube in cases in which the infant has a heart rate less than 100 beats per minute, absent respirations, or poor muscle tone
- Arterial blood gases to determine respiratory status and to guide treatment (Zukowsky, 2004)
- Chest x-ray exam
- Blood glucose monitoring
- Oxygen with or without assisted ventilation depending on the neonate's condition.
- Surfactant therapy to decrease risk of need for ECMO (Martin, Fanaroff, & Walsh, 2006)
- Sedatives or paralytic agents to relax neonates who are receiving ventilation (Martin, Fanaroff, & Walsh, 2006; Zukowsky, 2004)

Nursing Actions

- Assist with suctioning and resuscitation at the time of delivery.
- Perform a physical assessment to evaluate neonate for:
  - *Respiratory distress*
  - *Cyanosis*
  - *Complications of meconium aspiration syndrome such as acidosis, hypoglycemia, hypocalcemia, pneumonia, pneumothorax, bronchopulmonary dysplasia, and persistent pulmonary hypertension*
  - *Neurological problems secondary to asphyxia (Zukowsky, 2004)*
- Monitor blood glucose as per order.
- Administer oxygen and/or assisted ventilation as per order.
- Manage ECMO if ordered.

PERSISTENT PULMONARY HYPERTENSION OF THE NEWBORN

Normally after birth there is relaxation of the pulmonary vascular bed allowing blood circulation to the lungs. **Persistent pulmonary hypertension (PPHN)** results when the normal vasodilation and relaxation of the pulmonary vascular bed does not occur. This leads to elevated pulmonary vascular resistance, right ventricular hypertension, and right-to-left shunting of blood through the foramen ovale and ductus arteriosus (Martin, Fanaroff, & Walsh, 2006; Martin, Sosenko, & Bancalari, 2001). PPHN is predominantly a problem among term or near term neonates who experience hypoxia/asphyxia, RDS, meconium aspiration, sepsis, or congenital lung anomalies such as diaphragmatic hernia (Martin, Fanaroff, & Walsh, 2006). Even after the precipitating factor is treated, vasoconstriction and increased vascular resistance may persist, causing decreased pulmonary blood circulation, hypoxemia, lactic acidosis, and acidemia (Zukowsky, 2004).

- Risk factors for PPHN
  - *Hypoxia and asphyxia are the most common risk factors for PPHN*
  - *RDS, meconium aspiration, pneumonia*
  - *Bacterial sepsis*
  - *Delayed circulatory transition at birth caused by factors such as delayed resuscitation, central nervous system depression, hypothermia*
  - *Hypothermia or hypoglycemia leading to acidosis*
  - *Polycythemia or hyperviscosity of the blood which could cause blockages in the pulmonary vascular bed*
  - *Prenatal pulmonary hypertension associated with premature closure of the ductus arteriosus, or fetal systemic hypertension*
  - *Underdevelopment of pulmonary vessels associated with congenital anomalies of the lung or heart*
  - *Abnormal development of pulmonary vessels associated with intrauterine asphyxia or intrauterine meconium aspiration which leads to increased muscularization of pulmonary vessels which causes increased vascular resistance (Zukowsky, 2004)*

Assessment Findings

- Term or near term neonate
- Low Apgar scores
- Symptoms evident within 12 hours of birth
- Hypoxia and/or asphyxia at the time of birth
- Neonate depressed at birth, slow to breathe, difficulty with administering ventilation
- Tachypnea
- Chest retractions, grunting
- Low PaO_2, even with administration of high levels of oxygen
- Cyanosis
- Hypotension
- Heart murmur

- Pulmonary disorders such as air leaks, and bronchopulmonary dysplasia are possible complications of PPHN
- Echocardiogram shows pulmonary hypertension, and enlarged right side of the heart
- Congestive heart failure may occur.
- Hypoglycemia, hypocalcemia
- Metabolic acidosis
- Possible kidney damage, leading to decreased urine output, proteinuria, and hematuria
- Liver damage that may lead to blood clotting problems
- Hematologic problems such as hemorrhage, disseminated intravascular coagulation (DIC), and thrombocytopenia may occur as complications of PPHN
- Long-term outcomes after PPHN include:
  - *Hearing loss (sensorineural)*
  - *Neurological deficits*
  - *Chronic lung disease*
  - *Death (Martin, Fanaroff, & Walsh, 2006; Zukowsky, 2004)*

Medical Management

- Perform rapid and efficient resuscitation at birth to prevent hypoxia and acidosis.
- Treat acidosis if present.
- Measure preductal and postductal blood gas to distinguish structural heart problems from PPHN. If there is a difference of 10 mm Hg or more between the preductal and postductal PaO_2, then right to left shunting is suspected (Zukowsky, 2004).
- Order chest x-ray exam.
- Order echocardiogram to evaluate for cardiac anomalies, right to left shunting of blood, pulmonary resistance, and pulmonary artery pressures.
- Begin oxygen and conventional mechanical ventilation.
  - *Hyperoxygenation is often used to keep PaO_2 levels above 90 mm Hg, and hyperventilation is used to keep $PaCO_2$ levels in the low normal range, to prevent acidosis, and promote decreased pulmonary artery pressure. Hyperventilation causes alkalosis, which has been found to lower pulmonary resistance (Zukowsky, 2004).*
  - *If conventional mechanical ventilation is ineffective, high-frequency oscillatory ventilation may be instituted.*
  - *ECMO if other treatments are not effective.*
- Begin intravenous fluids.
- Begin antibiotic therapy.
- Order laboratory tests (complete blood count, glucose, electrolytes, calcium, arterial blood gases, blood cultures).
- Insert umbilical catheter to institute arterial and venous pressure monitoring, blood gas monitoring, and to administer vasopressors as indicated.
- Begin transcutaneous pulse oximetry monitoring.
- Begin surfactant therapy.
- Administer inhaled nitric oxide and wean gradually. Nitric oxide induces vasodilation and reduces pulmonary resistance. Use of nitric oxide has reduced the percentage of neonates with PPHN being placed on ECMO.
- Medications:
  - *Vasopressors, such as dopamine and nitroprusside, to decrease right to left shunting by maintaining systemic vascular pressure above pulmonary vascular pressure*
  - *Vasodilators, such as prostaglandins and isoproterenol, to promote pulmonary artery dilation*
  - *Muscle relaxants, such as Pavulon, to induce paralysis among neonates who resist ventilation*
  - *Sedatives and analgesics, such as morphine and Versed (midazolam)*
  - *Antibiotic therapy to decrease risk of and/or treat infection*

Nursing Actions

- Review maternal prenatal, intrapartal, and neonatal history.
- Assess the neonate for respiratory distress, meconium aspiration, and clinical manifestations of PPHN.
- Monitor vital signs and pulse oximetry.
- Keep handling, treatments, suctioning, and stimulation to a minimum, as these can result in decreased PaO_2 levels, and vasoconstriction.
- Administer IV fluids as per order.
- Administer medications as per order.
- Administer oxygen and mechanical ventilation as ordered.
- Anticipate the placement of umbilical catheters.
- Obtain and monitor results of laboratory tests.
- Provide emotional support for parents, incorporate them in care of their infant, keep them informed of their infant's condition.

SMALL FOR GESTATIONAL AGE AND INTRAUTERINE GROWTH RETARDATION

A **small for gestational age (SGA)** infant is one whose weight is less than the 10th percentile for his or her gestational age. Neonates whose growth is not consistent with gestational age may be affected by **intrauterine growth restriction (IUGR)**. IUGR is due to a decrease in cell production related to chronic malnutrition. There are two types of IUGR:

- **Symmetric IUGR,** a generalized proportional reduction in the size of all structures and organs except for heart and brain, is the result of a condition that occurs early in pregnancy and affects general growth. When a complication occurs very early in pregnancy, fewer cells develop, leading to smaller organ size (Furdon & Benjamin, 2004).
  - *Conditions that may result in symmetric IUGR include exposure to teratogenic substances, congenital infections, and genetic problems (Furdon & Benjamin, 2004).*
  - *Symmetric IUGR can be identified by ultrasound in the early part of the second trimester.*
- **Asymmetric IUGR,** a disproportional reduction in the size of structures and organs, results from maternal or placental conditions that occur later in pregnancy and impede placental blood flow.
  - *Examples of conditions that may result in asymmetric IUGR include preeclampsia, placental infarcts, or severe maternal malnutrition (Furdon & Benjamin, 2004).*
- Risk factors
  - *Include maternal, fetal, and placental factors (Table 17-3).*
- Neonates with IUGR are at risk for:
  - *Labor intolerance related to placental insufficiency and inadequate nutritional and oxygen reserves*
  - *Meconium aspiration related to asphyxia during labor (Zukowsky, 2004)*
  - *Hypoglycemia related to inadequate glycogen stores and reduced gluconeogenesis, and an increase in metabolic demands from heat loss which diminishes glucose stores (Levine, Tudehope, & Thearle, 2000)*
  - *Hypocalcemia, defined as serum calcium levels less than 7.5 mg/dL, related to birth asphyxia (Levine, Tudehope, & Thearle, 2001)*
    - Signs of hypocalcemia are often similar to those of hypoglycemia and include jitteriness, tetany, and seizures.

TABLE 17–3   FACTORS CONTRIBUTING TO INTRAUTERINE GROWTH RESTRICTION

MATERNAL	FETAL	PLACENTAL	ENVIRONMENTAL
Multiple gestation	Female sex	Small placenta	High altitude
Primiparity	Discordant twins	Abnormal cord insertion	Excessive exercise
Grand multiparity	Congenital anomalies	Placental previa	Exposure to x-ray
Black race	Chromosomal syndromes	Chronic abruptio placenta	Exposure to toxins
Age <15 years	Congenital infections	Thrombosis	
Age >45 years	Rubella		
No prenatal care	Toxoplasmosis		
Low socioeconomic status	Cytomegalovirus		
Nutritional status	Inborn errors of metabolism		
Low pre-pregnancy weight			
Low weight gain			
Substance abuse			
Smoking			
Vascular disease			
Renal disease			
Cardiac disease			
Preeclampsia			
Chronic hypertension			
Advanced diabetes			
Sickle cell anemia			
Phenylketonuria			
Medications			
Anticonvulsants			
History of stillbirth			
History of preterm birth			
History of IUGR/LBW baby			
Maternal short stature			

Source: Southgate & Pittard (2001)

Assessment Findings

- Physical characteristics of the IUGR neonate include:
  - *Large head in relationship to the body*
  - *Long nails*
  - *Large anterior fontanel*
  - *Decreased amounts of Wharton's jelly present in the umbilical cord*
  - *Thin extremities and trunk*
  - *Loose skin due to a lack of subcutaneous fat*
  - *Skin that may be dry, flaky, and meconium stained (Southgate & Pittard, 2000)*
- Weight, head circumference, and length are all below the 10th percentile for gestational age in symmetric IUGR (Furdon & Benjamin, 2004).
- Head circumference and length are appropriate for gestational age; however, the weight is below the 10th percentile for the baby's gestational age in asymmetric IUGR (Furdon & Benjamin, 2004).
- RDS may occur in SGA neonates who are born prematurely, or have aspirated meconium-stained amniotic fluid (Southgate & Pittard, 2001).
- Hypothermia related to decreased subcutaneous fat and glucose supply, impaired lipid metabolism, and depleted brown fat stores (Southgate & Pittard, 2001).
- Polycythemia

- Congenital anomalies are 20 times more prevalent among neonates who are IUGR as compared to babies whose weight is in the normal range (Southgate & Pittard, 2001).

Medical Management

- Identify IUGR during pregnancy and intervene based on the cause.
- Assess for congenital anomalies.
- Administer oxygen therapy for perinatal depression and respiratory distress.
- Order laboratory tests.
  - *Blood glucose monitoring*
  - *Hematocrit if polycythemia is suspected*
  - *Serum calcium levels*

Nursing Actions

- Review prenatal and intrapartal records for risk factors.
- Perform a gestational age assessment.
- Assess the neonate for gross anomalies.
- Assess for respiratory distress.
- Assess the skin for color and signs of meconium staining.
- Assess for signs of hypocalcemia and hypoglycemia.
- Monitor vital signs and daily weights.
- Monitor blood glucose per agency protocol.
- Provide early and frequent feedings to prevent hypoglycemia, if respiratory distress is not present.

■ Obtain laboratory tests as per orders.
■ Maintain a neutral thermal environment.
■ Teach parents the importance of keeping the baby warm and providing frequent feedings.

LARGE FOR GESTATIONAL AGE

A large for gestational age (LGA) infant is a neonate whose weight is above the 90th percentile for his or her gestational age. Characteristically LGA infants are macrosomic, and have greater body length and head circumference compared to infants who are appropriate for gestational age (AGA) (Fig. 17-6).

■ Risk factors for LGA
 ■ *Maternal diabetes*
 ■ *Multiparity*
 ■ *Previous macrosomic baby*
 ■ *Prolonged pregnancy (Klaus & Fanaroff, 2001)*
■ LGA fetuses and neonates are at risk for:
 ■ *Cesarean births*
 ■ *Operative vaginal delivery*
 ■ *Shoulder dystocia*
 ■ *Breech presentation*
 ■ *Cephalopelvic disproportion*
 ■ *Hypoglycemia*
 ■ *Hyperbilirubinemia*

Assessment Findings

■ Birth trauma related to shoulder dystocia or breech presentation. These birth traumas include:
 ■ *Fractured clavicle*
 ■ *Brachial nerve damage*
 ■ *Facial nerve damage*
 ■ *Depressed skull fractures*
 ■ *Cephalohematoma*
 ■ *Intracranial hemorrhage*
 ■ *Asphyxia (Furdon & Benjamin, 2004)*
■ Poor feeding behavior
■ Hypoglycemia
■ Polycythemia in neonates of diabetic mothers related to a decrease in extracellular fluid and/or fetal hypoxia

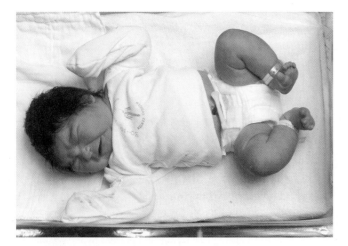

Figure 17-6   Large for gestational age (LGA) neonate.

■ Hyperbilirubinemia that occurs 48 to 72 hours after delivery related to polycythemia, decreased extracellular fluid, or bruising or hemorrhage from birth trauma

Medical Management

■ Assess for birth trauma, hypoglycemia, and respiratory distress.
■ Order laboratory tests:
 ■ *Blood glucose*
 ■ *Hematocrit*
 ■ *Bilirubin levels when indicated for jaundice*

Nursing Actions

■ Review prenatal and intrapartal records for risk factors.
■ Perform a gestational age assessment.
■ Assess neonates for birth traumas such as fractured clavicles, brachial nerve damage, facial nerve damage, and cephalohematoma.
■ Assess respiratory status.
■ Observe for signs of hypoglycemia.
■ Assess skin color for signs of polycythemia that appears as a red, ruddy skin color.
■ Observe for jaundice.
■ Obtain and monitor blood glucose per agency protocol.
■ Obtain and monitor hematocrit as per orders.
■ Provide frequent feedings to decrease risk for hypoglycemia.

HYPERBILIRUBINEMIA

Hyperbilirubinemia, high levels bilirubin in the blood, is common among neonates (AWHONN, 2006). When serum bilirubin levels are greater than 6 to 7 mg/dL, neonates will exhibit visible signs of jaundice (Watson, 2004). Approximately 50% of term neonates and 85% of preterm neonates are jaundiced during the first week after birth (Levene, Tudehope, & Thearle, 2000). The clinical significance of jaundice is based on the age of the neonate in hours and the total serum bilirubin level (Klaus & Fanaroff, 2001). Prematurity may result in greater severity of physiological jaundice, and any jaundice among preterm neonates must be evaluated (Martin, Fanaroff, & Walsh, 2006).

A complication of hyperbilirubinemia is kernicterus. **Kernicterus** is an abnormal accumulation of unconjugated bilirubin in the brain cells. Bilirubin accumulates within the brain and becomes toxic to the brain tissue, which causes neurological disorders such as deafness, delayed motor skills, hypotonia, and intellectual deficits (Klaus & Fanaroff, 2001; Walker, 2004). A goal of medical and nursing actions is to prevent kernicterus through early identification and treatment of hyperbilirubinemia.

Hyperbilirubinemia is categorized into physiological jaundice and pathological jaundice.

Physiologic Jaundice

Physiologic jaundice results from hyperbilirubinemia that commonly occurs after the first 24 hours of birth and during the first week of life (Watson, 2004). Common physiological characteristics of the neonate place the neonate at risk for physiological jaundice:

■ Neonates have an increased red blood cell volume.
■ Neonatal red blood cells have a life span of 70 to 90 days, compared to 120 days in adults.
■ Neonates produce more bilirubin (6–8 mg/kg/day) than adults.

■ Neonates reabsorb increased amounts of unconjugated bilirubin in the intestine due to lack of intestinal bacteria, decreased gastrointestinal motility, and increased β-glucuronidase (a deconjugating enzyme).

■ Neonates have a decreased hepatic uptake of bilirubin from the plasma due to a deficiency of ligandin, the primary bilirubin binding protein in hepatocytes.

■ Neonates have a diminished conjugation of bilirubin in the liver due to decreased glucuronyl transferase activity (Klaus & Fanaroff, 2001; Walker, 2004).

Risk Factors for Physiologic Jaundice

■ Asian, Native American, and Greek ethnicity.
■ Fetal hypoxia.
■ ABO incompatibility (the woman is blood type O and the neonate is blood type A or B)
■ Rh incompatibility (the woman is Rh negative and the neonate is Rh positive).
■ Use of oxytocin during labor.
■ Delayed cord clamping, which increases red blood cell volume.
■ Breastfeeding (Table 17-4).
■ Delayed feedings, caloric deprivation, or large weight loss
■ Bruising or cephalohematoma
■ Gestational age of 35 to 38 weeks.
■ Maternal diabetes with macrosomia
■ Epidural bupivacaine
■ Asphyxia
■ Older sibling with jaundice

Assessment Findings

■ Physiologic jaundice is typically visible after 24 hours of life (Klaus & Fanaroff, 2001).
■ Jaundice is characterized by a yellowish tint to the skin and sclera of the eyes.
  ■ *As total serum bilirubin levels rise, jaundice will progress from the newborn's head, downward toward the trunk and lower extremities.*
■ Mean peak total serum bilirubin level is 5 to 6 mg/dL of full-term neonates between 48 and 120 hours of life among white and African American neonates, and 10-14 mg/dL between

72 and 120 hours among Asian American newborns (Martin & Fanaroff, 2001; Walsh, 2006).
■ Declines to 3 mg/dL by the 5th day of life for white and African American babies, and by 7 to 10 days of life for Asian American neonates (Martin, Fanaroff, & Walsh, 2006).

Pathological Jaundice

Pathological jaundice results when various disorders exacerbate physiological processes that lead to hyperbilirubinemia of the newborn. Such disorders can result in pathologic unconjugated or conjugated hyperbilirubinemia (Table 17-5).

Assessment Findings

■ Jaundice that occurs within the first 24 hours of life (Klaus & Fanaroff, 2001; Walker, 2004)
■ Total serum bilirubin levels above 12.9 mg/dL in a term neonate or 15 mg/dL in a preterm baby (Walker, 2004)
■ Total serum bilirubin levels that increase by more than 5 mg/dL per day (Walker, 2004)
■ Jaundice lasting more than 1 week in a term newborn, or more than 2 weeks in a premature neonate (Walker, 2004)

Medical Management for Hyperbilirubinemia

■ Diagnostic tests
  ■ *Total serum bilirubin, with fractionation of serum bilirubin into direct (conjugated bilirubin) and indirect (unconjugated bilirubin) reacting pigments (Martin, Fanaroff, & Walsh, 2006)*
  ■ *Antiglobulin (Coombs') test: Test used to determine hemolytic disease of the newborn related to Rh or ABO incompatibility.*
    ■ Direct antiglobulin (Coombs') test is used to detect abnormal in vivo coating of the neonate's red blood cells with antibody globulin (maternal antibodies); when present, the test is considered positive.
  ■ *Transcutaneous bilirubinometry, a noninvasive method to estimate total serum bilirubin levels among term and near term neonates, is used to identify neonates at risk for developing hyperbilirubinemia (Klaus & Fanaroff, 2001; Walker, 2004).*
  ■ *Complete blood count assists in management of pathological jaundice.*

TABLE 17–4 HYPERBILIRUBINEMIA ASSOCIATED WITH BREASTFEEDING: A COMPARISON OF BREASTFEEDING VERSUS BREAST MILK JAUNDICE

BREASTFEEDING JAUNDICE	BREAST MILK JAUNDICE
Early onset of jaundice (within the first few days of life)	Late onset (after 3–5 days)
Associated with ineffective breastfeeding	Gradual increase in bilirubin that peaks at 2 weeks of age
Dehydration can occur.	Associated with breast milk composition in some women that increases the enterohepatic circulation of bilirubin
Delayed passage of meconium stool promotes reabsorption of bilirubin in the gut.	Treatment: Continued breastfeeding in most infants. In some cases where bilirubin levels are excessively high, breastfeeding may be interrupted and formula feedings can be given for several days. This typically results in a decline of the bilirubin level. Breastfeeding is resumed when bilirubin levels decline.
Treatment: Encourage early effective breastfeeding without supplementation of glucose water or other fluids.	

Source: Reiser (2001).

TABLE 17–5   CAUSES OF PATHOLOGIC HYPERBILIRUBINEMIA

CAUSES OF PATHOLOGICAL UNCONJUGATED HYPERBILIRUBINEMIA	CAUSES OF CONJUGATED HYPERBILIRUBINEMIA (ALWAYS PATHOLOGIC)
HEMOLYSIS OF RBCS Rh/ABO incompatibilities Bacterial and viral infections Inherited disorders of red blood cell/bilirubin metabolism Glucose-6-phospate dehydrogenase deficiency	**HEPATITIS** Neonatal idiopathic hepatitis Infectious hepatitis Toxic hepatitis Intestinal obstruction Ischemic necrosis Parenteral alimentation

SEQUESTERED BLOOD:
Cephalohematoma
Bruising
Hemangiomas
Cerebral, pulmonary, retroperitoneal bleeding
Decreased hepatic uptake of bilirubin
Decreased hepatic function/perfusion
  ■ Hypoxia
  ■ Asphyxia
  ■ Sepsis
Increased enterohepatic circulation
  ■ Delayed feedings
  ■ Breastfeeding jaundice
  ■ Breast milk jaundice
  ■ Intestinal obstructions
Polycythemia
Swallowed blood
Hypothyroidism
Hypopituitarism
	Metabolic disorders
	
	Hematologic disorders
	
	Ductal disturbances in bilirubin excretion:
	  ■ Extrahepatic biliary atresia
	  ■ Intrahepatic biliary atresia
	  ■ Bile plug syndrome
	  ■ Tumors of the liver and biliary tract

Source: Martin, Fanaroff, & Walsh (2006).

- Treatment is determined by the level of bilirubin and the age of the neonate in hours (Table 17-6).
- Phototherapy
  - *Phototherapy is the most widely used and effective treatment for hyperbilirubinemia.*
  - *Various types of phototherapy delivery systems are available, including blue lights, white lamps, halogen lamps and fiberoptic blankets, and blue light emitting diodes (LED).*

TABLE 17–6   MANAGEMENT OF HYPERBILIRUBINEMIA IN THE HEALTHY TERM AND NEAR TERM NEONATE

AGE (HR)	CONSIDER PHOTOTHERAPY	PHOTOTHERAPY
≤24	–	–
25–48	≥12	≥15
49–72	≥15	≥18
>72	≥17	≥20

Source: American Academy of Pediatrics (2004b).

- Evidence suggests blue lights are the most effective (Martin, Fanaroff, & Walsh, 2006).
- *Phototherapy results in photoisomerization and photo-oxidation, which promotes the conversion of bilirubin to photobilirubin (Klaus & Fanaroff, 2001; Watson, 2004).*
  - Photobilirubin can be excreted from the body in urine without undergoing conjugation in the liver (Klaus & Fanaroff, 2001).
- *Total serum bilirubin levels should drop 1 to 2 mg/dL within 4 to 6 hours after the initiation of phototherapy.*
- *Phototherapy should be administered continuously, except during feeding times or parental visits, when eye patches are removed to allow for bonding (Klaus & Fanaroff, 2001).*
- Exchange transfusion is used in cases where phototherapy is not effective or severe hemolytic disease is present (Martin, Fanaroff, & Walsh, 2006; Walker, 2004).
  - *In this procedure, approximately 85% of the neonate's red blood cells are replaced with donor cells.*
  - *This procedure reduces bilirubin, removes red blood cells coated with maternal antibody, corrects anemia, and removes other toxins associated with hemolysis (Klaus & Fanaroff, 2001).*
  - *Efforts to prevent Rh hemolytic disease with Rh immunoglobulin (Rhogam) administered to Rh-negative women, and the use of phototherapy, have diminished the need for exchange transfusion (Klaus & Fanaroff, 2001).*

■ Infants discharged before 72 hours of life should be seen for follow-up by a health care provider within 1 to 2 days to assess the neonate's health status and to assess for jaundice.

    ■ *Timely identification of significant hyperbilirubinemia is key to preventing acute bilirubin encephalopathy (American Academy of Pediatrics [AAP], 2004b).*

Nursing Actions for Hyperbilirubinemia

■ Review maternal and neonatal record for risk factors.

■ Review laboratory findings such as neonatal blood type; Rh factor; and indirect and, direct Coombs'.

■ Assess degree of jaundice every shift with the use of a transcutaneous meter (AAP, 2004b).

    ■ *When meter is not available, in a well lit area, use your fingers to blanch the neonate's skin on the face, upper trunk, abdomen, thigh, and lower leg and feet. The skin will appear yellow after the pressure is released and before return of normal skin color.*

■ Document the assessment findings.

■ Notify the physician if jaundice is present.

■ Obtain serum bilirubin levels.

■ Ensure adequate hydration by feeding neonate every 2 to 3 hours to promote excretion of bilirubin in the urine, and to compensate for insensible water loss due to phototherapy (Klaus & Fanaroff, 2001).

    ■ *Early feedings decrease the enterohepatic circulation of bilirubin, which decreases bilirubin levels (Walker, 2004).*

■ Implement phototherapy as ordered and provide related nursing care.

■ Assess for side effects of phototherapy:

    ■ *Eye damage*
    ■ *Loose stools*
    ■ *Dehydration*
    ■ *Hyperthermia*
    ■ *Lethargy*
    ■ *Skin rashes*
    ■ *Abdominal distention*
    ■ *Hypocalcemia*
    ■ *Lactose intolerance*
    ■ *Thrombocytopenia*
    ■ *Bronze baby syndrome*

■ Include the following in discharge teaching: verbal and written instructions about how to identify signs of jaundice in an infant; notify the physician if jaundice is present.

CENTRAL NERVOUS SYSTEM INJURIES

Various types of central nervous system (CNS) injuries can occur among term and premature neonates. Injury can be the result of intracranial hemorrhage (Table 17-7); hypoxia and ischemia during the prenatal and intrapartal periods, and post-birth; systemic chronic fetal compromise such as IUGR; or hypotension that leads to a decreased cerebral profusion resulting in preventricular leukomalacia (Table 17-8).

Depending on the extent and location of the injury, CNS injuries may result in normal outcomes or serious long-term problems such as seizures, neurological deficits, developmental disability, motor deficits, visual impairments, or death (Lynam & Verklan, 2004).

■ Risk factors for CNS injuries

    ■ *Prematurity*
    ■ *Birth trauma*

CRITICAL COMPONENTS

Care of the Neonate Receiving Phototherapy

■ Fluorescent "bili lights" should be positioned 45 to 50 cm from the infant.

■ Fluorescent lights should be positioned 2 inches from the top of an incubator

■ A photometer should be used to measure irradiance of lamps to facilitate optimal treatment.

■ Banks of lights should be covered by Plexiglas.

■ The neonate should be placed under lights with only a diaper in place, for maximal exposure to light.

■ Eye patches are placed on infant to protect eyes from the effects of the light.

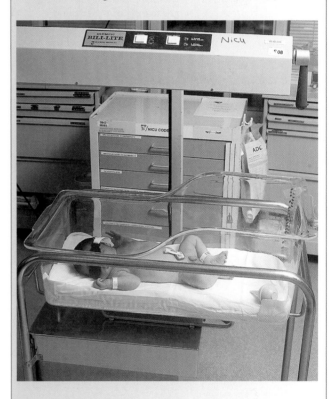

■ During feedings, eye patches are removed and the neonate should be held by a parent or the nurse.

■ Change the neonate's position frequently to facilitate increased exposure to the light.

■ Vital signs including temperature monitoring should be done per agency protocol.

■ Closely monitor intake and output. Phototherapy results in increased insensible fluid loss.

■ Feedings every 2 to 3 hours are important to provide adequate fluids to compensate for insensible fluid loss, and promote excretion of bilirubin in the urine.

■ Closely monitor newborn for side effects of phototherapy.

(Martin, Fanaroff, & Walsh, 2006)

    ■ *Breech delivery or other malpresentations*
    ■ *Precipitous labor*
    ■ *Difficult labor, traumatic delivery, and use of forceps*
    ■ *Hypoxia, asphyxia, hypotension, ischemia, respiratory distress.*

TABLE 17–7 TYPES OF CENTRAL NERVOUS SYSTEM INJURIES: HEMORRHAGES

	SUBDURAL HEMORRHAGE	SUBARACHNOID HEMORRHAGE	INTRACEREBELLAR HEMORRHAGE
DEFINITION	Tear of the dura overlying the cerebellum or cerebral hemispheres	Intracranial hemorrhage into the cerebrospinal fluid filled space between the pial and arachnoid membranes on the surface of the brain. Most common neonatal intracranial hemorrhage.	Hemorrhage in the cerebellum from primary bleeding or from extension of intraventricular or subarachnoid hemorrhage into the cerebellum. Occurs more commonly in preterm, low birth weight neonates.
PATHOPHYSIOLOGY	Excessive molding, stretching, or tearing of the falx and tentorium. Stretching or tearing of the vein of Galen or cerebellar bridging veins	May occur because of trauma in a term neonate or hypoxia in a preterm neonate. Venous bleeding in the subarachnoid space related to ruptured small vessels in the leptomeningeal plexus or bridging veins in the subarachnoid space.	Breech presentation, difficult forceps delivery, external pressure over the occiput. History of a hypoxic–ischemic insult. Vitamin K deficiency. Vascular factors.
MANIFESTATIONS	Symptoms may be delayed for first 24 hours, then: Seizures Decreased level of consciousness Asymmetrical motor function Full fontanel Irritability Lethargy Respiratory abnormalities Facial paralysis	Commonly there are no symptoms. Seizures may occur, starting on day 2 of life. Apnea may occur in preterm neonates.	Manifestations occur within the first 2 days to 3 weeks of life. Apnea Bradycardia Decreasing hematocrit. Bloody cerebrospinal fluid
PROGNOSIS	Hydrocephalus Mortality rate 45% Hypoxic–ischemic injury	90% of babies with seizures will have normal follow up. Abnormal outcome is rare.	Poorer outcome in preterm neonates than in term newborns. Neurologic deficits probable.

Source: Lynam & Verklan (2004).

Hypoxic events may be related to:

■ Maternal causes such as cardiac arrest and hypovolemic shock.
  ■ Uteroplacental causes such as placental abruption, cord prolapse, and uterine hyperstimulation.
  ■ Fetal causes such as cardiac arrhythmia (Martin, Fanaroff, & Walsh, 2006).

Assessment Findings

■ Clinical manifestations are specific to the type and extent of the CNS injury (see Tables 17-7 and 17-8).

Medical Management

■ Prevent hypoxia, ischemia, and asphyxia during the perinatal and intrapartal periods.
  ■ *Identification and treatment of a compromised fetus may prevent asphyxiation and multiorgan damage (Lynam & Verklan, 2004; Martin, Fanaroff, & Walsh, 2006).*

■ Evaluate neurological and behavioral status.
■ Order laboratory tests:
  ■ *Serum glucose level*
  ■ *Electrolyte levels*
  ■ *Arterial blood gas analysis*
  ■ *Blood, urine, cerebrospinal fluid (CSF) cultures*
  ■ *Complete blood count with differential*
■ Obtain computed tomography (CT) scan, ultrasonography, magnetic resonance image (MRI), and skull radiographs as indicated.
■ Perform lumbar puncture for CSF analysis if clinically indicated.
■ Obtain electroencephalography to confirm occurrence of seizures, and to identify presence and severity of brain damage if clinically indicated.
■ Evoked potentials to predict neurodevelopmental outcomes in cases of hypoxic–ischemic encephalopathy (Martin, Fanaroff, & Walsh, 2006).

TABLE 17-8   TYPES OF CENTRAL NERVOUS SYSTEM INJURY: HYPOXIC-ISCHEMIC ENCEPHALOPATHY

	HYPOXIC-ISCHEMIC ENCEPHALOPATHY	PERIVENTRICULAR LEUKOMALACIA
DEFINITION	Abnormal neonatal neurologic behavior resulting from a hypoxic–ischemic event. Brain edema and massive cellular necrosis. Intraventricular, subdural, or intracerebral hemorrhage.	Necrosis of periventricular white matter resulting from ischemia. Ischemic lesion of arterial origin. Multicystic encephalomalacia with/without hemorrhage into ischemic area.
RISK FACTORS	Hypoxia, anoxia, decreased blood supply to the brain (ischemia). Acute birth asphyxia (e.g., cord compression) Chronic subacute asphyxia (prenatal or intrapartum) Systemic hypotension Multiorgan system failure may occur.	Systemic hypotension leading to decreased cerebral blood flow. Apnea and bradycardia, secondary to poor cerebral perfusion. Chorioamnionitis
CLINICAL MANIFESTATIONS	Clinical manifestations depend on extent of encephalopathy Stage I: Mild encephalopathy Hyperalert state Hyper-responsiveness Normal muscle tone and reflexes Increased tendon reflexes Myoclonus present Tachycardia Dilated pupils EEG normal Usually no seizure activity Stage II: Moderate encephalopathy Lethargy and hypotonia Increased tendon reflexes Myoclonus Weak suck Strong grasp Incomplete moro reflex Seizures Pupils constrict and reactive Abnormal EEG findings Stage III: Severe encephalopathy Level of consciousness deteriorates to comatose. Apnea, bradycardia Mechanical ventilation needed. Seizures occur within 12 hours of life. Severe hypotonia, absent Moro, grasp, and suck reflexes. Pupils unequal; poor light reflex and variable reactivity. Deterioration may occur within 24–72 hours. Death may follow.	Acute phase: Lethargy, central nervous system depression, and hypotension. After 6-10 weeks: Frequent tremors, and startle reflex. Abnormal Moro reflex. Hypertonia, irritability, extension of legs, increased flexion of arms.

Continued

TABLE 17–8	TYPES OF CENTRAL NERVOUS SYSTEM INJURY: HYPOXIC-ISCHEMIC ENCEPHALOPATHY—CONT'D	
	HYPOXIC–ISCHEMIC ENCEPHALOPATHY	**PERIVENTRICULAR LEUKOMALACIA**
PROGNOSIS	Outcome depends on severity of encephalopathy. 20-50% of asphyxiated babies with hypoxic-ischemic encephalopathy (HIE) will die. Early seizure activity associated with poorer outcome. Less severe HIE associated with hyperactivity and attention deficit problems. Normal outcome may occur	Outcome depends on location and extent of injury. Motor deficits Spastic diplegia Visual impairments Lower limb weakness Intellectual deficits more common when there is upper arm involvement.

Sources: Lynam & Verklan (2004); Klaus & Fanaroff (2001).

■ Consult the neurologist as indicated.
■ Administer medications to treat seizure activity.
■ Infants with hypoxic–ischemic encephalopathy may require the following medical management and treatment (Lynam & Verklan, 2004):
    ■ *Resuscitation at the time of delivery*
    ■ *Oxygen and ventilator support*
    ■ *Monitoring of fluids, electrolytes, and acid–base balance*
    ■ *Monitoring of blood volume and blood pressure*
    ■ *Maintaining perfusion and preventing/treating hypotension*
    ■ *Evaluating and supporting the renal, hepatic, gastrointestinal, pulmonary, and cardiovascular systems*

Nursing Actions

■ Review maternal prenatal and intrapartal history for risk factors.
■ Perform physical assessment of the neonate, including evaluation of tone, reflexes, and behavior.
■ Notify physician of abnormal findings.
■ Obtain laboratory tests as per order.
■ Ensure that ordered diagnostic tests are completed.
■ Assist with diagnostic procedures such as lumbar puncture.
■ Administer oxygen as per order.
■ Administer medications as per order.
■ Provide the family with support and information about their infant's status, treatment, and follow-up.

INFANTS OF MOTHERS WITH TYPE 1 DIABETES

Diabetes is the most common chronic medical problem affecting pregnant women (Dunne, Brydon, Smith, & Gee, 2003). Maternal diabetes during pregnancy is associated with poor outcomes for the fetus and neonate (Armentrout, 2004; Dunne, Brydon, Smith, & Gee, 2003). Complications of high maternal levels of glucose during pregnancy are:

■ Congenital anomalies:
    ■ *Cardiac anomalies, such as transposition of the great vessels, ventricular septal defect, and left to right ventricular wall hypertrophy*
    ■ *Skeletal defects, such as sacral agenesis and neural tube defects*
    ■ *Small left colon syndrome and renal anomalies (Gilbert, 2007)*

■ IUGR, perinatal asphyxia, and SGA neonates due to placental insufficiency related to maternal vascular disease in woman with type 1 diabetes of long duration (Gilbert, 2007)
■ Risk for RDS due to delay in surfactant production related to the high maternal glucose levels and fetal hyperstimulation (Armentrout, 2004)
■ Risk of hypoglycemia during the first few hours of life due to increased levels of fetal and neonatal insulin and decreased circulating glucose after delivery
■ Neurological damage and seizures related to inadequate glucose supply to the brain due to neonatal hyperinsulinism
■ Risk for hyperbilirubinemia related to polycythemia due to insulin-induced increases in metabolism that leads to hypoxia (Armentrout, 2004).
■ Risk of shoulder dystocia during the birthing process related to macrosomia
■ Risk of childhood obesity and type 2 diabetes (Gilbert, 2007)

Assessment Findings

■ Macrosomia due to fetal exposure to elevated maternal glucose levels. In response to high glucose levels, the fetal pancreas produces insulin. Hyperinsulinemia results in increased fat production and growth (Gilbert, 2007).
■ Fractured clavicle and brachial nerve damage related to shoulder dystocia (Armentrout, 2004)
■ Hypoglycemia
■ Hypocalcemia and hypomagnesemia
■ Polycythemia
■ Hyperbilirubinemia

Medical Management

■ Assess for complications associated with maternal diabetes.
■ Order laboratory tests such as hematocrit and calcium and magnesium levels.
■ Order x-ray exams if clinically indicated for birth trauma related to shoulder dystocia.
■ Consult the cardiologist if cardiac anomalies are suspected.
■ Monitor blood glucose. Abnormal results are confirmed by laboratory analysis of plasma glucose (Armentrout, 2004; Kliegman, 2001). If the neonate is hypoglycemic, blood glucose

levels should be monitored 30 minutes after feeding to evaluate response to treatment (Kliegman, 2001).

■ Order early (by 1–2 hours of age) and frequent oral feedings of breast milk or formula unless the neonate feeds poorly or is too sick to be fed orally. If oral feedings are contraindicated and/or the neonate is hypoglycemic, 10% dextrose and water is administered intravenously (Kliegman, 2001).

Nursing Actions

■ Assess neonate for signs of respiratory distress, birth trauma, congenital anomalies, hypoglycemia, hypocalcemia, polycythemia, and hyperbilirubinemia.
■ Monitor blood glucose per agency protocol.
■ Provide early and frequent feedings to treat and prevent hypoglycemia.
■ Obtain laboratory tests as per orders.
■ Maintain a neutral thermal environment to reduce energy needs (Kliegman, 2001).

NEONATAL INFECTION

Infections among neonates are a leading cause of morbidity and mortality. Neonates can be exposed to infection via vertical or horizontal transmission (Horns, 2004). The immune system of a neonate is immature, placing the newborn at risk for infection during the first several months of life (Martin, Fanaroff, & Walsh, 2006). **Vertical transmission** of infection, the passing of infection from the mother to the baby, can occur in several ways:

■ Transplacental transfer: Infection is transmitted to the fetus through the placenta such as syphilis.
■ Ascending infection: Infection ascends into the uterus related to prolonged rupture of membranes.

■ Intrapartal exposure: The neonate is exposed to infection during the birth process (e.g., herpes virus).

Horizontal transmission (nosocomial infection) is an infection that is transmitted from hospital equipment or staff to the neonate (Horns, 2004).

Infections may be caused by bacteria, viruses, fungus, yeast, spirochetes (syphilis), and protozoa (Table 17-9).

Infections may affect specific organ systems such as respiratory, urinary tract, brain, gastrointestinal tract, and skin; or local sites such as the umbilical stump and eyes. Neonates may develop systemic infections (sepsis) (Martin, Fanaroff, & Walsh, 2006).

■ Early-onset sepsis occurs within the first 7 days of life. It is a serious, overwhelming infection that is typically acquired through vertical transmission from the mother (Martin, Fanaroff, & Walsh, 2006).
■ Late-onset sepsis occurs after 7 days of life and is associated with a lower mortality rate than early-onset sepsis.
■ Very late onset sepsis affects premature, very low birth weight babies, after 3 months of age. This sepsis is related to long-term use of equipment such as indwelling catheters and endotracheal tubes (Martin, Fanaroff, & Walsh, 2006).
■ Risk factors
  ■ *There are several maternal, neonatal, and environmental factors that predispose a neonate to infection (Table 17-10).*

Group B *Streptococcus*

Group B *Streptococcus* (GBS) is the primary cause of neonatal meningitis and sepsis in the United States (Himmelberger, 2002). Approximately 10% to 30% of all women are asymptomatic carriers of GBS, which is found in the urogenital and lower gastrointestinal tract (Himmelberger, 2002). Evidence supports the use of antibiotics

TABLE 17–9   CAUSES OF NEONATAL INFECTION

BACTERIAL	VIRAL	FUNGAL	OTHER
Group B *Streptococcus*	Rubella	*Candida albicans*	Syphilis
Escherichia coli	Cytomegalovirus (CMV)	Candidiasis	*Treponema pallidum* (spirochete)
Coagulase-negative	Respiratory syncytial virus (RSV)		Toxoplasmosis
Staphylococcus	Herpes simplex (HSV)		Protozoan parasite
Staphylococcus aureus	Hepatitis B		
Viridans streptococci	Human immunodeficiency virus (HIV)		
Enterococcus species	Varicella-zoster (Chickenpox)		
Group D *Streptococcus*			
Pseudomonas species			
Klebsiella			
Listeria monocytogenes			
Hemophilus influenzae			
Neisseria gonorrhea			
C. trachomatis			
Chlamydia			
Mycobacterium tuberculosis			

TABLE 17–10   RISK FACTORS FOR NEONATAL INFECTION

MATERNAL FACTORS	NEONATAL FACTORS	ENVIRONMENTAL FACTORS
Poor prenatal nutrition	Prematurity	Length of stay in hospital
Low socioeconomic status	Birth weight <2,500 g	Invasive procedures
Substance abuse	Difficult delivery	Use of humidification in incubator or ventilatory care
History of sexually transmitted infection	Birth asphyxia	Routine use of broad-spectrum antibiotics
Recurrent abortion	Meconium staining	
Lack of prenatal care	Need for resuscitation	
Prolonged rupture of membranes (>12–18 hours)	Congenital anomalies	
Vaginal Group B *Streptococcus* colonization	Black neonates	
Chorioamnionitis	Male neonates	
Maternal temperature during labor and delivery	Multiple gestation	
Premature labor		
Difficult or prolonged labor		
Maternal urinary tract infection		
Invasive procedures during labor and delivery		
Maternal and/or fetal tachycardia		
Fetal scalp electrode use		

Sources: Horn (2004); Martin, Fanaroff, & Walsh (2006).

during labor among women who have positive cultures for GBS during pregnancy in reducing vertical transmission of GBS, and early-onset GBS sepsis (AAP, 1997). The following are recommendations established by the Centers for Disease Control and Prevention (CDC, 2002) to prevent perinatal Group B streptococcal disease:

■ All pregnant women should be routinely screened for vaginal and rectal GBS colonization at 35 to 37 weeks' gestation. Women who are positive for GBS should be given prophylactic antibiotics at the time of labor or rupture of membranes.

■ Women who were GBS positive during pregnancy, or have delivered a previous baby with GBS infection, or women with membranes rupture before 37 weeks gestation, should be given penicillin during the intrapartum period without obtaining a GBS culture.

■ If GBS status is not known at the time of rupture of membranes or labor onset, prophylactic antibiotics should be administered if: (a) membranes have been ruptured for 18 hours or more, (b) gestational age is less than 37 weeks, or (c) maternal temperature is 100.4°F (38°C) or higher.

■ Women with positive GBS cultures who have a planned cesarean section before rupture of membranes or the onset of labor should not receive routine prophylaxis for perinatal GBS prevention.

■ For intrapartum chemoprophylaxis, penicillin G is recommended at an initial dose of 5 million units intravenously (IV), followed by 2.5 million units every 4 hours until delivery. Ampicillin can be used as an alternative, and is given at an initial dose of 2 g IV followed by 1 g IV every 4 hours until delivery. Women who are allergic to penicillin but are not at high risk for anaphylaxis are given cefazolin IV. Erythromycin or clindamycin IV may also be used if the GBS isolate is not resistant to these medications.

■ Neonates of women who received intrapartum chemoprophylaxis do not require routine antibiotic administration, unless they exhibit signs of sepsis.

■ The American Academy of Pediatrics (1997) recommends that asymptomatic infants of mothers who received prophylactic antibiotics and who are less than 35 weeks' gestation at the time of delivery, should be evaluated with a complete blood count with differential, and blood cultures. These neonates should be observed in the hospital for at least 48 hours.

■ Infants at any gestational age who exhibit signs of infection should have a complete blood count (CBC) with a differential, blood cultures and a chest x-ray exam if respiratory symptoms are present (AAP, 1997). Antibiotics (ampicillin and gentamicin) should be started immediately after blood cultures are obtained.

■ Neonates who are term, who appear to be healthy, and whose mothers received 4 or more hours of antibiotic prophylaxis can be discharged after 24 hours if they meet all other discharge criteria.

Assessment Findings for Neonatal Infections

■ Signs of infection in a newborn are often nonspecific and subtle (Table 17-11).

■ Laboratory findings suggestive of infection include:

■ *Leukocytosis: An elevated white blood cell count (WBC >25,000/mm³)*

■ *Leukopenia: A low white blood cell count (WBC <1750/mm³)*

■ *Neutrophilia: Increased neutrophil count*

■ *Neutropenia: Decreased neutrophil count (<1,500/mm³) is strongly predictive of infection.*

■ *An immature to total neutrophil ratio greater than 0.20 is suggestive of infection.*

■ *Thrombocytopenia: Platelet count <100,000/mm³ can be related to viral infection or bacterial sepsis (Horns, 2004).*

Medical Management

■ Monitor for clinical signs of infection.

■ Order laboratory tests if the neonate exhibits manifestations of infection or is at risk for infection:

■ *CBC including a differential to evaluate white blood cell counts*

TABLE 17–11   SIGNS OF NEONATAL INFECTION

RESPIRATORY	THERMO-REGULATION	CARDIO-VASCULAR	NEUROLOGICAL	GASTROINTESTINAL	SKIN	METABOLIC
Apnea Grunting Retractions Tachypnea Cyanosis	Hypothermia Fever Temperature instability	Bradycardia Tachycardia Arrhythmias Hypotension Hypertension Decreased perfusion	Tremors Lethargy Irritability High pitched cry Hypertonia Hypotonia Seizures Bulging fontanelles	Poor feeding Vomiting Diarrhea Abdominal distention Enlarged liver/spleen	Rash Pustules Vesicles Pallor Jaundice Petechiae Vasomotor instability	Glucose instability Metabolic acidosis

Source: Horns (2004).

■ *Microbial cultures of the blood, urine, and CSF*
  ■ Neonatal sepsis can be diagnosed definitively only with a positive blood culture (Martin, Fanaroff, & Walsh, 2006). Urine and CSF cultures may also be obtained when sepsis is suspected. Other cultures are obtained as clinically indicated (e.g., skin).
  ■ *C-reactive protein levels (CRP) may be measured every 12 hours to detect inflammation associated with infection (Horns, 2004).*
  ■ *Polymerase chain reaction (PCR) testing for bacterial or viral DNA allows for identification of a specific bacterial or viral gene segment (Horns, 2004).*
■ Begin antibiotic therapy, if indicated for suspected sepsis after cultures are obtained (Martin, Fanaroff, & Walsh, 2006).
  ■ *Antibiotics, such as ampicillin and aminoglycosides, that provide broad-spectrum coverage are often started initially (Horns, 2004; Martin, Fanaroff, & Walsh, 2006).*
  ■ *If culture results are negative, antibiotics will be stopped after 48 to 72 hours.*
  ■ *If sepsis is confirmed, antibiotics continue for 10 to 14 days, and 21 days for meningitis (Horns, 2004).*
  ■ *If it is determined the infection is not bacterial in nature, appropriate antiviral or antifungal medications are ordered (Martin, Fanaroff, & Walsh, 2006).*
  ■ *The dosage and frequency of medication administration are dependent on the neonate's weight, gestational age, postnatal age, and liver and kidney function (Martin, Fanaroff, & Walsh, 2006).*
■ Administer intravenous fluid and parenteral nutrition.
■ Monitor glucose and electrolytes
■ Use ventilatory support if indicated (Horns, 2004; Martin, Fanaroff, & Walsh, 2006).

Nursing Actions

■ Assess maternal and neonatal history for factors that may place a neonate at risk for infection such as maternal Group B *Streptococcus* status.
■ Assess vital signs and adequacy of feedings, and monitor intake and output and weight, per agency protocol.
■ Assess neonate for signs of infection (see Table 17-11).
■ Notify the physician if the neonate demonstrates signs of infection. Early recognition and treatment of neonatal infection is important in preventing morbidity and mortality.
■ Obtain laboratory tests as per order.

■ Assist with diagnostic tests such as lumbar puncture for CSF.
■ Administer antibiotics as per orders.
■ Administer intravenous fluid and parenteral nutrition as per orders.
■ Monitor glucose and electrolytes.
■ Provide respiratory support as per orders.
■ Wash hands before handling equipment and caring for the neonate.
■ Provide parents with information about the neonate's status, infection prevention strategies such as hand-washing before contact with the baby, and diagnostic tests and treatments as appropriate.
■ Include the following in discharge teaching for parents: identification of signs and symptoms of infection, what signs/symptoms should be reported to the physician, how to prevent infection, scheduling a follow-up appointment before discharge.

SUBSTANCE ABUSE EXPOSURE

In the United States, 3.9% of pregnant women report use of illicit drugs, 12.1% report use of alcohol, and 16.6% report use of tobacco (SAMHSA, 2006). Perinatal use of illicit drugs, alcohol, and tobacco has both short-term and long-term effects on the developing fetus (Table 17-12).

Women who use illicit drugs, alcohol, and tobacco are at higher risk for:

■ No or inadequate prenatal care
■ Inadequate prenatal weight gain
■ Sexually transmitted infections
■ Obstetrical complications (e.g., preterm labor and abruptio placenta)
■ Severe mood swings

Assessment Findings

■ Effects of perinatal maternal substance use on the neonate are specific to the substance that has been used (see Table 17-12).
■ **Neonatal abstinence syndrome** (neonatal withdrawal) may result from intrauterine exposure to various substances including opioids such as heroin, methadone, oxycodone, and Demerol; alcohol; Valium; caffeine; and barbiturates (AAP, 1998).
  ■ *The extent to which a newborn exhibits drug withdrawal is dependent on several factors (e.g., timing of the last exposure, type of substance, and the half life of the substance; AAP, 1998).*

TABLE 17–12   SUBSTANCES COMMONLY USED DURING PREGNANCY: SIGNS OF WITHDRAWAL AND SHORT- AND LONG-TERM EFFECTS

SUBSTANCE	POST-BIRTH EFFECTS/ SIGNS OF WITHDRAWAL	SHORT- AND LONG-TERM EFFECTS
TOBACCO	None known	Low birth weight Intrauterine growth restriction Smaller head circumference Increased stillbirth Cleft palate/lip Childhood cancer Lower IQ Learning difficulties Attention deficit disorder Increased risk for sudden infant death syndrome Increased risk for asthma/respiratory infections Inner ear infections

ALCOHOL	Onset of withdrawal 12 hours after birth
	Hypertonia
	Tremors
	Weak suck
	Poor feeding
	Crying
	Increased wakefulness
	Increased mouthing behavior
		Facial anomalies:
		    Flat upper lip
		    Flat philtrum
		    Short eye openings
		Low birth weight
		Failure to thrive
		Microcephaly
		Mental retardation
		Poor fine motor skills
		Aggressiveness
		Attention deficit disorder
		Poor short-term memory
		Problem solving difficulties
		Neurosensory hearing losses
		Gait problems
		Hand–eye coordination problems
		Increased risk of infection
		Lack of understanding of consequences
		Impulsive behavior
		Poor judgment
		Short attention span
		Social interaction problems

MARIJUANA	Tremors Altered sleep patterns High pitched cry Exaggerated startle reflex	Low birth weight Preterm birth Intrauterine growth restriction Attention deficit disorder Impulsiveness Poor self directed responses Lower scores on verbal and memory assessments Increased risk for sudden infant death syndrome with paternal use Congenital anomalies
COCAINE	Tremors Hyperreflexia Hypotonia Abnormal state patterns-Prolonged periods of being awake/crying Extreme sensitivity to stimuli/ easily distressed Depressed interactive behaviors Poor response to comforting Short attention to stimuli Poor suck leading to feeding problems	Prematurity Intrauterine growth restriction Decreased head circumference Low birth weight Congenital anomalies Fetal distress during labor may lead to meconium aspiration Cerebrovascular accident, intraventricular hemorrhage Increased risk for sudden infant death syndrome Attention deficit and behavioral problems Cognitive delays

TABLE 17–12   SUBSTANCES COMMONLY USED DURING PREGNANCY: SIGNS OF WITHDRAWAL AND SHORT- AND LONG-TERM EFFECTS —CONT'D

SUBSTANCE	POST-BIRTH EFFECTS/ SIGNS OF WITHDRAWAL	SHORT- AND LONG-TERM EFFECTS

METHAMPHETAMINES	Abnormal sleep patterns
	Tremors
	Poor feeding
	State disorganization
	Agitation/lethargy
	Weight gain problems
	Sweating
	Vomiting
	With methamphetamine and cocaine use:
	   Frantic first sucking
	   High pitched cry
	   Loose stools
	   Yawning
	   Fever
	   Hyperreflexia
	   Excoriation
		Intrauterine growth restriction
		Reduced brain growth
		Developmental effects
		Congenital anomalies
		Increased risk for sudden infant death syndrome

NARCOTICS/OPIOIDS
 	
Heroin
 	
Methadone
 	
Morphine
 	
OxyContin
	Hypertonia
	Tremors
	Hyperreflexia
	Seizures
	Irritability/restlessness
	High pitched cry
	Excessive crying
	Sleep problems
	Wakefulness
	Yawning
	Nasal congestion
	Sneezing
	Lacrimation
	Sweating
	Fever
	Skin mottling
	Diarrhea
	Vomiting
	Poor feeding
	Dysmature swallowing
	Excessive/frantic sucking
	Tachypnea
	Apnea
	Excoriated skin
	Behavior irregularities
	Weight loss or failure to gain weight
		Prematurity
		Hypoxia/low Apgar scores
		Intrauterine growth restriction
		Low birth weight
		Microcephaly
		Increased risk for meconium stained fluid/
		  meconium aspiration
		Congenital infections
		Increased risk for sudden infant death syndrome
		Increased chromosomal abnormalities
		  (heroin exposure)

INHALANTS	Fetal dysmorphogenesis syndrome–similar to fetal alcohol syndrome Small for gestational age Microcephaly Deep-set eyes Small face Low-set ears Micrognathia Spoon shaped fingertips/small fingernails	Developmental delay Language problems Cerebellar dysfunction Hyperactivity

Sources: Gilbert (2007); Pitts (2004).

■ *Neonates exposed to alcohol in utero may demonstrate withdrawal symptoms within 3 to 12 hours after birth (AAP, 1998).*

■ *Neonates exposed to narcotics in utero exhibit withdrawal within 48 to 72 hours after birth.*

■ *Neonates exposed to barbiturates in utero exhibit withdrawal between days 1 and 14 (AAP, 1998).*

CRITICAL COMPONENT

Signs of Neonatal Withdrawal

Hypertonia	Nasal congestion
Tremors	Sneezing
Hyperreflexia	Lacrimation
Seizures	Sweating
Irritability/restlessness	Fever
High pitched cry	Skin mottling
Excessive crying	Diarrhea
Sleep problems	Tachypnea
Wakefulness	Apnea
Yawning	Excoriated skin
Vomiting	Behavior irregularities
Poor feeding	Weight loss or failure to gain weight
Dysmature swallowing	
Excessive/frantic sucking	

(Pitts, 2004)

■ Alcohol use during pregnancy can cause a wide range of problems from no effect to major long-term disabilities (Gilbert, 2007). The following are conditions resulting from alcohol exposure during pregnancy:

■ ***Fetal alcohol syndrome (FAS):*** *A wide array and spectrum of physical, cognitive and behavioral abnormalities associated with maternal alcohol use during pregnancy (AAP, 2000). Signs of FAS include:*

■ Distinctive facial features: small eyes, thin upper lip, and short nose

■ Heart defects

■ Joint, limbs, and finger deformities

■ Delayed physical growth both intrauterine and post-birth

■ Vision problems

■ Hearing problems

■ Mental retardation

■ Behavior disturbances such as short attention span, hyperactivity, and poor impulse control (Mayo Clinic Staff, 2007)

■ ***Alcohol related birth defects (ARBD):*** *Congenital anomalies associated with alcohol use during pregnancy that may affect the heart, skeleton, kidneys, eyes, and ears*

■ ***Alcohol related neurodevelopmental disorder (ARND):*** *Abnormalities of the central nervous system that are associated with prenatal alcohol exposure:*

■ Neurological problems (e.g., poor hand–eye coordination and fine motor skills, and neurosensory hearing loss)

■ Decreased cranial size, brain abnormalities

■ Cognitive and behavioral problems (Pitts, 2004)

Medical Management

■ Review the maternal history for substance use, prescription drug use, and risk factors for substance use.

■ Perform physical assessment of the neonate, including observation for physical and behavioral effects of prenatal substance use.

■ Obtain toxicology screening of the neonate's urine and/or meconium.

■ Order diagnostic tests such as cranial ultrasound and EEG, if indicated by clinical manifestations of withdrawal symptoms.

■ *Problems such as infection and hypoglycemia may manifest symptoms similar to those of neonatal withdrawal, and should be ruled out by the appropriate diagnostic tests (AAP, 1998).*

■ Use an assessment tool to determine signs of neonatal abstinence syndrome (Fig. 17-7).

■ *Use of the tool should be initiated within 2 hours of birth and neonates should be assessed for signs of withdrawal every 4 hours (Pitts, 2004).*

■ *Use tool to guide decisions about when a neonate should be evaluated for treatment with medication (Pitts, 2004).*

■ Pharmacological therapy should be considered if seizures, excessive weight loss, dehydration, poor feeding, diarrhea, vomiting, fever, and inability to sleep occur (AAP, 1998).

■ Medications used to treat withdrawal in neonates include:

■ *Methadone, morphine, paregoric, tincture of opium, clonidine, and diazepam, for opioid withdrawal*

■ *Benzodiazepines to treat withdrawal from alcohol*

■ *Phenobarbital for hyperactive behavior associated with narcotic withdrawal, also used for withdrawal from non-narcotic agents*

■ *Chlorpromazine for babies exhibiting gastrointestinal and CNS effects of narcotic withdrawal (AAP, 1998; Pitts, 2004)*

■ Give frequent, small feedings with a high calorie formula (24 calories/oz.).

■ Monitor feedings, output, and weight daily.

■ Educate mothers about substance use and breastfeeding.

■ *Breastfeeding is contraindicated if a woman is actively using any of the following substances: cocaine, methamphetamines, alcohol, heroin, and/or marijuana (Pitts, 2004).*

■ *Breastfeeding is not contraindicated with methadone use (AAP, 1998). Infants of mothers on methadone must be weaned gradually to avoid withdrawal (Pitts, 2004).*

■ *Women who smoke cigarettes should be advised to quit and be given information about cessation resources. Women who choose to continue to smoke should be taught to avoid smoking around the baby, to smoke immediately after breastfeeding and not before, and to cut down on the number of cigarettes that they smoke (Pitts, 2004).*

■ Arrange for comprehensive follow-up care for the mother of the baby or the foster mother before discharge. Infants exposed to substances prenatally often need long-term interdisciplinary physical and developmental care (Pitts, 2004).

■ *Referrals must be made to the appropriate departments and agencies (Pitts, 2004). In many health care settings, health care providers obtain a social service consult for women who have a history of substance use. Notification of agencies such as Child Protective Services is dependent on laws of each state. In some states, neonates who are positive for prenatal substance exposure are placed in foster care.*

Nursing Actions

■ Review maternal history including risk factors of substance use and history of current or past substance use.

■ Assess the neonate, including gestational age.

■ Assess for congenital anomalies and physical and behavioral signs of withdrawal/neonatal abstinence syndrome.

■ Monitor vital signs.

- Obtain toxicology screening as per order.
- Use a scoring tool to assess for signs of withdrawal on neonates who are at high risk for neonatal abstinence syndrome (see Fig. 17-7).
  - *Notify the physician if the score is outside of what is considered normal.*
- Care for neonates experiencing neonatal abstinence syndrome:
  - *Assess feedings and daily weights: Increased activity, decreased sleep, irritability, loose stools, vomiting, and poor feeding behavior may all result in increased caloric needs.*
  - *Provide frequent and small feedings: A higher calorie formula (24 cal/oz.) can be used to support increased caloric needs.*
    - Allow the neonate to rest during feedings.
    - Position the neonate upright during feedings.
  - *Provide a pacifier to the neonate.*
- *Bathe the baby in warm water to treat increased tone and irritability.*
- *Swaddle neonate with arms close to the body.*
- *Provide a quiet environment, with lights dimmed, and minimize stimuli.*
- *Be sensitive to infant cues that indicate stress; minimize stress-inducing activities.*
- *Rock the neonate gently (AAP, 1998; Pitts, 2004).*
- Care for the mother of a neonates with neonatal abstinence syndrome:
  - *Provide nonjudgmental, honest, supportive care.*
  - *Teach what to expect in regard to the neonate's behavior. Educate about strategies that will provide comfort to her infant during withdrawal.*
  - *Teach her how to feed her infant.*

System	Signs and symptoms	Date Time							Comments
		Score							
CENTRAL NERVOUS SYSTEM DISTURBANCES	Crying: Excessive high-pitched	2							
	Crying: Continuous high-pitched	3							
	Sleeps less than 1 hour after feeding	3							
	Sleeps less than 2 hours after feeding	2							
	Sleeps less than 3 hours after feeding	1							
	Hyperactive Moro reflex	2							
	Markedly hyperactive Moro reflex	3							
	Mild tremors: Disturbed	1							
	Moderate-severe tremors: Disturbed	2							
	Mild tremors: Undisturbed	3							
	Moderate-severe tremors: Undisturbed	4							
	Increased muscle tone	2							
	Excoriation (specify area)	1							
	Myoclonic jerks	3							
	Generalized convulsions	5							
METABOLIC, VASOMOTOR, AND RESPIRATORY DISTURBANCES	Sweating	1							
	Fever less than or equal to 101 (37.2–38.3°C)	1							
	Fever greater than 101 (38.4°C)	2							
	Frequent yawning (greater than 3)	1							
	Mottling	1							
	Nasal stuffiness	1							
	Sneezing (greater than 3)	1							
	Nasal flaring	2							
	Respiratory rate (greater than 60/min)	1							
	Respiratory rate (greater than 60/min with retractions)	2							
GASTROINTESTINAL DISTURBANCES	Excessive suckling	1							
	Poor feeding	2							
	Regurgitation	2							
	Projectile vomiting	3							
	Loose stools	2							
	Watery stools	3							
	TOTAL SCORE								

Figure 17-7 Neonatal Abstinence Scoring Tool.

- *Observe maternal–newborn interactions and involve the mother in the care of her newborn.*
  - Neonates who have been exposed to substances during the prenatal period often exhibit behaviors that interfere with the maternal-newborn relationship such as irritability, resistance to being comforted, arching while being held, altered sleep states, poor feeding behavior, easily agitated when stimulated, and difficult transitions from one state to another.
  - Characteristics of mothers with a history of substance abuse that may impair the maternal-newborn relationship include lack of sensitivity to infant cues, lack of emotional stability, lack of communication with the infant, and inconsistent/unavailable caregiving.
  - Document all assessments and observations in the medical record per agency protocol (Pitts, 2004).

CONGENITAL ABNORMALITIES

Congenital anomalies or birth defects occur in approximately 20% of infant deaths in the United States (March of Dimes, 2007b; Sterk, 2004). Abnormalities range from being undetectable at birth, to major and life threatening.

- Risk factors
  - *Chromosomal abnormalities*
- Environmental factors: Teratogens such as radiation, illicit substances, alcohol, diseases (diabetes) medications, and infections such as TORCH (**T**oxoplasmosis, **O**ther infections, **R**ubella, **C**ytomegalovirus, **H**erpes simplex virus)
  - *Multifactorial disorders: Abnormalities that result in a combination of environmental and genetic factors (Sterk, 2004)*

Assessment Findings

- See Table 17-13 for common congenital anomalies.
- See Table 17-14 for common cardiac anomalies.
- See Table 17-15 for common metabolic disorders.

Nursing Actions

- Nursing care is determined by the type and severity of anomaly.
- Genetic disease screening is obtained before discharge of the neonate. The test is repeated if the initial test is done before 48 hours of age.
- Provide emotional support for parents and family.
- Provide information on support groups.
- Provide information on need for follow-up care.

REGIONAL CENTERS

Women experiencing a high-risk pregnancy may require transfer to a facility that can provide the appropriate level of care to them and their neonate after delivery. Many facilities/communities lack the resources to provide care to high-risk mothers and high-risk neonates; thus, regional centers were developed to provide services such as high-risk perinatal care and neonatal intensive care. Transport of a high-risk neonate to a center with a neonatal intensive care unit (NICU) requires coordination between the transferring and receiving hospitals, appropriate preparation, a highly skilled

team, and the appropriate equipment (Fig. 17-8). Key considerations of neonatal transport are:

- During the transport process, the transport team provides care that is an extension of the NICU. The aim is to provide the appropriate amount of support to the neonate to maintain stable condition. The transport process should minimize adverse effects of transfer on the neonate, and be carried out in a way that protects the safety of the patient and the transport team (Bowen, 2004).
- The transport team must be knowledgeable about high-risk neonatal care and assessment. Members of the team may include a neonatal nurse practitioner, neonatologist, resident, fellow, registered nurse, respiratory therapist, and a paramedic or emergency medical technician (Bowen, 2004).
- The transport process includes the following:
  - *Once the need for NICU care is identified, arrangements are made to transfer the high-risk neonate.*
  - *Information pertaining to maternal and neonatal history is communicated during the referral call.*
  - *The appropriate team is dispatched with supplies and equipment needed to care for the neonate.*
  - *The neonate is stabilized before transport.*
  - *During transport the infant is kept in an incubator, thermoregulation is maintained, respiratory support and IV therapy are provided, and the following are monitored:*
    - Vital signs, oxygen saturation, blood glucose, the neonate's condition, pain status, and response to transport
  - *Strategies should be used to provide developmental care during transfer such as protecting the neonate's eyes from bright lights, using ear protection in noisy vehicles such as helicopters, using a gel mattress to prevent jarring, and using blankets to promote containment.*
  - *Notify parents when the infant arrives at the receiving facility (Bowen, 2004).*

Various vehicles may be used for transport such as ambulance, helicopter, or fixed wing aircraft. The type of vehicle that is used will be determined by factors such as the neonate's condition and diagnosis, distance of transport, weather, and cost. Appropriate supplies and equipment based on the neonate's condition must be stocked and checked regularly. Equipment includes:

- Monitoring devices such as a pulse oximeter, cardiorespiratory monitor, blood pressure monitors
- Oxygen tanks and other respiratory supplies such as endotracheal tubes, oxygen tubing and masks, oxygen hood, ventilator, and suctioning equipment
- Medications
- Intravenous therapy equipment
- Equipment to maintain and assess thermoregulation such as an incubator, thermometer, heat packs, and blankets
- Equipment to perform blood glucose, and blood gas monitoring
- Personal protective equipment such as gloves and gowns

DISCHARGE PLANNING

Discharge planning for high-risk neonates involves many considerations since these neonates often require special care and follow-up after release from the hospital. In some cases, infants require long-term evaluation to monitor health issues, growth, and neurodevelopment. Many high-risk conditions such as prematurity and related complications, perinatal substance use, and congenital anomalies

TABLE 17–13 COMMON CONGENITAL ANOMALIES

TYPE OF ANOMALY	INCIDENCE	DESCRIPTION	TREATMENT
TRACHEOESOPHAGEAL FISTULA	1 in 4,500 live births	Abnormal opening between the trachea and esophagus	Surgical repair
CHOANAL ATRESIA	2–4 in 10,000 live births	Obstruction of the nasal passages	Surgical repair
DIAPHRAGMATIC HERNIA	1 in 1,000–6,000 live births	Herniation of abdominal organs through a hole in the diaphragm into the thoracic cavity	Gastric decompression Stabilization Surgical repair
OMPHALOCELE	1 in 5,000–6,000 live births	Herniation of abdominal contents through the umbilicus which is covered by the peritoneal sac	Surgical repair. Staged surgical repair for large defects (abdominal contents returned gradually)
GASTROSCHISIS	1 in 30,000–50,000 live births	Herniation of abdominal contents through a hole in the abdomen often to the right of the umbilicus	Surgical repair Staged surgical repair for large defects
CLEFT LIP	1 in 1,000 live births	Failure of the mesenchymal masses of the nasal and maxillary prominences to come together	Surgical repair
CLEFT PALATE	1 in 2,500 live births	Failure of the mesenchymal masses in the palate to fuse	Surgical repair
SPINA BIFIDA: Meningocele	1 in 20,000 live births	A sac with meninges and cerebral spinal fluid bulge through defect in undeveloped vertebrae	Surgical repair
Myelomeningocele	1 in 1,000 live births	A sac with meninges and nerve tissue bulge through a defect in the spinal column	Surgical repair
ANENCEPHALY	1 in 1,000 live births	Incomplete formation of the cranium and brain	Most babies die within a few days of birth
DEVELOPMENTAL DYSPLASIA OF THE HIP	1–2 in 1,000 live births	Dislocation of the femoral head from the acetabulum	Pavlik harness to promote abduction/flexion to stabilize hip Surgery if Pavlik harness is not successful
POLYDACTYLY		Extra digits on the hand or foot	Surgery or ligation
SYNDACTYLY	1 in 2,200 live births	Fusion of digits of hand or foot	Surgery depending on extent of anomaly
TALIPES EQUINOVARUS	1 in 1,000 live births	Sole of the foot is turned in; the back part of the foot is deformed. Also called "clubfoot," usually bilateral.	Casting/splinting Surgery Treatment depends on severity.

Source: Sterk (2004).

TABLE 17–14   COMMON CARDIAC ANOMALIES

TYPE OF ANOMALY	INCIDENCE	DESCRIPTION	TREATMENT
VENTRICULAR SEPTAL DEFECT (VSD)	1 in 3,000 live births	Opening in the septum between the right and left ventricles of the heart.	Up to 75% of VSDs close without treatment. Treat with digoxin and diuretics if congestive heart failure is present. Surgical repair.
ATRIAL SEPTAL DEFECT (ASD)	1 in 5,000 live births	Opening in the septum between the right and left atria.	ASDs may close without treatment. Treat congestive heart failure with medication. Surgical repair may be needed.
COARCTATION OF THE AORTA	1 in 10,000 live births	Narrowing of the aorta at the transverse aortic arch or in the area of the ductus arteriosus	Medical management of congestive heart failure. Surgical repair.
TETRALOGY OF FALLOT	1 in 5,000 live births	Consists of four defects: 1. VSD 2. Aorta overriding VSD 3. Pulmonary stenosis 4. Hypertrophy of the right ventricle	Medical management includes propranolol for cyanotic infants. Prostaglandin E1 may be administered to maintain a patent ductus arteriosus until surgery, for infants with a severe tetralogy of Fallot. Surgical repair.
TRANSPOSITION OF GREAT VESSELS	1 in 5,000 live births	The positions of the great arteries are reversed from the normal position. Aorta emerges from the right ventricle and the pulmonary artery emerges from the left ventricle.	This defect results in a medical emergency. Stabilization-treat acidosis. Administer prostaglandin E1 to maintain a patent ductus arteriosus until surgery is performed.

Source: Sadowski (2004).

may have long-term, even lifelong, physical, cognitive, and behavioral consequences. The following are critical components of the discharge process for high-risk neonates (Gracey, 2004):

■ When a high-risk neonate is admitted, planning for discharge begins. Parents should be encouraged to be involved with the care of their infant from the time of admission. Care-related teaching with parents should begin as soon after delivery as possible.

■ Interdisciplinary teams are often involved in the discharge process. The team may consist of physicians, nurse practitioners, nurses, social workers, occupational therapist, case manager, lactation consultant, respiratory therapist, nutritionist, pharmacist, and home health agency/nursing staff.

■ Readiness for discharge is assessed.
  ■ *The neonate's condition must be stable (e.g., weight gain, temperature stability, able to tolerate feedings, stable respiratory status; Fig. 17-9).*
  ■ *All appropriate examinations and screenings are completed such as an eye exam, genetic disease/metabolic disease screening.*

  ■ *The neonate is able to sit in a car seat and maintain adequate oxygenation.*
  ■ *Family's readiness to take their infant home is assessed.*
    ■ The family's willingness and ability to provide care to their infant with special needs is evaluated, as are their financial resources. In addition, the home setting assessed for safety and adequacy.
  ■ *The educational needs of the family are meet. Discharge teaching includes:*
    ■ General infant care such as bathing, feeding schedule, diapering, skin care
    ■ Safety issues such as car seat safety, positioning the infant on the back to sleep, infant CPR, baby proofing the house
    ■ Instructions on use of required equipment (e.g., apnea monitoring)
    ■ Information on treatments (e.g., oxygen, suctioning) and medications ordered

TABLE 17–15 COMMON GENETIC DISORDERS OF METABOLISM

TYPE OF DISORDER	INCIDENCE	DESCRIPTION	TREATMENT
PHENYLKETONURIA	1 in 10,000-15,000 live births	Lack of the enzyme needed to convert phenylalanine to tyrosine. If untreated causes cognitive and physical problems.	Diet that restricts intake of phenylalanine.
DISORDERS OF FATTY ACID OXIDATION (e.g., medium chain acyl-CoA-deficiency)	1 in 15,000 live births	18 disorders identified. Impaired fat metabolism leads to hypoglycemia and organ failure.	Hypoglycemia is treated. Fasting is avoided.
CONGENITAL ADRENAL HYPERPLASIA	1 in 5,000 live births	Cortisol production is inhibited. Adrenal hypertrophy results, with excessive production of adrenal androgens. Electrolyte imbalances common, female infants exhibit ambiguous genitalia.	Steroid administration Corrective surgery for ambiguous genitalia.
MAPLE SYRUP URINE DISEASE	1 in 150,000	Lack of enzymes needed to metabolize leucine, valine, and isoleucine. These amino acids build up in the blood. Disease is fatal if untreated.	Peritoneal dialysis Low protein diet
GALACTOSEMIA	1 in 40,000-60,000 live births	Lack of enzyme that converts galactose to glucose. Inability to metabolize lactose. If untreated results in liver disease, mental retardation, and cataracts.	Lactose-free or soy formula.

Source: Strek (2004).

■ Signs and symptoms of illnesses that need to be reported to the primary care provider
■ Infant growth and developmental milestones
■ Follow-up information including visits with the pediatrician, immunization schedules, and referrals to the appropriate medical and developmental specialists

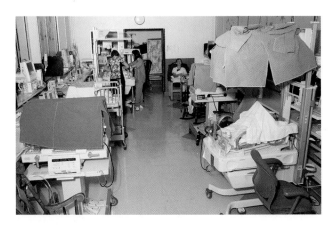

Figure 17-8 Neonatal Intensive Care Unit (NICU).

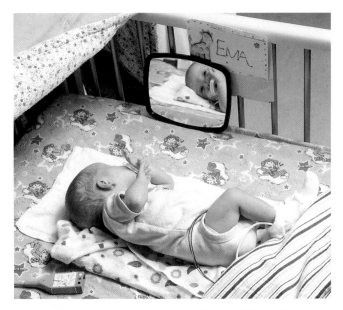

Figure 17-9 A 10-week-old neonate, born at 27 weeks' gestation, who will soon be going home.

PSYCHOSOCIAL NEEDS OF PARENTS WITH HIGH-RISK NEONATES

The birth of a baby who is premature, or who has conditions that place him or her at risk for illness or even death is a significant stressor for the family. Parents may grieve over the loss of an ideal baby, and find the experience of having a baby with complications overwhelming. It is devastating for most parents when the woman is discharged and their baby must remain in the hospital.

Common effects on the parents and family are:

■ Delay of attachment process due to the separation of parent and newborn, which can place the newborn at risk for abuse and neglect.
■ Guilt feelings by the woman, who may feel she did something wrong to cause her newborn to be ill.
■ Emotional distancing of parents from their newborn as a protective mechanism due to fear of losing their child
■ Disruption of family life; parents needing to return to work, caring for other child, and at the same time wanting to spend time in the hospital with their neonate

Nursing actions that support parents of high-risk neonates are:

■ Assess parents comfort level with the NICU environment.
■ Orient parents to the NICU environment by explaining equipment/monitors used for their neonate.
■ Provide opportunities for parents to share their concerns and frustrations by developing a trusting rapport with the parents and through active listening skills.
■ Provide opportunities for parents to talk about their experiences by asking parents how they are coping with the experience and by use of active listening.
■ Provide information regarding their neonate's status to both parents at a level they can understand.
■ Inform parents that they should ask any question they have regarding the condition and care of their neonate.
■ Inform parents that they can talk to their neonate's nurse at any time.
■ Assess the parents' readiness to care for their neonate and provide opportunities for them to participate in the care of their neonate.
■ Encourage parents to touch and hold neonate as indicated by the neonate's health status.
■ Encourage the woman to pump her breast and bring the milk to the NICU to be used for feeding.
   ■ *Review breast milk storage and provide equipment as needed.*
■ Provide a private area for woman to breastfeed when the neonate is able to nurse.

■ Encourage parents to take photos to share with their family and friends.
■ Praise parents for their involvement in the neonate's care.
■ Provide information on support groups for parents of preterm infants or infants with disabilities.

LOSS AND GRIEF

When a baby dies, parents must work through profound grief associated with the loss of their child, and the loss of their hopes and dreams for that child and their family. Grief is a process that is individual in nature. Often members of the family experience grief in different ways and in varied time lines. The stages of grief include:

■ Avoidance, disbelief, shock
■ Pain, physical discomforts, depression, difficulty concentrating, anger at self or partner, guilt
■ Acceptance and adaptation. Grief persists, but a sense of balance is achieved (Kenner, 2004; March of Dimes, 2007a).

It is important that nurses keep in mind that each person experiences and expresses grief in his or her own way. Culture, religion, and personal experience and beliefs will impact how individuals and families respond to loss. Nurses can help families that are grieving the death of their baby by carrying out various interventions including:

■ Allow parents to express their feelings by being present and listening.
■ Express empathy and condolences. Avoid clichés such as "at least you are young; you can have another baby." If the baby has been named, refer to the baby by that name.
■ Provide information about the process of grieving and what to expect physically and emotionally.
■ Provide ample opportunity for the parents to spend time with the baby before and after he or she dies.
■ Provide parents with memorabilia associated with their baby such as pictures, blankets, a cap, a lock of hair, ID bracelet, footprints, and crib card.
■ Offer to contact the hospital chaplain. Encourage the family to contact their own clergy. Explore the family's desire for baptism or other religious rites.
■ Discuss the family's plan for autopsy, a memorial or funeral, burial/cremation.
■ Encourage the family to accept help and support from others.
■ Refer parents to community services and support groups that may assist in facilitating the grief process (Kenner, 2004).

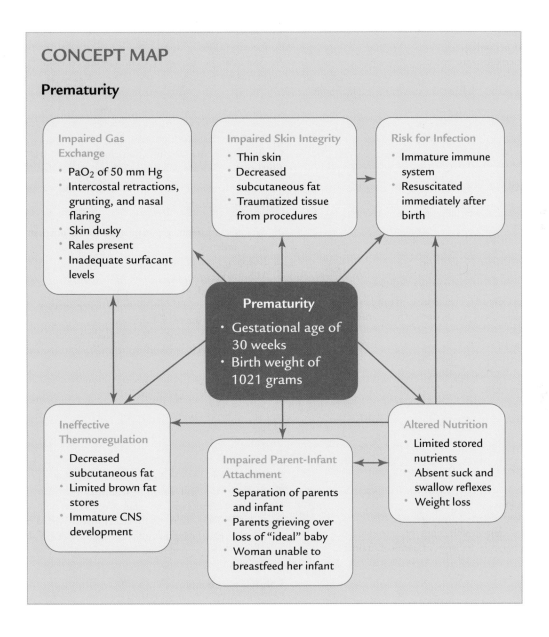

CONCEPT MAP

Prematurity

Impaired Gas Exchange
- PaO₂ of 50 mm Hg
- Intercostal retractions, grunting, and nasal flaring
- Skin dusky
- Rales present
- Inadequate surfacant levels

Impaired Skin Integrity
- Thin skin
- Decreased subcutaneous fat
- Traumatized tissue from procedures

Risk for Infection
- Immature immune system
- Resuscitated immediately after birth

Prematurity
- Gestational age of 30 weeks
- Birth weight of 1021 grams

Ineffective Thermoregulation
- Decreased subcutaneous fat
- Limited brown fat stores
- Immature CNS development

Impaired Parent-Infant Attachment
- Separation of parents and infant
- Parents grieving over loss of "ideal" baby
- Woman unable to breastfeed her infant

Altered Nutrition
- Limited stored nutrients
- Absent suck and swallow reflexes
- Weight loss

Problem No. 1: Impaired gas exchange
Goal: Adequate gas exchange
Outcome: PaO₂ is 60–70 mm Hg; PaCO₂ is 35-45 mm Hg; skin color is pink; lung sounds are clear; and no signs of retractions, grunting, or nasal flaring.

Nursing Actions

1. Monitor vital signs, oxygen saturation, and arterial blood gases.
2. Maintain patent airway.
3. Suction airway as indicated.
4. Administer oxygen as per orders.
5. Maintain a neutral thermal environment.
6. Cluster nursing activities.
7. Monitor for adverse effects related to surfactant replacement therapy.

Problem No. 2: Impaired skin integrity
Goal: Intact skin
Outcome: The neonate's skin will be intact and without signs of skin irritation.

Nursing Actions

1. Assess skin for redness, dryness, breakdown, and rashes.
2. Use a neutral pH cleanser and sterile water when bathing. Bathe only soiled body parts.
3. Use adhesives sparingly.
4. Apply emollient to dry areas.
5. Change diapers frequently and apply zinc-oxide.
6. Change positions frequently.
7. Use water, air, or gelled mattresses as indicated.

Problem No. 3: Risk of infection
Goal: Be free of infection
Outcome: Neonates will not exhibit signs of infection such as elevated temperature, lethargy, or purulent drainage.

Nursing Actions

1. Promote hand washing for staff and parents.
2. Assess for signs of infection.
3. Maintain intact skin.
4. Properly prepare sites for invasive procedures.
5. Properly care for invasive lines to maintain sterility.
6. Administer antibiotics as per orders.
7. Encourage use of breast milk for infant feedings.

Problem No. 4: Ineffective thermoregulation
Goal: Stable temperature within normal range
Outcome: Neonates temperature will be between 36.4° and 37.2°C (97.5°–99°F).

Nursing Actions

1. Keep the neonate dry.
2. Use plastic barriers when indicated.
3. Prewarm radiant warmers, incubators, and linens.
4. Encourage kangaroo care.
5. Keep area free of drafts.
6. Swaddle the neonate when holding outside of warmer or incubator.

Problem No. 5: Altered nutrition
Goal: Growth and weight gain within normal ranges
Outcome: Neonate will gain 20–30 grams per day.

Nursing Actions

1. Administer parenteral nutrition, enteral feedings, or oral feedings as per orders.
2. Encourage use of breast milk.
3. Monitor weight daily.
4. Monitor length and head circumference weekly.
5. Instill breast milk or formula, when gavage feeding, over 20 minutes at a rate of 1 mL/min.
6. Monitor the neonate during feedings for signs of feeding intolerance, such as vomiting, regurgitation, and excessive gastric residual.
7. Encourage breastfeeding when indicated.
8. Monitor intake and output.

Problem No. 6: Impaired parent–infant attachment
Goal: Positive parent–infant attachment
Outcome: Parents hold the infant close to the body and the infant appears calm and relaxed; parents spend time each day with the infant and participates in care of the infant; parents respond to infant cues.

Nursing Actions

1. Orient parents to the NICU environment
2. Provide opportunities for parents to share their concerns and frustrations.
3. Provide opportunities for parents to talk about their experiences of having a high-risk neonate.
4. Assess parent's readiness to care for their neonate and provide opportunities for participation in caring for their neonate.
5. Instruct parents on neonatal care.
6. Praise parents for their involvement.
7. Encourage the woman to pump her breast and bring her breast milk for use with infant feeding.
8. Encourage kangaroo holding by both parents.

TYING IT ALL TOGETHER

Baby girl Polk is a newly delivered 32 weeks' gestation neonate who is admitted to the NICU. Her mother, Mallory, is a 42-year-old African American single woman. Mallory is a G2 P0 who conceived after three attempts at in vitro fertilization. Mallory was admitted to the birthing unit for preterm labor. She was given magnesium sulfate, ampicillin, and two doses of betamethasone. Her labor contraction continued. When her cervix was 5 cm dilated, a decision was made to discontinue the magnesium sulfate. A few hours after the magnesium sulfate was discontinued, Mallory gave birth spontaneously to a baby girl. The 1- and 5-minute Apgar scores were 7 and 8, respectively. Baby Polk weighed 2010 grams and was assessed at 32 weeks based on Ballard score.

Detail the aspects of your initial nursing assessment.
List the nursing diagnosis for this neonate.
What are the immediate priorities in the nursing care of Baby Polk?
Discuss the rationale for the selected priorities.
List the anticipated medical care for Baby Polk.

4 hours later:
Baby Polk is on NCPAP. There is an increase in intercostal retractions and expiratory grunting. The results of arterial blood gas (ABG) tests are P_{CO_2} of 70 and pH of 7.2. CBC indicates an increase in WBC.
Medical orders include initial dose of Survanta, IV of D10, glucose monitoring every 4 hours, ampicillin 50 mg/kg, and gentamicin 4 mg/kg.

Based on this additional information, list the nursing diagnosis for this neonate.
List the anticipated medical care.
Discuss the nursing are for this neonate and mother.

1 week later:
Baby Polk is extubated and is placed on high-flow nasal cannula at 1 liter. She is tolerating gavage feedings and gaining weight. She is experiencing occasional episodes of apnea and bradycardia.

Discuss the criteria for discharge from the NICU.
Describe the discharge teaching for the care of baby Polk.

■ ■ ■ Review Questions ■ ■ ■

1. A nurse is assessing a preterm baby with a gestational age of 32 weeks and birth weight of 1389 grams. Which of the following signs if present would be a possible indication of RSD?
   A. Expiratory grunting and intercostal retractions
   B. Respiratory rate of 46 breaths per minute and presence of acrocyanosis
   C. Mild nasal flaring and heart rate of 140 beats per minute
   D. Bradycardia and bounding pulse

2. The primary risk factor for necrotizing enterocolitis (NEC) is:
   A. Early oral feedings with formula
   B. Passage of meconium during labor
   C. Prematurity
   D. Low birth weight

3. A common characteristic of a premature infant is:
   A. Absence of lanugo
   B. Dry skin
   C. Increased flexion of arms and legs
   D. Transparent and red skin.

4. When gavage feeding a preterm neonate, the nurse should:
   A. Measure the tube before insertion from the mouth to the sternum.
   B. Check for placement by injecting a small amount of sterile water into the feeding tube and listen for a gurgling noise.
   C. Instill formula over a 20-minute period of time.
   D. Flush the tube at the end of feeding with dextrose water.

5. Which of the following statements is true regarding hyperbilirubinemia?
   A. Jaundice covers the entire body in pathological jaundice versus only the face in physiologic jaundice.
   B. Jaundice occurs within the first 24 hours post-birth in pathological jaundice versus after 24 hours in physiologic jaundice.
   C. Kernicterus only occurs in pathologic jaundice.
   D. Jaundice begins to appear in term neonates when the bilirubin level is 3 mg/dL.

References

Aher, S., & Ohlsson, A. (2006). Late erythropoietin for preventing red blood cell transfusion in preterm and/or low birth weight infants (Review). *Cochrane Database of Systematic Reviews*, Issue 3. Art. No.: CD004868. DOI: 10.1002/14651858.CD004868.pub2.

American Academy of Pediatrics (AAP). (1997). Revised guidelines for prevention of early-onset group B streptococcal (GBS) infection. *Pediatrics, 99*, 489–496.

American Academy of Pediatrics (AAP). (1998). Neonatal drug withdrawal. *Pediatrics, 6*, 1079–1088.

American Academy of Pediatrics (AAP). (2000). Fetal alcohol syndrome and alcohol related neurodevelopmental disorders. *Pediatrics, 106*, 358–361.

American Academy of Pediatrics (AAP). (2004a). An evidence-based review of important issues concerning neonatal hyperbilirubinemia. *Pediatrics, 114*, pe130–e153.

American Academy of Pediatrics (AAP). (2004b). Management of hyperbilirubinemia in the newborn infant 35 or more weeks of gestation. *Pediatrics, 114*, 297–316.

American Lung Association. (2006). *Respiratory distress syndrome of the newborn fact sheet* [on-line]. Retrieved from www.lungusa.org (Accessed July 6, 2009).

Anderson, G., Moore, E., Hepworth, J., & Bergman, N. (2003). Early skin to skin contact for mothers and their healthy newborn infants (Review). *Cochrane Database of Systematic Review*, Issue 2. Art. No.: CD003519. DOI: 10.1002/14651858.CD003519.

Armentrout, D. (2004). Glucose management. In M. Verklan & M. Walden (Eds.), *Core curriculum for neonatal intensive care nursing*. St. Louis, MO: Elsevier Saunders.

Askin, D., & Diehl-Jones, W. (2004). Assisted ventilation. In M. Verklan & M. Walden (Eds.), *Core curriculum for neonatal intensive care nursing*. St. Louis, MO: Elsevier Saunders.

Association of Women's Health, Obstetric, and Neonatal Nurses/National Association of Neonatal Nurses (AWHONN/NANN). (2001). *Neonatal skin care: Evidence based clinical practice guideline*. Washington, DC: Author.

Association of Women's Health, Obstetric and Neonatal Nurses (AWHONN). (2006). *The compendium of postpartum care* (2nd ed.). Philadelphia: Medical Broadcasting Company.

Badr, L., & Purdy, I. (2006). Brain injury in the infant: The old, the new, and the uncertain. *Journal of Perinatal and Neonatal Nursing, 20,* 163–175.

Bancalari, E. (2006). Bronchopulmonary dysplasia and neonatal chronic lung disease. In R. Martin, A. Fanaroff, & M. Walsh (Eds.), *Neonatal-perinatal medicine: Vol. 2. Diseases of the fetus and infant.* Philadelphia: Mosby Elsevier.

Bakewell-Sachs, S., & Brandes, A. (2004). Nutritional management. In M. Verklan & M. Walden (Eds.), *Core curriculum for neonatal intensive care nursing.* St. Louis, MO: Elsevier Saunders.

Bowen, S. (2004). Intrafacility and interfacility neonatal transport. In M. Verklan & M. Walden (Eds.), *Core curriculum for neonatal intensive care nursing.* St. Louis, MO: Elsevier Saunders.

Caplan, M. (2006). Neonatal necrotizing enterocolitis. In R. Martin, A. Fanaroff, & M. Walsh (Eds.), *Neonatal-perinatal medicine: Vol. 2. Diseases of the fetus and infant* (8th ed.). Philadelphia: Mosby Elsevier.

Carrier, C. (2004). Developmental support. In M. Verklan & M. Walden (Eds.), *Core curriculum for neonatal intensive care nursing.* St. Louis, MO: Elsevier Saunders.

Centers for Disease Control and Prevention (CDC). (2002). Prevention of perinatal group B streptococcal disease. *MMWR, 51,* 1-27.

Cincinnati Children's Hospital Medical Center. (2005). Evidence-based care guideline for necrotizing enterocolitis among very low birth weight infants. *National Guideline Clearinghouse.* Retrieved from www.guideline. gov/summary (Accessed September 4, 2009).

Conde-Agudelo, A., Diaz-Rossello, J., & Belizan, J. (2003). Kangaroo mother care to reduce morbidity and mortality in low birthweight infants (Review). *Cochrane Database of Systematic Reviews,* Issue 2. Art. No.: CD002771. DOI: 10.1002/14651858.CD002771.

Cramer, K., Wiebe, N., Hartling, L., Crumley, E., & Vohra, S. (2005). Heat loss prevention: A systemic review of occlusive skin wrap for premature neonates. *Journal of Perinatology, 25,* 763–769.

Dunn, R., Brydon, P., Smith, K., & Gee, H. (2003). Pregnancy in women with type 2 diabetes: 12 years outcome data 1990-2002. *Diabetic Medicine, 20,* 734–738.

Fowlie, P., & Davis, P. (2002). Prophylactic intravenous indomethacin for preventing mortality and morbidity in preterm infants. *Cochrane Database of Systematic Reviews,* Issue 3. Art.No.: CD000174.DOI: 10.1002/14651858.CD000174.

Furdon, S., & Benjamin, K. (2004). Physical assessment. In M. Verklan & M. Walden (Eds.), *Core curriculum for neonatal intensive care nursing.* St. Louis, MO: Elsevier Saunders.

Ghodrat, M. (2006). Lung surfactant. *American Journal of Health-Systems Pharmacology, 63,* 1504–1521.

Gilbert, E. S. (2007). *Manual of high risk pregnancy and delivery* (4th ed.). St. Louis, MO: Mosby.

Goodwin, M. (2004). Apnea. In M. Verklan & M. Walden (Eds.), *Core curriculum for neonatal intensive care nursing.* St. Louis, MO: Elsevier Saunders.

Gracey, K. (2004). Discharge planning and transition to home care. *Core curriculum for neonatal intensive care nursing.* St. Louis, MO: Elsevier Saunders.

Hamilton, B., Martin, J., & Ventura, S. (2006). Births: Preliminary data for 2005. *National Vital Statistics Reports* 55(11). Hyattsville, MD: National Center for Health Statistics.

Hendson, L., Phelps, D. L., & Andersen, C.C. (2002). Laser photocoagulation versus transscleral cryotherapy for threshold retinopathy of prematurity (Protocol). *Cochrane Database of Systematic Reviews,* Issue 3. [0]CD003847

Himmelberger, S. M. (2002). Preventing group B strep in newborns: Prenatal screening is critical to catching, curing, this deadly infection. *AWHONN Lifelines, 6,* 339–342.

Horns, K. (2004). Immunology and infectious disease. In M. Verklan & M. Walden (Eds.), *Core curriculum for neonatal intensive care nursing.* St. Louis, MO: Elsevier Saunders.

Kenner, C. (2004). Families in crisis. In M. Verklan & M. Walden (Eds.), *Core curriculum for neonatal intensive care nursing.* St. Louis, MO: Elsevier Saunders.

Klaus, M., & Fanaroff, A. (Eds.) (2001). *Care of the high risk neonate* (5th ed.). Philadelphia: W. B. Saunders.

Kliegman, R. (2001). Problems in metabolic adaptation: Glucose, calcium, and magnesium. In M. Klaus & A. Fanaroff (Eds.) *Care of the high risk neonate* (5th ed.). Philadelphia: W. B. Saunders.

Knobel, R., & Holditch-Davis, D. (2007). Thermoregulation and heat loss prevention after birth and during neonatal intensive-care unit stabilization of extremely low-birthweight infants. *JOGNN, 36,* 280–287.

Kochanek, K., & Martin, J. (2004). *Supplemental analyses of recent trend infant mortality. Health E-Stats* [online]. Retrieved from www.cdc/gov/nchs/products/pubs/pubd/hestats/infantmort/infantmort.htm (Accessed September 4, 2009).

Levene, M., Tudehope, D., & Thearle, M. (2000). *Essentials of neonatal medicine* (3rd ed.). London: Blackwell.

Lynam, L., & Verklan, M. (2004). Neurologic disorders. In M. Verklan & M. Walden (Eds.), *Core curriculum for neonatal intensive care nursing.* St. Louis, MO: Elsevier Saunders.

Maguire, D. (2004). Care of the extremely low birth weight infant. In M. Verklan & M. Walden (Eds.), *Core curriculum for neonatal intensive care nursing.* St. Louis, MO: Elsevier Saunders.

Malviya, M., Ohlsson, A., & Shah, S. (2003). Surgical versus medical treatment with cyclooxygenase inhibitors for symptomatic patent ductus arteriosus in preterm infants (Review). *Cochrane Database of Systematic Reviews,* Issue 3. Art.No.: CD003951. DOI: 10.1002/14651858.CD003951.

March of Dimes. (2007a). *Grieving is a process.* Retrieved from http://marchofdimes.com/572_15992.asp (Accessed September 4, 2009).

March of Dimes.(2007b). *Birth defects.* Retrieved from www.marchofdimes.com/572_15992.asp (Accessed September 4, 2009).

Martin, R., Fanaroff, A., & Walsh, M. (2006). *Neonatal-perinatal medicine:* Vol. 2: *Diseases of the fetus and infant* (8th ed.). Philadelphia: Mosby Elsevier.

Martin, R. J., Sosenko, I., & Bancalari, E. (2001). Respiratory problems. In M. Klaus & A. Fanaroff (Eds.), *Care of the high risk neonate* (5th ed). Philadelphia: W. B. Saunders.

Matthews, T., & MacDorman, M. (2008). Infant mortality statistics from the 2005 period linked birth/death data set. *National Vital Statistics Reports, 57,* 1–32.

Mayo Clinic Staff, 2007. *Fetal alcohol syndrome, Mayo Clinic.* Retrieved from www.mayoclinic.com/health/fetal-alcohol-syndrome/DS00184 (Accessed September 4, 2009).

McCall, E., Alderdice, F., Halladay, H., Jenkins, J., & Vohra, S. (2005). Interventions to prevent hypothermia at birth in preterm and/or low birthweight babies (Review). *Cochrane Database of Systematic Reviews,* Issue 1. Art.No.: CD004210.DOI: 10.1002/14651858.CD004210.pub2.

Mercer, J., Erickson-Owens, D., Graves, B., & Haley, M. (2007). Evidence based practices for the fetal to newborn transition. *Journal of Midwifery and Women's, Health, 52,* 262–272.

Minino, A., Heron, M., & Smith, B. (2006). *Deaths: Preliminary data for 2004. Health E-Stats* [on-line]. Retrieved from www.cdc.gov/nchs/data/nvsr/nvsr54/nvsr54_19.pdf (Accessed September 4, 2009).

Moore, M. (2003). Preterm labor and birth: What have we learned in the past two decades? *JOGNN, 32,* 638–649

Pinelli, J., & Symington, A. (2005). Non-nutritive sucking for promoting physiologic stability and nutrition in preterm infants (Review). *Cochrane Database of Systematic Reviews,* Issue 4. Art.No.: CD001071.DOI: 10.1002/14651858.CD001071.pub2.

Phelps, D. (2006). Retinopathy of prematurity. In R. Martin, A. Fanaroff, & M. Walsh (Eds.), *Neonatal-perinatal medicine: Vol. 2. Diseases of the fetus and infant* (8th ed.). Philadelphia: Mosby Elsevier.

Pitts, K. (2004). Perinatal substance abuse. In M. Verklan & M. Walden (Eds.), *Core curriculum for neonatal intensive care nursing.* St. Louis, MO: Elsevier Saunders.

Reiser, D. (2001). Hyperbilirubinemia: Exploring neonatal conditions related to bilirubin production. *AWHONN Lifelines, 5,* 55–61.

Roberts, D., & Dalziel, S. (2006). Antenatal corticosteroids for accelerating fetal lung maturation for women at risk for preterm birth (Review). *Cochrane Database of Systematic Reviews,* Issue 3. Art. No.: CD004454.DOI: 10.1002/14651858.CD004454.pub2.

Sadowski, S. (2004). Cardiovascular disorders. In M. Verklan & M. Walden (Eds.), *Core curriculum for neonatal intensive care nursing.* St. Louis, MO: Elsevier Saunders.

Scher, M. (2001). Brain disorders of the fetus and neonate. In M. Klaus & A. Fanaroff (Eds.), *Care of the high risk neonate* (5th ed.). Philadelphia: W. B. Saunders.

Sinclair, L., & Sinn, J. (2007). Higher versus lower humidity for the prevention of morbidity and mortality in preterm infants in incubators (Protocol). *Cochrane Database of Systematic Reviews, Issue 2. Art. No.: CD006472.DOI:* 10.1002/14651858.CD006472.

Southgate, W., & Pittard, W. (2001). Classification and physical examination of the newborn infant. In M. Klaus & A. Fanaroff (Eds.), *Care of the high risk neonate* (5th ed.). Philadelphia: W. B. Saunders.

Sterk, L. (2004). Congenital anomalies. In M. Verklan & M. Walden (Eds.), *Core curriculum for neonatal intensive care nursing*. St. Louis, MO: Elsevier Saunders.

Stevens, B., Yamada, J., & Ohlsson, A. (2007). Sucrose for analgesia in newborn infants undergoing painful procedures. *Cochrane Database of Systematic Reviews*, Issue 7.

Substance Abuse and Mental Health Services Administration (SAMHSA). (2006). *Results from the 2005 National Survey on Drug Use and Health: National Findings* (Office of Applied Studies, NSDUH Series H-30, DHHS Publication No. SMA 06-4184) Rockville, MD. Retrieved from www.oas.samhsa.gov/2k5/nsduh/2k5results.htm#2.6

Tyson, J., & Kennedy, K. (2005). Trophic feedings for parenterally fed infants (Review). *Cochrane Database of Systematic Reviews*, Issue 3. Art. No.: CD000504. DOI: 10.1002/14651858.CD000504.pub2.

Watson, R. (2004). Gastrointestinal disorders. In M. Verklan & M. Walden (Eds.), *Core curriculum for neonatal intensive care nursing*. St. Louis, MO: Elsevier Saunders.

Zukowsky, K. (2004). Respiratory distress. In M. Verklan & M. Walden (Eds.), *Core curriculum for neonatal intensive care nursing*. St. Louis, MO: Elsevier Saunders.

Answers to Chapter Review Questions

Chapter 1

1. C
2. D
3. A
4. C
5. B

Chapter 2

1. D
2. C
3. B
4. A
5. A

Chapter 3

1. A, B, and C
2. B
3. C
4. D
5. A, C, and D

Chapter 4

1. D
2. B
3. C
4. B
5. C
6. C
7. C
8. D

Chapter 5

1. A
2. B
3. B
4. B
5. A
6. C

Chapter 6

1. B
2. C
3. B
4. A
5. D

Chapter 7

1. C
2. D
3. D
4. C
5. B
6. A
7. C
8. B
9. A
10. C
11. B
12. A

Chapter 8

1. C
2. B
3. D
4. B
5. B
6. C and D
7. D
8. C
9. C
10. A

Chapter 9

1. B
2. C
3. A
4. A
5. D

Chapter 10

1. D
2. A
3. B
4. C
5. B

Chapter 11

1. C
2. A
3. B
4. D
5. C

Chapter 12

1. B and C
2. A
3. C
4. B, C, and D
5. A and D

Chapter 13

1. C
2. B
3. D
4. A, B, C, and D
5. A, B, C, and D

Chapter 14

1. B
2. A, B, C, and D
3. C
4. B
5. A, B, and D

Chapter 15

1. B
2. D
3. C
4. B
5. C

Chapter 16

1. A
2. C
3. A
4. C
5. A

Chapter 17

1. A
2. C
3. D
4. C
5. B

Appendices

Appendix A

AWHONN Quick Care Guide for Neonatal Skin Care

Association of Women's Health, Obstetric and Neonatal Nurses

QUICK CARE GUIDE

NEONATAL SKIN CARE

This Quick Care Guide is based on AWHONN's Neonatal Skin Care Evidence-Based Clinical Practice Guideline; it is meant to serve as a quick reference for the clinician. Detailed clinical practice guidelines, referenced rationales and evidence ratings are presented in the Guideline.

Newborn Skin Assessment
- assess skin condition daily
- identify risk factors for skin injury
- assess for erythema, dryness, flaking, breakdown, rashes
- try to determine cause of breakdown; skin culture per order if infection suspected

Bathing
Initial:
- stable temperature, at least 2–4 hours old
- universal precautions, wear gloves
- water or neutral pH cleanser, not necessary to remove all vernix
Routine:
- use neutral pH cleanser; daily soap bathing discouraged
- avoid rubbing; rinse with soft cloth or cotton balls
- < 32 weeks, use warm or sterile water only
Immersion:
- water depth approximately 5 inches or deep enough to cover infant's shoulders
- water temperature of 100.4° F
- immediately dry and wrap infant in warm blankets when bath completed
- after ten minutes, dress infant, change cap and wrap in dry, warmed blankets

Cord Care
- initially, clean cord and skin with neutral pH cleanser or sterile water
- keep cord area clean and dry
- keep diaper folded and under cord to allow drying
- cleanse with water if cord soiled with urine/stool

Circumcision Care
- povidone iodine or chlorhexidine for skin preparation
- remove prep completely with water post procedure
- cover circumcised penis: petrolatum or petrolatum gauze
- antimicrobial ointment may be unnecessary
- no lubricants if Plastibell™ used
- clean site with water only for 3–4 days

Disinfectants
- povidone iodine or chlorhexidine for disinfection before invasive procedures
- remove prep completely with sterile water post procedure
- avoid use of isopropyl alcohol for skin prep or removal of povidone iodine or chlorhexidine

Diaper Dermatitis
- frequent diaper changes, absorbent material to keep skin dry
- contact irritant dermatitis: apply thick layer of zinc-oxide barrier; if ineffective, use thick application alcohol-free pectin paste covered with petrolatum or zinc oxide
- treat underlying cause: malabsorption, opiate withdrawal
- assess for Candida diaper rash; antifungal ointment/cream as ordered
- avoid powders, antibiotic ointments

Emollients
- infants <1000 gm: apply preservative-free, petrolatum based emollient sparingly (0.5–1.5 ml) to body except face, head q12 hours or prn
- infants, all gestational ages: apply emollient to dry, flaking or fissured areas q12 hours or prn

Adhesives
- use adhesives sparingly
- use semipermeable dressings to secure silicone catheters, central lines, IVs, nasal cannulas, NG/OG tubes
- consider pectin barriers for better molding, adherence
- hydrogel adhesive EKG or limb electrodes
- stretchy wraps for pulse ox probes, electrodes; do not restrict blood flow
- avoid solvents, bonding agents, adhesive bandages
- remove adhesives slowly with water soaked cotton balls
- optional mineral oil or petrolatum for removal unless retaping

Transepidermal Water Loss
- risk of heat and fluid losses high in prematures < 30 weeks
- measure humidity regularly in the first weeks of life
- if humidity <40%, consider double walled incubator, plastic tent, water filled heating pad
- select one or more of the following techniques:
  - increase humidity to >70% with servo-regulated incubators, humidifiers
  - transparent adhesive dressings to body
  - emollient to body surfaces every 6 hours

Skin Breakdown
Prevention:
- water, air, gelled mattresses; cotton surfaces, sheepskin
- transparent dressings to prevent friction injury
- emollients to groin, thighs can reduce urine irritation
Treatment:
- irrigate with sterile water or diluted sterile saline, use 20 cc syringe/teflon catheter
- antifungal ointment for fungal rashes, breakdown per order
- petrolatum for uninfected or non-fungal breakdown
- transparent dressings, hydrogel, hydrocolloid dressings for discrete wounds

Intravenous Infiltration
Prevention:
- use insertion devices covered with plastic or silicone catheters
- avoid IV placement in areas difficult to immobilize whenever possible
- use transparent adhesive/clear tape so site is visible
Treatment:
- stop infusion/elevate site
- administer therapeutic agents/antidotes per order
- discourage application of silver sulfadiazene, heat, cold

Skin Nutrition
- appropriate protein and fat intake and caloric intake
- zinc deficiency risk with intestinal pathology and prematurity
- zinc supplementation: 400 mcg/kg/day prematures, 100 mcg/kg/day term
- lipids 0.5 gm/kg/day prevent essential fatty acid deficiency

Appendices

Appendix B

AWHONN Quick Guide to Breastfeeding

ASSOCIATION OF WOMEN'S HEALTH, OBSTETRIC AND NEONATAL NURSING

QUICK CARE GUIDE

Breastfeeding Support: Prenatal Care Through The First Year, Second Edition

This Quick Care Guide is based on AWHONN's Breastfeeding Support: Prenatal Care Through the First Year Evidence-Based Clinical Practice Guideline, second edition; it is meant to serve as a quick reference for the clinician. Detailed clinical practice guidelines, referenced rationales and evidence ratings are included in the Guideline. Evidence supporting the benefits of breastfeeding, critical messages, responsibilities and key assessment and teaching points summarized herein are presented in the Guideline.

BENEFITS OF BREASTFEEDING

Discussions with women who are considering or are undecided about breastfeeding should include description of the following benefits:

For infants:
- Natural source of nutrients necessary for optimal growth and development during the first 6 months
- Decreased incidence or severity of infections such as GI and respiratory infections, otitis media, necrotizing enterocolitis, gastroenteritis, meningitis and urinary tract infections
- Potential protective effect against sudden infant death syndrome (SIDS)
- Potential protective effect against childhood and adult-onset diseases such as insulin-dependent diabetes, allergies, asthma, lymphoma, ulcerative colitis, and adult-onset hypertension
- Less gastric reflux and constipation than formula feeding
- Potential for enhanced cognitive development

For women:
- Enhanced uterine involution resulting in less postpartum blood loss and reduced risk of infection
- Delayed resumption of ovulation that may facilitate family planning
- Association between earlier return to pre-pregnancy weight compared with women who do not breastfeed
- Reduced risk of osteoporosis, ovarian cancer and premenopausal breast cancer, and rheumatoid arthritis
- Enhanced mother-infant attachment, maternal role attainment and self-esteem

Breastfeeding is less expensive than formula feeding and can contribute to significant health care cost savings.

CRITICAL MESSAGES TO SHARE WITH WOMEN AND THEIR PARTNERS

- Breastfeeding is the optimal method of infant feeding.
- Most women can breastfeed successfully when they are given consistent information and support.
- Breastfeeding can be sustained upon return to work or school.
- Ideally, infants should breastfeed exclusively for the first year of life, i.e., during the first 6 months, the infant receives only breast milk; during the second 6 months, as other foods are introduced, the only source of milk given to the infant is breast milk.

RESPONSIBILITIES AND OPPORTUNITIES

- Deliberate integration of breastfeeding information into academic and professional education programs will help ensure that health care professionals gain the knowledge needed to promote and support breastfeeding.
- Nurses working with breastfeeding women should maintain current, evidence-based knowledge of breastfeeding practice and can be instrumental in initiating or participating in lactation research.
- Breastfeeding support programs should be culturally sensitive and age- and community-appropriate.
- Nurses and other health care professionals should relay consistent, supportive messages about breastfeeding.
- Nurses can be instrumental in promoting breastfeeding as our cultural norm by supporting legislation that promotes breastfeeding and educating society about the benefits of breastfeeding.

ASSOCIATION OF WOMEN'S HEALTH, OBSTETRIC AND NEONATAL NURSING QUICK CARE GUIDE
Breastfeeding Support: Prenatal Care Through The First Year

Key Assessment Parameters	Key Teaching Points
Preconception and Prenatal Care • During the first preconception or prenatal visit, ask the woman whether anyone has explained to her the benefits of breastfeeding for herself and her infant. Assess the woman's knowledge of and experiences with breastfeeding. • Explore the woman's beliefs and attitudes about breastfeeding. • For the woman who is undecided about breastfeeding, continue to explore her concerns and desires during subsequent contacts. • If the woman plans to breastfeed, ask how long she plans to do so and how long she plans to breastfeed exclusively. • Verify presence of support for the woman's decision to breastfeed. • Review the woman's history. Assess her breasts and nipples for risk factors and physical characteristics that may affect breastfeeding.	• Educate women about maternal and neonatal benefits of breastfeeding. • Previous breastfeeding experiences, positive or negative, influence choice of feeding method. Some factors, such as perceived insufficient milk supply, can be addressed by education and support that continue throughout pregnancy and the early postpartum period. • Discuss and correct misconceptions about breastfeeding. Address concerns or ambivalence. • Continue targeted, culturally appropriate education throughout pregnancy. Culture and beliefs can positively or negatively influence the woman's decision to initiate or continue breastfeeding. • Suggest that return to work or school does not mean that the woman must stop breastfeeding. Benefits continue as long as the infant is breastfeeding, even when the infant is being partially breastfed. • Discuss community resources that are available to the woman such as support groups, lactation consultants and La Leche League. • Explain that family, friends and health care providers (including peer counselors) can help a woman meet her breastfeeding goals. • Explain that many physical characteristics do not preclude breastfeeding. Share interventions to address identified problem(s). For example, infants are often able to grasp and pull out inverted nipples during early feedings at the breast. Some women who have had previous breast surgery are able to exclusively breastfeed their infants. Regardless of the amount of breast milk received by the infant, both mother and infant benefit.
Postpartum Care—First Two Weeks • Assess parental knowledge and ability to establish correct infant latch onto the breast. • Assess parental knowledge of infant states and ability to demonstrate caring for the infant as the infant transitions between states. • Assess parental knowledge of and ability to respond to infant feeding cues. • Assess parent's ability to identify signs of adequate milk intake.	• Instruct parents how to correctly position infant at breast. • Facilitate uninterrupted skin-to-skin contact at birth and during hospitalization. Ideally, the first feeding should occur within 1 hour of birth if mother and infant are stable. • Instruct mother how to identify a correct latch: infant's nose, cheeks and chin should touch the breast. The woman should feel tugging, not pinching or pain, when the infant sucks. The infant is usually held tummy-to-tummy with the mother, and the mother positions her fingers to ensure the lactiferous sinuses are not blocked. • Teach parents that infant may be sleepy for the first 24 hours. Try to wake the infant every 2–3 hours for feeding. Assure them that waking and feeding the infant should get progressively easier throughout the first 24 hours. • Teach parents about infant states and help parents identify how their infant transitions between states. • Teach early infant feeding cues: rooting, hand-to-mouth movements, sucking movement and sounds, mouth opening in response to tactile stimulation and quietly alert state. Crying is a late feeding cue. • Educate parents that infant should have at least one stool and one void in the first 24 hours, three or more voids and one to two stools per day by day 3 and six or more voids and three or more stools per day by day 4. Other signs include light colored urine, audible swallows and appropriate weight gain; a maternal sign of adequate intake is full breasts at the start of a feeding that become soft by the end.

ASSOCIATION OF WOMEN'S HEALTH, OBSTETRIC AND NEONATAL NURSING
QUICK CARE GUIDE
Breastfeeding Support: Prenatal Care Through The First Year

Key Assessment Parameters	Key Teaching Points
• Assess parents' ability to identify and respond to infant cues of satiety.	• Teach parents infant cues of satiety: a gradual decrease in the number of sucks, pursed lips, pulling away from breast and releasing the nipple, relaxed body, leg extension, absence of hunger cues, sleep and contented state.

• Assess parental knowledge about ways to support the mother-infant dyad in a successful breastfeeding experience.	• Parental education should include the following:
	  - Discourage the use of pacifiers until the baby is able to latch on and breastfeed successfully.
	  - The infant should receive only breast milk unless medically indicated.
	  - Discourage routine distribution of formula sample packs.
	• Provide parents with resources to contact after discharge, such as a lactation consultant, La Leche League or a breast-feeding support group.
	• Recommend follow-up with a health care provider within 3–5 days after discharge, or within 48 hours of discharge for infants discharged from the hospital prior to 48 hours of age.

Postpartum Care—Two Weeks Through First Year	
• Discuss how long the woman intends to breastfeed.	• Describe the association between an infant's age when first given formula and time of weaning. • Explain that internationally, many professional organizations agree that exclusive breastfeeding during the first 6 months of life (except when medical contraindications exist) provides adequate nutrition to facilitate optimal growth and development and protection against diarrhea and respiratory tract infections. • Define exclusive breastfeeding: the infant receives only breast milk and no other liquid or solid supplements except vitamins, minerals and medications. • Discuss feeding after 6 months, when other foods are introduced into the infant's diet. Exclusive breastfeeding during this time means that the only source of milk given to the infant continues to be breast milk. If a mother and infant desire, breastfeeding may continue for the first year of life and beyond.
• Assess for the presence of individuals in the woman's life who support her decision to breastfeed.	• Describe the influence that support from partners, maternal grandmother, employers and fellow employees may have on the duration of breastfeeding.

• Identify factors that may decrease duration of breastfeeding.	• Discuss factors that may negatively influence duration of breastfeeding:
	  - Perceived insufficient milk supply
	  - Returning to work before 2 months postpartum
	  - Wanting to leave the infant or have someone else feed
	  - Born outside the United States
	  - Postpartum depression
	• Engage adolescent women in discussions about unique concerns, e.g., relatives' advice to quit, embarrassment, modesty and concern about breastfeeding in public.
	• Explain that early introduction of pacifiers may be associated with decreased duration of breastfeeding. As an intervention to decrease the risk of SIDS, pacifiers should be introduced to breastfeeding infants after 1 month of age when breastfeeding is well established.

• Identify challenges to breastfeeding.	• Discuss challenges to breastfeeding, including lack of support and returning to work. • Provide the breastfeeding woman with resources for her employer that describe how the employer and the work environment can support breastfeeding. • Describe periods of rapid infant growth (2 weeks, 6 weeks and 3 months) when women may perceive that their milk supply has decreased because their infant is breastfeeding more often. • Explain that "stabbing" or "burning" pain or pruritus on the surface of the breast may be associated with a fungal infection such as *Candida albicans*. Should these occur, consultation with a health care provider is important to rule out other sources of infection and to treat both the mother and the infant as indicated.

ASSOCIATION OF WOMEN'S HEALTH, OBSTETRIC AND NEONATAL NURSING
QUICK CARE GUIDE
Breastfeeding Support: Prenatal Care Through The First Year

Key Assessment Parameters	Key Teaching Points
• Assess the woman's knowledge of available professional and community resources.	• Encourage participation in breastfeeding support groups, regular visits to Women, Infants, and Children (WIC) program office (if the mother participates in WIC) and follow-up phone calls to registered nurses, lactation consultants or the primary health care provider, all of which may help increase the duration of breastfeeding.
• Discuss options to support continued breastfeeding after returning to work.	• Encourage use of a double rather than a single pump to decrease the length of time needed to pump. • Encourage women to begin pumping before returning to work. The more experience a woman has with pumping the more efficient she becomes and the less time pumping will take.
• Assess the breastfeeding woman's understanding of techniques to wean her infant.	• Describe weaning techniques, such as replacing one feeding during the day with solid food, a bottle or cup depending on the infant's age and stage of development. After the infant has adjusted, replace a second feeding at the opposite time of day. Generally, the first morning and last evening feedings are the last to be stopped.
Vulnerable and Preterm Infants	

• Assess woman's beliefs, attitudes and knowledge about providing own mother's milk for her vulnerable/preterm infant.	• Explain that human milk affords unique advantages for the vulnerable/preterm infant (such as protection from necrotizing enterocolitis, better gastric function and reduced incidence of infection), as well as for the woman.
	• Teach the woman to optimize milk yield using the following suggested techniques:
	  - Begin milk expression within 6 hours after delivery, using an electric, hospital-grade breast pump with double collection kit whenever possible.
	  - Express milk at the infant's bedside.
	  - Engage in skin-to-skin contact at least 30 minutes daily, whenever feasible.
	  - Mechanically express approximately 8–10 times daily during the first week to 10 days postpartum.
	  - Individualize the frequency of mechanical expression on the basis of milk output.
	  - Continue mechanical expression for 2 minutes after milk droplets cease flowing.

• Determine woman's willingness to provide human milk via various options.	• Instruct that human milk may be provided to the infant via tube feeding (gavage), cup- or finger-feedings, as well as by bottle. • Instruct parents how to properly collect, store and transport human milk to the hospital. • Assist parents to identify resources necessary to collect, store and transport milk.
• Assess woman's and infant's readiness for oral feeding at breast.	• When the infant is medically stable, teach mothers who desire to transition the infant to feeding at breast to put the infant to breast following milk expression to help him or her acclimate to suckling. • Demonstrate positions that provide head and shoulder support of the infant, such as the football hold, when infant suction if compromised. • Remind the mother to express remaining milk after each breastfeeding session. • Suggest that thin silicone nipple shields may increase milk transfer with this infant population. • Explain that infant test-weighing provides an accurate estimate of infant milk intake.
• Assess parental knowledge related to the vulnerable/preterm infant's milk intake after discharge.	• Discuss that modified demand feedings will likely be needed, coupled with infant test-weighing for a period of time. • Emphasize the difference between insufficient milk supply and the infant's ability to consume adequate milk volume. • Teach that appropriate follow-up after discharge is critical for mother of a vulnerable/preterm infant.

Appendices

Appendix C

Laboratory Values

LABORATORY VALUE	NONPREGNANT	PREGNANT	NEWBORN
Hemoglobin, g/dL	12–16	11–13	13.5–20.5
Hematocrit, %	37–47	33–39	45–65
Red cell count, 10^6cells/mm^3	4.2–5.4	3.8–4.4	5.33–5.47
White blood cell count, 10^3cells/mm^3	4.5–11.0	5.0–12.0	9.4–34.0
Platelets, mm^3	150,000–400,000	No significant change	150,000–450,000
Fibrinogen, mg/dL	200–400	↑ levels late in pregnancy	125–300
Serum cholesterol, mg/dL	110–330	↑ 60%	Rises rapidly after birth reaching adult levels by day 1
Blood glucose, mg/dL		↓ 10–20%	≥40
Fasting	65–99	≤95	
2-hour postprandial	≤105	≤120	
Total bilirubin, mg/dL	0.3–1.2	No significant change	<24 hours: <6.0 1–2 days: <10 3–5 days: <12

Appendices

Appendix D

Conversions: Approximate Temperature Equivalents

FAHRENHEIT	CENTIGRADE
104°	40°
103°	39.44°
102°	38.89°
101°	38.33°
100°	37.78°
99°	37.22°
98.6°	37°
98°	36.67°
97°	36.11°
96°	35.56°

Fahrenheit–Centigrade Conversions

F = (C × 9/5) + 32
C = (F − 32) × 5/9

Appendices

Appendix E

Cervical Dilation Chart

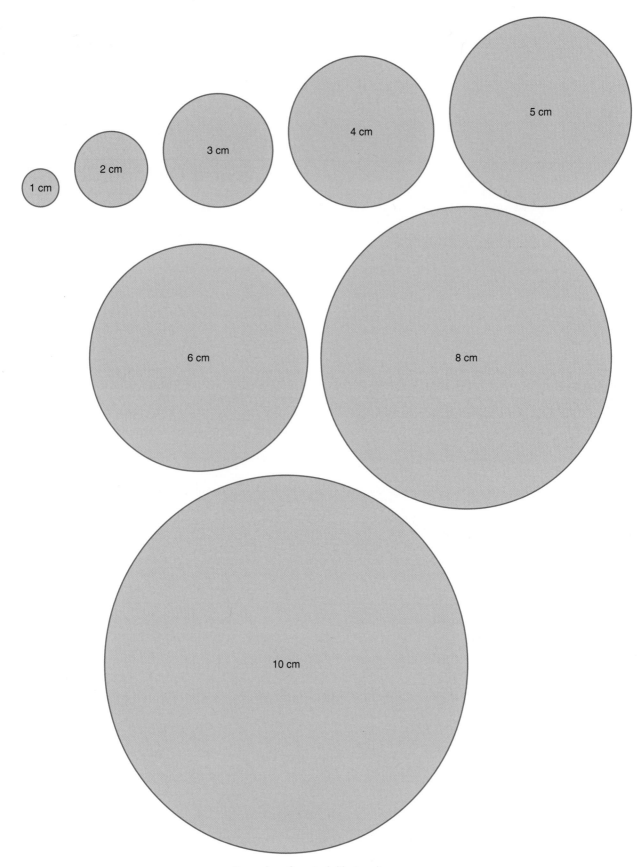

Examples of cervical dilation diameters.

Abortion (AB)   The spontaneous or induced termination of a pregnancy before 20 weeks of gestation

Abruptio placenta   The separation of the placenta from its site of implantation before delivery

Acceleration   An abrupt transitory increase in the fetal heart rate from the baseline rate; associated with sympathetic nervous stimulation; when using EFM to assess FHR data in the term fetus, an acceleration is a visually apparent abrupt increase in FHR peaking at least 15 beats per minute above the FHR baseline, lasting at least 15 seconds from onset to return to baseline; in the fetus under 32 completed weeks gestation an acceleration increases at least 10 beats per minute above baseline and lasts at least 10 seconds from onset to return to baseline.

Acme phase   The peak of intensity of a contraction

Acrocyanosis   Cyanosis of hands and feet in newborn

Active phase   Second phase of labor; cervical dilation from 4 to 7 cm

Advocacy   An action taken in response to our ethical responsibility to intervene on behalf of those in our care

Afterpains   Moderate to severe cramp-like pain caused by uterine contractions during the first few postpartum days

Alcohol-related birth defects (ARBDs)   Congenital anomalies associated with alcohol use during pregnancy

Alcohol-related neurodevelopmental disorder (ARND)   Abnormalities of the central nervous system that are associated with prenatal alcohol exposure

Alpha-fetoprotein (AFP)/α_1-Fetoprotein/Maternal serum alpha-fetoprotein (MSAFP)   A glycoprotein produced by the fetus used for assessing for the levels of AFP in the maternal blood as a screening tool for certain developmental defects in the fetus such as fetal neural tube defects (NTDs) and ventral abdominal wall defects

Amenorrhea   Absence of menstruation

Amniocentesis   Diagnostic procedure in which a needle is inserted through the maternal abdominal wall into the uterine cavity to obtain amniotic fluid

Amniotic fluid   Fluid contained within the amniotic sac

Amniotic fluid embolism (AFE)/Anaphylactoid syndrome   A rare but often fatal complication that occurs during pregnancy, labor and birth, or postpartum in which amniotic fluid that contains fetal cells, lanugo, and vernix enters the maternal vascular system and initiates a cascading process that leads to maternal cardiorespiratory collapse and disseminated intravascular coagulation (DIC)

Amniotic fluid index (AFI)   Screening tool that measures the volume of amniotic fluid with ultrasound to assess fetal well-being and placental function

Amniotomy (AROM)   The artificial rupture of membranes

Amplitude   The distance between high and low points of the FHR tracing oscillations; describes the range of variation in fetal heart rate changes from peak to trough

ANA Code of Ethics   Makes explicit the primary goals, values, and obligations of the profession of nursing

Antepartum/antepartal   The time period beginning with conception and ending with the onset of labor

Anticipatory guidance   The provision of information and guidance to women and their families that promotes being informed about and prepared for events to come

Apgar score   A rapid assessment of five physiological signs that indicate the physiological status of the newborn at birth

Asphyxia   Decrease in oxygen in body tissue (hypoxia), increase in CO_2 level (hypercapnia), and decrease in pH (metabolic and/or respiratory acidosis) with buildup of lactic acid in the tissue

Assessment   A systematic, dynamic process by which the nurse, through interaction with women, newborns and families, significant others, and health care providers, collects, monitors, and analyzes data; data may include the following dimensions: psychological, biotechnological, physical, sociocultural, spiritual, cognitive, developmental, and economic, as well as functional abilities and lifestyle

Asymmetric intrauterine growth restriction   A disproportional reduction in the size of structures and organs; results from maternal or placental conditions that occur later in pregnancy related to impeded placental blood flow

Attachment   Emotional connection that forms between the infant and his or her parents; it is bidirectional from parent to infant and infant to parent

Augmentation of labor   Stimulation of ineffective uterine contractions after labor has started

Auscultation   Use of the Doppler or fetoscope (a listening device) to assess the fetal heart rate by listening

Autonomy   Refers to two concepts that operate as a whole; one is the right of self-determination or the right of the individual to make his or her own choice to accept or reject treatment; the ability to exercise autonomous rights requires and is related to elements in informed consent; the second aspect is concerned with respect of persons, that is, to respect the patient's decision irrespective of the nurses' own values

Ballard maturational score (BMS)   Standardized test to calculate the gestational age of the neonate

Baroreceptors   Pressure-sensitive stretch receptors in carotid sinus and aortic arch that detect changes in blood pressure; stimulation of fetal baroreceptors alters the FHR by stimulating the autonomic nervous system to increase or decrease the FHR via the sympathetic or parasympathetic branch

Baseline fetal heart rate   The average fetal heart rate (FHR) rounded to increments of 5 beats per minute (bpm) during a 10-minute segment between uterine contractions, accelerations or decelerations

Baseline fetal heart rate variability   Fluctuations in the baseline FHR that are irregular in amplitude and frequency; the fluctuations are visually quantitated as the amplitude of the peak-to-trough in bpm; variability is a characteristic of the baseline: it is determined in a 10-minute period excluding accelerations and decelerations, and quantified as absent (visually undetectable), minimal (visually detectable but >5 bpm), moderate (6-25 bpm), or marked (< 25 bpm)

Beneficence   The obligation to do good; beneficence is concerned not only with doing good but also with removing harm and preventing harm

Betamimetic drugs   Medications that mimic stimulation of the sympathetic nervous system; specifically in myometrial cells they have a relaxant or depressant effect on uterine contractility; (sometimes referred to as sympathomimetic or betasympathomimetic)

Bilirubin   The yellow pigmentation derived from the breakdown of red blood cells

Biochemical assessment   Involves biological examination and chemical determination

Biophysical profile (BPP)   An antenatal assessment of fetal well-being that combines NST results with multiple physiologic parameters observed with real-time ultrasound; the BPP includes the assessment of five parameters: fetal breathing movement, gross body movement, fetal tone, amniotic fluid volume, and fetal heart rate reactivity (NST)

Biophysical risk factors   Factors that originate from the mother or fetus and impact the development or function of the mother or fetus; they include genetic, nutritional, medical, and obstetric issues.

Biparietal diameter (BPD)   The largest transverse measurement and an important indicator of head size (9.25 cm average measurement)

Birth rate   Number of live births per 1,000 people

Bishop score   A method for determining cervical readiness for induction of labor by scoring 5 components: cervical dilation, effacement, consistency, position, and station of the presenting part. Higher scores (<6) are associated with successful induction of labor

Blastocyst   Stage of embryo development that follows the morula stage; the blastocyst is composed of an inner cell mass referred to as the embryoblast and an outer cell layer referred to as the trophoblast

Bloody show   Brownish or blood-tinged cervical mucus discharge.

Body Mass Index (BMI)   A tool for determining appropriate body weight compared to height

Bonding   Emotional feelings between parent and newborn that begin during pregnancy or shortly after birth; it is unidirectional from parent to newborn

Bradycardia   Baseline FHR of less than 110 bpm lasting for 10 minutes or longer

Braxton-Hicks contractions   Intermittent, painless, and physiological uterine contractions occurring in some pregnancies in the second and third trimesters that do not result in cervical change and are associated with false labor

Breech presentation   The presenting part of the fetus is the buttock and/or feet

Bronchopulmonary dysplasia (BPD)   A chronic lung condition that affects neonates that have been treated with mechanical ventilation and oxygen for problems such as respiratory distress syndrome

Brow presentation   When the fetal head presents in a position midway between full flexion and extreme extension

Brown fat   Also referred to as brown adipose tissue or nonshivering thermogenesis; a highly dense and vascular adipose tissue that is unique to neonates

Cardinal movements of labor   The positional changes that the fetus goes through to best navigate the birth process

Category I FHR patterns   FHR tracings demonstrating normal baseline rate, moderate variability, and the absence of late or variable decelerations; accelerations and early decelerations may or may not be present; tracings with these features are strongly predictive of normal fetal acid-base status at the time of observation

Category II FHR patterns   Tracings which cannot be classified as either category I or category III patterns; these tracings are not predictive of abnormal acid-base status, but there is not enough evidence to classify them in category I or III

Category III FHR patterns   Tracings exhibiting a sinusoidal pattern or exhibiting absent variability in conjunction with bradycardia or recurrent late or variable decelerations; these tracings are predictive of abnormal fetal acid-base status at the time of observation

Cephalic presentation   The presenting part is the head

Cephalopelvic disproportion (CPD)   A condition in which the size, shape, or position of the fetal head prevents it from passing through the lateral aspect of the maternal pelvis or when the maternal pelvis is of a size or shape that prevents the descent of the fetus through the pelvis; term used when the maternal bony pelvis is not large enough or appropriately shaped to allow for fetal descent

Cervical dilation   A measurement that estimates the dilation of the cervical opening by sweeping the examining finger from the margin of the cervical opening on one side to that on the other

Cervical effacement   A measurement that estimates the shortening of the cervix from 2 cm to paper thin measured by palpation of cervical length with fingertips

Cervical ripening   The process of physical softening and opening of the cervix in preparation for labor and birth

Cervix   The neck or lowest part of the uterus; interfaces with the vagina

Cesarean birth   Also referred to as cesarean section or C-section (C/S); an operative procedure in which the fetus is delivered through an incision in the abdominal wall and the uterus

Cesarean delivery on maternal request (CDMR)   A cesarean section that is performed at the request of the woman before the beginning of labor and in the absence of maternal or fetal medical condition that presents a risk for labor

Chadwick's sign   Bluish-purple coloration of the vagina and cervix evident in the first trimester of pregnancy

Chain of command or authority   Definition of the lines of authority and responsibility for clinical problem resolution within an organization; describes the persons to contact and the order in which to contact them when differences of opinion about clinical management of patients cannot be resolved directly between providers

Chemoreceptor   Sensory nerve endings or cells stimulated by increased or decreased blood concentrations of a chemical substance; sensitive to change in oxygen, carbon dioxide and pH levels in the blood; chemoreceptors are located in the aortic and carotid bodies and in the medulla

Childbearing and newborn health care   A model of care addressing the health promotion, maintenance, and restoration needs of women from the preconception through the postpartum period; and low-risk, high-risk, and critically ill newborns from birth through discharge and follow-up, within the social, political, economic, and environmental context of the mother's, her newborn's, and the family's lives

Cholasma   Increased pigmentation over bridge of nose and cheeks of pregnant woman; also called mask of pregnancy

Cholelithiasis   Presence of gall stones in the gall bladder

Chorionic villi   Projections from the chorion that embed into the decidua basalis and later form the fetal blood vessels of the placenta

Chorionic villus sampling (CVS)   Aspiration of a small amount of placental tissue (chorion) for chromosomal, metabolic, or DNA testing

Circumcision   An elective surgery to remove the foreskin of the penis

Classical cesarean delivery   A vertical midline incision made into the abdominal wall with a vertical incision in the upper segment of the uterus performed for cesarean births

Cleavage   Mitotic cell division of the zygote, fertilized oocyte

Clinical pelvimetry   Measurements of the dimensions of the bony pelvis during an internal pelvic examination for determination of adequacy of the pelvis for a vaginal birth

Clonus   Spasmodic alternation of muscular contraction and relaxation; tested in the foot and counted in beats

Cold stress   A term used when there is excessive heat loss that leads to hypothermia and results in the utilization of compensatory mechanisms to maintain the neonate's body temperature

Colic   A term used to describe uncontrollable crying in healthy infants younger than the age of 5 months

Collaborative working relationships   Working together with mutual respect for the accountability of each profession to the shared goal of quality patient outcomes

Colostrum   Clear, yellowish breast fluid, which precedes milk production; it contains proteins, nutrients, and immune globulins; produced prenatally as early as the second trimester and before lactation in the first days after birth

Combined decelerations   A deceleration pattern that has combined features, such as a variable deceleration that is also a late deceleration

Combined spinal epidural analgesia (CSE)   Involves the injection of local anesthetic and/or analgesic into the subarachnoid space

Compensatory response to hypoxemia   Describes the ability of the fetus to adjust to low blood oxygen levels by drawing on fetal reserves and mobilizing physiologic responses to maintain central oxygenation; the presence of moderate variability implies adequate physiologic compensation and fetal reserves

Complete abortion   Products of conception are totally expelled from uterus

Complete breech   Where there is complete flexion of thighs and legs and a buttocks presentation of the fetus

Compound presentation   The fetus assumes a unique posture, usually with the arm or hand presenting alongside the presenting part

Conception   Also known as fertilization; occurs when a sperm nucleus enters the nucleus of the oocyte

Conduction   Transfer of heat to a cooler surface by direct skin contact such as cold hands of caregivers or cold equipment

Conjugated bilirubin   The conjugated form of bilirubin (direct bilirubin) is soluble and excretable

Contraction stress test (CST)   Screening tool to assess fetal well-being with electronic fetal monitoring (EFM) in women with a nonreactive non-stress test (NST) at term gestation; the purpose of the CST is to identify a fetus that is at risk for compromise through observation of the fetal response to intermittent reduction in utero placental blood flow associated with stimulated uterine contractions (UCs)

Convection   Loss of heat from the neonate's warm body surface to cooler air currents such as air conditioners or oxygen masks

Cotyledons   Rounded portions, lobes, of the maternal side of the placenta

Couvade syndrome   The occurrence in the mate of a pregnant woman of symptoms related to pregnancy, such as nausea, vomiting, and abdominal pain

Crowning   Stage of birth when the top of the fetal head can be seen on the maternal perineum

Cultural stereotyping   The practice of making generalizations about a person based on his or her culture

Culturally competent care   Providing care to patients and their families that is effective, understandable, and respectful in a manner that is compatible with their cultural beliefs, practices, and preferred language

Cystitis   Infection of the bladder

Cystocele   Bulging of the bladder into the vagina

Daily fetal movement count (kick counts)   Maternal assessment of fetal movement by counting fetal movements in a period of time to identify a potentially hypoxic fetus

Deceleration   A transitory decrease in the FHR from the baseline rate

Decidua basalis   The portion of the decidua that forms the maternal portion of the placenta

Decrement phase   The descending or relaxation of the uterine muscle

Descent   The movement of the fetus through the birth canal during the first and second stages of labor

Diabetes mellitus (DM)   A chronic metabolic disease characterized by hyperglycemia as a result of limited or no insulin production

Diagnosis   A clinical judgment about the patient's response to actual or potential health conditions or needs; diagnoses provide the basis for determination of a plan of nursing care to achieve expected outcomes

Diagnostic tests   Tests that help to identify a particular disease or provide information that aids in the making of a diagnosis

Diastasis recti   A separation of the two rectus abdominis muscle bands at the midline

Diastasis recti abdominis   Separation of the rectus muscle

Dilation   The enlargement or opening of the cervical os

Direct bilirubin   Conjugated bilirubin

Direct obstetric death   Death of a woman resulting from complications during pregnancy, labor/birth, and/or postpartum, and from interventions, omission of interventions, or incorrect treatment

Disseminated intravascular coagulation (DIC)   Syndrome in which the coagulation pathways are hyperstimulated; occurs when the body is breaking down blood clots faster than it can form a clot, thus quickly depleting the body of clotting factors and leading to hemorrhage

Diversity   A quality that encompasses acceptance and respect related to but not limited to age, class, culture, disability, education level, ethnicity, family structure, gender, ideologies, political beliefs, race, religion, sexual orientation, style, and values

Dizygotic   Pertaining to or derived from two separate zygotes (fertilized ova), as in twin gestation occurring from two fertilized ova; results in fraternal twins

Doppler   An instrument that emits ultrasound waves and receives a return signal; in the context of FHR monitoring, a Doppler usually refers to a hand-held ultrasound device used to detect the FHR; it converts the sound waves reflected from the motion of the heart valves into a fetal heart rate

Doula   A Greek word meaning "woman's servant"; an assistant hired to give the woman support during pregnancy, labor and birth, and postpartum

Dubowitz neurological exam   Standardized tool to assess gestational age of neonate

Ductus arteriosus   Structure in fetal circulation that connects the pulmonary artery with the descending aorta; the majority of the oxygenated blood is shunted to the aorta via the ductus arteriosus with smaller amounts going to the lungs

Ductus venosus   Structure in fetal circulation that connects the umbilical vein to the inferior vena cava. This allows the majority of the high levels of oxygenated blood to enter the right atrium

Duration of contractions   Length of a contraction measured by counting from the beginning to the end of one contraction and measured in seconds

Dysfunctional labor   Abnormal uterine contractions that prevent the normal progress of cervical dilation or descent of the fetus

Dystocia   A long, a difficult or an abnormal labor

Early decelerations   A gradual decrease in FHR, 20 to 30 bpm below baseline, generally the onset, nadir, and the recovery mirror the contraction

Eclampsia   Preeclampsia with the onset of tonic–clonic seizure/convulsions that place the mother and fetus at risk for death

Ectoderm   The outer layer of cells in the developing embryo

Ectopic pregnancy   A pregnancy that develops as a result of the blastocyst implanting somewhere other than the endometrial lining of the uterus; implantation of a fertilized ovum outside the uterus

Effacement   The shortening and thinning of the cervix

Effleurage   A massage technique using a very light touch of the fingers in two repetitive circular patterns over the gravid abdomen; done by lightly stroking the abdomen in rhythm with breathing during contractions

Elective abortion (EAB)   Termination of pregnancy before viability at the request of the woman but not for reasons of the impaired health of the maternal health or fetal disease

Electronic fetal monitoring (EFM)   An auditory and visual assessment of the FHR and uterine activity with data generated by fetal monitor technology; the data generated includes an auditory FHR signal, a digital or graphic display of FHR and UA data, and a permanent record on paper or computerized storage

Embryo   Term used for the developing human from the time of implantation through 8 weeks of gestation

Embryoblast   The inner cell mass of the blastocyst which develops into the embryo

Embryonic membranes   Two membranes, amnion and chorion, that form the amniotic sac; the chorionic membrane (outer membrane) develops from the trophoblast; the amniotic membrane (inner membrane) develops from the embryoblast; the embryo and amniotic fluid are contained within the amniotic sac

En face   Position in which the mother and newborn are face-to-face with eye contact

Endoderm   The inner layer of cells in the developing embryo

Endometrial biopsy   A biopsy of the endometrial tissue of the uterus to assess for the response of the uterus to hormonal signals that occur during the menstrual cycle

Endometrial cycle   Pertains to the changes in the endometrium of the uterus in response to the hormonal changes that occur during the ovarian cycle; consist of three phases: proliferative phase, secretory phase, and menstrual phase

Endometritis   An infection of the endometrium that usually starts at the placental site and can spread to encompass the entire endometrium

Endometrium   The mucous membrane lining the interior of the uterus

Engagement   Occurs when the greatest diameter of the fetal head passes through the pelvic inlet

Engrossment   Phenomenon experienced by new fathers who have an intense preoccupation about and interest in their newborn

Entrainment   Phenomenon in which the newborn and infant moves his or her arms and legs in rhythm with speech patterns of an adult

Environmental risk factors   Risks in the workplace or the general environment that impact pregnancy outcomes; various environmental substances can affect fetal development, for example, exposure to chemicals, radiation, and pollutants

Epidural anesthesia   Involves the placement of a very small catheter and injection of local anesthesia and or analgesia between the 4th and 5th vertebrae into the epidural space

Epidural block   An anesthetic injected in the epidural space; located outside the dura mater between the dura and spinal canal via an epidural catheter

Episiotomy   An incision in the perineum to provide more space for the fetal presenting part at delivery

Episodic changes   Accelerations or decelerations of the FHR which are not associated with uterine contractions

Epispadias   An abnormality in which the urethral opening is on dorsal side of penis

Ethical dilemma   A choice that has the potential to violate ethical principals

Ethics   Based in philosophical discussions of ancient Greek scholars about the nature of good and evil or right and wrong.

Ethnocentrism   The belief that the customs and values of the dominant culture are preferred or superior in some way

Evaluation   The process of determining the patient's progress toward attainment of expected outcomes and the effectiveness of nursing care

Evaporation   Loss of heat that occurs when water on neonate's skin is converted to vapors such as during bathing or directly after birth

Evidence-based nursing (EBN)   Combining the best research evidence with clinical expertise while taking into account patients' preferences and their situation in the context of the available resources part of nursing practice

Evidence-based practice (EBP)   The integration of best research evidence, clinical expertise, and patient values in making decisions about the care of patients

Expulsion   Movement during which the shoulders and remainder of the body are delivered

Extension   The movement, which is facilitated by resistance of the pelvic floor, that causes the presenting part to pivot beneath the pubic symphysis and the head to be delivered; occurs during the second stage of labor

External fetal monitoring   Collection and assessment of FHR and UA data using an ultrasound transducer to monitor the fetal heart rate and a tocodynamometer to monitor uterine contractions

External rotation   Movement during which the sagittal suture moves to a transverse diameter and the shoulders align in the anteroposterior diameter; the sagittal suture maintains alignment with the fetal trunk as the trunk navigates through the pelvis

Extremely low birth weight infant (ELBW)   An infant who weighs less than 1,000 grams at birth

Face presentation   When the fetal head is in extension rather than flexion as it enters the pelvis

Failure to progress   An arrest in dilation

False labor   Irregular contractions with little or no cervical changes

False positive   When an assessment incorrectly identify a healthy fetus as compromised

Family-centered maternity care   A model of obstetric care that views pregnancy and childbirth as a normal life event or life transition that is not primarily medical but rather developmental; health care is provided in an inclusive manner, with family and significant others, including children, as an active part of the process; the emphasis is on holistic care, with the focus on the pregnant woman and her well-being, including emotional and psychosocial considerations

Favorable physiologic response   An FHR response predictive of a fetus that is able to respond appropriately to the environment and maintain fetal reserves

Ferguson's reflex   A physiological response of the woman, activated when the presenting part of the fetus is at least at +1 station; it is usually accompanied by spontaneous bearing-down efforts

Ferning   When a sample of fluid in the upper vaginal area is obtained the fluid is placed on a slide and assessed for "ferning pattern" under a microscope to confirm rupture of membranes

Fertility rate   Total number of live births, regardless of age of mother, per 1,000 women of reproductive age, 15 to 44 years

Fetal alcohol syndrome (FAS)   Refers to a wide array and spectrum of physical, cognitive and behavioral abnormalities associated with maternal alcohol use during pregnancy

Fetal asphyxia   A condition of fetal hypoxemia, hypercapnia, and respiratory and metabolic acidosis that may occur in utero

Fetal attitude or posture   The relationship of the fetal parts to one another; this is noted by the flexion or extension of the fetal joints

Fetal bradycardia   Baseline FHR of less than 110 bpm lasting for 10 minutes or longer

Fetal compromise   Evidence of a fetal heart rate pattern that indicates the fetus may be in jeopardy

Fetal dystocia   May be caused by excessive fetal size, malpresentation, multifetal pregnancy, or fetal anomalies

Fetal fibronectin (fFN)   A protein detected via immunoassay; a positive test is greater than 50 ng/mL

Fetal heart rate accelerations   The visually abrupt, transient increases (onset to peak <30 sec) in the FHR above the baseline, 15 beats above the baseline, and last from 15 seconds to less than 2 minutes

Fetal heart rate decelerations   Transitory decreases in the FHR baseline; they are classified as early, variable, or late decelerations

Fetal lie   The relationship of the fetal body to the maternal body; fetal lie may be longitudinal (fetal body is parallel to maternal spine), transverse (fetal body is perpendicular to maternal spine), or oblique (fetal body is at an angle between longitudinal and transverse lie)

Fetal position   Location of the presenting part and specific fetal structures to determine fetal position in relation to maternal pelvis; relation of the denominator or reference point to the maternal pelvis

Fetal presentation   The lowest part of the fetus that comes out of the uterus first; most often the presentation is vertex (occiput first), but it can also be breech (buttocks or feet first), shoulder (shoulder first), face or brow (face or brow first) or compound (hand with head or foot with buttocks)

Fetal reserve   The ability to maintain tissue oxygenation and essential physiologic function in response to decreased availability of oxygen or other physiologic stressors; this term is also used to refer to the excess amount of oxygen available to the fetus beyond that normally required for metabolism

Fetal scalp stimulation   An indirect method of assessing acid-base status of the fetus by rubbing the fetal head to elicit acceleration; can be performed with or without ruptured membranes; scalp stimulation is performed during a period of baseline FHR; it is not a resuscitative measure, and should not be performed during decelerations

Fetal surveillance   Assessment of fetal well-being via indirect methods such as auscultation, electronic fetal monitoring and antepartum testing

Fetoscope   Stethoscope used to auscultate fetal heart rate

Fetus   Term used for the developing human from 9 weeks of gestation to birth

Fidelity   Refers to the faithfulness or obligation to keep promises

First-degree laceration   Laceration that involves the perineal skin and vaginal mucous membrane

First stage of labor   Begins with onset of labor and ends with complete cervical dilation

Flexion   When the chin of the fetus moves toward the fetal chest; flexion occurs when the descending head meets resistance from maternal tissues

Follicular phase   Part of the ovarian cycle; it begins the first day of menstruation and lasts 12 to 14 days; during this phase, the graafian follicle is maturing

Footling breech   When either one (single footling) or both (double footling) feet of the fetus present first in the pelvis

Foramen ovale   A structure in fetal circulation; it is an opening between the right and left atria; blood high in oxygen is shunted to the left atrium via the foramen ovale

Forceps   An instrument used to assist with delivery of the fetal head, typically done to improve the health of the woman or the fetus

Foremilk   The milk that is produced and stored between feedings and released at the beginning of the feeding session; it has higher water content

Fourth-degree laceration   Laceration that extends into the rectal mucosa and to expose the lumen of the rectum

Fourth stage of labor   Begins with the delivery of the placenta and typically ends within 4 hours or with the stabilization of the mother postpartum

Frank breech   Where there is complete flexion of the thighs and the legs extend over the anterior surfaces of the body with the fetal buttocks as the presenting part

Frequency of contractions   Determined by counting number of contractions in a 10-minute period, counting from the start of one contraction to the start of the next contraction in minutes

Fundus   The upper portion of the uterus

Gate control theory of pain   States that sensation of pain is transmitted from the periphery of the body along ascending nerve pathways to the brain; due to the limited number of sensations that can travel along these pathways at any given time, an alternate activity can replace travel of the pain sensation, thus closing the gate control at the spinal cord and reducing pain impulses traveling to the brain

General anesthesia   The use of IV injection and/or inhalation of anesthetic agents that render the woman unconscious

Genital fistulas   An abnormal connection between the vagina and bladder, rectum, and/or urethra; the fistula provides a pathway for fecal material and/or urine to enter the vagina

Genome   An organism's complete set of DNA

Gestation   Period of intrauterine development from conception to birth

Gestational diabetes mellitus (GDM)   Any degree of glucose intolerance with the onset or first recognition in pregnancy.

Gestational hypertension   A relatively benign disorder without underlying physiological changes in the mother; high blood pressure detected for the first time after mid-pregnancy, without proteinuria; diagnosis is made postpartum

Glans penis   Tip of the penis

Gonadotoxins   Factors, such as drugs, infections, illness, and heat exposure, that can have an adverse effect on spermatogenesis

Goodell's sign   Softening of the cervix in the first trimester of pregnancy

Gradual   Timing from onset to nadir or peak of FHR change is >30 seconds; refers to characteristics of periodic and episodic changes in the FHR

Gravida   A pregnant woman; also, the number of times a woman has been pregnant (Gravida/Para notation)

Hegar's sign   Softening of the lower uterine segment (isthmus) in the first trimester of pregnancy

HELLP syndrome   (**H**emolysis, **E**levated **L**iver enzymes, and **L**ow **P**latelets) Acronym used to designate the variant changes in laboratory values that is sometimes a complication of severe preeclampsia

Hematomas   Collection of blood within the connective tissues; common sites in the postpartum woman are the vagina and perineal areas

Hind milk   The milk produced during the feeding session and released at the end of the session; it has a higher fat content

Hydatiform mole   A benign proliferate growth of the trophoblast in which the chorionic villi develop into edematous, cystic, vascular transparent vesicles that hang in grapelike clusters without a viable fetus

Hydrocele   Enlarged scrotum due to excess fluid

Hyperbilirubinemia   Term used when there is a high level of unconjugated bilirubin in the neonate's blood

Hyperemesis gravidarum   Vomiting during pregnancy that is so severe it leads to dehydration, electrolyte and acid–base imbalance, and starvation ketosis

Hyperstimulation   Excessive uterine activity

Hypertonic uterine dysfunction   Uncoordinated uterine activity

Hypospadias   An abnormality in which the urethral opening is on ventral surface of penis

Hypotonic uterine dysfunction   Occurs when the pressure of the uterine contraction (UC) is insufficient (<25 mm Hg) to promote cervical dilation and effacement

Hypoxemia   Low levels of oxygen in the blood

Hypoxia   Low levels of oxygen in the tissue, oxygen levels inadequate to meet metabolic needs of the tissue

Hysterosalpingogram   A radiologic examination that provides information about the endocervical canal, uterine cavity, and the fallopian tubes

Implantation   The embedding of the blastocyst into the endometrium of the uterus

Implementation   The process of taking action by intervening, delegating, and/or coordinating; women, newborns, families, significant others, or health care providers may direct the implementation of interventions within the plan of care

Inadequate expulsive forces   Occurs in the second stage of labor when the woman is not able to push or bear-down effectively

Incompetent cervix   A mechanical defect in the cervix that results in painless cervical dilation and ballooning of the membranes into the vagina followed by expulsion of an immature fetus in the second trimester

Incomplete abortion   Fragments of products of conception are expelled and tissue parts are retained in the uterus

Increment phase   The ascending or buildup of the contraction which begins in the fundus and spreads throughout the uterus

Indeterminate   Not definitely or precisely determined or fixed; not leading to a definite end or result; category II FHR patterns are indeterminate: they are not predictive of abnormal fetal acid-base status, yet there is not adequate evidence at present to classify these as category I or category III; category II FHR tracings require evaluation and continued surveillance and reevaluation, taking into account the entire associated clinical circumstances

Indirect bilirubin   Unconjugated bilirubin

Indirect obstetrical death   Death of a woman that is due to a preexisting disease or a disease that develops during pregnancy that is not directly related to obstetrical cause, but is aggravated by the changes of pregnancy

Induced abortion   The medical or surgical termination of pregnancy before viability

Induction   The deliberate stimulation of UCs before the onset of spontaneous labor

Inevitable abortion   Termination of pregnancy is in progress

Infant mortality   Infant death before the first birthday

Infertility   The inability to conceive and maintain a pregnancy after 12 months (6 months for woman older than 35 years of age) of unprotected sexual intercourse

Intensity   Strength of the contraction and measured by palpation, or internally by an intrauterine pressure catheter (IUPC) in mm Hg

Interconceptional interval   The period of time in between pregnancies

Intermittent auscultation   Auditory assessment of the FHR at intervals either by fetoscope or hand-held Doppler

Intermittent decelerations   Occur with fewer than 50% of contractions in a 20-minute period.

Internal fetal monitoring   An invasive assessment of the FHR or uterine contractions or both; a fetal spiral electrode provides auditory and visual fetal heart ECG data; an intrauterine pressure catheter provides visual intrauterine pressure measurements during and between contractions

Internal rotation   This movement, the rotation of the fetal head, aligns the long axis of the fetal head with the long axis of the maternal pelvis; occurs mainly during second stage of labor

Interval   Period between uterine contractions, timed from the end of one contraction to the beginning of the next

Intrapartum period   Begins with the onset of regular uterine contractions and lasts until the expulsion of the placenta

Intrauterine growth restriction (IUGR)   A decreased rate of fetal growth usually due to a decreased in cell production related to chronic malnutrition; there are two types of IUGR, symmetric and asymmetric

Intrauterine pressure catheter (IUPC)   A catheter used to directly measure intrauterine pressure during and between uterine contractions

Intrauterine resuscitation   Interventions initiated when indeterminant or abnormal FHR patterns occur

Intrinsic factors   Internal fetal regulatory mechanisms that controls the heart rate, including sympathetic, parasympathetic, and central nervous systems, baroreceptors, chemoreceptor and hormonal responses.

Involution   The process by which the uterus returns to a prepregnant size, shape, and location; and the placental site heals

Isthmus   The narrower, lower segment of the uterus

Justice   The principle of or equal treatment of others or that others be treated fairly; justice refers to fairness

Kernicterus An abnormal accumulation of unconjugated bilirubin in the neonates' brain cells

Labor The process in which the fetus, placenta, and membranes are expelled through the uterus

Labor augmentation The stimulation of ineffective uterine contractions (UCs) after the onset of spontaneous labor to manage labor dystocia

Lacerations Tears in the perineum that may occur at delivery

Lactation The production of breast milk

Large for gestational age (LGA) Term used for neonates whose weight is above the 90th percentile for gestational age

Latching-on Refers to the newborn's ability to grasp the breast and to effectively suckle

Late deceleration Late decelerations are visually apparent gradual decreases in the FHR that is associated with uterine contractions; late decelerations are delayed in timing, meaning the deceleration reaches its nadir (lowest point) after the peak of the contraction; in most cases the onset, nadir, and recovery of the deceleration occur after the respective onset, peak, and resolution of the contraction as well; late decelerations are typically symmetrical in shape

Late maternal death Death of a woman that occurs more than 42 days after termination of pregnancy from a direct or indirect obstetrical cause

Late premature/late preterm Neonate born between 34 and 36 weeks of gestation

Latent phase First phase of labor; the early and slower part of labor with cervical dilation from 0 to 3 cm

Leopold's maneuvers A systematic method of abdominal palpation to assess fetal position, attitude, and lie

Let-down reflex Also referred to as milk ejection reflex; results in milk being ejected into and through the lactiferous duct system

Leukorrhea A white, odorless, physiological vaginal discharge; increases in pregnancy due to increased mucus secretion by cervical glands

Lightening Term used to describe the descent of the fetus into the true pelvis which occurs approximately 2 weeks before term in first-time pregnancies

Local An anesthetic injected into perineum at episiotomy site

Lochia Bloody discharge from the uterus that contains sloughed off tissue; it undergoes changes that reflect the healing stages of the uterine placental site

Long-term variability (LTV) The changes in fetal heart rate (FHR) range or fluctuations in the FHR baseline

Low birth weight infant (LBW) An infant who weighs less than 2,500 grams at birth, regardless of gestational age

Low-lying placenta The placenta is implanted in the lower uterine segment in close proximity to the internal cervical os

Luteal phase Part of the ovarian cycle; It begins after ovulation and lasts approximately 14 days

Macrocephaly Head circumference greater than the 90th percentile

Macrosomia Birth weight above 4,000 to 4,500 grams

Magnetic resonance imaging (MRI) Diagnostic radiologic evaluation of tissue and organs from multiple planes

Marginal placenta previa The placenta is at the margin of the internal cervical os

Mastitis Inflammation/infection of the breast

Maternal death Death of a woman during pregnancy or within 42 days of termination of pregnancy; the death is related to the pregnancy or aggravated by pregnancy, or management of the pregnancy; it excludes death from accidents or injuries

Maternal phases A process, defined by Reva Rubin, that occurs during the first few weeks of the postpartum period; this process includes three phases: Taking-in, Taking-hold, and Letting-go

Maternal tasks of pregnancy Psychological work done by the pregnant woman toward the development of a positive adaptation to pregnancy and the establishment of a maternal identity

Maternal touch A process, described by Reva Rubin, that new mothers transition through beginning with the first physical contact with their newborns

Meconium stool The first stool eliminated by the neonate; it is sticky, thick, black, and odorless

Medical nutritional therapy (MNT) A cornerstone of diabetes management for all diabetic women with the goal of providing adequate nutrition and preventing diabetic ketoacidosis and postprandial euglycemia

Menstrual phase Part of the endometrial cycle; it occurs in response to hormonal changes and results in the sloughing off of the endometrial tissue

Mesoderm The middle layer of cells in the developing embryo

Microcephaly Head circumference below the 10th percentile of normal for the newborn's gestational age

Missed abortion Embryo or fetus dies during first 20 weeks of gestation but is retained in the uterus

Mitotic cell division or mitosis Occurs when a cell (parent cell) divides and forms two daughter cells that contain the same number of chromosomes as the parent cell

Moderately premature Neonate born between 32 and 34 weeks of gestation

Moderately preterm Neonate born between 32 and 36 completed weeks of gestation

Modified BPP Combines a non-stress test with an amniotic fluid index (AFI) as an indicator of short-term fetal well-being and AFI as an indicator of long-term placental function to evaluate fetal well-being

Molding The ability of the fetal head to change shape to accommodate/fit through the maternal pelvis

Monozygotic Pertaining to or derived from a single zygote (fertilized ovum), as in twin gestation occurring from a single fertilized ovum; results in identical twins.

Montevideo units (MVU) Total pressure in mm Hg for all uterine contractions within a 10-minute time frame; calculated by measuring the peak intensity or amplitude (in mm Hg) for each contraction occurring in a 10-minute period and adding the numbers together; contraction amplitude is the difference between the resting tone and the peak of the contraction (in mm Hg); it is important to note that these calculations are dependent on the accuracy of IUPC data.

Morula Sixteen-cell solid sphere that forms 3 days after fertilization as a result of mitotic cell division of the zygote

Multigravida A woman who has been pregnant multiple times

Multipara A woman who has given birth after 20 weeks of gestation multiple times

Multiple gestation A pregnancy with more than one fetus

Myomectomy Surgical removal of fibroids

Myometrium The smooth muscle layer of the uterus

Nadir The lowest FHR value in a deceleration; with electronic monitoring, it is visually the lowest point in the deceleration curve.

Naegele's rule The standard formula for calculating an estimated date of birth based on last menstrual period (LMP; LMP minus 3 months plus 7 days)

Natural childbirth   Labor and delivery acccomplished with little or no medical intervention

Necrotizing enterocolitis (NEC)   A gastrointestinal disease that affects neonates; this disease results in inflammation and necrosis of the bowel, usually the proximal colon or terminal ileum

Neonatal abstinence syndrome   Also referred to as neonatal withdrawal; may result from intrauterine exposure to various substances including opioids such as heroin, methadone, oxycodone, and Demerol; alcohol; Valium; caffeine; and barbiturates

Neonatal period   The time period from birth through the first 28 days of life

Neutral thermal environment (NTE)   Refers to an environment that maintains body temperature with minimal metabolic changes and/or oxygen consumption

Nonmaleficence   The obligation to do no harm

Nonreassuring FHR   An abnormal FHR pattern that reflects an unfavorable physiological response to the maternal–fetal environment

Non-stress Test (NST)   Antepartum fetal assessment test used to assess fetal well-being; the FHR is monitored for 2 accelerations (in a term fetus, FHR increases at least 15 bpm above baseline lasting for 15 seconds from the time the FHR leaves the baseline to the time it returns to the baseline) in 20 minutes; in a fetus under 32 weeks gestation accelerations are increases of at least 10 bpm for 10 bpm duration; the presence of accelerations indicates adequate fetal oxygenation

Nulligravida   A woman who has never been pregnant

Nullipara   A woman who has never given birth after 20 weeks of gestation

Obstetrical emergency   An urgent clinical situation that places either the maternal or fetal status at risk for increased morbidity and mortality

Occiput   Back part of the head or skull

Occiput posterior   When the occiput of the fetus is in the posterior portion of the pelvis rather than the anterior

Occult prolapse   When the cord is palpated through the membranes but does not drop into the vagina

Oligohydramnios   Decreased amounts of amniotic fluid (<500 mL at term or 50% reduction of normal amounts) during pregnancy

Ominous FHR patterns   Fetal heart rates (FHRs) associated with increased risk of fetal acidemia

Open glottis   Refers to spontaneous, involuntary bearing down accompanying the forces of the uterine contraction and is usually characterized by expiratory grunting or vocalizations by a woman during pushing

Operative vaginal delivery   A vaginal birth that is assisted by a vacuum extraction or forceps

Organogenesis   The formation and development of body organs that occurs during the first trimester of pregnancy

Orthostatic hypotension   A sudden drop in the blood pressure when the woman stands up from a sitting or laying position

Outcome   A measurable individual, family, or community state, behavior, or perception that is responsive to nursing interventions

Ovarian cycle   Pertains to the maturation of ova and consists of three phases: follicular phase, ovulatory phase, and luteal phase

Ovulatory phase   Part of the ovarian cycle; it begins when estrogen levels peak and ends with the release of the oocyte (egg) from the mature graafian follicle; the release of the oocyte is referred to as ovulation

Oxytocin induction   Pharmacological method for induction of labor with oxytocin

Papanicolaou smear   A screening test used to identify cervical cancer

Para   A woman who has given birth to an infant after 20 weeks of gestation; also, the number of births that occurred after 20 weeks of gestation (Gravida/Para notation) or the number of infants born after 20 weeks of gestation (TPAL notation)

Parasympathetic nervous system   Part of autonomic nervous system; includes the vagus nerve which decreases the heart rate when stimulated.

Partial placenta previa   The placenta partially covers the internal cervical os

Parturition   (or labor) The process in which the fetus, placenta, and membranes are expelled through the uterus

Passage   Includes the bony pelvis and the soft tissues of cervix, pelvic floor, vagina, and introitus (external opening to the vagina)

Passenger   The fetus

Patent ductus arteriosus (PDA)   Occurs when the ductus arteriosus remains open or remains open after birth

Peak pressure   The maximum uterine pressure during a contraction measured with an IUPC

Pelvic dystocia   Related to the contraction of one or more of the three planes of the pelvis

Pelvic inflammatory disease (PID)   A general term that refers to an infection of the uterus, fallopian tubes, and other reproductive organs

Percutaneous umbilical blood sampling (PUBS)   The removal of fetal blood from the umbilical cord for fetal blood sampling; also referred to as cordocentesis

Perinatal   The time period "around" the birth of a baby; generally refers to the weeks before and after a baby is born, from 28 weeks of gestation to 28 days after birth

Perineum   Area between the vagina and rectum

Periodic and nonperiodic changes   Accelerations or decelerations in the fetal heart rate (FHR) that are related to uterine contractions and persist over time

Periodic changes   Accelerations or decelerations of the FHR that are associated with uterine contractions

Persistent pulmonary hypertension (PPHN)   Results when the normal vasodilation and relaxation of the pulmonary vascular bed does not occur

Pfannenstiel incision or "bikini cut"   A transverse skin incision at the level of the mons pubis with a transverse incision in the lower uterine segment performed for cesarean births

Phenotype   Refers to how the genes are outwardly expressed (i.e., eye color, hair color, height)

Phenylketonuria (PKU)   An inborn error of metabolism that affects the neonate's ability to metabolize phenylalanine, an amino acid commonly found in many foods such as breast milk and formula

Physiologic anemia of pregnancy   A relative anemia in mid- to late pregnancy due to physiologic hypervolemia without a correspondingly proportionate increase in erythrocytes in the maternal system

Pica   A craving for and consumption of nonfood substances such as starch and clay; can result in toxicity due to ingested substances or malnutrition from replacing nutritious foods with nonfood substances

Pilonidal dimple   A small pit or sinus in the sacral area at the top of the crease between the buttocks

Placenta   A specialized vascular disk-shaped organ for maternal-fetal gas and nutrient exchange; normally it implants in the thick muscular wall of the upper uterine segment; postpartum it may be referred to as the afterbirth

Placenta accreta   An abnormality of implantation defined by degree of invasion into the uterine wall of the trophoblast of the placenta; invasion of the trophoblast beyond the normal boundary

Placenta increta   Invasion of the trophoblast that extends into myometrium

Placenta percreta   Invasion of the trophoblast beyond the serosa

Placenta previa   Occurs when the placenta attaches to the lower uterine segment of the uterus, near or over the internal cervical os, instead of in the body or fundus of the uterus

Placental reserve   Describes the reserve oxygen available to the fetus to withstand the transient changes in blood flow and oxygen during labor

Polydactyly   Extra digits of hands or feet

Polyhydramnios or hydramnios   Increased amounts of amniotic fluid (1,500–2,000 mL)

Position of cervix   Relationship of the cervical os to the fetal head and is characterized as posterior, mid, or anterior position

Postpartum   The 6-week period of time after childbirth

Postpartum blues   Also known as baby blues; occurs during the first few weeks postpartum and lasts for a few days; it is a time of heightened maternal emotions with the woman being tearful and irritable with emotional swings

Postpartum chills   Episode of shaking and feeling cold that most women experience during the first few hours after birth

Postpartum depression (PPD)   A mood disorder characterized by severe depression that occurs within the first 6 to 12 months postpartum

Postpartum psychosis (PPP)   A variant of bipolar disorder and is the most serious form of postpartum mood disorders

Post term   Born after 42 weeks of gestation

Post term pregnancy   Pregnancy that has a gestational period of 42 completed weeks

Powers   Refers to the involuntary uterine contractions of labor and the voluntary pushing or bearing-down powers that combine to propel and deliver the fetus and placenta from the uterus

Practice standards   Standards that help to guide professional nursing practice; they summarize the nursing profession's best judgment and optimal practice based on current research and clinical practice

Precipitous labor   Labor that lasts less than 3 hours from onset of labor to birth

Preconception care   Well-woman health care focusing on preparation for and anticipation of a pregnancy, including health promotion, risk screening, and implementation of interventions before pregnancy, the goal being to modify risk factors that could negatively impact a pregnancy in order to optimize perinatal outcomes

Preeclampsia   Hypertension accompanied by underlying systemic pathology that can have severe maternal and fetal impact; a systemic disease with hypertension accompanied by proteinuria after the 20th week of gestation

Preeclampsia superimposed on chronic hypertension   Occurs with hypertensive women who develop new onset proteinuria; proteinuria before the 20th week of gestation or sudden uncontrolled hypertension

Pregestational diabetes   Diabetes type I or type II that exists before pregnancy

Premature rupture of membranes   Rupture of the chorioamniotic membranes before the onset of labor

Prenatal   The entire time period during which a woman is pregnant; includes the antepartum/antepartal and the intrapartal periods

Prenatal care   Health care relating to pregnancy that a woman receives during the pregnancy and before the onset of labor

Prescriptive behavior   Expected behavior of the pregnant woman during the childbearing period

Presenting part   The specific fetal structure lying nearest to the cervix

Preterm birth   Any birth that occurs after 20 weeks and before 37 completed weeks of pregnancy

Preterm labor   Labor that occurs prior to 37 weeks gestation

Preterm/premature infant   Infant born after 20 weeks and before 37 completed weeks of gestation

Preterm premature rupture of membranes (PPROM)   Rupture of membranes with a premature gestation (<37 weeks)

Primary engorgement   An increase in the vascular and lymphatic system of the breasts, which precedes the initiation of milk production; the woman's breasts become larger, firm, warm, and tender and the woman may feel a throbbing pain in the breasts

Primigravida   A woman who is pregnant for the first time

Primipara   A woman who has given birth after 20 weeks of gestation one time

Prodromal labor   When contractions are frequent and painful in early labor but ineffective in promoting dilation and effacement

Prolactin   The primary hormone responsible for lactation

Prolapse of the umbilical cord   When the cord lies below the presenting part of the fetus

Proliferative phase   Part of the endometrial cycle; it follows menstruation and ends with ovulation; during this phase the endometrium is preparing for implantation by becoming thicker and more vascular

Prolonged deceleration   A visually apparent abrupt decrease in fetal heart rate (FHR) below baseline that lasts more than 2 minutes and less than 10 minutes

Prolonged rupture of membranes (PROM)   Rupture of membranes greater than 24 hours

Psychosocial risk factors   Maternal behaviors or lifestyles that have a negative response to the mother or fetus; examples include smoking, caffeine, alcohol/drugs, and psychological status

Pudendal block   An anesthetic injected in the pudendal nerve (close to the ischial spines) via needle guide known as "trumpet"

Pulmonary surfactant   A substance that is composed of 90% phospholipids and 10% proteins that is used in the treatment of respiratory distress syndrome of the neonate

Quad screen   Adds inhibin-A to the triple marker screen to increase detection of trisomy 21 to 80%

Quickening   A woman's first awareness/perception of fetal movement within her uterus

Radiation   Transfer of heat from neonate to cooler objects that are not in direct contact with neonate such as cold walls of isolate or cold equipment near the neonate

Reassuring fetal heart rate   Normal fetal heart rate (FHR) pattern that reflects a favorable physiological response to the maternal–fetal environment

Rectoceles   Bulging of the rectum into the vagina

Recurrent abortion   Condition in which two or more successive pregnancies have ended in spontaneous abortion

Recurrent decelerations   Occurring with at least 50% of the contractions in a 20-minute period

Respect for others   The principle that all persons are equally valued

Respiratory distress syndrome (RDS)   A life-threatening lung disorder that results from underdeveloped and small alveoli and insufficient levels of pulmonary surfactant

Resting tone   The pressure in the uterus between contractions

Restrictive behavior   Activities during the childbearing period that are limited for the woman based on cultural practices

Review of systems (ROS)   A component of the health history that includes systematic questioning about health status by body system, typically in a head-to-toe sequence, in order to gather information about current and past medical experiences.

Rh factor   A type of antigen on the surface of red blood cells; if a woman's red blood cells have the antigen, she is Rh positive and if they do not have the antigen, she is Rh negative; this is significant and can cause isoimmunization from blood incompatibility if fetal blood enters the maternal system in an Rh-positive fetus and an Rh-negative mother

Rights approach   The focus is on the individual's right to choose; includes the right to privacy, to know the truth, and to be free from injury or harm

Risk factors   Assessment findings that can contribute to a negative outcome for woman or fetus

Risk management   A systems approach to the prevention of litigation; it involves the identification of system problems, analysis, and treatment of risks before a suit is brought

Rupture of the uterus   When there is a partial or complete tear in the uterine muscle

Screening test   Test designed to identify those who are not affected by a disease or abnormality

Second-degree laceration   Laceration involves skin, mucous membrane, and fascia of perineal body

Second stage of labor   Begins at complete dilation of cervix and ends with delivery of the neonate

Secretory phase   Part of the endometrial cycle; it begins after ovulation and ends with the onset of menstruation; during this phase the endometrium continues to thicken

Septic abortion   Condition in which products of conception become infected during abortion process

Short-term variability (STV)   Changes in the FHR from one beat to the next; measures the R-to-R intervals of subsequent fetal cardiac cycles (QRS); historically, short-term variability and long-term variability were assessed independently of each other and an internal electrode was necessary for assessment of short-term variability; in current clinical practice FHR variability is visually assessed as a unit by peak-to-trough amplitude fluctuations regardless of electronic monitoring method; no distinction is made between short-term and long-term FHR variation

Shoulder dystocia   Refers to difficulty encountered during delivery of the shoulders after the birth of the head

Shoulder presentation   The presenting part is the shoulder; when the fetal spine is vertical to the maternal pelvis

Sibling rivalry   Negative behaviors exhibited by siblings in response to a new baby in the family

Sinusoidal pattern   A sinusoidal fetal heart rate pattern is a visually apparent undulating smooth sine wave like pattern in FHR baseline with a cycle frequency of 3-5 per minute which persists for at least 20 minutes; there is an absence of accelerations and no response to uterine contractions, fetal movement, or stimulation

Small for gestational age (SGA)   A term used for neonate whose weight is below the 10th percentile for gestational age

Social support   Support given by someone with whom the expectant mother has a personal relationship, involving the primary groups of most importance to the individual woman

Sociodemographic risk factors   Variables that pertain to the woman and her family and place an increased risk to the mother and the fetus; examples include income, access to prenatal care, age, parity, marital status, and ethnicity

Sperm antibodies   An immunological reaction against the sperm that causes a decrease in sperm motility

Spermatogenesis   The process in which mature functional sperm are formed

Spinal block   An anesthetic injected in the subarachnoid space

Spiral electrode/fetal scalp electrode (FSE)   An internal device for recording the FHR that is applied directly to the fetal presenting part and receives signals from the electrocardiac impulses of the fetal heart; used to directly determine FHR based on changes in the R-to-R intervals in successive QRS complexes

Spontaneous abortion (SAB)   Abortion occurring without medical or mechanical means; also called miscarriage

Spontaneous rupture of the membranes (SROM)   Rupture of the membranes that occurs naturally

Standard   An authoritative statement enunciated and promulgated by the profession and by which the quality of practice, service, or education can be judged

Standards of care   Authoritative statements that describe competent clinical nursing practice for women and newborns demonstrated through assessment, diagnosis, outcome identification, planning, implementation, and evaluation

Standards of nursing practice   Authoritative statements that describe the scope of care or performance common to the profession of nursing and by which the quality of nursing practice can be judged; standards of nursing practice for women and newborns include both standards of care and standards of professional performance

Standards of professional performance   Authoritative statements that describe competent behavior in the professional role, including activities related to quality of care, performance appraisal, resource utilization, education, collegiality, ethics, collaboration, research, and research utilization

Station   Level of the presenting part in the birth canal in relationship to the ischial spines; refers to the relationship of the ischial spines to the presenting part of the fetus and assists in assessing for fetal descent during labor

Sterile vaginal exam (SVE)   Assessment of cervix by feeling the cervix in the vagina

Striae   A band of depressed tissue most commonly seen on abdomen, thighs, buttocks, or breasts due to stretching of the skin; synonymous with stretch marks

Stripping the membranes   Digital separation of the chorionic membrane from the wall of the cervix and lower uterine segment during a vaginal exam done by a primary care provider to stimulate labor

Subinvolution of the uterus   A term used when the uterus does not decrease in size and does not descend into the pelvis

Supine hypotensive syndrome   Hypotension resulting from compression of the vena cava when a woman lies supine and the gravid uterus exerts pressure on the inferior vena cava

Symmetric intrauterine growth restriction   A generalized proportional reduction in the size of all structures and organs except for the heart and brain

Sympathetic nervous system   A part of the autonomic nervous system; stimulation results in FHR increase

Syndactyly   Webbed digits of hands or feet

Taboos   Cultural restrictions believed to have serious consequences

Tachycardia   Baseline FHR of greater than 160 bpm for a period of 10 minutes or more

Tachycardia   Baseline FHR above 160 beats per minute for a period of ten minutes or more.

Tachysystole   Abnormally frequent contractions; 5 or more contractions in 10 minutes

Teratogens   Any drug, virus, infection, or other exposures that can cause embryo/fetal developmental abnormality

Term birth   A birth that occurs between 37 and 42 weeks of gestation

Therapeutic abortion (TAB)   Termination of pregnancy for serious maternal medical indications or serious fetal anomalies

Third-degree laceration   Laceration involves skin, mucous membrane, and muscle of perineal body and extends to the rectal sphincter

Third stage of labor   Begins immediately after the delivery of the fetus and involves separation and expulsion of the placenta and membranes

Threatened abortion   Continuation of pregnancy is in doubt as symptoms indicate termination of pregnancy is in progress

Thrombosis   Blood clot within the vascular system

Tocodynamometer (tocotransducer) (toco)   The transducer on an electronic fetal monitor that externally detects abdominal pressure or contour changes resulting from uterine contractions and transmits this information to the monitor to be displayed in graphic form

Tocolytic   A medication that diminishes or stops uterine activity by altering smooth muscle activity

Tonus   Intensity of uterine tone or intrauterine pressure between uterine contractions (resting tone)

TORCH   An acronym that stands for **T**oxoplasmosis, **O**ther (hepatitis B), **R**ubella, **C**ytomegalovirus, and **H**erpes Simplex virus

Total placenta previa   The placenta completely covers the internal cervical os

Transepidermal water loss (TEWL)   Water loss that can occur through the neonate's immature skin

Transition phase   Third phase of labor; dilation from 8 to 10 cm

Transitional stool   Neonatal stools that begin around the 3rd day and can continue for 3 or 4 days; the stool transitions from black to greenish black, to greenish brown, to greenish yellow

Transverse presentation   The presenting part is usually the shoulder

Trial of labor after cesarean (TOLAC)   When a trial of labor and vaginal birth is attempted in a woman who has had a prior cesarean birth

Trimester   One of three periods of about 3 months into which the pregnancy is divided

Triple marker   A screening that combines all three chemical markers (alpha-fetoprotein [AFP], human chorionic gonadotropin [hCG], and estriol levels) with maternal age to detect some trisomies and neural tube defects

Trophic feedings   Small-volume enteral feedings that are administered to neonates

Trophoblast   Outer cell mass of the blastocyst that assists in implantation and becomes part of the placenta

True labor   Contractions occur at regular intervals and increase in frequency, duration, and intensity; true labor contractions bring about changes in cervical effacement and dilation

Turtle sign   A retraction of the fetal head against the maternal perineum after delivery of the head

Type 1 diabetes mellitus   A result of autoimmunity of beta cells of the pancreas resulting in absolute insulin deficiency

Type 2 diabetes mellitus   Characterized by insulin resistance and inadequate insulin production

Ultrasonography   The use of high-frequency sound waves to produce an image of an organ or tissue

Ultrasound transducer (US)   An external monitor that detects movement of the fetal heart valves opening and closing through transmission of a sound wave and Doppler shift; monitor processor converts reflected sound waves into an electronic signal corresponding to the FHR

Umbilical artery Doppler flow   Studies assess the rate and volume of blood flow through placenta and umbilical cord vessels using ultrasound

Umbilical cord   The structure that connects the fetus to the placenta; it consists of two arteries and one vein and is surrounded by Wharton's Jelly

Unconjugated bilirubin   A relatively insoluble bilirubin and mostly bound to albumin; also called indirect bilirubin

Undescended testes   An abnormality in which testes are not in the scrotum

Urinary incontinence   Loss of bladder control

Uterine atony   A decreased tone of the uterine muscle postpartum that is the primary cause of immediate postpartum hemorrhage

Uterine fibroids   Benign growths of the muscular wall of the uterus

Uterine hypertonus   An increasing resting tone greater than 20 to 25 mm Hg, peak pressure greater than 80 mm Hg or Montevideo units greater than 400

Uterine prolapse   Occurs when there is a weakening of the pelvic connective tissue, pubococcygeus muscle, and uterine ligaments which allows the uterus to descend into the vagina

Utero placental insufficiency   Decline in placental function–a decrease in exchange of gases, nutrients and wastes–potentially leading to fetal hypoxia and acidosis

Uterus   The muscular reproductive organ that contains and supports a pregnancy

Utilitarian approach   This approach suggests that ethical actions are those that provide the greatest balance of good over evil and provides for the greatest good for the greatest number

Utility   The greatest good for the individual or an action that is valued; utility is concerned with the evaluation of risk and benefit or benefit versus burden

Vacuum-assisted delivery   Is a birth involving the use of a vacuum cup on the fetal head to assist with delivery of the fetal head

Vaginal birth after a cesarean (VBAC)   When a trial of labor and vaginal birth is attempted in a woman who has had a prior cesarean birth

Valsalva maneuver   Method of breath holding, closed-glottis pushing

Variable deceleration   Visually apparent, abrupt (onset to nadir < 30 seconds) decrease in the FHR below baseline; the decrease is calculated from onset to the beginning of the nadir of the deceleration; the FHR decreases > 15 bpm, lasting > 15 seconds and < 2 minutes in duration; may occur with or without relationship to uterine contractions; when variable decelerations are associated with uterine contractions, their onset, depth, and duration typically vary with successive uterine contractions

Veracity   The obligation to tell the truth

Very low birth weight infant (VLBW)   An infant who weighs less than 1,500 grams at birth

Very premature/preterm   Neonate born at less than 32 weeks of gestation

Vibroacoustic stimulation (VAS)   Screening tool that uses auditory stimulation (using an artificial larynx) to assess fetal wellbeing with electronic fetal monitoring when the non-stress test (NST) is nonreactive

Wharton's Jelly   A collagen substance that surrounds the vessels of the umbilical cord and protects the vessels from compression

Zygote   A fertilized oocyte that contains the diploid number of chromosomes (46)

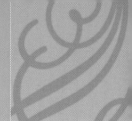

Photo and Illustration Credits

Chapter 3

Figure 3-1 Scanlon V., & Sanders T. (2007). *Essentials of anatomy and physiology* (5th ed., p. 469). Philadelphia: F. A. Davis.

Figure 3-2 Scanlon V., & Sanders T. (2007). *Essentials of anatomy and physiology* (5th ed., p. 478). Philadelphia: F. A. Davis.

Figure 3-3 Scanlon V., & Sanders T. (2007). *Essentials of anatomy and physiology* (5th ed., p. 479). Philadelphia: F. A. Davis.

Figure 3-4 Scanlon V., & Sanders T. (2007). *Essentials of anatomy and physiology* (5th ed., p. 305). Philadelphia: F. A. Davis.

Figure 3-5 Scanlon V., & Sanders T. (2007). *Essentials of anatomy and physiology* (5th ed., p. 484). Philadelphia: F. A. Davis.

Figure 3-6 Scanlon V., & Sanders T. (2007). *Essentials of anatomy and physiology* (5th ed., p. 485). Philadelphia: F. A. Davis.

Chapter 4

Figure 4-1 Ward S., & Hisley S. (2009). *Maternal-child nursing care: Optimizing outcomes for mothers, children, & families* (p. 264). Philadelphia: F. A. Davis.

Figure 4-3 Ward S., & Hisley S. (2009). *Maternal-child nursing care: Optimizing outcomes for mothers, children, & families* (p. 121). Philadelphia: F. A. Davis.

Figure 4-4 Ward S., & Hisley S. (2009). *Maternal-child nursing care: Optimizing outcomes for mothers, children, & families* (p. 195). Philadelphia: F. A. Davis.

Figure 4-5 Ward S., & Hisley S. (2009). *Maternal-child nursing care: Optimizing outcomes for mothers, children, & families* (p. 201). Philadelphia: F. A. Davis.

Figure 4-6 Ward S., & Hisley S. (2009). *Maternal-child nursing care: Optimizing outcomes for mothers, children, & families* (p. 198). Philadelphia: F. A. Davis.

Figure 4-8 U.S. Department of Agriculture, 2005.

Chapter 5

Figure 5-2 Courtesy of Randi Willis and Gwen Ortiz.

Figure 5-3 Courtesy of Gwen Ortiz and Randi Willis.

Chapter 6

Figure 6-3 Ward S., & Hisley S. (2009). *Maternal-child nursing care: Optimizing outcomes for mothers, children, & families* (p. 340). Philadelphia: F. A. Davis.

Chapter 7

Figure 7-5 Ward S., & Hisley S. (2009). *Maternal-child nursing care: Optimizing outcomes for mothers, children, & families* (p. 185). Philadelphia: F. A. Davis.

Figure 7-9 Dillon P. (2007). *Nursing health assessment: A critical thinking, case studies approach* (2nd ed., p. 841). Philadelphia: F. A. Davis.

Figure 7-10 Ward S., & Hisley S. (2009). *Maternal-child nursing care: Optimizing outcomes for mothers, children, & families* (p. 298). Philadelphia: F. A. Davis.

Figure 7-11 Holloway B., Moredich C., & Aduddell K. (2006). *OB peds women's health notes: Nurse's clinical pocket guide* (p. 45). Philadelphia: F. A. Davis.

Figure 7-13 Ward S., & Hisley S. (2009). *Maternal-child nursing care: Optimizing outcomes for mothers, children, & families* (p. 294). Philadelphia: F. A. Davis.

Chapter 8

Figure 8-1 Ward S., & Hisley S. (2009). *Maternal-child nursing care: Optimizing outcomes for mothers, children, & families* (p. 294). Philadelphia: F. A. Davis.

Figure 8-2 Ward S., & Hisley S. (2009). *Maternal-child nursing care: Optimizing outcomes for mothers, children, & families* (p. 359). Philadelphia: F. A. Davis.

Figure 8-3 Ward S., & Hisley S. (2009). *Maternal-child nursing care: Optimizing outcomes for mothers, children, & families* (p. 123). Philadelphia: F. A. Davis.

Figure 8-4 Ward S., & Hisley S. (2009). *Maternal-child nursing care: Optimizing outcomes for mothers, children, & families* (p. 122). Philadelphia: F. A. Davis.

Figure 8-5 Holloway B., Moredich C., & Aduddell K. (2006). *OB peds women's health notes: Nurse's clinical pocket guide* (p. 53). Philadelphia: F. A. Davis.

Figure 8-6 Ward S., & Hisley S. (2009). *Maternal-child nursing care: Optimizing outcomes for mothers, children, & families* (p. 361). Philadelphia: F. A. Davis.

Figure 8-6 Ward S., & Hisley S. (2009). *Maternal-child nursing care: Optimizing outcomes for mothers, children, & families* (p. 361). Philadelphia: F. A. Davis.

Figure 8-7 Ward S., & Hisley S. (2009). *Maternal-child nursing care: Optimizing outcomes for mothers, children, & families* (p. 362). Philadelphia: F. A. Davis.

Figure 8-8 Ward S., & Hisley S. (2009). *Maternal-child nursing care: Optimizing outcomes for mothers, children, & families* (p. 361). Philadelphia: F. A. Davis.

Figure 8-9 Ward S., & Hisley S. (2009). *Maternal-child nursing care: Optimizing outcomes for mothers, children, & families* (pp. 361, 363, 364). Philadelphia: F. A. Davis.

Figure 8-10 Ward S., & Hisley S. (2009). *Maternal-child nursing care: Optimizing outcomes for mothers, children, & families* (p. 362). Philadelphia: F. A. Davis.

Figure 8-10 Ward S., & Hisley S. (2009). *Maternal-child nursing care: Optimizing outcomes for mothers, children, & families* (p. 362). Philadelphia: F. A. Davis.

Figure 8-11 Ward S., & Hisley S. (2009). *Maternal-child nursing care: Optimizing outcomes for mothers, children, & families* (p. 363). Philadelphia: F. A. Davis.

Figure 8-12 Adapted from Ward S., & Hisley S. (2009). *Maternal-child nursing care: Optimizing outcomes for mothers, children, & families* (p. 364). Philadelphia: F. A. Davis.

Figure 8-13 Ward S., & Hisley S. (2009). *Maternal-child nursing care: Optimizing outcomes for mothers, children, & families* (p. 365). Philadelphia: F. A. Davis.

Figure 8-16 Ward S., & Hisley S. (2009). *Maternal-child nursing care: Optimizing outcomes for mothers, children, & families* (p. 374). Philadelphia: F. A. Davis.

Figure 8-17 Ward S., & Hisley S. (2009). *Maternal-child nursing care: Optimizing outcomes for mothers, children, & families* (p. 388). Philadelphia: F. A. Davis.

Figure 8-20 Dillon P. (2007). *Nursing health assessment: A critical thinking, case studies approach* (2nd ed., p. 631). Philadelphia: F. A. Davis.

Figure 8-21 Dillon P. (2007). *Nursing health assessment: A critical thinking, case studies approach* (2nd ed., p. 838). Philadelphia: F. A. Davis.

Figure 8-22 Ward S., & Hisley S. (2009). *Maternal-child nursing care: Optimizing outcomes for mothers, children, & families* (p. 390). Philadelphia: F. A. Davis.

Figure 8-23 Ward S., & Hisley S. (2009). *Maternal-child nursing care: Optimizing outcomes for mothers, children, & families* (p. 387). Philadelphia: F. A. Davis.

Figure 8-29 Dillon P. (2007). *Nursing health assessment: A critical thinking, case studies approach* (2nd ed., p. 90). Philadelphia: F. A. Davis.

Figure 8-30 Ward S., & Hisley S. (2009). *Maternal-child nursing care: Optimizing outcomes for mothers, children, & families* (p. 417). Philadelphia: F. A. Davis.

Figure 8-31 Ward S., & Hisley S. (2009). *Maternal-child nursing care: Optimizing outcomes for mothers, children, & families* (p. 409). Philadelphia: F. A. Davis.

Chapter 9

Figure 9-1 Dillon P. (2007). *Nursing health assessment: A critical thinking, case studies approach* (2nd ed., p. 837). Philadelphia: F. A. Davis.

Figure 9-2 Ward S., & Hisley S. (2009). *Maternal-child nursing care: Optimizing outcomes for mothers, children, & families* (p. 381). Philadelphia: F. A. Davis.

Figure 9-3 Ward S., & Hisley S. (2009). *Maternal-child nursing care: Optimizing outcomes for mothers, children, & families* (p. 381). Philadelphia: F. A. Davis.

Figure 9-5 Lyndon A., & Ali L. U. (2009). *Fetal heart rate monitoring: Principles and practice* (4th ed.). Dubuque, IA: Kendal/Hunt.

Figure 9-7 Holloway B., Moredich C., & Aduddell K. (2006). *OB peds women's health notes: Nurse's clinical pocket guide* (p. 57). Philadelphia: F. A. Davis.

Figure 9-14 Holloway B., Moredich C., & Aduddell K. (2006). *OB peds women's health notes: Nurse's clinical pocket guide* (p. 59). Philadelphia: F. A. Davis.

Figure 9-15 Holloway B., Moredich C., & Aduddell K. (2006). *OB peds women's health notes: Nurse's clinical pocket guide* (p. 60). Philadelphia: F. A. Davis.

Figure 9-17 Holloway B., Moredich C., & Aduddell K. (2006). *OB peds women's health notes: Nurse's clinical pocket guide* (p. 61). Philadelphia: F. A. Davis.

Figure 9-18 Holloway B., Moredich C., & Aduddell K. (2006). *OB peds women's health notes: Nurse's clinical pocket guide* (p. 60). Philadelphia: F. A. Davis.

Chapter 10

Figure 10-5 Ward S., & Hisley S. (2009). *Maternal-child nursing care: Optimizing outcomes for mothers, children, & families* (p. 359). Philadelphia: F. A. Davis.

Figure 10-6 Ward S., & Hisley S. (2009). *Maternal-child nursing care: Optimizing outcomes for mothers, children, & families* (p. 433). Philadelphia: F. A. Davis.

Figure 10-8 Ward S., & Hisley S. (2009). *Maternal-child nursing care: Optimizing outcomes for mothers, children, & families*

(p. 439). Philadelphia: F. A. Davis.

Figure 10-9 Ward S., & Hisley S. (2009). *Maternal-child nursing care: Optimizing outcomes for mothers, children, & families* (p. 439). Philadelphia: F. A. Davis.

Figure 10-10 Ward S., & Hisley S. (2009). *Maternal-child nursing care: Optimizing outcomes for mothers, children, & families* (p. 438). Philadelphia: F. A. Davis.

Figure 10-11 Ward S., & Hisley S. (2009). *Maternal-child nursing care: Optimizing outcomes for mothers, children, & families* (p. 438). Philadelphia: F. A. Davis.

Figure 10-13 Ward S., & Hisley S. (2009). *Maternal-child nursing care: Optimizing outcomes for mothers, children, & families* (p. 459). Philadelphia: F. A. Davis.

Figure 10-15 Ward S., & Hisley S. (2009). *Maternal-child nursing care: Optimizing outcomes for mothers, children, & families* (p. 445). Philadelphia: F. A. Davis.

Figure 10-16 Ward S., & Hisley S. (2009). *Maternal-child nursing care: Optimizing outcomes for mothers, children, & families* (p. 445). Philadelphia: F. A. Davis.

Figure 10-17 Ward S., & Hisley S. (2009). *Maternal-child nursing care: Optimizing outcomes for mothers, children, & families* (p. 453). Philadelphia: F. A. Davis.

Figure 10-18 Ward S., & Hisley S. (2009). *Maternal-child nursing care: Optimizing outcomes for mothers, children, & families* (p. 454). Philadelphia: F. A. Davis.

Figure 10-19 Ward S., & Hisley S. (2009). *Maternal-child nursing care: Optimizing outcomes for mothers, children, & families* (p. 454). Philadelphia: F. A. Davis.

LOP. Ward S., & Hisley S. (2009). *Maternal-child nursing care: Optimizing outcomes for mothers, children, & families* (p. 365). Philadelphia: F. A. Davis.

ROP. Ward S., & Hisley S. (2009). *Maternal-child nursing care: Optimizing outcomes for mothers, children, & families* (p. 365). Philadelphia: F. A. Davis.

Face presentation. Ward S., & Hisley S. (2009). *Maternal-child nursing care: Optimizing outcomes for mothers, children, & families* (p. 362). Philadelphia: F. A. Davis.

Shoulder presentation. Ward S., & Hisley S. (2009). *Maternal-child nursing care: Optimizing outcomes for mothers, children, & families* (p. 364). Philadelphia: F. A. Davis.

Frank breech. Ward S., & Hisley S. (2009). *Maternal-child nursing care: Optimizing outcomes for mothers, children, & families* (p. 363). Philadelphia: F. A. Davis.

Complete breech. Ward S., & Hisley S. (2009). *Maternal-child nursing care: Optimizing outcomes for mothers, children, & families* (p. 363). Philadelphia: F. A. Davis.

Single footing breech. Ward S., & Hisley S. (2009). *Maternal-child nursing care: Optimizing outcomes for mothers, children, & families* (p. 363). Philadelphia: F. A. Davis.

Chapter 11

Figure 11-2 Ward S., & Hisley S. (2009). *Maternal-child nursing care: Optimizing outcomes for mothers, children, & families* (p. 417). Philadelphia: F. A. Davis.

Figure 11-3 Ward S., & Hisley S. (2009). *Maternal-child nursing care: Optimizing outcomes for mothers, children, & families* (p. 459). Philadelphia: F. A. Davis.

Chapter 12

Figure 12-2 Dillon P. (2007). *Nursing health assessment: A critical thinking, case studies approach* (2nd ed., p. 844). Philadelphia: F. A. Davis.

Figure 12-3 Ward S., & Hisley S. (2009). *Maternal-child nursing care: Optimizing outcomes for mothers, children, & families* (p. 478). Philadelphia: F. A. Davis.

Chapter 14

Figure 14-1 Holloway B., Moredich C., & Aduddell K. (2006). *OB peds women's health notes: Nurse's clinical pocket guide* (p. 83). Philadelphia: F. A. Davis.

Figure 14-2 Ward S., & Hisley S. (2009). *Maternal-child nursing care: Optimizing outcomes for mothers, children, & families* (pp. 518, 519). Philadelphia: F. A. Davis.

Chapter 15

Figure 15-5 Reprinted from *Journal of Pediatrics*, 119:418, Ballard J, et al. Copyright 1991, with permission from Elsevier.

Figure 15-7 Ward S., & Hisley S. (2009). *Maternal-child nursing care: Optimizing outcomes for mothers, children, & families* (p. 597). Philadelphia: F. A. Davis.

Head circumference. Dillon P. (2007). *Nursing health assessment: A critical thinking, case studies approach* (2nd ed., p. 856). Philadelphia: F. A. Davis.

Chest circumference. Dillon P. (2007). *Nursing health assessment: A critical thinking, case studies approach* (2nd ed., p. 856). Philadelphia: F. A. Davis.

Length. Dillon P. (2007). *Nursing health assessment: A critical thinking, case studies approach* (2nd ed., p. 857). Philadelphia: F. A. Davis.

Cardiac. Dillon P. (2007). *Nursing health assessment: A critical thinking, case studies approach* (2nd ed., p. 864). Philadelphia: F. A. Davis.

Stork bite. Dillon P. (2007). *Nursing health assessment: A critical thinking, case studies approach* (2nd ed., p. 859). Philadelphia: F. A. Davis.

Palpating fontanel. Dillon P. (2007). *Nursing health assessment: A critical thinking, case studies approach* (2nd ed., p. 860). Philadelphia: F. A. Davis.

Normal eye line. Dillon P. (2007). *Nursing health assessment: A critical thinking, case studies approach* (2nd ed., p. 861). Philadelphia: F. A. Davis.

Thrush. Dillon P. (2007). *Nursing health assessment: A critical thinking, case studies approach* (2nd ed., p. 862). Philadelphia: F. A. Davis.

Auscultating lungs posteriorly. Dillon P. (2007). *Nursing health assessment: A critical thinking, case studies approach* (2nd ed., p. 863). Philadelphia: F. A. Davis.

Auscultating lungs anteriorly. Dillon P. (2007). *Nursing health assessment: A critical thinking, case studies approach* (2nd ed., p. 863). Philadelphia: F. A. Davis.

Auscultating the heart. Dillon P. (2007). *Nursing health assessment: A critical thinking, case studies approach* (2nd ed., p. 864). Philadelphia: F. A. Davis.

Palpating the scrotum. Dillon P. (2007). *Nursing health assessment: A critical thinking, case studies approach* (2nd ed., p. 865). Philadelphia: F. A. Davis.

Barlow-Ortolani maneuver no. 1. Dillon P. (2007). *Nursing health assessment: A critical thinking, case studies approach* (2nd ed., p. 866). Philadelphia: F. A. Davis.

Barlow-Ortolani maneuver no. 2. Dillon P. (2007). *Nursing health assessment: A critical thinking, case studies approach* (2nd ed., p. 866). Philadelphia: F. A. Davis.

Barlow-Ortolani maneuver no. 3. Dillon P. (2007). *Nursing health assessment: A critical thinking, case studies approach* (2nd ed., p. 866). Philadelphia: F. A. Davis.

Caput succedaneum. Ward S., & Hisley S. (2009). *Maternal-child nursing care: Optimizing outcomes for mothers, children, & families* (p. 579). Philadelphia: F. A. Davis.

Cephalhematoma. Ward S., & Hisley S. (2009). *Maternal-child nursing care: Optimizing outcomes for mothers, children, & families* (p. 579). Philadelphia: F. A. Davis.

Epstein's pearls. Dillon P. (2007). *Nursing health assessment: A critical thinking, case studies approach* (2nd ed., p. 862). Philadelphia: F. A. Davis.

Natal teeth. Dillon P. (2007). *Nursing health assessment: A critical thinking, case studies approach* (2nd ed., p. 861). Philadelphia: F. A. Davis.

Moro reflex. Dillon P. (2007). *Nursing health assessment: A critical thinking, case studies approach* (2nd ed., p. 868). Philadelphia: F. A. Davis.

Startle reflex. Dillon P. (2007). *Nursing health assessment: A critical thinking, case studies approach* (2nd ed., p. 868). Philadelphia: F. A. Davis.

Tonic neck reflex. Dillon P. (2007). *Nursing health assessment: A critical thinking, case studies approach* (2nd ed., p. 868). Philadelphia: F. A. Davis.

Rooting reflex. Dillon P. (2007). *Nursing health assessment: A critical thinking, case studies approach* (2nd ed., p. 870). Philadelphia: F. A. Davis.

Palmar grasp reflex. Dillon P. (2007). *Nursing health assessment: A critical thinking, case studies approach* (2nd ed., p. 869). Philadelphia: F. A. Davis.

Plantar grasp reflex. Dillon P. (2007). *Nursing health assessment: A critical thinking, case studies approach* (2nd ed., p. 869). Philadelphia: F. A. Davis.

Babinski reflex. Dillon P. (2007). *Nursing health assessment: A critical thinking, case studies approach* (2nd ed., p. 869). Philadelphia: F. A. Davis.

Stepping or dancing reflex. Dillon P. (2007). *Nursing health assessment: A critical thinking, case studies approach* (2nd ed., p. 870). Philadelphia: F. A. Davis.

Heel stick. Ward S., & Hisley S. (2009). *Maternal-child nursing care: Optimizing outcomes for mothers, children, & families* (p. 610). Philadelphia: F. A. Davis.

Chapter 16

Figure 16-2 Scanlon V., & Sanders T. (2007). *Essentials of anatomy and physiology* (5th ed., p. 467). Philadelphia: F. A. Davis.

Chapter 17

Figure 17-7 Adapted from Finnegan L. P. (1986). Neonatal abstinence syndrome; assessment and pharmacotherapy. In F. F. Rubatelli & B. Gradadi (Eds.), *Neonatal therapy: An update*. New York: Excerpta Medica.

Index

Note: Page numbers followed by f refer to figures; page numbers followed by t refer to tables; page numbers followed by b refer to boxes.